PSYCHOSOCIAL TREATMENT
FOR MEDICAL CONDITIONS:
PRINCIPLES AND TECHNIQUES

Psychosocial Treatment for Medical Conditions:
Principles and Techniques

Edited by

Leon A. Schein
Harold S. Bernard
Henry I. Spitz
Philip R. Muskin

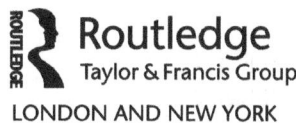

Routledge
Taylor & Francis Group

LONDON AND NEW YORK

First published 2003 by Brunner-Routledge

Published 2018 by Routledge
2 Park Square, Milton Park, Abingdon, Oxon OX14 4RN
52 Vanderbilt Avenue, New York, NY 10017

Fisrt issued in paperback 2018

Routledge is an imprint of the Taylor & Francis Group, an informa business

Library of Congress Cataloging-in-Publication Data
Psychosocial treatment for medical conditions : principles and techniques / edited by Leon A. Schein . . . (et al.).
        p. ; cm.
Includes bibliographical references and index.
    ISBN 1-58391-366-1 (hardback : alk. paper)
1. Clinical health psychology. 2. Medicine, Psychosomatic. 3. Physician and patient. 4. Stress (Psychology)
    [DNLM: 1. Psychophysiology. 2. Chronic Disease—psychology. 3. Health Behavior. 4. Stress, Psychological. WL 103 P9745 2002]
    I. Schein, Leon A.

R726.7 .P7956 2002
616'.0019—dc 21   2002007320

ISBN 13: 978-1-138-86962-2 (pbk)
ISBN 13: 978-1-58391-366-6 (hbk)

To Suzanne, for her love and encouragement from the seeds of the idea for this book nine years ago to its fruition.

To Bonnie, Nicole, and Bradley, whose love and understanding give me room to do what I need to do and be who I need to be.

To Susan, Becky, and Jake, for their abiding love and unwavering devotion.

To Matthew and Marlene, who provide daily love and inspiration.

Contents

Contributors   ix

Foreword: Mind Matters   xiii
David Spiegel

Preface   xv

SECTION I   INTRODUCTION

1 *Significance of Psychosocial Factors to Health and Disease*   3
       Charles L. Sheridan and Sally A. Radmacher

2 *Psychosocial Factors Affecting Medical Conditions*   27
       Kenneth S. Gorfinkle and Felice Tager

SECTION II   MEDICAL CONDITIONS

3 *Psychosocial Sequelae of Cancer Diagnosis and Treatment*   79
       Michael A. Andrykowski, Janet S. Carpenter, and Rita K. Munn

4 *Psychosocial Considerations in Essential Hypertension,*
       Coronary Heart Disease, and End-Stage Renal Disease   133
       Timothy W. Smith and Paul N. Hopkins

5 *Psychosocial Dimensions of Gastrointestinal Disorders*   181
       Kevin W. Olden and Philip R. Muskin

6 *Endocrine Disorders*   201
       Elbert F. Sholar, Susan G. Kornstein, and David F. Gardner

7 *Neurological Illnesses*   231
       Laurie Stevens and Julie K. Schulman

8   *Infectious Diseases*   267
       Jenifer A. Nields and John A. R. Grimaldi, Jr.

9   *Women's Health*   333
       Mindy E. Weiss, Elizabeth H. W. Ricanati, and
       Elsa-Grace V. Giardina

SECTION III   TREATMENT

10 *The Impact of Stress and the Objectives of Psychosocial*
       Interventions   373
       Luiz R. A. Gazzola and Philip R. Muskin

11 *Treatment*   407
       Kathleen Ulman

SECTION IV   SUMMARY

12 *Summary and Future Directions*   431
       Harold S. Bernard, Henry I. Spitz, Leon A. Schein,
       and Philip R. Muskin

       Index   443

Contributors

Editors

Leon A. Schein, Ed.D., Clinical Assistant Professor of Psychiatry, Department of Psychiatry, New York University School of Medicine, and Co-Director and Dean of Curriculum, Eastern Group Psychotherapy Society Training Program, New York, NY

Harold S. Bernard, Ph.D., President, American Group Psychotherapy Association, and Clinical Associate Professor, Department of Psychiatry, New York University School of Medicine, New York, NY

Henry I. Spitz, M.D., Clinical Professor of Psychiatry, Department of Psychiatry, Columbia University, College of Physicians & Surgeons, and Director, Training Programs in Group & Family Therapy, New York State Psychiatric Institute, New York, NY

Philip R. Muskin, M.D., Professor of Clinical Psychiatry, Department of Psychiatry, Columbia University, College of Physicians & Surgeons, and Chief of Service, Consultation-Liaison Psychiatry, New York-Presbyterian Hospital, New York, NY

Chapter Authors

Michael A. Andrykowski, Ph.D., Professor of Behavioral Science, Department of Behavioral Science, University of Kentucky College of Medicine, Lexington, KY

Janet S. Carpenter, R.N., Ph.D., Assistant Professor of Nursing, Vanderbilt University School of Nursing, Nashville, TN

David F. Gardner, M.D., Professor of Medicine, Department of Endocrinology, Medical College of Virginia Campus/Virginia Commonwealth University, Richmond, VA

Luiz R. A. Gazzola, M.D., Ph.D., Assistant Professor of Clinical Psychiatry, Department of Psychiatry, Columbia University, College of Physicians & Surgeons, New York, NY

Elsa-Grace V. Giardina, M.D., Professor of Clinical Medicine, Columbia University, College of Physicians & Surgeons, New York, NY

Kenneth S. Gorfinkle, Ph.D., Assistant Clinical Professor of Medical Psychology (in Psychiatry), Department of Behavioral Medicine, Columbia University, College of Physicians & Surgeons, New York, NY

John A. R. Grimaldi, Jr., M.D., Assistant Professor of Clinical Psychiatry, Center for Special Studies, New York-Presbyterian Hospital, New York, NY

Paul N. Hopkins, M.D., Associate Professor of Internal Medicine, Division of Cardiovascular Genetics, University of Utah, Salt Lake City, UT

Susan G. Kornstein, M.D., Associate Professor of Psychiatry, and Obstetrics and Gynecology and Chair, Division of Ambulatory Care Psychiatry, Medical College of Virginia Campus/Virginia Commonwealth University, Richmond, VA

Rita K. Munn, M.D., Associate Professor of Medicine, Roswell Park Cancer Institute, Department of Medicine, Buffalo, NY

Jenifer A. Nields, M.D., Assistant Professor of Psychiatry, Department of Psychiatry, Yale University School of Medicine, New Haven, CT

Kevin W. Olden, M.D., Division of Gastroenterology, Mayo Clinic Scottsdale, Scottsdale, AZ

Sally A. Radmacher, Ph.D., Professor of Psychology, Department of Psychology, Missouri Western State College, St. Joseph, MO

Elizabeth H. W. Ricanati, M.D., Instructor of Clinical Medicine, Columbia University, College of Physicians & Surgeons, New York, NY

Julie K. Schulman, M.D., Clinical Instructor, Department of Psychiatry, Columbia University, College of Physicians & Surgeons, New York, NY

Charles L. Sheridan, Ph.D., Professor Emeritus, Department of Psychology, University of Missouri-Kansas City, and Former Clinical Director UMKC-Bloch Cancer Center, Kansas City, MO

Elbert F. Sholar, M.D., Associate Professor of Psychiatry, Medical College of Virginia Campus/Virginia Commonwealth University, Richmond, VA

Timothy W. Smith, Ph.D., Professor and Chair, Department of Psychology, University of Utah, Salt Lake City, UT

David Spiegel, M.D., Professor and Associate Chair of Psychiatry and Behavioral Sciences, Stanford University School of Medicine, Stanford, CA

Laurie Stevens, M.D., Associate Clinical Professor of Psychiatry, Department of Psychiatry, Columbia University College of Physicians & Surgeons, New York, NY

Felice Tager, Ph.D., Instructor in Clinical Psychology, Department of Psychiatry, Columbia University College of Physicians & Surgeons, New York, NY

Kathleen Ulman, Ph.D., Instructor, Department of Psychiatry, Harvard Medical School, Cambridge, MA

Mindy E. Weiss, M.D., Instructor in Clinical Medicine, Columbia University, College of Physicians & Surgeons, New York, NY

Foreword
Mind Matters

The very success of modern biotechnological medicine has brought to the fore its greatest weakness: The better we get at extending survival with serious illness, the more people we have with chronic illness. Cancer, once thought of as a uniformly terminal illness, is now seen as a chronic illness, as only 50% of people diagnosed with a cancer will die from it. Mortality from heart disease is decreasing, due to a combination of more effective prevention, early detection, and more effective treatments. Nowhere is this picture clearer than in the case of HIV infection, which has gone in just a decade from being a death sentence to a chronic disease, with the help of antiretroviral treatment.

Despite these many successes, growing numbers of people are seeking alternative or complementary treatments. Forty-two percent of Americans did so in 1997, up from 32% in 1990. Why do they turn from the medical treatment that so palpably helps them? Medicine has become trapped by its own success. We have focused on cure rather than care, medication and surgery rather than management. The average doctor now spends 7 minutes per patient; the average alternative practitioner, 30 minutes. We can do the math—patients want and need someone who treats them as a person, someone who helps them cope.

Psychosocial Treatment for Medical Conditions: Principles and Techniques fills the gap between what modern medicine is and what it needs to be. This book makes it clear that the best medical treatment is a combination of emotional and social support along with somatic treatment. Indeed, the authors reconceptualize a variety of medical illnesses as a series of stressors: fears of mortality, the rigors of treatment, loss of social roles, the need to make treatment decisions, reorienting life priorities. There are circumstances in which stress may cause disease. In almost all cases, disease causes stress, and stress and the person's reaction to it may well contribute to the progression of the disease: viral infection, cancer, and heart disease, among others.

There is frequent and appropriate reference in this book to group support as an effective treatment modality. Groups have many advantages. Not only are they cost-effective, but they provide a new network of social support, pulling together those with common problems. This helps them to normalize their own experiences and utilize what they have learned about coping with their illness to help others, enhancing their own sense of competence. Both group and individual support also provide an occasion for patients to ventilate and thus better manage their emotional reactions to illness. Emotion is often viewed as a nuisance factor in medical treatment. We treat crying as if it were bleeding—we apply direct pressure until it stops. This message forces patients to take their misery elsewhere, which leaves them alienated. Patients deeply appreciate the caring shown by health care professionals who demonstrate acceptance and understanding of their distress.

With the growing pressure of increasingly complex technological medicine and the predations of managed care, doctors can still do it better, but they cannot do it all. This book provides incisive discussions of the psychosocial complications of a variety of important medical illnesses, and integrative chapters on stress and group therapy provide further presentation of the needs and methods of intervention. The book reinforces the importance of improving communication between physicians and mental health providers working together to diminish the psychological-psychosocial sequelae accompanying a serious illness and to enhance patients' quality of life. Sophisticated attention to the biopsychosocial aspects of medical illness is not just a useful addition to medicine—it is good medicine.

DAVID SPIEGEL, M.D.

Preface

New diagnostic and treatment protocols for medical conditions have increased the life expectancy of patients and have shifted previously imminent life-threatening diseases to a more chronic status. The psychosocial and psychological sequelae associated with medical conditions have not received concomitant attention nor been adequately integrated with medical treatment.

This volume provides a comprehensive practice focus for psychiatrists, psychologists, social workers, nurses, and others who conduct psychosocial treatment interventions for chronic or life-threatening medical conditions. We will provide information about the principles of psychosocial individual, group, and family interventions and their application to a variety of medical conditions. Basic information with regard to various medical conditions will be presented, including a concise description of the medical condition, treatments, side effects, prognosis, and expectable psychological sequelae. The psychosocial reactions about which clinicians should be aware to enable an optimal understanding of the concerns of patients and their families are reviewed. Understanding their reactions is central in order to conduct effective psychosocial interventions. Psychosocial individual, group, or family intervention offers an excellent vehicle for mental health practitioners in hospitals, in social service agencies, and in private practice to meet the varied treatment needs of a large population. Among the concerns to be considered are race, cultural implications, women's health, and the implications of working within the medical culture. Few medical institutions have yet developed comprehensive and integrated programs that incorporate knowledge about, and sensitivity to, these factors.

Specifically, psychosocial support group treatment can contribute to a reduction in behaviors that affect risk factors for various illnesses or enhance the progression of illness; diminish depression, anxiety, and stress; enhance a sense of feeling understood; clarify information; assist patients in assuming an active participant position with their physician and in their treatment; sustain the medical and lifestyle recommendations of patients' physicians; help discuss concerns of self-image, self-esteem, and body-image; help patients cope with their condition; and mobilize maximum support from family and friends. These groups can improve the patients' quality of life and enhance adherence to medical treatment protocols. The book will describe the special adaptations that are required in technique for working with individuals with specific medical conditions.

In some instances contradictory studies are presented. The purpose is not to confuse the reader, but to reinforce the perspective that we are involved in a process in which, at the present time, hypotheses rather than conclusions are more appropriate.

The medical conditions included in this book were selected, after a thorough review of the literature and consultation with medical specialists, as being more representative of the illnesses currently treated by medical practitioners and offering potential opportunities for psychosocial interventions. What follows is an overview of the unique aspects of each chapter.

In Chapter 1, Sheridan and Radmacher emphasize the influence of psychosocial interventions on health-related behaviors and on the effectiveness of medical treatment. The authors examine the lack of adherence to medical treatment, especially where there are significant side effects or discomfort. They present the importance of patients' participation in treatment decisions and the concomitant role of assessing patients' capacity to process information. Coordination between mental health practitioners and physicians concerning the most effective way to discuss treatment decisions with patients is critical.

Though the research is contradictory, Sheridan and Radmacher note the lack of a clear definition of the "difficult" patient, and the possible inadvertent influences on the quality of medical care. The authors cogently address a major concern that has generally received little attention: the psychosocial obstacles that contribute to delaying medical treatment.

Gorfinkle and Tager, in Chapter 2, discuss historical and contemporary perspectives about the influence of personality and emotional styles on the development of illness and disease. They emphasize the importance of the clinician's knowledge about the relationship between stress, somatic illness, and psychological sequelae. The physician's role is complex; it requires having a knowledge base in his or her speciality and understanding the impact of illness from the patient's perspective. Gorfinkle and Tager review the environmental and work stressors that contribute to illness and disease, and consider the emotional components that may inhibit changes in lifestyle practices. The authors discuss the role of spiritual practices and their effects, though with the caution that substantial validated research has not been developed. The authors provide a caveat worthy of emphasis: Disease entities are complex and it is more constructive to consider what we now know as hypotheses rather than conclusions.

Chapter 3, by Andrykowski, Carpenter, and Munn, considers the psychological and psychosocial sequelae associated with different forms of cancer. The authors note that the reluctance of patients, families, partners, companions, and children to discuss mutual concerns and emotional responses is an impediment to a patient adapting to the implications of the diagnosis. Pain is a major concern for patients diagnosed with cancer. Although adequate pain relief can enhance the patients' quality of life and reduce psychological distress, the authors note that many patients do not receive such treatment as a result of physicians' unfounded fear of addiction and/or inadequate training in pain management.

Andrykowski, Carpenter, and Munn suggest that some patients may develop post-traumatic stress disorder without psychosocial intervention, an observation that may explain earlier research findings that some patients develop intense fears of a cancer recurrence. Even years after completion of treatment, this may trigger reactions to medical follow-up. Patients' subjective interpretation of the chances of recurrence may cause psychological distress.

The authors consider the effect of hospitalization on children and adolescents who are often most distressed by external changes such as hair or weight loss. Behavioral changes are more likely to be seen in children and adolescents, in contrast to more clearly defined emotional responses in adults. They report that mothers and fathers appear to have differential reactions for which different interventions would be constructive. The chapter also reviews the emerging research that reflects the association between emotional and social support with longer post-diagnosis survival and a more extended period before recurrence. Coping strategies thus seem to be related not only to psychological adjustment but to clinical outcomes.

In Chapter 4, Smith and Hopkins review the clinical manifestations of coronary heart disease. They address the modifiable psychosocial lifestyle factors associated with the development of coronary heart disease including myocardial infarction and recurrent coronary episodes. They present both unmodifiable physical risk factors (age, sex, family history) and those which are modifiable (high cholesterol levels, hypertension, smoking). Significant studies point to the contribution of individual and cumulative psychosocial factors in the development of coronary heart disease and the recurrence of cardiac events, including inadequate social support, isolation, Type A behavior, anger and hostility, depression, stress, and anxiety. The authors offer the caveat that there is presently a lack of clarity about whether these psychosocial factors influence the development of coronary artery disease itself, precipitate clinical manifestations, or both. They also caution that the control of lifestyle behaviors does not dissipate the effects of psychosocial factors on the development of coronary heart disease. They contrast the cumulative effect of stressful responses (anger, depression, anxiety, hostility) to the reduction of stress associated with social support. The authors focus upon the contribution of effective psychosocial interventions in reducing recurrent cardiac events, and mortality and morbidity.

In the management of a coronary crisis Smith and Hopkins review studies differentiating the surprising benefits of denial. They discuss how the presentation and course of coronary heart disease varies across racial, ethnic, and gender groups. The abundance of research on the subject clearly indicates that psychosocial interventions are successful in reducing rehospitalization and recurrence of cardiac events. An outline is provided of the appropriate psychosocial interventions during diagnostic procedures, before surgery, after myocardial infarction, and during rehabilitation.

The second section of the chapter discusses the psychological stressors and emotional factors associated with the development of hypertension. The authors emphasize the importance of reliable assessment to identify risk factors that may influence prognosis while at the same time encourage the implementation of lifestyle modifications. In reviewing the literature they note the absence of consistent results in the efficacy and effectiveness of psychosocial interventions. Specifically, they emphasize the importance of psychosocial interventions in the significant rate of nonadherence to medical regimens.

In the final section of the chapter, Smith and Hopkins discuss diagnosis, treatment and the multiple psychosocial considerations of end-stage renal disease. Among the issues examined are the identification of variables related to patient compliance and adaptation and the conflicting empirical studies that considered the relationship of depression to decreased life-expectancy.

In Chapter 5, Olden and Muskin discuss the relationship between psychosocial sequelae and gastrointestinal disorders. The authors cite many studies to support the importance of collaboration between physicians and mental health providers. They note that there might be a temptation to conclude that gastrointestinal diseases derive from similar psychological or psychosocial sequelae, but the literature does not support this perspective.

The authors discuss the importance of obtaining a history of trauma and abuse in evaluating patients with functional gastrointestinal disorders. Numerous researchers indicate that patients who have been abused are more likely to have a functional GI disorder. The authors also encourage evaluation of the psychosocial factors most affecting patients diagnosed with gastrointestinal disorders, as obtaining this information can assist providers in understanding why some patients seek treatment and others do not. For these disorders, the combination of medical management and psychotherapeutic approaches is more useful than medical treatment alone.

Patients suffering from metabolic or endocrine conditions frequently present with psychological symptoms. In Chapter 6, Sholar, Kornstein, and Gardner present a summary of the psychosocial and psychological sequelae of endocrine disorders. As endocrine conditions may be misdiagnosed as psychiatric disorders, particularly in the early stages, knowledge in this area is particularly important for mental health professionals. They note that the physician can limit misdiagnoses and excessive laboratory tests by conducting an in-depth, though often time-consuming, medical history. The authors discuss the limited research into the psychiatric and psychological factors that can trigger endocrine disorders. Although they note the contribution that stress may play in a number of illnesses, they caution that the methodology has raised questions as to the applicability of the results. Although psychosocial factors have been shown to be inclusive in the onset of endocrine conditions, these factors seem to influence many endocrine conditions once there is a diagnosis.

In Chapter 7, Stevens and Schulman outline the major neurological conditions and describe representative illnesses within each category. The indication for psychosocial intervention with patients following a stroke is the high incidence of depression and dysthymia. They note that what is often overlooked is that the duration of depression is associated with the location of the injury to the brain, and the concomitant limitations imposed on the individual's lifestyle. The chapter reviews the psychosocial sequelae and psychiatric symptoms that accompany the surgical removal of a brain tumor, Parkinson's disease, and multiple sclerosis.

In Chapter 8, Nields and Grimaldi discuss infectious diseases and focus specifically on HIV, AIDS, Lyme Disease, and Chronic Fatigue Syndrome. Psychological issues among patients diagnosed HIV-positive often impede the motivation to go for testing. Psychological factors predispose individuals to adaptive or nonadaptive responses to their illnesses.

The authors address the ongoing uncertainties and controversies that continue to surround the diagnosis and treatment of Lyme Disease. Patients often experience alienation from family and friends, and a pervasive feeling of not being believed. Intervention both prior to diagnosis and during medical treatment can reduce diminished psychosocial functioning.

The inclusion of Chronic Fatigue Syndrome is somewhat controversial. Some believe this condition is a result of a post-viral infection, immune system dysregulation, or connective tissue or hormonal disorder. Attention to psychosocial factors can decrease feelings of self-blame, diminish depression, improve cognitive functioning, increase socialization, enhance social support, improve physical conditioning, and improve the capacity to work.

Chapter 9 by Weiss, Ricanati, and Giardini on women's health is a minitext that could stand on its own. Though much of the information appears in other chapters, the material presented is unique to women's health and their treatment. Most clinical trials, until recently, were conducted with men, with the assumption that the results would be similar in women and therefore were applicable to women. The authors outline specific areas that require attention to enhance the health of women, not only from physicians but also mental health practitioners. They highlight differences between male and female practitioners that have profound effects on the care that female patients receive. Throughout the chapter, the authors emphasize the use of a multidisciplinary model to enhance more successful outcomes.

Chapter 10, written by Muskin and Gazzola, reviews the impact of stress on people in general, and the special effects of medical illness as a stressor. Psychosocial factors such as support resources, vulnerability to stress, control issues, and coping ability influence illness and treatment response. Health care workers possess a variety of strategies and tools that can be used to minimize the negative impact of some of these psychosocial factors. Patients can learn to use the therapeutic properties of personal, professional, and social relationships. The objectives of psychosocial interventions are to increase patients' experience of control, reduce stress, enhance resilience, enable the use of the most effective coping skills, and maximize the support available from family and friends. Gazzola and Muskin describe the various components of stress reeducation and review the research in each of these areas. They examine the reasons for treatment failures and recommend some techniques that are useful to improve the likelihood of successful outcomes.

In Chapter 11, Ulman provides a summary of psychosocial interventions for medical patients. She elucidates the initial preparation for a psychosocial referral by the physician, including discussing with the patient the rationale for the suggested intervention. This step is often overlooked because of time constraints, and frequently results in patients' failure to follow the recommended intervention. Ulman also focuses on the evaluation of patients' capacity to cope, attitude and emotional responses toward their illness, and expectations. Consultation by mental health practitioners with the referring physician is useful in discerning the reason for the referral as well as the physician's expectations. For example, patients who resist the physician's recommendations or who call too frequently due to anxiety may be referred with the hope of alleviating some of the pressures they are experiencing. Ulman discusses the variety of efficacious psychosocial interventions that may be chosen. These include psychoeducation, supportive psychotherapy, cognitive and/or behavioral psychotherapy, and insight-oriented psychotherapy. Psychological interventions such as stress management, visualization, and relaxation techniques are also appropriate for motivated patients. Groups can often be utilized for these adjunctive interventions. Psychosocial-psychological evaluations of patients and their illnesses are necessary prior to beginning treatment. Combining interventions is often most effective, depending upon the patient's wishes, psychosocial situation, and type of illness.

In the final chapter, the editors conclude that psychotherapeutic and psychosocial interventions are crucial components in the treatment of medical conditions. Despite the numerous studies cited, they note the difficulty in comprehensively validating the efficacy of the positive effect of psychosocial interventions (in combination with medical treatment) in affecting the course of patients' illnesses. Managed care companies and the concerns of insurers in financing medical costs have continued to impact the patient–provider relationship as well as the introduction and expansion of psychosocial interventions. An ethical concern and dilemma for mental health practitioners, in dealing with insurers, is the protection of patient information in order to diminish prejudicial actions in the workplace or by the insurer. As a result, a fuller integration of the efforts of physicians and mental health clinicians, in providing comprehensive care for the patient, has thus far eluded us. The authors describe the benefits of conducting psychosocial interventions in groups, including responses such as a diminished sense of feeling alone, direct emotional support, observing others who struggle with similar issues, receiving useful suggestions and resources from others, and enhancing self-esteem by being of help to others.

Increasingly, physicians and mental health clinicians have become cognizant of the relationship between illness and the psychosocial sequelae that influence patients' responses, and in some instances, the course of the disease. It is our hope that this volume will reinforce and influence this awareness. We are optimistic that collaborative efforts between physicians and mental health clinicians will enhance the integration of medical treatment and psychosocial interventions, and thus improve the quality of care that is offered to our patients.

LEON A. SCHEIN
HAROLD S. BERNARD
HENRY I. SPITZ
PHILIP R. MUSKIN

Introduction

1

Significance of Psychosocial Factors to Health and Disease

CHARLES L. SHERIDAN
SALLY A. RADMACHER

Despite the many successes of our standard way of treating disease, Engel (1977) proposed a change in our fundamental model of health care. The traditional, "biomedical" model has focused on the application of biological science to maintain health and treating disease. Engel in no way wanted to lose the obvious advantages of this approach. He pointed toward an additional set of factors that are highly significant to health and the course of disease. We now have a considerable body of knowledge that we did not have at the turn of the century, when the biomedical model was put in place. The model Engel proposed continues the emphasis on biological knowledge in medicine, but also encompasses the utilization of psychosocial knowledge. He called this combined approach the "biopsychosocial model." In this chapter, we provide an introduction to Engel's broader approach to health care, along with what we hope will be examples of how psychosocial knowledge can be combined with biomedicine to foster health and treat disease.

BACKGROUND

Scholars commonly credit the philosopher Rene Descartes (1596–1650) with introducing the rule of reason to scientific thinking; he was also responsible for the radical conceptual separation of mind and body. Descartes held that mind and body were separate entities, of entirely different realms, and that the body was a mere machine. Though entirely speculative, he believed the mind could influence the body only to a modest degree, by exerting an influence over the brain's pineal gland.

Despite four centuries of scientific discoveries and revolutionary developments in medicine and psychiatry, we still struggle with what has come to be known as the "mind-body problem." The influence of Descartes' defining schema is found in medicine's historical tendency to minimize the role of the mind and focus exclusively on the "machinery" of the body. Today, that separation between mind and body is diminishing. In psychiatry, patients are being treated with biochemical interventions. Similarly, in many other branches of medicine there is a growing realization that patients' maintaining treatment protocols often depend on their psychological state. Cardiologists are increasingly aware of the frequency of depression following heart attacks and its effects on recovery. In one major study, patients with depression in the period immediately following a myocardial infarction were 3.5 times more likely to die than nondepressed patients (Frasure-Smith, Lesperance, & Talajic, 1993). The trend to treat somatic illness through modification of mental processes is based on evidence from extensive studies and clinical trials that have examined the physiological mechanisms of the brain as they influence somatic health. For example, it is now well established that the brain has an intimate relationship to the immune system, demonstrated by studies in the field of psychoneuroimmunology (Kiecolt-Glaser & Glaser, 1989).

RELATIVE IMPORTANCE OF PSYCHOSOCIAL FACTORS IN HEALTH

As noted above, Descartes posited only limited influence of the mind upon the body. Since his time, significant evidence has accumulated suggesting that the mind can play a much more important role in body regulation than Descartes' model suggests (Barber, 1984).

The ability to control emotions and appetites is a matter of ordinary experience. Deep-lying assumptions, as well as views reflecting the social systems in which we live exert great influence over our bodies. For example, Antonovsky (1979, 1987) found that individuals with a strong "sense of coherence" tended to be less likely to get sick compared with those whose sense of coherence was weak. Sense of coherence involves an abiding tendency to see one's experiences as meaningful, manageable, and comprehensible. This kind of deep-seated worldview is obviously something quite different from an individual's willpower.

As Antonovsky (1979, 1987) noted, the development of a sense of coherence results from being raised in an environment that fosters it. Hence, investigators of the mind-body relationship find themselves studying both psychosocial influences and psychological ones. When examining the importance of psychosocial influences on health, the tendency to compare their impact to factors taken more seriously in traditional biological medicine is probably inevitable. In this comparison, however, real-world applications of biomedicine are often idealized. Emphasis is placed in published research on the efficacy of individual treatments, and it is assumed that the success of these treatments will generalize to the overall impact of medicine. It is important to look at empirical evidence concerning the overall influence of the technological approach to treatment as it is applied in the real world. For example, a treatment cannot be effective if patients fail to utilize it, or its effectiveness may be reduced by actions taken by patients or by the failure of professionals to administer the treatment appropriately. Much available research indicates that in order to fulfill the potential of medical treatment, a scientific understanding and utilization of psychosocial influences is required.

PSYCHOSOCIAL FACTORS ARE POWERFUL INFLUENCES ON HEALTH

Although a core factor in fostering health and avoiding disease is access to medical care, the influence of psychosocial factors should not be underestimated. A substantial body of research also indicates that psychosocial factors have a far greater impact on health than might have been anticipated (see, for example, Dubos, 1959; Illich, 1976; Sagan, 1987; and Wilkinson, 1996). Lynch (1977) summarized compelling evidence that social support is crucial to resisting and surviving heart disease. Lynch reported several studies showing that surviving heart disease depends heavily on marital status. He also linked reductions in a wide range of other diseases to marital status. Findings consistent with those of Lynch were obtained in the Alameda County Study, a major community-based study of the relationships between social networks and mortality that included research on close to 5,000 people over the span of a decade (Belloc & Breslow, 1972). The study found that those who lacked social ties had about twice the mortality rate of those with the strongest social bonds. Here too, many of the deaths were due to cardiovascular disease, but other causes of death including cancer, infectious diseases, respiratory diseases, and all other causes combined, were linked to the psychosocial factors. The quality of one's marriage is also relevant to health (Kiecolt-Glaser et al., 1993), since behaviors associated with conflict tend to affect the immune system. Another study, of 1,368 cardiac catheterization patients, found that those who were unmarried or lacked a confidant were more than three times as likely to die within five years as compared to patients with strong social ties (Woloshin et al., 1997).

In the classic Roseto Study, it was first found that death rates in Roseto, Pennsylvania, were much lower than those in comparable neighboring towns. Roseto was a close-knit Italian community in which it was considered shameful for people to put themselves above others. Social cohesion was a central emphasis in Roseto. Death rates due to heart disease were on average 40% lower than those of comparable communities even after traditional risk factors such as diet, smoking, and exercise were taken into account. Bruhn and Wolf (1979) noted that "[t]hroughout the years of study of this community the indications were that the strength of unconditional interpersonal support and family and community cohesiveness had served to counteract the effects of life stress and thereby were a protection against fatal myocardial infarction" (p. 136). In the 1960s and 1970s, social cohesion diminished and the health advantage disappeared.

PSYCHOSOCIAL INTERVENTION AS A MAJOR FACTOR IN COPING WITH AND RECOVERING FROM DISEASE

Much evidence has been amassed in support of the significant role of the mind in somatic health and disease. One of the earliest attempts to investigate this role was made by proponents of "psychosomatic" medicine. Most of these early proponents were heavily influenced by Freudian theories and viewed somatic symptoms as manifestations of unconscious wishes or conflicts. Not every physical ailment was seen as stemming from such a source. Rather, psychosomatic theorists tended to view only certain diseases as "psychosomatic" expressions of the unconscious. Asthma, colitis, duodenal ulcers, hives, and essential hypertension were among the classic examples in this category.

Treatments for cancer also commonly make great demands on the patient, and the ability to cope with these circumstances plays a significant role in recovery. For patients undergoing chemotherapy, nausea and vomiting tend to be very high on the list of distressing side effects of such therapy (Fallowfield, 1992), despite the routine administration of antiemetic agents (de Boer-Dennert et al., 1997). The fact that patients rate these symptoms as highly distressing clearly indicates a large impact on their quality of life. There may also be an impact on survival due to total or partial refusal of treatment.

A second example of the impact of psychosocial interventions in coping with physical illness has to do with surgical preparation. Dreher (1998) recently reviewed the literature on such preparation, including meta-analyses of almost 200 prior studies. Methods of preparation ranged from simple psychoeducational efforts (giving information about the procedure, comforting words, and instructions on how to cope) to rather elaborate suggestions and imagery. The interventions were intended to optimize the body's cooperation and quick recovery from the surgery (e.g., directing blood flow adaptively during and after surgery, stimulating gastrointestinal movement after gut surgery). Statistical analyses indicated that these interventions had significant effects, and the size of those effects was moderate to large. Improved outcomes included such things as decrease of blood loss, more rapid return of gastric motility after gut surgery, swifter wound healing, less need for pain medication, and shorter hospital stays. The studies indicate that these kinds of interventions are likely to result in physical benefits for the patient as well as lower costs.

It is hard to imagine that a psychological intervention could have a notable impact on what appear to be basic physiological reactions to chemicals. Yet the utilization of relaxation techniques, imagery, and biofeedback with cancer patients undergoing such treatment tends to have an impact on symptoms typically encountered by medical patients. Research evidence indicates that a small number of sessions of relaxation training, with or without imagery, hypnosis, or biofeedback, routinely reduces treatment-induced nausea, as measured by ratings done independently by patients and nurses (Carey & Burish, 1988; Burish & Jenkins, 1992).

THE STRESS MODEL

Perhaps the most useful psychosomatic framework was the "stress model." Walter Cannon (1932) and Hans Selye (1936) identified two major facets of stress response. Cannon showed that stressful events result in the "fight or flight" reaction, which is appropriate for survival in the wild, but often unhealthy in civilized environments where physical attacks and running for one's life are rarely required. The "fight or flight" response is mediated by the hypothalamus, the sympathetic nervous system, and the core or "medulla" of the adrenal glands. It produces such things as elevations of blood pressure, speeding of the heart, and increased blood clotting. These examples illustrate that stress reactions, if chronic, can have serious health consequences. For example, chronically elevated blood pressure can stimulate thickening of arterial walls, resulting in the blockage of blood flow through the narrowed arteries and potentially leading to a heart attack.

The hypothalamus, pituitary gland, and the outer layers ("cortex") of the adrenal glands mediate the second facet of stress, discovered by Selye (1936). Selye argued that any "stress" produces the same initial reaction, which he called "The General Adaptation Syndrome." Specifically related to the health consequences of stress is the inclusion in this syndrome of increases in cortisol, which result in suppression of immunity. This suppression of immunity can result in susceptibility to infectious disease (Cohen, Tyrell, & Smith, 1993) and possibly also in many types of cancer (Antoni, 1987; Greenberg, 1987). Unlike the earlier psychosomatic model, which limited itself to a special subset of diseases, in these models stress can be seen as having implications for disease in general.

Recently there has been a great increase in research on stress reactions. Changes in the immune system in response to stress are now very well established. We also know now that, even after removal of the adrenal glands, immune suppression occurs in response to stress (Vernikos-Danellis & Heybach, 1980). There appears to be an alternative path, other than through the adrenals, for the brain to influence immune response. In fact, the relationship of the immune system to the brain appears to be much more intimate and elaborate than Selye realized. Exploration of these interconnections has burgeoned, and we now have a new field called *psychoneuroimmunology*.

THE SIGNIFICANCE OF PSYCHONEUROIMMUNOLOGY

The field of psychoneuroimmunology came into being as a result of the serendipitous discovery of conditioned immune suppression by Ader and Cohen (1975). Years before, Pavlov had shown that physiological reactions, such as salivation, could be elicited by previously neutral stimuli, such as sounds or lights, simply by pairing the "neutral stimuli" with stimuli that naturally elicited the physiological response. Ader and Cohen (1975) discovered that immune suppression produced by a chemical agent could also be brought under the control of neutral stimuli by using the Pavlovian method. It seemed that reactivity of the immune system was subject to a learning process.

The early finding of Ader and Cohen (1975) indicated that a process we usually consider "mental" (i.e., learning) could exert at least some control over the nervous system. The Ader-Cohen finding was especially remarkable because it persisted after the adrenal glands had been removed. This means that conditioning of the stress hormones produced by the adrenal cortex, and known to produce immune suppression, could not be used to explain the finding. There had to be another pathway between the nervous and immune systems.

A number of investigators have now demonstrated close relationships between the nervous system and the immune system. For example, Bulloch (1981) published anatomical work showing a direct relationship between the brain and the thymus, some of which suggested that the brain might play a role in the development of the thymus. Other work had shown that anaphylactic reactions are influenced by experimentally induced damage to specific regions of the hypothalamus (Keller, Shapiro, Schliefer, & Stein, 1982; Foldes, Nemethy, Szalay, & Kovacs, 2000).

Research has shown that the Ader-Cohen findings are replicable. They demonstrated that the interrelationships between the nervous and immune systems are extensive, that they are activated in response to actions of the immune system, and that the immune system reacts to psychological stressors, often by being less active.

Questions remain about how significant these influences might be for health. From the beginning, it has been recognized that immune system changes in response to psychological reactions are small (Ader & Cohen, 1975). However, evidence of the clinical significance of these variations has grown in the past several years. For example, highly stressed spousal caregivers of dementia patients have been shown to have diminished antibody-and virus-specific T cell responses to an influenza virus when compared to controls, and they also produce fewer antibodies in response to pneumococcal pneumonia vaccine as measured months after the vaccination (Glaser, Sheridan, Malarkey, MacCallum, & Kiecolt-Glaser, 2000). Also, stressed caregivers display modified activity of immune cellular signaling mechanisms, as reflected in levels of interleukin-1, and also heal more slowly in response to an experimentally induced, standardized wound (Kiecolt-Glaser, Marucha, Malarkey, Mercado, & Glaser, 1995).

Observation that health-relevant immune reactions occur in response to psychological influences is important in its own right. It is of particular importance because it provides at least an understanding of a physiological mechanism capable of mediating between psychosocial influences and disease. It also reinforces evidence for a model of health and disease that fully incorporates such influences. For many years research has supported the idea that psychosocial factors have a substantial influence on health, but known mechanisms of mediation between the brain and the immune system have been sparse. Psychoneuroimmunology opens a new panorama in which such things as "mind-body medicine" have the potential to be integrated with the more familiar form of scientifically based medicine.

SHOULD RECENT ADVANCES IN BIOMEDICAL KNOWLEDGE LEAD US TO DISCOUNT PSYCHOSOCIAL FACTORS?

In some instances, research and treatment have moved away from inclusion of the mind or brain as influences on health. Current views of the etiology and treatment of peptic ulcers illustrate this opposing trend very well. Early on, peptic ulcers were included in the core group of psychosomatic diseases. More recently, evidence has come forth indicating that these ulcers are due to a bacterium, *Helicobacter pylori*, and that they can successfully be treated with antibiotics.

If correct, this account would challenge the theory that the brain directly influences bodily functions. It suggests that a great deal of research can be done on mind-body influences, only to be undermined eventually by evidence that reality is in line with a very simple biomedical model—germs cause diseases, and getting rid of germs with medicine cures those diseases.

The facts are not so simple. Weiner (1996) pointed out that, though 70–90% of patients with ulcers have *H. pylori,* some 80% of people without the disease also have it. In addition, 10–30% of ulcer patients do not have *H. pylori* at all. Furthermore, though antibiotics are effective in treating ulcers, many patients do not respond, and the rate of cure is only modestly better than that for placebo (Overmier and Murison, 1997). Overmier and Murison argue that something besides bacteria is modulating the vulnerability of the stomach wall, and they provide notable evidence from animal research that stress is the source of variations in vulnerability. It has long been known that stress can induce ulcers in rats in a matter of hours. Restraining rats in water at room temperature for about an hour induces substantial gastric erosions, but only if the rats are conscious. Furthermore, prior experiences of uncontrollable, though moderate, stress increase the vulnerability of rats to the water restraint and result in more ulceration.

The model implicit in the work of Overmier and Murison (1997) is not consistent with a biomedical model. While the biological influences such as bacteria are of central importance to disease, and management of those biological influences goes a long way toward treating the disease, the realities of health and disease are more complex and require inclusion of factors from the psychosocial sphere.

Andersen, Kiecolt-Glaser and Glaser (1994), working in the area of cancer treatment, have developed an important model that places psychosocial interventions in an appropriate context. They point out that there are many ways in which psychological treatment can influence the outcome of cancer treatment. Some of these may involve the mind's direct control over the body. For example, a high-stress load with poor coping skills is likely to produce immune suppression and thus impair the body's resources for dealing with cancer. Stress-management training can help the patient neutralize or at least diminish the impact of the many distressing aspects of dealing with cancer, and some of this effect may be due to direct mind-body influences. However, some of the effect may be due simply to adaptive stress-coping behaviors, such as getting enough sleep, eating properly, or dealing effectively with people in situations where there is potential for conflict. In fact, psychological influences on treatment outcomes may sometimes account for an enhanced ability to endure difficult medical treatments.

THE INFLUENCE OF CONCEPTUALIZATIONS OF HEALTH AND DISEASE ON PSYCHOSOCIAL FACTORS

Though medical tests are certainly scored with a range of gradations, the ultimate issue tends to be whether one has a diagnosis or not. Medical sociologists have referred to this as being assigned a "sick role." Many have objected to this view. Thus, an alternative, called the "Wellness Continuum," has been proposed.

The wellness continuum is anchored at one end by disease, disability, and death, and at the other end by a mode of human functioning in which one's potential is more or less fully realized (Sheridan & Radmacher, 1992). At the "well" end of the continuum, the person is maximally healthy, with resources for resisting disease optimized, and is also capable of experiencing the joy and fullness of life. The wellness focus is not so much on the distinction between being healthy versus sick but rather is on optimal health and full functioning of a multidimensional human being.

The shift from the dichotomous health/disease model to the wellness model encourages inclusion of the psychological, social, and spiritual dimensions, and thus results necessarily in an enhancement of the role of psychosocial factors in health. Within such a model, our goal is not just to fight a somatic disease, though that is part of it. Rather the goal is to enhance the capacity of patients to move beyond the disease to find a way of life that fulfills their potential for living as psychologically healthy, socially connected, spiritually fulfilled people. Medical tests, prescriptions, and surgical interventions obviously play a role in reaching that goal, but only a partial one.

Illich (1976), in his classic work, *Medical Nemesis*, took a position very similar to the wellness model, specifically with respect to the concept of *iatrogenesis*. Traditionally we think of iatrogenesis as physical harm caused by medical treatment. But if a human being exists at various levels, including the somatic, the psychological, the social, and the spiritual, treatments can be iatrogenic at any of those levels. Illich argued that technological medicine that ignores everything about the patient except the body creates another range of iatrogenic problems by encouraging passivity and dependency on the part of patients and their families. Furthermore, this kind of treatment can intrude upon patients and their loved ones during times in which social and spiritual meanings and their accompanying rituals are of central importance.

The wellness model points toward an expanded conceptualization of successful treatment outcomes. For example, a very talkative person whose business is sales and who has laryngeal cancer cannot be adequately treated by a laryngectomy. Removal of the larynx is crucial and may permit continuation of somatic existence, but other dimensions of the person's life have been severely damaged due to the loss of normal speech. The wellness model directs us toward the formidable task of restoring such things as the person's social and economic standing, insofar as that is possible.

If we were to accept a wellness model, cancer support groups would have a larger role in treatment than they currently do. There is evidence that support group participation may extend life, although most of us would agree that the evidence is not yet definitive. But the evidence that support groups and other psychosocial interventions enhance the quality of life is quite good. Meyer and Mark (1995) did a meta-analysis of studies on this topic and concluded that the case had been so clearly made that there is no need for further studies asking whether these interventions improve quality of life; rather we should investigate which types of interventions work best.

PATIENT PARTICIPATION AND TREATMENT DECISIONS

Various social and legal shifts and trends have given increased significance to patients playing an active role in their medical decisions. Mechanic (1996) has noted that there has been a general erosion of trust in our society to which medical settings have not been immune. Further, there are pressures to increase the level and quality of information about treatment options before concluding that a patient has given "informed" consent. In addition, many patients have an ideological commitment to being active, informed participants in their care.

There is evidence that patients weigh costs and benefits differently than their physicians do. For example, Turner, Maher, Young, Young, and Vaughn (1996) examined retrospective treatment decisions of former cancer patients and found that unexpected importance was placed on side effects such as weight gain, fatigue, and infertility. This makes it all the more important that physicians encourage patients to discuss their concerns about prospective treatment plans.

Unfortunately, there are serious barriers to full inclusion of patients in their medical treatment. For one thing, many patients prefer the more traditional passive role. Demographics suggest who will and will not want to participate fully in their medical decisions. The elderly, the young, less-educated patients, and Asian patients are among those less likely to want to participate (Kaplan, Gandek, Greenfield, Rogers, & Ware, 1995). However, such generalizations may not permit us to make a judgment about the wishes of any given patient. On the other hand, Kaplan, Greenfield, Rogers, & Ware (1996) found that doctors who have ratings in the bottom 25% with respect to participatory style are considerably more likely to have patients leave their practices within the following year, compared with more participatory physicians.

A number of studies have demonstrated that simple preconsultation interventions with patients can lead them to be more active during the consultation. These interventions have included (a) providing a simple pamphlet that encourages participation (McCann & Weinman, 1996); (b) giving patients an audiotape of their previous consultation (Ford, Fallowfield, & Lewis, 1994); and (c) having an assistant meet with the patient for a 20-minute session of what might reasonably be called "cognitive-behavioral" training on medical decisions relevant to their health problems and on effective inquiries to be made during the physician visit, including rehearsal of participatory behaviors to be used during the consultation (Greenfield, Kaplan, & Ware, 1985; Greenfield, Kaplan, Ware, Yano, & Frank, 1988).

Most interventions increased participation but did not necessarily result in greater satisfaction with the care received, or better health outcomes. The work of Greenfield et al. (1985, 1988) was an exception. They found greater patient participation was significantly related to better health outcomes (i.e., fewer functional limitations and, for patients with diabetes, lower follow-up blood glucose levels). Much more work needs to be done using their approach to determine how broadly applicable their findings may be.

LIMITATIONS OF HUMAN INFORMATION PROCESSING

Students of human cognition have identified limitations on information processing that are very fundamental to the way the brain operates and highly relevant to the health care provider. One of these basic limitations lies in the amount of information the brain can process per unit of time, which is commonly referred to as its *channel capacity*.

We are used to hearing about the magnificent capacities of the brain, with its virtually boundless memory and its incredibly clever strategies for getting at the crucial aspects of a body of information. However, its channel capacity is very limited. In a classic paper, George Miller (1956) showed that over a wide range of functions, including judgments of various dimensions of stimuli from several different senses as well as immediate perception and immediate memory, the average adult brain's information processing is limited to the information in approximately five, plus or minus two, equally likely alternatives. In the language of information theory, this is 2.5 bits. We can get a sense of what this means by contrasting it to the capacity of an average desktop computer. A typical computer might have a 32-bit capacity and operates millions of times faster than the brain.

Research has repeatedly confirmed Miller's original findings (Shiffrin & Nosofsky, 1994). Moreover, our limited capacity becomes even more limited when we are stressed. It may be a surprise to learn that the largest inflow of information to the brain comes from sensory systems in our muscles (Sheridan, 1986). As a result, stress and tension tend to overload our information-processing capacity. Dollard and Miller (1950) rather colorfully referred to the resulting condition as "neurotic stupidity."

Despite the dramatic limitation of our channel capacity, we do quite well in dealing with even complex aspects of the world because we use various clever strategies to compensate for our deficiencies. Unfortunately, the strategies tend to simplify the information and lose parts of it that seem, though they may not always be, nonessential. These can lead to failures of both practitioner and patient.

Technical skills rest on the health care provider's ability to process information accurately and efficiently. To arrive at a correct diagnosis and treatment plan, health care providers must ask the right questions, give the right tests, and use the resulting information effectively. They are often under great time pressures, flooded with information, and working in very distracting environments. Consequently, their capacity to process information may be stretched to its limits. Patients are also subjected to very high demands to process information under stressful conditions. For most patients, medical information is very high in information content because of its unfamiliarity. Tension and anxiety add still more to the information flow into the patient's "channel." They must take in information and instructions that are presented using medical language that is very high in information content. At the same time, they may be coping with intense emotional reactions to their diagnoses and also to potential diagnoses they imagine. The limitations of human channel capacity suggest that functioning and communicating in the typical health care setting is very challenging for patients and professionals alike. Fortunately, there are ways of dealing with these limitations so that the proper procedures are more likely to be effectively implemented.

Perhaps the most important step lies in realizing how important it is to deal with problems of information processing. Practitioners must carefully disperse the information content of communications important to health outcomes. Sensitivity to the timing of communications can help. If a previous communication has put a patient on overload, repeating the communication or asking the patient to summarize it in his or her own words could benefit the patient. Redundancy is one of the best tools for maximizing information-processing capacity. It is best to be repetitious and to present materials in more than one modality. A good way to do this is to tell the needed information to the patient and then also provide it in writing (Boyd, Covington, Stanaszek, & Coussons, 1974). Communicating in settings where distractions are at a minimum can also reduce the total information load for practitioner and patient.

IMPACT OF HEURISTICS ON HEALTH CARE

Human beings are cognitive misers. Since we routinely want to think of more things than our brains will allow, we have developed strategies to deal with the "great, blooming, buzzing confusion" of the outer world (James, 1890, p. 488). These strategies, or mental shortcuts, are called *heuristics*, and they have been well studied by investigators of human cognition.

Most of the time, these heuristics work reasonably well or we would not continue to use them. However, they cause us to ignore other relevant information (Myers, 1999). One of the most commonly used is the "availability heuristic." The availability heuristic involves judging the probability of something based on how readily we can imagine or recall it. The availability influences health-related judgments by making us overestimate the likelihood of serious diseases (Elstein & Bordage, 1979). Serious diseases are readily available to the mind because they tend to be vividly imagined; therefore, we tend to overestimate their chances of occurring.

People are likely to exaggerate the likelihood of anything that is easily imagined or recalled. To illustrate, people tend to estimate that they are more likely to die in an airplane crash than to die of asthma. The opposite is the case. Because of media interest in plane crashes, we have many vivid images of them that we can call to mind, whereas most of us have few, if any, images of death due to asthma.

Health care providers also rely on the availability heuristic. An example of this may be the sharp increase in the incidence of hospitalized toxic shock syndrome in 1983. Researchers (Petitti, Reingold, & Chin, 1986) found that an increase in the incidence of toxic shock syndrome appeared by 1977 with the rate peaking in 1980 and decreasing by 1982. However, there was a sharp increase in the rate in 1983. The temporal trend in the increase between the years of 1977 through 1982 was consistent with the patterns of use of tampons containing higher-absorbency materials; however, the increase in 1983 remains unexplained. It is possible that toxic shock was being overdiagnosed because of the high number of journal articles on toxic shock and resulting media attention. Any syndrome is a collection of symptoms; physicians, because of the availability heuristic, may have attended selectively to symptoms associated with toxic shock.

The "representative heuristic" is another commonly used mental shortcut that may lead us to make errors in judgments. It involves making judgments about the likelihood of things by how well they represent particular prototypes. For example, people who enter a hospital emergency room may assume that a woman who greets them with a stethoscope around her neck is a nurse, when in fact she may be a physician.

TREATMENT COMPLIANCE

Medicine invests a great deal of energy and ingenuity in developing biomedical treatments. However, it is useless to have state-of-the-art medical technology and treatment if patients fail to implement prescribed treatments. Massive studies are conducted to evaluate the effectiveness of medications, but they all assume that the drugs are being taken in the prescribed manner. Unfortunately, there is consistent and strong evidence that treatment compliance is not high (Sackett & Snow, 1979; Murphy and Coster, 1997). Murphy and Coster report that poor compliance is the most common cause of nonresponse to medication regimens.

There is evidence that physicians are unaware of the degree of noncompliance in patients. An early study found that 89% of physicians believed that virtually all of their patients were complying with the prescribed treatment, when in reality, only about 50% were doing so (Davis, 1966). In 1982, DiMatteo and DiNicola reported a study that found physicians did no better than chance in judging which of their patients was compliant. A more recent study (Goldberg, Cohen, & Rubin, 1998) found no significant relationship between practitioner evaluations of compliance and the self-reports of 138 adult patients. Furthermore, it seems that patients are not very accurate in assessing their own compliance. One study found that patient-kept diaries statistically overestimated actual compliance for treatment of ischemic heart disease when compared to electronic monitoring (Straka, Fish, Benson, & Suh, 1997).

The following is a list of principles for encouraging compliance summarized by Sheridan and Radmacher (1992), based to some degree on the recommendations made by Levy (1987) and by Dunbar and Agras (1980):

1. Behave in a warm, empathic manner with patients by listening to them and following common courtesies, e.g., introducing yourself and shaking hands. Interact actively with patients by viewing them as key members of the treatment team.
2. Give specific details about what you want the patient to do and why you want them to do it. Remember that they may be distressed and this limits their ability to process information. Present the material verbally and visually and make sure your instructions are understood.
3. Provide skill training when necessary. This may include oral and written instructions as well as modeling by the health care provider. For example, patients may be trained to take their own blood pressure in this way.
4. Explain the rationale behind the treatment plan and the evidence that it will be effective. Patients are more likely to adhere to the treatment plan if they have positive expectations about its efficacy and their abilities to carry it out.
5. Social support and reward for compliance should be arranged. If possible, solicit the support of families or friends or recommend support groups. To some extent, this kind of care may have to be provided by health care professionals. When rewarding patients, it is important to be sincere because many patients will be repelled by insincerity.
6. Provide at-home reminders that will help patients carry out their treatment plan. Written reminders that can be posted and pill containers are good examples of this kind of intervention.

7. Anticipate the possible barriers to compliance and the negative effects they may have. Patients should be informed of the various kinds of inconvenience, discomfort, or pain they may experience, and specific instructions should be provided to help patients cope with these barriers.
8. Remember how prevalent noncompliance is and monitor it as much as possible. However, monitoring should not be carried to the point that it impairs the health care provider's relationship with the patient.

DELAY IN SEEKING MEDICAL HELP

The problem of patient delay in seeking health care is a familiar one. How do we decide when to seek medical care? It would be hard to point to a topic more germane to recognizing the significance of psychosocial factors in health care outcomes. If patients fail to make appropriate decisions about seeking medical care, their lives or well-being may be placed in jeopardy. When referring to judgments, decisions, and actions, we are talking about psychological factors. Furthermore, these factors are always influenced by social circumstances, so we inevitably find ourselves back to the biopsychosocial model. In order to gain an understanding of the variables that influence delay in seeking health care, it is useful to discuss some broader conceptual issues that pertain to detection, judgment, and decision-making in general.

In the early history of scientific psychology, late in the nineteenth century, much emphasis was placed on determining the point at which stimuli of low intensity could first be detected. This point was termed the "absolute threshold." Additionally, early investigators took an interest in measuring the smallest amount of change that could be noted in a detectable stimulus. The latter was called the "difference threshold" or the "just noticeable difference." Both the absolute and the difference thresholds were thought to be fixed. Later, in the twentieth century, research and theory led to the recognition that there really were no fixed points at which we detect stimuli or changes in them.

Detection of stimuli as well as deciding how to categorize them depends on many factors, including the discriminability of the stimuli, but also their baseline frequency, the benefits and costs for various possible decisions about the stimuli, our expectations and motivations, and also various social influences. There are many steps from noting some indicator in one's body that might be a symptom and the implementation of a decision to seek medical care.

The decision to seek medical care is a highly complex one, and each step in it is a multiply determined task of signal detection and categorization. We have to detect subjective sensations or objective signs in our bodies, and even this original detection task will be influenced by such factors as the degree to which our channel capacity is overloaded. Pennebaker (1982) has done some interesting research in which he showed that exercisers report far fewer distressing symptoms when they are distracted by an attractive, changing environment than when they are exercising in a monotonous one. Whether we detect signs or sensations will depend on our context and the informational load contained in it as well as other factors.

The first step is the detection of sensations or signs, followed by the decision of whether those sensations and signs fall outside the ordinary range of experience and should be categorized as "symptoms." The presence of atypical signs and sensations is not enough to trigger the decision to seek medical care (Cameron, Leventhal, & Leventhal, 1993). Rather, the decision will be influenced by a range of factors, perhaps most notably the availability of alternative interpretations. For example, menopausal women can readily attribute abnormal vaginal bleeding to their menopausal status (Cochran, Hacker, & Berek, 1986) and conclude that although they have observable signs those signs should not be interpreted as symptoms.

Once it is decided that a symptom is present, the next step is to determine whether the symptom is enough to merit seeking medical help. Probably most of the symptoms we experience are not seen as calling for medical consultation. Often we discuss them with family or friends and are influenced by our supporters' assessments of seriousness. The views of these informal sources of medical care can even outweigh more objective medical information (Aspinwall, 1998).

Care-seeking is driven by advice to seek care, representations of a serious health threat, and perceptions of ability or inability to cope with the threat (Cameron et al., 1993). We have to appraise the symptom as important enough to require medical help but not so deadly as to make treatment useless (Safer, Tharps, Jackson, & Leventhal, 1979).

There are probably hundreds of variables that determine what we do at each of the decision-making points. In many cases, there is considerable overlap between affective and somatic symptoms, and it can be difficult to decide which we have. Pennebaker (1982) has pointed out how the same symptoms may easily be interpreted either as depression or physical illness. In addition, there is some evidence that stressors, especially those that correspond in time to disease onset, can make it difficult to recognize the need to seek medical care rather than attribute symptoms to natural responses to stress (Cameron, Leventhal, & Leventhal, 1995).

Simplistic conceptualizations, such as those that divide people into those who are "normal" or "realistic," those who are "hypochondriacs" or "crocks," and those who are "avoidants" or "deniers," hardly do justice to complex realities. Indeed, these realities are complex enough to make it very difficult to make definitive statements about the factors that result in delay in seeking medical care. Nonetheless, delay is very important, and we must come to grips with it. Research indicates that delay can be expected to result in worse outcomes, yet it is common. In one study, 30% of breast cancer patients delayed seeking help for a period of three months or more after detecting signs of tumors (Facione, 1993). Figures for delays in general are consistent with these; approximately 30% of patients fail to seek warranted treatment in a timely way (Keith, 1987).

Perhaps most significant are the reported levels of delay in patients with coronary heart disease. These cases are especially significant because (1) heart disease kills more people than any other disease and (2) there are effective interventions that we now know can significantly improve outcomes but that must be applied very quickly, preferably within the first hour after onset of symptoms, and that are probably useless if too much time (around 6–12 h) has elapsed. Studies vary in their estimates of typical delay time, but they commonly indicate that delays are too long for optimal care. If we rely on the exceptionally well done study of Goff, Feldman, McGovern, et al. (1999), we have to conclude that over half of patients delay more than 2 h and 15 min before starting treatment. As these investigators point out, "Given a median pre-hospital delay of two hours and an optimistic door-to-needle time (the time needed to evaluate a chest pain patient and begin thrombolysis if appropriate) of 15 minutes, fewer than half of all heart attack patients will receive the maximal efficacy of thrombolysis. . . . The 10% of patients who delay more than 12 hours will receive little if any benefit of thrombolysis" (p. 8).

There are some factors that have been reported to influence delay. First are external resources, both material and social. People who are financially distressed tend to delay (Keith, 1987). Lack of social support also encourages delay. For example, those who are dissatisfied with their marriage or who report a lack of emotional support are more likely to delay (Cochran et al., 1986). Readily available pathways to medical care in the form of having a regular health care provider reduce delay (Lauver & Ho, 1993).

Cognitions are important in determining whether people delay. Whether people correctly classify their signs and sensations as symptoms requiring professional consultation is highly important. In particular, the availability of an alternative explanation for the signs, sensations, and symptoms determines how difficult it will be to discriminate between those that are minor and those that require care. Patients who have recently experienced the onset of a new stressor tend to delay because they attribute their symptoms to the stressor (Cameron et al., 1995). People who have rectal bleeding and see it as a minor illness that will clear up by itself are delayers (Byles, Redman, Hennrikus, et al., 1992). Women who experience abnormal bleeding tend to attribute this symptom to their menopausal status (Cochran et al., 1986). In each of these cases the ready availability of an alternative explanation no doubt makes it hard to decide whether symptoms merit medical attention.

Representativeness also influences cognitive processing of symptoms and can lead to delay. As we pointed out earlier, people tend to judge probabilities by using certain heuristics, and representativeness is one of them. In this context, representativeness refers to the extent to which something is typically associated with a certain diagnosis. Thus, if an African American has symptoms that seem to fit sickle cell anemia, representativeness is high, but for a Caucasian it would be low. A Caucasian with symptoms of sickle cell anemia might delay taking action because of the implausibility of the diagnosis (assuming they understand that sickle cell anemia is unusual in Caucasians). Phenomena of this kind have been found in the published literature. For example, people with symptoms of sexually transmitted disease have been found to delay if they are heterosexual and believe themselves to be in a monogamous relationship. Those who are homosexual and have had anonymous sex partners are less likely to delay when experiencing such symptoms (Leemaurs, Rombouts, & Kok, 1993).

Another cognitive factor that influences delay has to do with expected payoffs and costs of alternative actions. A person who decides to seek care may have to expend considerable effort in such things as getting an appointment and finding ways to deal with personal obligations. The longer delays of those who do not have a regular health care provider may well have to do with their being burdened with the added task of deciding whom to call and arranging an appointment. In addition they may or may not believe that medical treatment will actually help them. Low expectations for medical outcome are associated with longer delay (Safer et al., 1979).

Motivation also influences delay. For example, in a retrospective study of patients seeking treatment for a particular symptom for the first time, Safer et al. (1979) found that more painful symptoms are associated with shorter delay.

WHAT IS TO BE DONE ABOUT DELAY?

Mikulincer and his colleagues have done a great deal of research on the influence of attachment styles on coping with stress, including disastrous stress (Mikulincer & Florian, 1998). The standard attachment style categories are "securely attached," "anxious-ambivalent," and "avoidant." The securely attached tend to grow up optimistic, confident, and ready to ask for help. The anxious-ambivalents are not so optimistic and confident; in fact they are much more likely to worry and be in conflict over asking for help. The avoidants tend to rely solely on their personal resources to deal with challenging situations.

Mikulincer and Florian (1998) and his colleagues used well-established measures of attachment style and then observed how people dealt with various stressful challenges. Their work was done in Israel, and they looked at military recruits facing the demands of basic training, as well as people who had endured missile attacks during the Persian Gulf War. True to their hypotheses, securely attached people tended to cope better than others. Yet there were perplexing instances in which people ran counter to their attachment style. For example, soldiers in training sought help whether they were classified as securely attached or avoidant. The investigators realized how obvious it was that people trained in well-developed, institutionalized coping strategies are likely to use those strategies regardless of their personal characteristics.

Mikulincer is not alone in having noted the impact of strategic planning and training on coping with challenges. Others have pointed out how important it is in coping with disasters to have a well-developed strategic plan and to thoroughly train people at risk in how to implement that plan (Gist & Lubin, 1989).

It is essential that a strategy be developed for coping with challenging situations and that people likely to face those challenges be well informed and even well trained in the use of those strategies. If such strategies are developed, taught, and reinforced in various ways, they can increase the likelihood that people will function effectively in challenging situations, even against their personal inclinations.

People, particularly those at special risk, should be educated and trained in a strategy for dealing with major health problems. They should know what signs and sensations to look for and especially know which ones require immediate action. The decision-making algorithms that are used in deciding on medical actions need not be complex, and there is no reason why lay people cannot be helped to understand a set of principles that would equip them to make better judgments and take more adaptive actions.

Furthermore, a clear pathway to appropriate care should be worked out, at least for people at relatively high risk. This would no doubt mean having a regular health care provider or somehow knowing where to call in order to minimize the delays due to factors out of the patient's control. They should be trained to develop and even rehearse a plan of action, including, where possible, arranging for help from significant others.

To implement such a concept fully would require a great commitment from society. On the other hand, each of us is likely to have opportunities to guide patients toward greater clarity about distinguishing symptoms that require professional attention and developing a strategy for coping with them. In one study comparing patients with or without a history of heart disease, it was found that those with such a history actually delayed longer. The authors of that paper make a very significant point, with which we will close this section. "The unexpected observation that patients with known ischaemic heart disease delay longer before seeking help in spite of their frequent contact with doctors suggests that opportunities for educating patients are being wasted" (Mumford, Warr, Owen, & Fraser, 1999).

CONCLUSION

At the beginning of this chapter we described the historical influences that contributed to the "personality" of modern medicine. These influences gave us scientific medicine, with its emphasis on treatments capable of being justified by scientific evidence and biological science. This approach has been of immeasurable value, but it was created before psychological and social sciences had adequately developed. It must now be expanded to include psychological and social factors if it is to realize its full potential. Evidence indicates that scientific medicine may be surprisingly limited when this larger context is neglected. Health care will be enhanced by recognizing the addition of psychosocial factors to the customary biological ones.

Throughout this chapter we have presented but a few examples of psychosocial interventions enhancing traditional treatment outcomes. There is far more related evidence than could be included in this short chapter. Moreover, renewed emphasis on psychosocial factors highlights the many facets of the person of the patient for which the traditional medical model allows little room. We are multidimensional beings, existing not only at the physical level but also in psychological, social, and spiritual realms, which necessarily interact, so that healing of any one of them tends to effect the others, with treatment of the right combination being optimal for full healing or even healing of the body alone. The psychological, social, and spiritual dimensions of the patient may require healing as much as the body does, and harm may be done when the body is treated in isolation.

Finally, as emphasized earlier, although there is convincing scientific evidence that the mind does influence the body, the rationale for the utility of psychosocial interventions does not rest only on this foundation. Whether the mind has direct control over the body or not, these interventions can help the healing professional deliver traditional services more effectively. For example, the patient undergoing repeated chemotherapy for cancer whose nausea and vomiting are not being adequately controlled by medicine has a good chance of enhancing that control through such things as relaxation training. The scientific evidence for this is good. The result may well be better adherence to the treatment regimen and thus improved outcome. When psychosocial influences are addressed, a broad range of skills and support systems may be cultivated and directed toward the production of greater treatment efficacy.

REFERENCES

Ader, R., & Cohen, N. (1975). Behaviorally conditioned immune suppression. *Psychosomatic Medicine, 37*, 333–340.

Andersen, B. L., Kiecolt-Glaser, J. K., & Glaser, R. (1994). A biobehavioral model of cancer stress and disease course. *American Psychologist, 49*(5), 389–404.

Antoni, M. H. (1987). Neuroendocrine influences in psychoimmunology and neoplasia: A review. *Psychology and Health, 1*, 3–24.

Antonovsky, A. (1979). *Health, stress, and coping.* San Francisco: Jossey-Bass.

Antonovsky, A. (1987). *Unravelling the mystery of health: How people manage stress and stay well.* San Francisco: Jossey-Bass.

Aspinwall, L. G. (1998). Social comparison. In E. A. Blechman & K. D. Brownel (Eds.), *Behavioral medicine and women: A comprehensive handbook* (pp. 176–182). New York: Guilford.

Barber, T. X. (1984). Changing "unchangeable" bodily processes by (hypnotic) suggestions: A new look at hypnosis, cognitions, imagining, and the mind-body problem.

In A. A. Sheikh (Ed.), *Imagination and healing* (pp. 69–127). New York: Baywood.

Belloc, N. D., & Breslow, L. (1972). Relationship of physical health status and family practices. *Preventive Medicine, 1,* 409–421.

Boyd, J., Covington, T., Stanaszek, W., & Coussons, R. (1974). Drug defaulting—Part I: Determinants of compliance. *American Journal of Hospital Pharmacy, 31,* 362–364.

Bruhn, J. G., & Wolf, S. (1979). *The Roseto story.* Norman, OK: University of Oklahoma Press.

Bulloch, K. (1981). Neuroendocrine-immune circuitry: Pathways involved with the induction and persistence of humoral immunity. *Dissertation Abstracts International, 41,* 4447-B.

Burish, T. G., & Jenkins, R. A. (1992). Effectiveness of biofeedback and relaxation training in reducing the side effects of cancer chemotherapy. *Health Psychology, 11,* 17–23.

Byles, J. E., Redman, S., Hennrikus, D., Sanson-Fisher, R. W., & Dickinson, J. (1992). Delay in consulting a medical practitioner about rectal bleeding. *Journal of Epidemiology & Community Health, 46,* 241–244.

Cameron, L., Leventhal, E. A., & Leventhal, H. (1993). Symptom representations and affect as determinants of care seeking in a community-dwelling adult sample population. *Health Psychology, 12,* 171–179.

Cameron, L., Leventhal, E. A., & Leventhal, H. (1995). Seeking medical care in response to symptoms and life stress. *Psychosomatic Medicine, 57,* 48–49.

Cannon, W. B. (1932). *The wisdom of the body.* New York: W.W. Norton.

Carey, M. P., & Burish, T. G. (1988). Etiology and treatment of the psychological side effects associated with cancer chemotherapy: A critical review and discussion. *Psychological Bulletin, 104,* 307–325.

Cochran, S. D., Hacker, N. F., & Berek, J. (1986). Correlates of delay in seeking treatment for endometrial cancer. *Journal of Psychosomatic Obstetrics & Gynecology, 5,* 245–252.

Cohen, S., Tyrell, D., & Smith, A. (1993). Negative life events, perceived stress, negative affect, and susceptibility to the common cold. *Journal of Personality and Social Psychology, 64,* 131–140.

Davis, M. S. (1966). Variations in patients' compliance with doctors' analysis of congruence between survey responses and results of empirical observations. *Journal of Medical Education, 41,* 1037–1048.

de Boer-Dennert, M., de Wit, R., Schmitz, P. I., Djontono, J., Beurden, V., Stoter, G., et al. (1997). Patient perceptions of the side-effects of chemotherapy: The influence of 5HT3 antagonists. *British Journal of Cancer, 76,* 1055–1061.

DiMatteo, M. R., & DiNicola, D. D. (1982). *Achieving patient compliance: The psychology of the medical practitioner's role.* New York: Pergamon Press.

Dollard, J., & Miller, N. E. (1950). *Personality and psychotherapy: An analysis in terms of learning, thinking, and culture.* New York: McGraw Hill.

Dreher, H. (1998). Mind-body interventions for surgery: evidence and exigency. *Advances in Mind-Body Medicine, 14,* 207–222.

Dubos, R. (1959). *Mirage of health: Utopias, progress, and biological change.* New York: Harper Colophon.

Dunbar, J., & Agras, S. (1980). Compliance with medical instructions. In J. Ferguson, & C. B. Taylor (Eds.), *The comprehensive handbook of behavioral medicine* (Vol. 3, pp. 115–145). New York: SP Medical & Scientific Books.

Elstein, A. S., & Bordage, G. (1979). Psychology of clinical reasoning. In G. C. Stone, F. Cohen, & N. E. Adler (Eds.), *Health psychology* (pp. 333–368). San Francisco: Jossey-Bass.

Engel, G. L. (1977). The need for a new medical model: A challenge for biomedicine. *Science, 196,* 129–135.

Facione, N. C. (1993). Delay versus help seeking for breast cancer symptoms: A critical review of the literature on patient and provider delay. *Social Science and Medicine, 36,* 1521–1534.

Fallowfield, L. J. (1992). Behavioural interventions and psychological aspects of care during chemotherapy. *European Journal of Cancer,* 28A (Suppl 1), S39–41.

Foldes, A., Nemethy, Z., Szalay, O., & Kovacs, K. J. (2000). Anaphylactoid reactions activate hypothalamo-pituitary-adrenocortical axis: Comparison with endotoxic reactions. *Brain Research Bulletin, 52,* 573–579.

Ford, S., Fallowfield, L., & Lewis, S. (1994). Can oncologists detect distress in their outpatients and how satisfied are they with their performance during bad news consultation? *British Journal of Cancer, 70,* 767–770.

Frasure-Smith, N., Lesperance, F., & Talajic, M. (1993). Depression following myocardial infarction: Impact on 6-month survival. *Journal of the American Medical Association, 270,* 1819–1825.

Gist, R., & Lubin, B. (1989). *Psychosocial aspects of disaster.* New York: Wiley.

Glaser, R., Sheridan, J. F., Malarkey, W. B., MacCallum, R. C., & Kiecolt-Glaser, J. K. (2000). Chronic stress modulates the immune response to a pneumococcal pneumonia vaccine. *Psychosomatic Medicine, 62,* 804–807.

Goff, D. C., Jr., Feldman, H. A., McGovern, P. G., Goldberg, R. J., Simons-Morton, D. G., Cornell, C. E., et al. (1999). Prehospital delay in patients hospitalized with heart attack symptoms in the United States: The REACT trial. *The American Heart Journal, 138,* 1048–1057.

Goldberg, A. I., Cohen, G., & Rubin, A. H. (1998). Physician assessments of patient compliance with medical treatment. *Social Science Medicine, 47,* 1873–1876.

Greenberg, P. D. (1987). Tumor immunology. In D. P. Stites, J. D. Stobo, & J. V. Wells (Eds.), *Basic and clinical immunology* (6th ed.). Norwalk, CT: Appleton & Lange.

Greenfield, S., Kaplan, S. H., & Ware, J. E. (1985). Expanding patient involvement in care: Effects on patient outcomes, *Annals of Internal Medicine, 102*(4), 520–528.

Greenfield S., Kaplan, S. H., Ware, J. E., Yano, E. M., & Frank, H. J. (1988). Patient participation in medical care: Effects on blood sugar control and quality of life in diabetes. *Journal General Internal Medicine, 3,* 448–457.

Hamer, D., & Copeland, P. (1994). *The science of desire: The search for the gay gene and the biology of behavior.* New York: Simon & Schuster.

Illich, I. (1976). *Medical nemesis: The expropriation of health.* New York: Pantheon Books.

James, W. (1890). *The principles of psychology, Vol. 1.* New York: Henry Holt.

Kaplan, S. H., Gandek, B., Greenfield, S. Rogers, W., & Ware, J. E. (1995). Patient and visit characteristics related to physicians' participatory decision-making style. Results from the Medical Outcomes Study. *Medical Care, 33,* 1176–1187.

Kaplan, S. H., Greenfield, S. Rogers, W. H., & Ware, J. E. (1996). Characteristics of physicians with participatory decision-making styles. *Annals of Internal Medicine, 124,* 511–513.

Keith, P. M. (1987). Postponement of health care by widowed, divorced, and never-married older men. *Lifestyles, 8,* 70–81.

Keller, S. E., Shapiro, R., Schliefer, S. J., & Stein, M. (1982). Hypothalamic influences on anaphylaxis. (Abstract). *Psychosomatic Medicine, 44*, 302.

Kiecolt-Glaser, J., Malarkey, W. B., Chee, M., Newton, T., Cacioppo, J. T., Mao, H. Y., et al. (1993). Negative behavior during marital conflict is associated with immunological down-regulation. *Psychosomatic Medicine, 55*, 410–412.

Kiecolt-Glaser, J. K., & Glaser, R. (1989). Psychoneuroimmunology: Past, present, and future. *Health Psychology, 8*, 677–682.

Kiecolt-Glaser, J. K., Marucha, P. T., Malarkey, W. B., Mercado, A. M., & Glaser, R. (1995). Slowing of wound healing by psychological stress. *Lancet, 346*, 1194–1196.

Lauver, D., & Ho, C. (1993). Explaining delay in care-seeking for breast cancer symptoms. *Journal of Applied Social Psychology, 23*, 1806–1825.

Leemaurs, P. E., Rombouts, R., & Kok, G. (1993). *Psychology and Health, 8*, 17–32.

Levy, R. L. (1987). Compliance and clinical practice. In J. A. Blumenthal & D. C. McKee (Eds.), *Applications in behavioral medicine and health psychology: A clinician's source book* (pp. 567–587). Sarasota, FL: Resource Exchange, Inc.

Lynch, S. E. (1977). *The broken heart: The medical consequences of loneliness.* New York: Basic Books.

McCann, S., & Weinman, J. (1996). Encouraging patient participation in general practice consultations: effect on consultations length and content, patient satisfaction and health. *Psychology and Health, 11*, 857–869.

Mechanic, D. (1996). Changing medical organization and the erosion of trust. *The Milbank Quarterly, 74*, 171–189.

Meyer, T. J., & Mark, M. M. (1995). Effects of psychosocial interventions with adult cancer patients: A meta-analysis of randomized experiments. *Health Psychology, 14*(2), 101–108.

Mikulincer, M., & Florian, V. (1998). The relationships between adult attachment styles and emotional and cognitive reactions to stressful events. In J. Simpson & W. S. Rholes (Eds.), *Attachment theory and close relationships* (pp. 143–165). New York: Guilford.

Miller, G. (1956). The magical number seven plus or minus two. *Psychological Review, 63*, 81–97.

Mumford, A. D., Warr, K. V., Owen, S. J., & Fraser, A. G. (1999). Delays by patients in seeking treatment for acute chest pain: Implications for achieving earlier thrombolysis. *Postgraduate Medical Journal, 75*, 90–95.

Murphy, J., & Coster, G. (1997). Issues in patient compliance. *Drugs, 54*, 797–800.

Myers, D. G. (1999). *Social psychology* (6th ed.). Boston: McGraw-Hill.

O'Rourke, K. D., & deBlois, J. (1991). The right to know: Ethical issues related to mandatory testing of healthcare workers for HIV. *Health Progress, 72*(10), 39–43.

Overmier, B., & Murison, J. (1997). Animal models reveal the "psych" in the psychosomatics of peptic ulcers. *Current Directions in Psychological Science, 6*, 180–184.

Pennebaker, J. W. (1982). *The psychology of physical symptoms.* New York: Springer-Verlag.

Pennebaker, J. W. (1990). *Opening up: The healing power of confiding in others.* New York: William Morrow.

Pennebaker, J. W. (Ed.). (1995). *Emotion, disclosure, & health.* Washington, DC: APA.

Petitti, D. B., Reingold, A., & Chin, J. (1986). The incidence of toxic shock syndrome in Northern California: 1972 through 1983. *Journal of the American Medical Association, 255*, 368–372.

Sackett, D. L., & Snow, J. C. (1979). The magnitude of compliance and noncompliance. In R. B. Haynes, D. W. Taylor, & D. L. Sackett (Eds.), *Compliance in healthcare* (pp. 11–23). Baltimore: Johns Hopkins University Press.

Safer, M. A., Tharps, O. J., Jackson, T. C., & Leventhal, H. (1979). Determinants of three stages of delay in seeking care at a medical clinic. *Medical Care, 17,* 11–29.

Sagan, L. A. (1987). *The health of nations: True causes of sickness and well-being.* New York: Basic Books.

Scrimshaw, N. S., Behar, M., Guzman, M. A., & Gordon, J. E. (1969). Nutrition and infection field study in Guatemalan villages, 1959–1964, IX. An evaluation of medical, social, and public health benefits, with suggestions for future field study. *Archives of Environmental Health, 18,* 51–62.

Selye, H. (1936). A syndrome produced by diverse nocuous agents. *Nature, 138,* 32.

Sheridan, C. L. (1986). The role of muscular tension in the control of psychophysiological discharge phenomena. *Clinical Biofeedback and Health, 9,* 48–55.

Sheridan, C. L. (1989). Technological versus psychodynamic treatment of impaired stress management. *Dynamische Psychiatrie/Dynamic Psychiatry, 22,* 51–58.

Sheridan, C. L., & Radmacher, S. A. (1992). *Health psychology: Challenging the biomedical model.* New York: Wiley.

Shiffrin, R. M., & Nosofsky, R. M. (1994). Seven plus or minus two: A commentary on capacity limitations. *Psychological Review, 101,* 357–361.

Smallwood, K. G. (1992). The feasibility of mandatory HIV testing for health professionals and other special populations. *Journal of Oklahoma State Medical Association, 85*(2), 74–80.

Smith, C. S. (1968). Matter versus materials: A historical view. *Science, 162,* 637–644.

Straka, R. J., Fish, J. T., Benson, S. R., & Suh, J. T. (1997). Patient self-reporting of compliance does not correspond with electronic monitoring: An evaluation using isosorbide dinitrate as a model drug. *Pharmacotherapy, 17,* 126–132.

Turner, S., Maher, E. J., Young, T. Young, J., & Vaughan, H. G. (1996). What are the information priorities for cancer patients involved in treatment decisions? An experienced surrogate study in Hodgkin's disease. *British Journal of Cancer, 73,* 222–227.

Vernikos-Danellis, J., & Heybach, J. P. (1980). Psychophysiologic mechanisms regulating the hypothalamic-pituitary-adrenal response to stress. In H. Selye (Ed.), *Selye's guide to stress research* (Vol. 1, pp. 46–70). New York: Van Nostrand Reinhold.

Weiner, H. (1996). Use of animal models in peptic ulcer disease. *Psychosomatic Medicine, 58,* 525–545.

Wilkinson, R. G. (1996). *Unhealthy societies: The afflictions of inequality.* New York: Routledge.

Williams, R. B. (1992). Prognostic importance of social and economic resources among medically treated patients with angiographically documented coronary artery disease. *Journal of the American Medical Association, 276,* 520–524.

Woloshin, S., Schwartz, L. M., Tosteson, A. N., Chang, C. H. Wright, B., Plohman, J., et al. (1997). Perceived adequacy of tangible social support and health outcomes in patients with coronary artery disease. *Journal of General Internal Medicine, 12,* 613–618.

2

Psychosocial Factors
Affecting Medical Conditions

KENNETH S. GORFINKLE
FELICE TAGER

What is psychosomatic or behavioral medicine, and why should the mental health professional keep current with advances in research and clinical applications? In recent years, mental health professionals have begun to integrate an increasingly sophisticated understanding of the mind-body problem; pathways of action between mind and body are complex, bidirectional, and heavily traveled. This has been a hot topic in both medical and psychological literature. This chapter will outline a number of those pathways. Familiarity with recent research in psychosomatic medicine is a useful tool in communicating with patients presenting with complex health problems. Mental health specialists should have at their fingertips an evidence-based understanding of the rationale for a referral for psychotherapeutic treatment of patients with conditions affecting both psyche and soma.

What should mental health professionals know about the interplay between stress, psychological distress, and somatic illness, and why is this a necessary part of a clinician's knowledge base? Today's medical patient has access to an unprecedented flow of high quality information about his condition and its treatment. A patient with a chronic illness, for example, can achieve a level of sophistication about his treatment to put him on a par with both psychotherapist and physician. Furthermore, the public is bombarded with advertising and information from complementary and alternative medical fields. An individual with osteoarthritis may choose from multiple treatment options ranging from mainstream medical rheumatology and orthopedics and pain specialists who are trained in neurology, psychiatry, or anesthesiology to acupuncturists, nutritionists, homeopaths, and herbalists. A majority of chronically ill patients make use of one or more alternative and complementary approaches to healing and wellness, in addition to conventional care.

A different obstacle to optimum care for the medically ill patient is borne not of physicians' ignorance but more of collective amnesia. In the days when medical care was not nearly as sophisticated as it is now, the medical professional knew less about *treating* and more about *caring* for patients' medical conditions. The modern model follows a formal sequence:

- from *relevant* symptoms
- to assessment
- to disease diagnosis
- to treatment, usually with some combination of medicine, surgery, or radiation therapy
- to cure, remission, or death.

To be an excellent physician using this model, one must rely on technology, access to up-to-date research, and a keen ability to apply deductive reasoning to complex questions such as how to cure disease. To be an excellent caregiver, a physician needs to see disease from the patient's point of view. That entails an understanding of *illness* as experienced by the patient. Illness is only partly a function of disease. Illness subsumes the idea of loss of well-being, stigma, isolation, and change of existential condition. It is defined by the personal/historical context of the patient's predicament: When were symptoms first noticed? What kind of attention did they receive? How did the patient's sense of well-being change over time? What are the social supports for the patient? How much hope and optimism did the patient have for recovery? What was the quality of the care given by the health providers? Was it perfunctory and impersonal or empathic and thoughtful? How did the illness change the person's life circumstances? In comparison to disease, illness covers a broader sweep of a person's life. An illness model might follow an informal sequence:

- from the time when the person began to feel *any* symptoms, and
- from the time when others noticed that the person behaved differently
- to the time when the person became a patient; i.e. entered "the land of the sick"
- to the time period when the person and family learn of and come to terms with the impact of illness on his or her life and ability to function
- to the time when the person adjusts (or fails to adjust) to the changes in health, well-being, and prognosis.

Physicians hard pressed to keep up with the rigorous demands of treating patients with complex illnesses are becoming decreasingly available to provide care to the people with the illness. Ironically, the trend toward setting new, high standards for providing evidence-based medical care may be turning good physicians away from the art of medical care in favor of the burgeoning science of medical treatment. In the best of worlds, patients and people would get the best of both.

The remainder of this chapter will review some of the relevant literature on psychological factors that affect the onset, diagnosis, treatment, and cure of disease. However, if the goal were to be confined to disease only, and not to illness, some of our literature would be difficult to interpret.

The first section of this chapter will review factors that moderate both illness and disease. These include environmental, lifestyle, and personality factors. The next section reviews literature elaborating on several descriptive and explanatory models of health-related behavior in relation to risk of contracting specific diseases. The final section focuses on the relatively more recent work on psychological predictors of illness and illness behavior.

FACTORS THAT MODERATE ILLNESS AND DISEASE

Environmental and Work Factors

One of the fascinating challenges for psychotherapy today is to help the patient harness his or her own abilities and motivation to get and stay healthy.

Environmental and work conditions are significant contributors to health and illness. Poverty, sleep deprivation, dangerous work conditions, and exposure to hazardous materials can lead to health problems both for the individual and for family members. The astute clinician needs to know what physical and situational obstacles stand in the way of health and well-being so that he or she can guide the patient toward minimizing stress-related physical and emotional problems and getting the most out of the complex health care system.

Poverty

Although the United States is the richest nation in the world, millions of Americans live in poverty. Approximately 36 million people were reportedly living below the poverty line ($15,569 annual income for a family of four) in 1995 (Weinberg, 1996). Approximately 40% of the individuals living in poverty are children (Bolig et al., 1999). The risk of growing up in poverty is not equally distributed. Minorities have higher rates of poverty than nonminorities, and female-headed households are at a greater poverty risk than male- or two-parent-headed households (Weinberg, 1996). Factors that contribute to the large number of people currently living in poverty include unemployment, lower wages for women, an increase in female-headed households (Hardy & Hazelrigg, 1993), minimum wage jobs that do not provide health benefits (Tarnowski & Rohrbeck, 1993), and failure to complete high school (Schorr, 1989). Living in poverty is associated with inferior and even dangerous housing, limited access to health care, poor nutrition, increased access to drugs, and higher rates of depression (Bartlett, 1998; Murphey et al., 1991).

Living in poverty affects the cognitive, emotional, social, and physical well-being of an individual and can extend across the lifespan (Bolig et al., 1999). For the poor, health problems may begin even before birth (Sherman, 1994) because of a lack of prenatal care (Tarnowski & Rohrbeck, 1993). In the perinatal and infancy period, poverty has been associated with congenital syphilis (Klerman, 1996), perinatally contracted AIDS (Zuckerman, 1993), prenatal drug and/or alcohol exposure (Abel, 1995), low birth weight (Children's Defense Fund, 1993), sudden infant death syndrome (Sherman, 1994), stunted growth (Tarnowski & Rohrbeck, 1993), malnutrition (Brown & Pollitt, 1996), lead poisoning, and failure to thrive (Black & Dubowitz, 1991).

As children develop in poverty, growth retardation, anemia, poor nutrition, and lead toxicity plague them (Klerman, 1996). Additional health problems are related to poor dental health (Rosenbaum, 1992), insufficient access to immunizations, untreated illnesses (i.e., ear infections) (Klerman, 1996; Oberg et al., 1995), and exposure to toxic chemicals, lead paint, and pollution (Kozol, 1995). Child abuse, neglect, and maltreatment compound these risks. The adverse effects of early poverty are far-reaching and may be difficult or even impossible to overcome.

In adolescence and adulthood, poverty is associated with additional health problems. Higher rates of teen pregnancy (Merrick, 1995), sexually transmitted diseases (Koniak-Griffin, Nyamathi, Vasquez, & Russo, 1994), and AIDS (Rosenbaum, 1992) are found in disadvantaged adolescents. Many of these difficulties continue into adult life with additional health problems, such as hypertension (Gilligan, 1996), heart disease (Ward, 1993), diabetes, cancer, tuberculosis, and sexually transmitted diseases (Bolig et al., 1999).

Poor working conditions and excessively long hours are not conducive to gaining access to medical or psychological care. In addition, a daunting wall of red tape keeps needy people from obtaining care and besets clinicians who attempt to provide mental health care for this population. With a grasp of some of these risk factors, the clinician can guide the patient through the red tape and set priorities that take physical and emotional health into account. Mental health workers who serve the poor are beset with similar job stress related to poor funding and stressful working conditions. It is therefore imperative that such workers make every effort to set an example by combating their own sources of work stress.

Sleep Deprivation

A good diagnostic work-up always includes questions about sleep. It provides hints about the presence of depression as well as other medical conditions. A recently reported study presented research findings from the University of Chicago linking prolonged sleep deprivation (4 h per night over 6 nights) with serious health problems (Brody, 1999). A 1994 report of the National Commission of Sleep Disorders Research reported that 30 million adults and teenagers in the

United States are chronically sleep deprived (Report of the National Commission on Sleep Disorders Research, 1994). A 9-year follow-up of the Alameda County health outcome study (Wingard, Berkman, & Brand, 1982) found a strong relationship between health outcomes and sleep. Specifically, individuals who slept fewer than 6 h per night had poorer health and had a 70% higher mortality rate than those individuals who slept more, independent of smoking, alcohol consumption, age, gender, race, physical health, and physical activity. Mortality rates from heart disease, cancer, stroke, and all causes combined were lowest for those individuals sleeping 7–8 h per night (Wingard et al., 1982). The relationship between sleep deprivation and cardiovascular morbidity, functional disability, and mortality have been documented (Wingard & Berkman, 1983; Kripke, Simons, Garfinkel, & Hammond, 1979; Partinen, Putkonen, Kaprio, Koskenvuo, & Hilakivi, 1982; Pollak, Perlick, Linsner, Wenston, & Hsieh, 1990). The common symptom of exhaustion upon waking in the morning can be an indicator of depression, thyroid disease, sleep apnea, restless leg syndrome, and subclinical heart disease (Appels & Schouten, 1991). Research from Japan on *karoshi* (sudden death caused by overwork) has found that lack of sleep may increase the following day's sympathetic nervous system activity, leading to increased blood pressure and heart rate (Tochikubo, Ikeda, Miyajima, & Ishii, 1996). Corroborating these findings, Lusardi et al. (1999) reported that lack of sleep, particularly during the first part of the night, in never-treated hypertensive patients might increase sympathetic nervous activity during the night and the following day, leading to increased blood pressure and heart rate. They conclude that chronically sleep-deprived hypertensives may be at higher risk of target organ damage and cardiovascular morbidity and mortality.

In addition to physical health problems, sleep deprivation has been linked to increases in careless errors and problems with attention-sustained vigilance and decision making (Linde, Edland, & Bergstrom, 1999; Hockey, 1973), which could be particularly significant for doctors, military staff, pilots, and air-control personnel.

The clinician therefore needs to stay well-versed in assessment and treatment of sleep pathology, know when to refer patients for medical evaluation, and understand that the sleep-deprived patient may not benefit from psychotherapy until sufficient sleep is restored.

Work Environments and Hazardous Conditions

The patient presenting with emotional fallout from a work-related injury or illness is worried not only about a physical condition or an emotional condition alone. His or her very livelihood may be at stake. A good understanding of the emotional, physical, and financial issues is essential for providing good care.

Work-related illnesses are becoming more and more common, with a recent review suggesting that musculoskeletal disorders are the most common self-reported work-related illness in the United Kingdom (Muggleton, Allen, & Chappell, 1999). Upper limb disorders such as nerve compression disorders, carpal tunnel syndrome, tendon and tendon-related disorders, finger tendonitis, and rotator cuff syndrome rank only second to back problems. They categorize the occupational risk factors related to these conditions as load-related (vibration, mechanical shock, and hard/sharp edges), posture-related (wrist flexion/ extension, elbow and shoulder movements, repetitive movements, and exposure time), and environmental (temperature, humidity, and psychological stress). They propose ergonomic design changes to reduce the incidence of such disorders. Industries have begun to focus on workplace activities as related to task frequency and variability. Both physiological and psychological variability in tasks has been emphasized as important (Hagberg, 1996). However, more research is needed to better establish the incidence of these injuries as well as the occupational risks of many of these disorders.

Another aspect of working conditions pertains to exposure to hazardous agents such as lead and waste gases. Exposure to nitrous oxide has been linked with adverse effects on fertility as well as spontaneous abortion (Rowland et al., 1995). Hoerauf et al. (1999) studied the extent of genetic damage in veterinary surgeons working routinely in the operating room and regularly exposed to waste anesthetic gases as compared with nonexposed veterinary physicians. They found that exposure to trace concentrations of waste anesthetic gases might cause dose-dependent genetic damage. The differences in genetic markers detected in the exposed veterinarians were comparable with smoking 11–20 cigarettes per day. It is unclear whether these genetic changes will lead to adverse health outcomes in otherwise healthy individuals, but further investigation is warranted.

Work environments can lead to adverse health outcomes both for the workers themselves and family members. Approximately 890,000 children in the United States between the ages of 1 and 5 have elevated blood lead levels (CDC, 1997). The CDC has long recognized that parental exposure to lead in work-related activities is potentially a risk of lead exposure to their children. A meta-analysis of the existing studies indicates that approximately 50% of children living with household members occupationally exposed to lead have elevated blood lead levels (Roscoe, Gittleman, Deddens, Peterson, & Halpernin, 1999). They conclude that children of lead-exposed workers should be included in the group targeted for blood lead screening.

For the clinician treating a patient with a work- or environment-related medical condition, anger, fear, and frustration about having been placed at risk in the first place may be a focus of treatment. Once an illness or injury is diagnosed and defined as such, the clinician might be called upon to document the degree of disability and therapeutic improvement as a function of treatment. These demands add to the complexity of such cases, especially when emotional reactions to injury or illness compound and amplify the symptoms. One must be cautious, however, to identify the influence of secondary gain to the patient whose financial reimbursement is tied to remaining symptomatic.

Lifestyle: Health-Impairing and Health-Enhancing Behaviors

Another way in which psychological factors are related to health and disease pertains to modifiable behaviors that mediate the disease process. These behavior patterns are not often the focus of treatment and are left to the treating physician or to the family to take care of. Yet the patient's mental health may either be dependent on or a cause of health-impairing behavior.

Reports from the early 1980s estimated that approximately 50% of the mortality rate from the 10 foremost causes of death might be ascribed to lifestyle (Hamburg, Elliot, & Parron, 1982). Attributing deaths to lifestyle is a fancy way of saying that they are potentially preventable through specific behavior change. The potential benefits of psychotherapeutic interventions for protecting public health are immeasurable. A study correlated the personal health practices and subsequent health status of thousands of people (Belloc & Breslow, 1972). Performance of seven health related behaviors (sleeping 8 h per night, eating breakfast, not eating between meals, maintaining appropriate weight, active participation in physical activity, drinking only moderately, and not smoking) was associated with satisfactory health. Recent literature has focused on specific behaviors, distinguishing between health-enhancing and health-impairing behaviors. Baum and Posluszny (1999) define health-enhancing behaviors as actions that carry benefits to one's health or otherwise safeguard people from disease such as diet and exercise. In addition, they define health- impairing behaviors as "activities that have harmful effects on health," such as cigarette smoking, substance abuse, high-risk sexual behavior, and prolonged exposure to ultraviolet radiation in sunlight. Some of these behaviors, such as diet and exercise, may exert direct physiological influences on the body, leading to illness and disease, or may be modified by the effects of emotions or stress. However, these behaviors are not immediate causes of disease but are factors that place an individual at higher risk for developing medical problems.

Human behaviors are complex actions and reactions to multiple internal or external triggers. Human beings do not simply "do" a particular act, such as lighting a cigarette or eating a piece of chocolate cake. Rather, humans respond to some combination of physiological, environmental, and emotional factors. Eating, for example, can be understood as a response to these multiple factors. An individual will be cued to eat when he feels hunger pains, when his body is telling him that he is in need of caloric intake. The same person, after feeling sated from a large meal, will be cued to eat if his surroundings encourage it, for example, at a party or in a restaurant with friends, or alternately, if the surroundings have become "learned" cues, such as eating potato chips while sitting on the couch and watching television. Our hypothetical person will be more inclined to eat the piece of cake, despite the lack of any physiological or environmental cues, if he is feeling anxious or depressed (Hill, Weaver, & Blundell, 1991). These factors may exert their influences independently, or in intricate, overlapping, and cyclical interactions, creating behavior patterns that are difficult to extinguish.

Patients seek help to quit smoking, lose weight, or increase exercise and discover that underlying conditions such as depression and anxiety contributed to maintaining their problems. The role for psychotherapy is obvious. The therapist can have the greatest impact when lifestyle patterns and psychopathology are addressed together.

Diet and Weight

Weight-loss programs are big business with a reputation for less than professional standards of treatment. For this reason, it especially behooves the mental health professions to verse themselves in the potential benefits and limits of various weight programs. The quantity and kinds of food that people eat, as well as a person's weight, are to a large extent behaviorally mediated.

There is a well-documented genetic component to weight as well as to other aspects of diet such as cholesterol level. Eating behavior can abate or exacerbate these predisposing genetic risk factors. The links between diet and weight, particularly obesity, and onset of health problems have been firmly established. Obesity tends to be a chronic condition, beginning in childhood, associated either directly or indirectly with medical problems such as high blood cholesterol, hypertension, diabetes, and certain cancers. This has great public health implications given that in the United States 35% of women over the age of 20 and 31% of men over the age of 20 are overweight, and approximately 25% of children and adolescents are obese (Institute of Medicine, 1995). For this reason weight control and nutritional programs have increasingly become part of health promotion campaigns (Wing, 1995).

Research on cardiovascular disease has demonstrated one of the clearest links with dietary health behaviors. Obesity, high cholesterol, and high fat and salt consumption play a significant role in the development of hypertension (Blair, Goodyear, Gibbons, & Cooper, 1994), coronary heart disease (Scheidt, 1996), and stroke (Baum & Posluszny, 1999). Many of the aspects of food and diet that are associated with weight gain and obesity are also associated risk factors for heart disease, and therefore both can be addressed concurrently. For instance, foods that are high in fat tend to be less filling than high-carbohydrate foods (Golay & Bobbioni, 1997). As a consequence, individuals eating high-fat diets will tend to eat increased amounts of food. (Baum & Posluszny, 1999). The findings promoting diet as a risk for the development of cancer are currently indeterminate (Nordevang, Azavedo, Svane, Nilsson, & Holm, 1993; Negri et al., 1996) and need to be clearly defined for different types of cancers.

Because of the links between diet and health risks, particularly cardiovascular disease, weight management and diet control have been recommended as strategies for the prevention and treatment of certain conditions, such as high blood cholesterol. Along with this trend, government agencies have been highlighting and advocating dietary change as a means to reduce a variety of health risks (Expert Panel, National Cholesterol Education Program, National Academy of Sciences). Pharmacologic interventions have been found to be helpful in reducing serum cholesterol concentrations (Law, Wald, & Thompson, 1994). Interventions focused on diet have begun to yield comparable positive results in the area of reduced mortality (Renaud et al., 1995; Walden, Retzlaff, Buck, McCann, & Knopp, 1997) and lower cholesterol (Ornish, Brown, & Scherwitz, 1990; Watts et al., 1992; Brown, Zhao, Sacco, & Albers, 1993). A review of the research indicates that aggressive dietary treatments consisting of diets low in total and saturated fat are associated with lowered blood cholesterol levels and positive angiographic changes, and in addition may improve symptoms such as angina (Van Horn & Kavey, 1997). Despite the potential gains from diet change, long-term adherence has been difficult to accomplish. Methodological inconsistencies have made it hard to interpret the various studies looking at dietary adherence (Brownell & Cohen, 1995a). However, it appears that dietary change is possible with effective interventions focusing on the individual's perceptions, psychological and cultural factors, and providing the necessary education and skills (Brownell & Cohen, 1995b).

These possibilities notwithstanding, the clinician must overcome the legitimate doubts of the client before entering into serious weight management treatment. Armed with familiarity with some of the above research as well as an understanding of psychological factors (such as depression) that mediate eating behavior, the therapist can provide an intelligent, well-thought-out treatment approach to a difficult problem.

Exercise

Exercise, or physical activity, has been found to impact physical functioning in a variety of ways. Regular exercise can significantly prevent obesity, manage weight and stress, and has been found to alter endocrine and circulatory functioning as well as muscle tone (Baum & Posluszny, 1999). Approximately 12% of the total mortality in the United States (250,000 deaths per year) has been associated with physical inactivity (Pate et al., 1995). As with diet and obesity, the relationship between physical activity and heart disease has been well established (Powell, Thompson, Casperson, & Kendrick, 1987; Berlin & Colditz, 1990). In addition, physical activity has been found to have a protective effect against a number of medical conditions including diabetes, osteoporosis, and colon cancer (Sternfeld, 1992). Evidence for the relationship between breast cancer and some other reproductive cancers and physical activity has been mixed. Bernstein et al. (1994) found that premenopausal women who engaged in regular exercise had a reduced risk of developing breast cancer, which was possibly due to an alteration in the production of ovarian hormones. Dorgan et al.'s (1998) findings did not support a protective effect of physical activity during adulthood for breast cancer.

The Harvard Alumni Study (Paffenbarger Jr., Hyde, Wing, & Hsieh, 1986, 1993; Lee, Hsieh, & Paffenbarger Jr., 1995) found that men who were physically active at baseline (physical activity index of >2,000 kcal per week) demonstrated a 25% lower risk of death from any cause and a 36% lower rate of death from coronary heart disease compared to men who were less physically active. Exercise has been found to be related to positive health benefits including modestly modifying the lipid profile (Tran & Weltman, 1985; King, Haskell, Young, Oka, & Stefanick, 1995), lowering blood pressure (Arroll & Beaglehole, 1992), preventing the development of noninsulin-dependent diabetes mellitus (Lynch et al., 1996) and improving psychological functioning (Taylor et al., 1986; Wenger et al., 1995). In the cardiac rehabilitation setting, the effects of physical activity alone were similar to the use of other common interventions (e.g., beta-blockers) in relation to mortality rates (Miller et al., 1997). Comprehensive rehabilitation including exercise has been associated with a 20–25% reduction in overall mortality and cardiovascular mortality (O'Connor et al., 1989; Oldridge et al., 1988).

Given the health benefits related to activity level, current national guidelines advocate that individuals of all ages should be involved in moderately intense exercise (i.e., brisk walking, bicycling, swimming, gardening/yardwork) for 30–60 minutes, four to six times weekly or at least 30 min of moderately intense exercise almost every day (Fletcher et al., 1996). As with diet, despite the known benefits of exercise, adherence to consistent physical exercise is difficult. Miller et al. (1997), in their review of the literature, report that an important area of future research is identifying how to increase compliance with exercise programs.

Exercise and its mental health benefits are also recruited by therapists to combat conditions like depression and anxiety disorders. Armed with an understanding of the interplay between exercise, health, and emotional well-being, the therapist is in the best possible position to bring about positive behavior change.

Smoking and Substance Abuse

Tobacco use has been implicated as a primary risk factor for multiple medical problems. Nicotine, the psychoactive ingredient in tobacco, reaches its highest brain concentration within one minute of ingestion (Searight, 1999). Nicotine is associated with improved attention and memory (Kassel, 1997) as well as reduced negative affective states (Hughes, 1988). Given these "gains" of cigarette smoking, its use tends to become a well-established, desirable habit and therefore highly resistant to change.

In addition to sympathetic nervous system arousal, smoking and tobacco use are significant contributors to heart disease, hypertension, stroke, cancer, and respiratory and pulmonary disorders. Smoking also affects bodily resistance to infection (Gatchel et al., 1989). There is an increase in head and neck cancers in drinkers who also smoke (Andre, Schraub, Mercier, & Bontemps, 1995). Second-hand smoke and exposure to cigarette smoke is a health hazard that may be similar to actual nicotine exposure (Hausberg et al., 1997).

Although the prevalence of new smokers has decreased in the United States over the past decade, 20% of Americans are smokers (Searight, 1999), and adolescent smoking has been on the rise since 1992 (Botvin & Epstein, 1999). Regular cigarette smoking tends to begin in middle adolescence (Botvin & Epstein, 1999) and becomes a habit that is difficult to break, with 77% of adult smokers having been daily smokers before the age of 20 (U.S. Dept. of Health and Human Services, 1994). Therefore, smoking prevention programs have attempted to target children and adolescents. In the United States, adolescent smoking has been connected to the perceived availability of cigarettes, cost, social models, peer pressure, and stress, mental health, and ADHD (Robinson et al., 1997; Milberger et al., 1997; Viinamaki et al., 1997). The success of the earlier prevention programs has been small (Rooney & Murray, 1996). However, approaches that teach adolescents social resistance skills and antismoking norms, focusing on skills training rather than health information regarding the adverse effects of smoking, have been demonstrated to effectively deter smoking behavior (Botvin & Epstein, 1999).

Substance abuse and dependence, including alcohol and drugs, crosses SES, race, and gender barriers. Individuals between the ages of 18 and 24 have a relatively high prevalence rate for use of almost every substance (APA, 1994). Medical complications directly and indirectly related to chronic alcohol use include peptic ulcer disease, alcoholic liver disease (especially hepatitis), hypertension, and central nervous system damage. A study of drinking patterns and problems in primary care patients identified alcohol use disorders in up to 50% of male and 10% of female patients (Cherpitel, 1991). Of particular importance are the rising rates of alcohol use disorders and consequent medical complications in women (North, 1996).

With the drop in the social acceptance of tobacco and other drugs in recent years, the therapist is more likely to intervene with patients' substance use. In doing so, the interplay between health risks and addictive behavior demand that the therapist be aware of both in providing comprehensive treatment.

High-Risk Sexual Behavior

Sexual practices and behaviors are directly associated with the development of sexually transmitted diseases (STDs), herpes, and HIV/AIDS. Psychotherapeutic approaches to patients vulnerable to STDs must face the issues surrounding use of social judgment and awareness of risk. Addressing this topic with sexually active teens is as much of a professional responsibility as assessing suicidal risk.

Young, sexually active women are at a significant risk for STDs such as chlamydia and gonorrhea which can have serious consequences, including pelvic inflammatory disease and sterility (Masters et al., 1992). Gay men, injection drug users, and minorities are at risk for developing HIV and AIDS (Ekstrand, 1992; Vanichseni et al., 1993; Catania et al., 1992). A number of approaches have been put forward to prevent HIV infection, ranging from advocacy of total abstinence from sex, monogamous relationships, and practice of "safe" sex through limiting the number of sexual partners. The use of protection during sex, e.g., condom use, has been promoted in order to prevent the exchange of bodily fluids, thereby greatly reducing the risk of infection (Francis & Chin, 1987). Reviews of the AIDS risk reduction literature and evaluation of interventions have found that these interventions generally have been unsuccessful in reducing AIDS risk behaviors (Choi & Coates, 1994; Fisher & Fisher, 1992). However, an intervention with college students focusing on information, motivation, and behavioral skills found an increase in AIDS risk behaviors, such as condom accessibility, safer sex negotiation, and condom use (Fisher et al., 1996). Targeted interventions have been found to be effective in promoting safer sexual behavior in college women as well (Bryan et al., 1996). In addition, risky sexual behavior among gay men has declined (Martin, 1986). However, more research is needed to determine the best risk-reducing interventions for specific populations.

The therapist needs to develop a comfort with opening frank discussion of risky sexual behavior with vulnerable patients. To this end, many find training in sex therapy to be a helpful tool. Treatment approaches require an understanding of cultural context of sexual behavior for the client, combined with detailed knowledge of the implications of specific sexual practices for risk.

Exposure to Ultraviolet Sunlight

Sun exposure is another behavior that has been linked to significant health consequences. Many skin cancers are caused by exposure to ultraviolet radiation from the sun. Currently, skin cancer accounts for approximately 40% of all cancers, and about 20% of Americans will develop skin cancer. One of the best ways to prevent skin cancer is to reduce exposure to the sun, specifically at an early age. This can be accomplished by wearing sun-protective clothing such as hats, using waterproof sunscreen with a sun protection factor (SPF) of 15 or above, and reapplying the sunscreen throughout the time spent outside (Council on Scientific Affairs, 1989). Moreover, constant use of sunscreen throughout childhood and adolescence may diminish the lifetime incidence of basal and squamous cell carcinomas by up to 78% (Stern, Weinstein, & Baker, 1986). Thus, adults with skin cancers may feel anger toward their parents for not adequately protecting them, and parents may feel guilt.

Despite the known risks, many people do not protect themselves from prolonged sun exposure and parents do not adequately protect their children from harmful sun exposure. Reports have described that fewer than 50% of sunbathers use sunscreen, and of those who do, many do not use sunscreen that provides adequate protection (Bak et al., 1992; Banks et al., 1992). Convictions that sun exposure is healthy and tanned skin is more attractive tend to outweigh the long-term risk of disease (Baum & Cohen, 1998). Although educational interventions focusing on the risks of increased sun exposure have led to heightened awareness and knowledge of skin cancer, there is little indication that this has been translated into actual behavior changes (Katz & Jernigan, 1991) and reduction in skin cancer morbidity (Baum & Cohen, 1998). In addition, further research is necessary to evaluate the interventions associated with long-term behavior change.

Religious/Spiritual Practices

A body of literature suggests that religious affiliation may be a health protector. Areas with higher concentrations of religious participants have been found to be associated with lower mortality rates for all malignancies (Dwyer et al., 1990). Religious affiliation has been linked with lower use of hospital services by medically ill older adults (Koenig & Larson, 1998). A recent comprehensive review of the empirical research linking religion and spirituality with better health outcomes (Sloan et al., 1999) pointed out many of the methodological flaws in the available literature. They concluded that any empirical evidence for a relationship between religion, spirituality, and health is weak and inconclusive. What this means is that asserting that an individual's illness was caused by lack of religious or spiritual involvement and/or prescribing religion for medically ill patients is premature and potentially harmful. Although more research is needed in this area, it seems evident that a clear understanding of the patient's religious beliefs and supporting religious practices that bring comfort to some can be an invaluable aid to the clinician.

PSYCHOSOCIAL FACTORS PREDICTIVE OF DISEASE

Personality and Illness

Historical Background

Among those factors long thought to influence the predisposition toward health or illness are various aspects of personality and emotional style. Aristotle wrote that pain is an emotion (Salisbury, 1990). Hippocrates described the healthy body as a delicately balanced organization of four "humors," and attributed the onset of disease to an imbalance of these characterological substances in the body. Freud and others working in the late nineteenth century continued to explore the relationship of psychological life to physical disease. Although he did not use the term "psychosomatic" in his writings (Taylor, 1987), psyche and soma were inextricably linked for Freud, who believed that somatic symptoms often emerged as a consequence of the repression of painful emotions (Freud, 1955; Friedman, 1990).

Freud's work on the relationship of unconscious emotional life and symptom formation opened the door to a new wave of theorizing about the relationship of mental state to health and illness. In the 1940s and 1950s, Dunbar and others sought to refashion early psychoanalytic hypotheses and attempted to link specific personality styles with particular symptoms (Dunbar, 1946). Dunbar argued that coronary conditions were likely to occur in people with ambitious, driving personality styles (Taylor, 1987). Dunbar's analyses, however, included no explanation of how these personality styles were related to disease processes. Grinker & Robbins (1953) argued that these analyses were superficial. Thus, both the medical and analytic communities discounted Dunbar's work.

By contrast, Alexander (1950) conducted extensive psychoanalytic investigations of his patients and developed his own multifactorial model of psychosomatic illness in which specific unconscious conflicts interact with somatic vulnerability to determine disease choice and symptom formation (Taylor, 1987).

While clinically interesting, the work of the early psychosomaticists was not substantiated by well-controlled studies. Psychosomatic theories fell into disfavor in the face of medical advances in cellular research, diagnosis, and treatment during the 1960s.

Contemporary Views

Engel (1977) attempted to bridge the gap between the medical and psychological models of disease when he proposed a biopsychosocial model of health. This approach is considered more "holistic" (Friedman, 1990) in that various aspects of an individual's life experience were recognized as having possible roles in the initiation of and response to disease processes. Personality was defined in this paradigm as the manifestation of an individual's stable patterns of thinking and behaving (Suls et al., 1990). According to this model, personality factors interact in a nonlinear fashion with environmental and physiological processes in ways that may either predispose one to disease, or conversely act as a protective buffer against illness. Current thinking owes much to the early pioneers of psychosomatic medicine. Engel's model, in particular, has had a profound influence on health psychology and related areas of research over the last two decades. It recognizes that a broader range of factors may influence health and disease, and introduces the concept of nonlinear directionality among factors.

Current research on the relationship of personality factors to disease has expanded to include a broader definition of psychological factors such as depression, anxiety, and coping styles which may predispose individuals to health (Kobasa, 1990) or disease (Friedman, 1990; Suls & Rittenhouse, 1990). Along with this expansion, researchers have delineated three areas of personality and psychological functioning which may influence disease onset and progression (Ricci Bitti, 1995). These areas include the management of *affect* (e.g., emotional expression versus emotional constriction), *behaviors* that correspond to affect states (e.g., health-promoting versus dangerous behaviors related to stress, anxiety, depression, or neuroticism), and finally, *cognitions* that correspond to a given affect state (e.g., hostile and contemptuous thoughts about others which may be associated with an angry and agitated state).

This model has spawned a burgeoning field of clinical research into the complex relationships that may exist among an individual's personality traits (affects, behaviors, and cognition), and the many other factors that affect one's life, such as social supports, environmental challenges, and biological predispositions. Numerous studies have found both positive and negative evidence supporting the theory that personality and psychological factors may play key roles in the onset and progression of disease processes.

A recent editorial (Angell, 1985) rejected the idea of "disease as a direct reflection of mental state." This statement seems to assume a simplistic and linear model of personality's influence on health and illness. In fact, current research assumes a "nonlinear and multifactoral" model (Temoshok, 1990). Working with this model, there is evidence pointing to the conclusion that some version of a biopsychosocial model best describes the complex relationship between personality factors, health, and disease.

Three Proposed Models

1. The Direct Impact Model: Certain personality styles may have a direct impact on pathophysiological processes. While the pathophysiological mechanisms of this Direct Impact Model are not fully known, studies have begun to identify some of the ways in which personality factors may act as causal cofactors in the pathogenesis of disease (Friedman, 1990; Levy, 1990). For example, hostility has been found to be associated with decreased vagal modulation of the heart (Sloan et al., 1994) and diminished autonomic control of the heart, which, in turn, may disinhibit pathogenic blood pressure variability and thereby contribute to CHD (Sloan, Shapiro, et al., 1999). Similarly, individuals showing tendencies for the "hostility component" (Williams, 1987) exhibit larger heart rate and blood pressure responses to behavioral and physical stressors (Dembroski, 1979).

2. The Constitutional Predisposition Model: It suggests that personality styles are simply markers for innate weaknesses or abnormalities that increases one's susceptibility to a particular disease (Suls et al., 1990). There is some research indicating that loudness of speech and potential for hostility (aspects of Type A behavior pattern) may be inherited (Matthews, 1984). We do not know the pathophysiological pathways by which these inherited traits might influence disease susceptibility (Suls et al., 1990).

3. The Dangerous Behaviors Model: It proposes that personality factors may predispose individuals to certain risky behaviors. Depressed patients (Persky et al., 1987) and stoic personality types may be less likely to seek medical care when confronted with symptoms of disease, thus putting them at greater risk due to late diagnosis and delayed introduction of treatment interventions; Type A personalities may engage in risky behaviors such as excessive physical exertion or smoking (Suls et al., 1990) which increase their risk for coronary disease.

Issues for the Clinician to Consider

There are several important issues to keep in mind when considering the relationship between personality factors and disease (Friedman, 1990). One's opinion on these issues may help determine their clinical approach to treating patients with somaticizing conditions. First, of critical importance in evaluating studies is the question of causality. Is a certain personality style or set of psychological characteristics a function of the disease itself, or do these factors predate (and somehow cause) the onset of disease? Retrospective and quasi-prospective studies are unable to determine causal relationships.

Second, how do we define stress (or, for that matter, any cluster of personality traits)? Is stress something external, an immediate precipitant that comes from daily life, or is it an endogenous factor related to psychological functioning?

Third, what magnitude of relationship is evident between personality factors and disease? Are the size effects strong enough to say with confidence that personality factors are necessary, if not sufficient, factors in the onset and/or progression of a disease state?

Fourth, what types of interventions are appropriate if personality factors are found to be relevant for various diseases? Do we intervene at the level of personality functioning, on the level of behavior, or at the level of physiological processes?

Finally, we must keep in mind the various ways that any given set of personality factors may operate within the specific life context of an individual. The varying nature of two individuals' social supports, socioeconomic level, age, gender, and other factors may all interact in complex ways with the so-called same personality and psychological profile.

Personality Factors and Disease

In what follows, we will give a brief overview of current views on the role of four constellations of personality traits and psychological factors, which have historically been linked with disease. Coronary heart disease (CHD), breast cancer, and ulcerative disease of the upper gastrointestinal tract have been the focus of attention in psychosomatic research. For each area, we will review the current thinking about the relationship of these psychosocial factors to health and disease processes. Possible psychophysiological mechanisms by which these factors may influence disease onset and/or progression will be reviewed.

The Type A Behavior Pattern and the Hostility Complex: Shifting Paradigms

Strong emotions have long been associated with coronary heart disease and sudden cardiac death (Sloan, Shapiro, et al., 1999). During the 1960s and 1970s, research focused on several psychological factors, including depression, anxiety, and personality traits (Delunas, 1996). By the 1970s, clinical impressions led researchers to speculate that personality traits of aggression, anger, and drivenness were dominant in individuals presenting with coronary heart disease. Friedman and Rosenman (1974) developed the concept of the Type A Behavior Pattern (TABP) to describe this cluster of traits, and mounted an ambitious prospective study (Rosenman et al., 1975) to determine whether in fact TABP is a risk factor for CHD. Positive findings from the Western Collaborative Group Study showed that Type A personalities are twice as likely as Type B personalities to develop coronary artery disease, which led to the conclusion that TABP is an independent risk factor for coronary artery disease (Review Panel on Coronary-Prone Behaviors and Coronary Heart Disease, 1981). To the extent that these findings would be clinically significant, the cost to society and industry would be enormous, and the potential benefit derived from addressing Type A-related risk behavior would be equally significant.

Numerous studies since have examined the relationship between TABP and CHD (Jenkins, 1976). Subsequent research has shown, however, that the 1981 conclusion was premature (Williams, 1987). Several studies which have examined the relationship between TABP and angiographic data have found little or no positive relation between Type A and the severity of CAD (Williams, 1987; Williams et al., 1988). Over the last decade, the Type A thesis has been refined, as additional studies have highlighted more specific aspects of TABP that may be more predictive of CHD. Most studies have focused on the personality trait of hostility (Williams, 1987; Barefoot et al., 1994; Sloan, 1994; Ricci Bitti, 1995; Delunas, 1996; Sloan, Shapiro, et al., 1999). The "hostility complex," as it is now called (Williams, 1987), refers to a more specific and stable tendency to react to a broad range of provocative and frustration-inducing events with myriad signs of anger, annoyance, disgust, disdain, and rancor (Williams, 1987).

Studies have found positive relationships between hostility and CAD. The Western Collaborative Group found that those with higher Hostility scores were more likely to have developed CAD over a 10-year follow-up period, and were also more likely to die from any cause than those with low hostility scores (Shekelle et al., 1983). More recently, hostility has been linked repeatedly with heart disease (Smith, 1992).

In sum, there is considerable evidence that personality factors may be influential in modulating important coronary processes such as heart rate variability (Sloan, Shapiro, et al., 1999), as well as in mediating unhealthy practices such as smoking. The precise mechanisms by which personality factors affect coronary health need further elaboration through rigorous empirical research. Which model the therapist espouses will likely determine choice and direction for psychotherapeutic treatment of conditions arising out of stress-induced health conditions.

A Breast Cancer Personality?

As difficult as it is to receive a cancer diagnosis, many patients compound their grief and distress with a fear that their lifestyle, behavior patterns, or coping style have contributed to their risk. The mental health clinician is in a good position to provide perspective and reassurance to the patient in the face of contradictory messages from friends and physicians alike.

Cancer, like heart disease, has long been associated with the vicissitudes of emotional life. The psychological factors associated with breast cancer, in particular, have been examined extensively, and for this reason breast cancer is the focus of our discussion here. Coping styles, anxiety and depression, and early childhood antecedents have all been implicated in the onset and progression of breast cancer (McKenna et al., 1999). Until recently, however, little systematic work has been done to identify the complex nature of these relationships.

In 1926, Evans (1926) observed that cancer patients tend to turn their psychic energy inside, against their own innate body defenses (Faragher & Cooper, 1990). Several early breast cancer studies had similar findings: Women with breast cancer had difficulty dealing with anger and hostility, and showed a marked inability to express these emotions (Tarlau & Smalheiser, 1951; Bacon et al., 1952).

Following the lead of Type A research, researchers attempted to isolate a single personality type associated with breast cancer. Numerous studies have found that breast cancer is associated with extreme suppression of emotions (Greer & Morris, 1975) and the suppression of anger and hostility in particular (Wirsching et al., 1985). In a study of 121 women with breast lesion biopsy, Cheang and Cooper (1985) found no significant relationship between cancer risk and Type A behavior. The subjects with breast cancer tended to suppress rather than vent their negative emotions, but they were less time-pressured and more easygoing than Type A personalities. The breast cancer subjects were dubbed Type B personality types, by default.

Faragher and Cooper (1990) found that breast cancer subjects did not conform perfectly to pure type characteristics. Even when controlling for age, subjects with breast cancer demonstrated many Type B characteristics (e.g., low ambition, low competitiveness, suppression of negative emotions), but some Type A characteristics as well (e.g., a strong desire for personal satisfaction). The concept of the Type C, or Cancer Personality, was developed to describe this style and to reflect the idea that suppression of negative emotions does not mean absence of negative emotions (Temoshok et al., 1985). Type C individuals are characterized as nice, friendly, unassertive, but often silently simmering with low denigrating attitudes toward others which cannot safely be expressed, often feeling physically aroused but reporting little emotional distress (Anagnostopoulos et al., 1993).

A recent meta-analysis found a modest connection between specific personality factors and breast cancer (McKenna et al., 1999). Strongest support was found for a relationship between disease and the tendency to use denial-repression as a coping strategy. Strong associations were also found between the incidence of breast cancer and a history of stressful life events, and profound loss or separation. A significant but weaker association was found between the conflict-avoidant personality and breast cancer incidence. With the exception of stressful life events, all of the other personality factors identified cluster together around a general personality type which relies heavily on repression and denial as a coping mechanism (Type C) (McKenna et al., 1999). When these various factors were combined, they proved less robust than the single predictor of the denial-repression factor did alone.

In the research examining the suppression versus expression of negative emotions, it is not clear whether subjects were actually suppressing emotions or whether they were not aware of feeling negative emotions (Levy & Heiden, 1990).

As with CHD, the precise psychophysiological mechanisms of breast cancer are unknown. There is experimental and clinical evidence that immunological and hormonal mechanisms may each play a role in tumor growth (Levy & Heiden, 1990). Further research is needed to specify the nature of these mechanisms and to highlight the ways in which psychological and physiological adaptations to stress may paradoxically lead to sickness as well.

The field of psycho-oncology has grown out of the increasing awareness of the emotional needs of cancer patients and ex-cancer patients. As their numbers in psychotherapeutic care increase, patients will rely on the therapist to help them negotiate the difficult course of coping with life- threatening disease. If supported by continued research, the Type C hypothesis might lead to psychotherapeutic interventions designed to counteract these risk factors. At this time, while the lay public has already taken these findings to heart, it is too soon to tell whether such clinical approaches are in any way protective.

Peptic Ulcers: Psychosomatic or Infectious?

As with the other ailments we have discussed, physicians have long speculated about the influence of emotional state on gastrointestinal ailments. Nineteenth century observers noted that emotional distress was associated with the development of peptic ulceration (Beaumont, 1833). During the 1940s, the early psychosomaticists viewed the peptic ulcer as a classic psychosomatic disease resulting from unconscious conflicts of dependency and longing (Alexander, 1950; Taylor, 1987; Lewin & Lewis, 1995). Alexander believed, for instance, that ulcers resulted from an autonomic imbalance due to the effects of harmful and defensive considerations (Lewin & Lewis, 1995) of psychosocial origin.

Numerous early studies were conducted in attempts to isolate the specific personality factors thought to be etiologically responsible for the development of peptic ulcers. Several studies found that patients with peptic ulcers were often conscientious, hard-driving, urgent, and anxious (Draper, 1942; Gainesborough & Slater, 1946). These findings must be viewed with caution, however, as most of the early research consists of case histories without controlled comparison groups.

Research grew more systematic during the 1960s with the introduction of standardized instruments such as the Maudsley Personality Inventory (Rotter et al., 1979), the Eysenck Personality Questionnaire (Eysenck & Eysenck, 1975), and the MMPI (Graham, 1981). Kanter & Hazelton (1964) found that peptic ulcer subjects had higher neuroticism scores and lower extroversion scores than normative subjects. The absence of well-matched control groups and small sample sizes, however, make the scientific import of these findings questionable (Lewin & Lewis, 1995).

In spite of serious methodological flaws such as unmatched control groups, low numbers of subjects (Lewin & Lewis, 1995), and retrospective research designs (Levenstein et al., 1995), findings from these studies spawned a third wave of peptic ulcer/personality research. During the 1970s, researchers tried to implicate the TABP in the etiology of the peptic ulcer. Findings were equivocal. Wrezesniewski et al. (1988) found personality traits in peptic ulcer subjects similar to those subjects, with circulatory disorders, but used only a small number of male subjects, and did not describe subject or control recruitment (Lewin & Lewis, 1995). However, Tennant et al. (1986) found that CHD subjects had higher mean scores of Type A behaviors than subjects with ulcers, and that the ulcer patients' scores did not differ from normative subjects. The association between TABP and peptic ulcer disease remains unproven (Lewin & Lewis, 1995).

The role of stress in the etiology of peptic ulcer disease was also examined, with mixed results. Numerous studies found evidence for a relationship between psychosocial factors (especially stress and shifting mood states) and human susceptibility to bacterial and viral infections (see Biondi & Zannino, 1997, for a review). Some studies, however, did not find a significant effect of stress on the pathogenesis of peptic ulcers (Thomas et al., 1980; Piper et al., 1981). By contrast, Levenstein et al. (1995) found that peptic ulcer patients who had few conventional risk factors were more likely to have more psychological risk factors (defined as stressful life events, abnormal MMPI scores, or mood disturbances). Neuroticism and anxiety have also been associated with incidence of peptic ulcers (McIntosh et al., 1983).

The discovery in 1983 of *Helicobacter pylori* changed the field of ulcer research completely. What was for decades considered a disorder of primarily psychosocial etiology was suddenly perceived to be an infectious disease caused by the action of *Helicobacter* on the secretion of gastrin and acid and their regulation. Peptic ulcers respond well to antimicrobial treatment, and recurrence is less in patients treated with antimicrobial therapy (Melmed & Gelpin, 1996). Since the emergence of *H. pylori*, there has been a 28% decrease in published articles examining the role of psychosocial stress in the etiology of peptic ulcers (Melmed & Gelpin, 1996). Although there are other well-documented predisposing factors such as O Blood Type, genetic predisposition, increased acid secretory capacity (Melmed, 1996), smoking, alcohol, and caffeine consumption (Levenstein et al., 1995), *H. pylori* is now believed to play a central role in the development of peptic ulcers.

Clearly, psychological factors alone no longer explain the pathogenesis of peptic ulcer. As Melmed and Gelpin (1996), Levenstein et al. (1995), and others point out, however, *H. pylori* should not be considered a sufficient factor for the development of ulcerative disease. By the age of 70, over half of the population has been exposed to *Helicobacter*, but only 20% will eventually develop peptic ulcers (Levenstein et al., 1995; Melmed & Gelpin, 1996). Levenstein et al. (1995) argue for the recognition of psychological factors as "etiologic cofactors" in the development of peptic ulcers. Melmed and Gelpin (1996) also argue for a more "holistic" evaluation of *Helicobacter*-host interactions which takes into account the more complex and multifactorial nature of host resistance factors and psychophysiological processes. Future research is needed for a definitive explication of the precise ways in which psychological factors interact with *H. pylori* and the relative importance of each factor in determining exactly who will develop ulcerative disease.

The long history of the search for an etiology for peptic ulcer is an object lesson on the danger of seeking to explain aspects of human pathophysiology or psychopathology with overly simplistic models. Results thus far point to a complex, multifactorial etiology for peptic ulcer. Neither an explanation emphasizing the psychogenic etiology nor a pure biological cause is sufficient alone. The same complexity appears to hold true for many disease entities.

This point of view has important implications for psychotherapy and mental health care. The sick patient seeks solace for his worries, often requesting answers to big questions like, "Why did I get sick?" The savvy clinician can be relatively objective about the likelihood that the patient either caused the illness, or alternatively that the patient has absolutely no control over the outcome. Clearly so far, the research suggests that the answer lies somewhere between the two extremes.

Somatization: An Evolving Interactional View

It is common in primary care settings for children, adolescents, and adults to present with physical symptoms for which there are inadequate medical explanations. "Medically unexplained symptoms" may account for nearly 40% of all primary care visits made by adults (Kroenke & Mangelsdorff, 1989; Garber et al., 1991). Most common symptoms among children and adults include headache, recurrent abdominal pain, and fatigue (Stewart et al., 1992; Walker et al., 1993; Campo & Fritsch, 1994; Katon & Walker, 1998). Doctor-patient relationships with these individuals often become strained (Katon & Walker, 1998), and mental health referrals are frequently dismissed by patients as irrelevant, especially for children (Campo & Fritsch, 1999).

The symptom picture of somatizing individuals is complex. At its most extreme, somatization is viewed as a full-blown psychiatric disorder. Grouped together with the related Somatoform Disorders, Somatization Disorder (SD), as defined by the *DSM-IV* (APA, 1994), is "a pattern of recurring, multiple, clinically significant somatic complaints" (p. 446). In practice, however, it tends to be a term used to cover an extensive range of widespread and general clinical conditions and circumstances (Kirmayer, 1991). Individuals with SD (or its subclinical counterpart, Undifferentiated Somatoform Disorder) frequently seek numerous medical opinions for their various and changing physical problems and often undergo repeated and unnecessary medical procedures. The combined effects of symptoms and related help-seeking behaviors can result in significant impairment in "social, occupational or other important areas of functioning" (APA, 1994, p. 446).

Of note is the fact that SD is more frequently found among women than men (APA, 1994), and among female children and adolescents than among males (Terre & Ghisell, 1997; Campo & Fritsch, 1999). Numerous studies have linked the relatively high incidence of SD in women to the incidence of sexual abuse among female children (Briere & Runtz, 1988; Morrison, 1989; Fry, 1993), which has been found in various studies to be significantly higher than among males (for a review, see Fry, 1993).

Historically, theorists have long hypothesized that functional symptoms for which there is no apparent organic etiology are the result of psychological factors (Escobar et al., 1991). In his *Treatise on Hysteria*, Paul Briquet (1859) wrote that hysteria is "a neurosis of the brain in which the observed phenomena consist chiefly of a perturbation of vital activities, which serve as the manifestation of affective feeling and passions" (cited in Mai & Merskey, 1980). Freud and Breuer originally described the somatic symptomatology of *hysteria* as the result of the "stimulation of a hysterogenic zone," which would produce neurological symptoms (Shorter, 1992) and would be caused by psychological trauma (Herman, 1992).

Unconscious conflict and strangulated affect (McDougall, 1989), alexithymia (Nemiah & Sifneos, 1970), and a tendency to internalize remain at the heart of the personality cluster associated with functional somatic symptoms since the nineteenth century. Although the psychophysiological mechanisms mediated by these factors remain largely unspecified by empirical research, some version of this thinking continues to dominate the theorizing around somatization and has not yet been supplanted by a more narrowly construed medical explanation.

In the absence of organic pathology, research efforts have continued to focus on the identification of associated psychological traits and psychiatric comorbidity. Somatization has been associated with personality disorders (Kernberg, 1984) and with various personality traits (Russo et al., 1994; Katon & Walker, 1998), such as neuroticism (Webb, 1983; Russo et al., 1994) and internalizing behaviors (Engel, 1959; Terre & Ghiselli, 1997; Campo et al., 1999). Children with multiple somatic complaints tend to be more fearful of novelty and demonstrate greater difficulties in areas of separation (Terre & Ghiselli, 1997; Campo et al., 1999). "Prepubertal children may experience affective distress as somatic sensations" (Fritz et al., 1997). Other predisposing risk factors include numerous psychosocial stressors such as early childhood sexual and/or physical abuse (Herman, 1992; Reilly et al., 1999), family dysfunction (Terre & Ghiselli, 1997), and a prior history of physical illness.

Empirical evidence suggests that individuals with medically unexplained somatic symptoms are more likely than those without somatic symptoms to have Axis I psychiatric disorders, especially anxiety and depression (Reilly et al., 1999; Katon & Walker, 1998). This is true for both adult and pediatric populations (Campo & Fritsch, 1994; Lavigne et al., 1998; Campo et al., 1999). A study of 1,617 adult primary care attenders found that somatization clustered with anxiety and would perhaps be better recognized and treated if diagnostic thresholds were lowered, thereby more accurately reflecting the prevalence of patients presenting with high numbers of functional symptoms but who do not meet the standard diagnostic threshold for SD (Piccinelli et al., 1999).

Attempts to identify the personality and psychosocial factors most associated with somatization have been hampered by several factors. Clinically, it is not simple, when presented with a patient with multiple physical symptoms, to rule out the presence of organic disease (Campo & Fritsch, 1994). In the realm of more systematic research, it has been difficult to establish reasonable control groups for comparison (Reilly et al., 1999), and studies have tended to rely on small samples (Cartmill & Betts, 1992). The development of standardized measures has also been problematic, particularly for use with children and adolescents (Campo & Fritsch, 1994; Campo et al., 1999). Most measures rely on self-report, and because of social stigma in various cultural contexts and in some primary care settings, some patients may tend to underreport their own symptoms and thereby be overlooked (Piccinelli et al., 1999). The prevalence of somatoform complaints has induced researchers to attempt to develop well-validated but abbreviated measures which may be more accurately able to identify the presence of a subthreshold disorder (Spitzer et al., 1994; Kroenke et al., 1997). Finally, it has been difficult to tease out the extent to which associated personality factors may be causal, mediating, or derivative of somatization symptoms.

The psychophysiological pathways by which psychosocial factors become manifest as physical symptoms remain open to discovery. Psychological distress may lead to somatic symptoms secondary to autonomic arousal (Katon & Walker, 1998). Psychological stress may induce risk-increasing behaviors such as smoking and alcohol consumption. What does emerge from the accumulation of research findings is that individuals who somatize seem to have coping styles and adjustment reactions which interact with their biological predispositions in complex ways. For people suffering with unexplained chronic somatic distress, the interaction between mind, emotions, and body may play a central and debilitating role in their lives. The presence of multiple unexplained physical symptoms should alert primary care physicians and mental health professionals to the possibility of a comorbid psychiatric disorder or significant psychological distress (Campo et al., 1999).

PSYCHOLOGICAL MODERATORS OF ILLNESS
AND ILLNESS BEHAVIORS

Despite continuing efforts to seek mind-body explanations for physical diseases, the field has come full circle, returning to the question of psychological functioning in relation to such factors as coping, quality of life, pain control, and maintenance of social support systems. A better understanding of such predictive factors will have specific implications for mental health care for the chronically ill.

Theoretical Concepts

Theoretical models ideally can provide consistency in operational definitions of phenomena under study, thereby allowing for cross-study comparisons to better assess the effects of intervention or the lack thereof (Curry & Emmons, 1994). Three models utilized to explain and predict health behavior changes will be presented: the Health Locus of Control model, the Health Beliefs model, and the Transtheoretical model. In addition to theoretical models, other factors that appear to determine whether an individual will engage in behavior change or adherence to change will be presented.

Health Belief Model (HBM)

The Health Belief Model (Rosenstock, 1966), a pioneering model for understanding health behavior change, stresses the role of cognitive factors in predicting health related behaviors. According to the constructs in this model, individuals go through a decision-making process taking into account (a) perceived susceptibility to disease, (b) perceived seriousness, and (c) the belief that specific behaviors will reduce the threat and the benefits of the behavior will outweigh the perceived costs. Practically, the model suggests that when an individual perceives a threat to be high and when the perception exists that the health benefits of a particular behavior outbalance any obstacles, then the person will engage in the behavior.

   When individuals hold irrational beliefs about health and illness or have a tendency to apprise circumstances in a distorted way, they may not adhere to a medical regimen (Meichenbaum & Turk, 1987). What this model suggests, then, is that a health practitioner may be able to help the patient by educating him or her about the condition as well as by ascertaining if any irrational general health beliefs exist and attempting to evaluate them.

Locus of Control Model

The Health Locus of Control Model (Wallston, Wallston, & DeVellis, 1978) is a cognitive-social model based on Rotter's (1954) social learning theory. Their

Multidimensional Health Locus of Control scales have been utilized to assess a person's perceived control in relation to his or her health. One assumption is that the source of reinforcement for health-related behaviors is internal, a matter of chance, or under the control of "powerful others" (Wallston & Smith, 1994). The model proposes that those individuals who believe that their health is largely within their control engage in health-promoting and health-maintaining behaviors. Those individuals who believe that their health is largely outside of their control are more likely to engage in health-impairing behaviors. A number of studies have confirmed these relationships, finding a positive relationship between scores on the internal scale and health-maintaining behaviors (Weiss & Larson, 1990) and a negative relationship between scores on the chance dimension and health-promoting behaviors (Steptoe et al., 1994).

Wallston & Smith (1994) suggested that a strong and consistent relationship between internal locus of control and health-promoting behaviors was only among individuals who place a high worth on their health. It may be important to differentiate between long-term and short-term health gains and the importance assigned to each one. For example, one study (Klesges et al., 1989) found that 5% of men and 19% of women smokers began smoking to help with weight control. Therefore, long-term health was jeopardized for the short-term perception of health. Future research should then focus on the short- and long-term health gains of different behaviors as well as the individual's health values. This model suggests that health care practitioners should work with patients to internalize their locus of control and increase the worth they place on their health. Practitioners should also evaluate the sense of the patient's long-term goals and how they compare with his or her short-term goals.

Transtheoretical Model

The Transtheoretical Model (Prochaska & DiClemente, 1983) is a model of behavioral change that provides a structure for examining not only the different stages of change but also the process of change. According to this model, individuals can be categorized into one of five categories on a continuum related to their stage of change: precontemplation, contemplation, preparation, action, and maintenance. Precontemplation refers to an unawareness of the problem with an individual exhibiting no desire to change the behavior. The contemplation stage is characterized by the beginning of awareness of the problem behavior and the initial decision-making process of weighing the pros and cons of potential change. The preparation stage reflects a continuation of the decision-making process with the addition of a more immediate timeframe as well as active measures to prepare for change, e.g., cutting back from two packs to one and a half packs of cigarettes per day. An individual in the action stage is actively involved in changing his or her behavior, e.g., has stopped smoking. The maintenance stage refers to long-term (> 6 months) adjustment to continuing and preserving the changes made in the previous stages. Future behavior change is thought to be predicted by the individual's stage. Interventions can be tailored to the individual's stage of change.

In addition to stages of change, the model includes 10 processes that individuals utilize when changing their behavior (DiClemente, 1993). These 10 processes, which are thought to operationalize varying coping mechanisms utilized in the process of change and can be used differentially across the varying stages of change, are grouped into two overarching categories: behavioral (changing response to stimuli, changing environment, changing reinforcers, and contingencies) and experiential (emotional reactions, changing appraisals, and creating new alternatives) (Prochaska et al., 1988).

This model has been utilized in smoking cessation research and has been extended to other addictive behaviors and health-impairing behaviors to predict behavioral change (Prochaska, DiClemente, & Norcross, 1992). Some research supports the hypothesis that successful stage transitions involve engaging in experiential processes in early stages and behavioral processes in the later stages (Perz et al., 1996). Other work has failed to find such a relationship (Herzog et al., 1999). The model has shown some promise in application to mammography screening (Rakowski et al., 1996). The model suggests that practitioners should assess a patient's stage of change in order to determine the best intervention.

More research is necessary to determine whether any one model can be utilized to consistently predict behavior change across various health behaviors or whether the diverse and individual challenges of different health behaviors preclude the utilization of only one model. Interactions between the various constructs of different models (Curry & Emmons, 1994) may be the key to understanding and predicting health behaviors and change in addition to looking at other factors that may not be included in a given model.

Other Factors Contributing to Health-Related Behavior Change

Social Support

Social support has been widely studied in all areas of the social sciences and increasingly as related to health care and health behaviors. Social support has been defined as various forms of aid and assistance provided by family, friends, and neighbors (Caplan, 1974). It has also been described as the belief that one is cared for, loved, valued, and part of a network of interaction and reciprocal responsibility (Cobb, 1976). Social support was hypothesized to have a direct beneficial impact on an individual's health by fulfilling a person's need for affiliation, information, and socialization (House, 1981). It predisposes an individual to engage in health-promoting behaviors (Hubbard et al., 1984), and buffers a person from the deleterious effects of stress (Cohen & Hoberman, 1983). Due to its perceived importance, social support has often been seen as an important aspect of any intervention to improve health outcomes.

A recent meta-analysis of the associations between social support and health outcomes (Smith et al., 1994) found only small associations between social support, as currently measured, and health outcomes. They point to the lack of attention given to situation-specific social support, seen as an individual's preference for type, amount, source, timing, and control over support given. It is important that clinicians realize that a better understanding of a person's desire for and acceptance of social support is imperative before utilizing the commonly recommended interventions (i.e., bereavement, marital therapy, and family therapy). Recommending that patients increase their social involvement or obtain aid from family members may actually have negative effects for some (Smith et al., 1994).

Knowledge and Understanding

Another factor related to behavior change and compliance with medical regimens is the patient's access to information and understanding of that information. Haynes et al. (1979) reported no consistent associations between knowledge and adherence. Under some conditions, provision of information has been found to influence compliance (Becker, 1979). For individuals who are motivated to comply but lack the proper information about the correct ways to comply, provision of information should enhance compliance. For individuals already knowledgeable but lacking in motivation, provision of additional information to increase knowledge will not increase compliance (Becker, 1979). Reading and language abilities, as well as disorganized and irrational thought patterns, can affect comprehension and interpretation of information conveyed, leading to potential misunderstandings and consequent unintentional noncompliance (Hussey & Gilliland, 1989).

The clinician must ensure that the patient has adequate information. The challenge that clinicians are faced with is how to convey the proper amount of information, in the proper way, at the most propitious time. Any important information should be given in the patient's primary language through the use of a proper translator who can adequately convey all of the information. Patient compliance is best achieved when information is conveyed in writing, in layperson's language, and in a clear and unambiguous fashion. In addition, information about treatment should be conveyed first and any important instructions should be stressed (DiMatteo & DiNicola, 1982). Immediate repetition by the patient is a good way to ensure that the information was adequately understood.

Emotional Moderators

When physical symptoms and the perception of illness are translated into a medical diagnosis or "disease entity," there can be a wide range of emotional reactions. In an instant, the individual is not the same person that he or she was before hearing the diagnosis, but is now a cancer patient or an individual with heart disease. Some have proposed a stage of adjustment to a medical diagnosis akin to the stages of adjustment to death and dying suggested by Kubler-Ross (1969). Mekarski (1999) proposed a seven-stage coping process defined by shock, denial, procrastination, bargaining, depression, anger, and adaptation/realistic coping. Although there is little empirical data to support the rigid sequence and progression from stage to stage, patients may experience one or all of these coping mechanisms. It is reasonable that patients coping with a relatively serious medical diagnosis will exhibit a wide variety of emotional reactions. These emotional reactions may have an impact on the course of treatment as well as outcome.

Initially individuals may grieve over the loss of their health. Playing a game of softball or walking up a flight of steps can no longer be taken for granted. Day to day activities such as being able to pay the bills or taking care of the children may prove to be too arduous and overwhelming. Most notably, being in a hospital, where an individual's sense of personal autonomy may be significantly compromised, can trigger depressive and anxious states.

Depression

Although medical patients may experience a wide range of psychiatric problems, much attention has been focused on depression in primary care due to its high prevalence, rates of impairment, and treatability (Schulberg et al., 1996). Patients with a chronic medical condition as well as a comorbid affective disorder tend to have increased medical utilization and costs, amplified symptoms, decreased quality of life, increased noncompliance with medical regimens, and increased mortality (Katon, 1996). A recent meta-analysis (Wulsin et al., 1999) found that depression does appear to increase the risk of death, particularly from unnatural causes and cardiovascular disease. The studies linking depression with increased rates of mortality tend to be poorly controlled and the correlation remains unclear. The relationship between heart disease and depression has been studied. Major depression at the time of a myocardial infarction has been associated with increased mortality independent of gender (Frasure-Smith et al., 1993; Frasure-Smith et al., 1999). Assessment of depression in the medically ill requires close attention to symptoms that could be explained by either physical or emotional causes. It is helpful at such times to assess whether thought patterns indicative of depression are present, so as not to attribute symptoms like fatigue and malaise to one specific cause.

Stress

The diagnosis of a serious or chronic medical condition may result in varying levels of distress. Patients may be concerned about family and financial matters as well as philosophical or existential matters. A number of anxiety disorders have been described in patients with somatic conditions, the most prevalent being adjustment disorders with anxiety, panic disorder, and generalized anxiety disorder (Stoudemire, 1996). The anxiety may manifest itself in all areas or may be particularly focused on a specific medical situation, for example anticipatory nausea prior to chemotherapy treatment. Both behavioral treatment as well as psychopharmacologic interventions may be helpful to these patients. Given the possibility of drug interactions, cognitive behavioral treatments may be particularly useful in this population. In addition to anxiety and distress before and during treatment, some research has found higher rates of posttraumatic stress symptoms in the medically ill, including cancer survivors (Alter et al., 1996) and heart transplant recipients (Stukas et al., 1999).

Cognitive Factors in Disease

Many diseases involve progressive brain tissue degeneration that may lead to temporary or permanent mental status and cognitive changes. In addition, some treatments and medications can also affect brain functioning . It is not unusual for these cognitive changes to be incorrectly perceived as depression or a response to the stress associated with medical illness. However, early recognition, work-up to ascertain the cause, and treatment can arrest the development of delirium and may slow the advancement of dementia (Fleishman & Lesko, 1989). In addition, cognitive dysfunction can impair overall functioning as well as impede health care compliance.

Patients with a number of infectious diseases and degenerative diseases may initially present with altered mental status or cognitive difficulties, such as memory or attention problems, confusion, or language problems. It is imperative that mental health professionals, who may see these patients first, rule out any medical or neurologic causes before giving a primary psychiatric or neuropsychiatric diagnosis.

Delirium

Delirium has been defined as an organic mental syndrome characterized by general cognitive impairment manifested by a relatively acute onset of clouded consciousness, disorientation, memory impairment, perceptual disturbances, incoherent speech, sleep-wake cycle disturbances, and increased or decreased psychomotor activity. These symptoms tend to fluctuate in intensity throughout the day (APA, 1994). Approximately 18–20% of patients admitted to general hospitals will exhibit symptoms of delirium, and it has been associated with both morbidity and mortality (Trzepacz, 1996). However, little research has been done to study delirium.

Delirium may be caused by a variety of conditions including, but not limited to, intracranial pathology, liver or kidney disease, hypoxia, electrolyte imbalance, anemia, dehydration, nutritional deficiencies, infection, and medications (Hanisch & Quirion, 1996). Delirium is commonly seen in patients with cancer (Fleishman & Lesko, 1989). Cytokine therapy to treat renal cell cancer, malignant melanomas, and leukemias, as well as HIV, hepatitis C, multiple sclerosis, and amyotrophic lateral sclerosis has been has been shown to have adverse effects on the central nervous system (Lerner et al., 1999). In particular, interleukin-2 (IL-2) has been associated with delirium (Lerner et al., 1999). Certain symptoms such as agitation and psychotic features may be a part of the 2–5 day course presentation of alcohol withdrawal delirium, but may also persist for weeks (Hersh et al., 1997; Miller, 1994). Transplant candidates, including patients waiting for a liver or heart, are especially at risk for delirium related to system failure, drug side effects, and infection (Riether & Libb, 1991).

Delirium may go unrecognized in up to 65% of patients (Levine, 1978). In one study (Massie et al., 1983), approximately 85% of patients with advanced or terminal cancer experienced delirium at some time during hospitalization. In cancer patients, delirium may present as early, or mild, being characterized by changed sleep patterns, increased irritability, withdrawal, and forgetfulness. Symptoms of later stage, severe delirium include refusal to cooperate, anger, demanding attitudes, illusions, delusions, and hallucinations (Fleishman & Lesko, 1989), which may be misdiagnosed as uncooperativeness, psychosis, or a personality disorder.

Dementia

Dementia is generally defined as a clinical syndrome distinguished by loss of function in various cognitive domains in an individual with prior intact intellectual abilities and current clear consciousness (Whitehouse et al., 1993). However, there have been several different criteria presented for the diagnosis of dementia to help differentiate it from other conditions, particularly delirium. The *DSM-IV* diagnostic criteria for dementia include "the development of multiple cognitive deficits related to focal neurological signs and symptoms, the direct effects of a general medical condition, or the effects of substance use as manifested by memory impairment, and one or more of the following: aphasia, apraxia, agnosia, or disturbance in executive functioning" (APA, 1994, p. 134). These deficits impair social or occupational functioning and represent a decline for the individual.

Dementia has been shown to be a major cause of morbidity and mortality in multiple countries, including the United States, and furthermore may account for a large segment of medical and health care expenses (Cross & Gurland, 1986). This is particularly true for the elderly, who are increasingly becoming a large segment of the population and are at greater risk for certain types of dementia.

The causes of dementia are manifold but include degenerative disorders of the central nervous system, metabolic disorders, cerebrovascular disease, deficiency disorders, toxins/drugs, brain tumors, head trauma, infections, and psychiatric syndromes, which may be broadly categorized into degenerative dementias and nondegenerative (or vascular) dementias (Whitehouse et al., 1993).

Doctor-Patient Relationship

The relationship between doctor and patient has been a topic of concern from the time of Hippocrates, generating approximately 8,000 articles, monographs, and books in the medical literature (Goold & Lipkin, 1999). Communication between doctor and patient appears to be a pivotal component to the relationship, with poor communication being one of the most prevalent components underlying medical malpractice claims (Gorney, 1999). Effective communication involves "mastering the art of listening" in addition to sensitivity and awareness of verbal and nonverbal signs from patients.

Over the past 50 years there has been much study of the most desirable types of physician-patient relationship, with no real consensus with respect to the superiority of any specific doctor-patient relationship model. In the traditional doctor-patient relationship the physician acts as protector and guardian of the patient, deciding what information will be presented and the best course of tréatment. Patients are expected to comply with the doctor's recommendations without question. Although this model may be adequate when dealing with acute problems, it is not suitable for long-term care of chronic conditions or disabilities. A new model of the doctor-patient relationship is being formed that takes this into account, with the doctor having less of an authoritative and paternalistic role and the patient having more autonomy. In addition, the role of the family as part of the doctor-patient relationship is being recognized as important.

Four ideal relationship types have been postulated by Emanuel and Emanuel (1992) representing four core differences related to the goals of the physician-patient interaction, the role of patients' values, conceptions of patient autonomy, and doctors' obligations toward their patients. In the paternalistic relationship, the physician decides the best course and treatment and delivers this in the role of the patient's guardian. The patient's values and concepts are assumed to be concordant with those of the physician, and patient autonomy is considered to be assent to the physician's recommendations. In the informative or consumerist relationship, a physician conveys the various biomedical information so that the patient can select the model or treatment he or she feels is most appropriate. While the patient's values are given little weight, autonomy is preserved. In the interpretive relationship the physician clarifies the goals and values of the patient to then help the patient choose the most suitable intervention. Finally, in a deliberative relationship, the physician presents technical information and helps to clarify the patient's values by using moral persuasion, suggesting why certain values are worthier than others. Emanuel and Emanuel (1992) claim that the ideal relationship is the physician with the caring attitude in the deliberative model, similar to the model of mutual participation (Laine & Davidoff, 1996). Physician satisfaction was highest in the consumerist model and lowest in the narrowly biomedical model, whereas patient satisfaction was greatest in the psychosocial pattern (Roter et al., 1997).

Although Emanuel and Emanuel (1992) have proposed an optimal model of the doctor–patient relationship, they and others have commented that one model may not fit every situation. Many doctors report the necessity of being flexible and shifting models depending on the patient's needs (Lagerlov et al., 1998). All of these various models represent a shift away from more traditional physician-centered medicine. The notion of patient-centered care that is more responsive to patients' wants, needs, and choices is practiced by more and more physicians (Laine & Davidoff, 1996). This increase in patient-centered care has been attributed to various factors, including the consumerist attitude of the newer utilizers of health care (Maloney & Paul, 1991) as well as a response to the increase in malpractice litigation (Laine & Davidoff, 1996). Participatory decision-making, where patients participate in their own treatment decisions, has been found to be desired by patients (Deber, 1994; Deber et al., 1996) and to lead to better health outcomes (Greenfield et al., 1985; Kaplan et al., 1995). Involving the family in planning and providing care to the patient has been recognized as important, particularly for children with special health care needs (Harrison, 1993; Desguin et al., 1994). In particular, the adaptive practice model (Feldman et al., 1999) provides a structure for analyzing clinical situations, choosing the clinical approach that is best suited to the family and the situation, and understanding any problems in the physician-family relationship when they arise in order to adjust the approach when necessary. This shift toward greater involvement of patients and their families in medical treatment involves changes in disclosure, medical decision-making, and end of life decision-making.

Disclosing Information to Patients and Decision-Making

Doctors, with the implicit assent of their patients, have traditionally withheld diagnostic and other medical information from their patients. In 1871, Oliver Wendell Holmes counseled medical students,

> Your patient has no more right to all the truth you know than he has to all the medicine in your saddlebags. . . . He should get only just so much as is good for him. . . . Some shrewd old physicians have a few phrases always on hand for patients who insist on knowing the pathology of their complaints without the slightest capacity of understanding the scientific explanation. I have known the term 'spinal irritation' to serve well on such occasions. (Holmes, 1883, in Lane & Davidoff, 1996, p. 152)

Today, medical ethics would dictate that this type of interaction with patients would be unacceptable and that patients have the right to be involved in and make decisions about their treatment (Childress, 1982). This transformation can be illustrated by the cancer diagnosis. In 1961, the majority of a sample of physicians reported that they would prefer not to inform patients of their cancer diagnosis, with only 12% stating that their usual policy was to inform patients of a cancer diagnosis (Oken, 1961). By 1979 this trend had reversed and almost all staff physicians at Strong Memorial Hospital preferred to inform patients of their cancer diagnosis (Novack et al., 1979). The law has changed as well. Prior to 1972, appropriate informed consent was determined by what a reasonable doctor would be expected to tell a patient. After a 1972 landmark case involving a man who suffered paralysis following surgery (who sued his physician for not informing him of the potential consequences of the surgery) informed consent was redefined to focus on what the patient has a right to know (Grant, 1992).

Patients' expectations regarding the amount of information they should receive, as well as their input in treatment decisions, have changed drastically. In part this is due to the amount of information on almost all health related subjects available via the Internet and other electronic information sources. Patients today may be more well-informed not only about their conditions but also about the various treatment alternatives, and consequently expect doctors to allow them to be involved in their care.

But do all patients truly wish to know all the information and be involved in all of the decision-making? Some studies suggest that many patients do not want to be actively involved in the decision-making process (Strull et al., 1984; Ende et al., 1989). Many of these studies fail to differentiate between the different types of "choice behaviors" inherent in medical situations. Patients may not want to be involved in problem-solving (i.e., making a diagnosis) as related to their health care but do not wish to yield decision-making control to their doctors (Deber et al., 1996).

It is important for doctors to take individual variables into account when determining the amount of information to give to patients. In many countries outside of the United States, it is still common practice for physicians to withhold diagnostic and treatment information from their patients (Surbonne, 1992). In Eastern Europe and Asia patients are not usually told of a fatal diagnosis (Levy, 1988). Due to cultural differences or age, certain patients may not wish to know any information and yield all decision-making to the doctor. Some families may not want school-aged children to know that they have cancer and ask that nurses and doctors refrain from using the word "cancer' in their child's presence. Sensitive doctors should explore the reasons why a patient or a family does not wish to be involved in treatment decisions or when a family does not want to disclose information to the patient. If there is any indication that the patient or family member is not making decisions in a rational manner, then a psychiatric consultation is required. However, when the concerns are culturally or religiously bound, doctors should be as respectful as possible, trying not to "pathologize" their patients' views.

Informing patients of a fatal illness is particularly difficult for many doctors. In part this reflects, on a more unconscious level, a way for the doctor to shield him or herself from any distress. The difficulties doctors face in having to give a poor diagnosis or break bad news may in actuality be a reflection of their own anxieties and fears (fear of being blamed, fear of the unknown, fear of unleashing a reaction, fear of expressing emotion, fear of not knowing all of the answers, and personal fear of illness and death) (Buckman, 1984). However, doctors are affected by the social milieu of the culture of the country and their particular hospital. When the "policy" is to be totally truthful and honest with patients, it is often difficult for patients not to be informed of their diagnosis (Levy, 1988). The emotional state and needs of the specific patient may be overlooked in giving a diagnosis possibly at a time when the person is not yet ready to hear it or in a way that is even callous or unfeeling. As with information-giving, it is important to take the individual needs of the patient into account, including the possible healthy utilization of the defense mechanism of denial. Doctors and medical students must be better trained in ways to convey difficult information to patients so that the focus is on the patient's needs rather than the doctor's feelings.

End-of-Life Decision-Making

One of the most critical times when the doctor-patient relationship can be most influential and helpful is during the end-of-life stage of disease. The physician plays a key role and can be helpful as both the initiator and conduit for continued discussions about end-of-life care. Zuckerman (1997) proposed three critical components for a paradigm of end-of-life decision-making, including recognizing and respecting the patient's goals, beliefs, and choices, open and empathic communication, and a multidisciplinary approach. Talking to patients and families about death and dying and walking them through the heart-wrenching decisions of stopping treatment or continuing with prophylactic treatment, hospice care, do not resuscitate (DNR) orders, and organ donation is facilitated when a trusting doctor-patient relationship exists.

Talking to patients and families about death is one of the most difficult challenges faced by practitioners, be it physicians or mental health professionals. Physicians, during their training, are rarely given opportunity to learn about death and dying and to speak candidly about this difficult topic (Bruhn et al., 1988). It is not unusual to find a "conspiracy of silence" surrounding the dying patient which is generally perpetuated by those around the patient rather than by the patient (Seeland, 1988). Many individuals, adults and children, know when they are dying intuitively, based on the verbal and nonverbal communications from their doctors, nurses, and families. Even children are aware of this, although parents may adamantly remain in denial of their child's knowledge. Often the dying patient would like to speak about death but is afraid of upsetting all of those caring people who are trying to "protect" him or her from the knowledge. Family members may feel that the patient will not "be able to handle it" and might break down or even commit suicide. Most terminally ill patients are not suicidal and families should be, in a sense, given permission to let the patient cry. They should also be counseled and advised that it is even healthy to cry with the patient. Parents of children or adolescents who are dying can be gently made aware of their child's knowledge and their child's needs at this time. Many dying patients need the opportunity to take care of practical matters such as wills, monetary matters, and personal relationships.

Patients and families need their doctor's help in making decisions about continued treatment, DNR, and hospice care. A recent chart review of patients who died in the hospital revealed that 77% of patients had DNR orders in their charts and 46% had comfort care plans (Fins et al., 1999). It has been found that doctors do not broach the subject of life-sustaining measures with patients while they are still able to make decisions. At the time when such decisions are needed the patient is usually unable to make them (Carmel, 1996; Kelner & Bourgeault, 1993). Communication styles and strategies used by physicians to discuss DNR have a direct effect on the outcomes as well as satisfaction with these discussions (Ventres et al., 1992). Consequently, communication difficulties between doctor, patient, and families may lead to DNR decisions that may not be truly reflective of each person's wishes (Ventres et al., 1992). Although many people prefer to die at home, families should be educated about the potential benefits of high-quality hospice care as a possible option that is not viewed as an admission of giving up hope (Johnson & Slaninka, 1999).

The communication, both amount and type, between a doctor, the patient, and the patient's family is influential in determining satisfaction with care. Although physicians are not trained in the art of communication, this must be recognized as a meaningful aspect of patient care. Deciding the proper amount of information to give and the type of patient involvement in decision-making should be based on the wants and needs of the individual patient and his or her family. Although never an easy task, talking with patients and families about chronic or fatal diseases as well as death and dying should be viewed as a part of the doctor's role and integrated into medical training.

CONCLUSIONS

The body of literature reviewed in this chapter offers the mental health professional a road map to a better understanding of the complex interplay between illness and disease, between mind and body; between patient and illness, and between doctor and patient. Today many diseases that once meant certain death are regarded as treatable chronic conditions. Perhaps for the first time in modern history, we are in the enviable position of caring for the emotional needs of the sick and of survivors of disease. What was once a luxury has become increasingly a social necessity, lest the chronically ill forego their potential as productive contributors to society. The mental health professional can play a key role in advocating for and maintaining a better quality of life for those who seek help in coping with their illness. To do this well, it is imperative that these clinicians keep abreast of the rapidly evolving fields of behavioral and psychosomatic medicine.

REFERENCES

Aaronson, L. (1989). Perceived and received support: Effects on health behavior during pregnancy. *Nursing Research, 38,* 4–8.

Abel, E. (1995). An update on incidence of FAS: FAS is not an equal opportunity birth defect. *Neurotoxicology and Teratology, 17,* 437–443.

Alexander, F. (1950). *Psychosomatic medicine.* New York: Norton.

Alter, C., Pelcovitz, D., Axelrod, A., Goldenberg, B., Harris, H., Meyers, B., et al. (1996). Identification of PTSD in cancer survivors. *Psychosomatics, 37* (2), 137–43.

American Psychiatric Association. (1994). *Diagnostic and statistical manual of the mental disorders-fourth edition.* Washington DC: APA.

Anagnostopoulos, F., Vaslamatzis, G., Markidis, M., Katsouyanni, K., Vassilaros, S., & Stafanis, C. (1993). An investigation of hostile and alexithymic characteristics in breast cancer patients. *Psychotherapy and Psychosomatics, 59,* 179-189.

Andre K., Schraub, S., Mercier, M., & Bontemps, P. (1995). Role of alcohol and tobacco in the aetiology of head and neck cancer: a case-control study in the Doubs region of France. *European Journal of Cancer. Part B, Oral Oncology, 31B*(5), 301–309.

Angell, M. (1985). Disease as a reflection of the psyche. *New England Journal of Medicine, 312,* 1570–1572.

Appels, A., & Schouten, E. (1991). Waking up exhausted as risk indicator of myocardial infarction. *American Journal of Cardiology, 68*(4), 395–398.

Arroll, B., & Beaglehole, R. (1992). Does physical activity lower blood pressure: A critical review of the clinical trials. *Journal of Clinical Epidemiology, 45,* 439–447.

Bacon, C. L., Renneker, R., & Cutler, M. (1952). A psychosomatic survey of cancer of the breast. *Psychosomatic Medicine, 14,* 453–460.

Bak, S., Koh, H., Howland, J., Mangiove, T., Hingson, R., & Levenson, S. (1992). Sunbathing habits and sunscreen use in 2485 Caucasian adults: Results of a national survey. In Progressive Abstract American Public Health Association Meeting, Washington, DC, Session 2052.

Banks, B., Silverman, R., Schwartz, R., & Tunnessen, W. (1992). Attitudes of teenagers toward sun exposure and sunscreen use. *Pediatrics, 89,* 40–42.

Barefoot, J. C., Patterson, J. C., Haney, T. L., Cayton, T. G., Hickman, J. R., & Williams, R. B. (1994). Hostility in asymptomatic men with angiographically confirmed coronary artery disease. *American Journal of Cardiology, 74,* 439–442.

Bartlett, S. (1998). Does inadequate housing perpetuate children's poverty? *Childhood, 5*(4), 403–420.

Baum, A., & Cohen, L. (1998). Successful behavioral interventions to prevent cancer: The example of skin cancer. *Annual Review of Public Health, 19,* 319–333.

Baum, A., & Posluszny, D. (1999). Health psychology: Mapping biobehavioral contributions to health and illness. *Annual Review of Psychology, 50,* 137–163.

Beaumont, W. (1833). *Experiments and observations on the gastric juice and physiology of digestion.* Plattburgh: F. P. Allen.

Becker, M. (1979). Understanding patient compliance. In S. Cohen (Ed.) *New directions in patient compliance.* Lexington MA: Lexington Books.

Belloc, N., & Breslow, L. (1972). Relationship of physical health status and health practices. *Preventive Medicine, 1*(3), 409–421.

Berlin, J., & Colditz, G. (1990). A meta-analysis of physical activity in the prevention of coronary heart disease. *American Journal of Epidemiology, 132,* 612–628.

Bernstein, L., Henderson, B., Hanisch, R., Sullivan-Halley, J., & Ross, R. (1994). Physical exercise and reduced risk of breast cancer in young women. *Journal of the National Cancer Institute, 86*(18), 1403–1408.

Biondi, M., & Zannino, L.G. (1997). Psychological stress, neuroimmunomodulation, and susceptibility to infectious diseases in animals and man: A review. *Psychotherapy and Psychosomatics, 66*(1), 3–26

Black, M., & Dubowitz, H. (1991). Failure-to-thrive: Lessons from animal models and developing countries. *Journal of Developmental and Behavioral Pediatrics, 12,* 259–267.

Blair, S., Goodyear, N., Gibbons, O., & Cooper, K. (1994). Physical fitness and incidence of hypertension in healthy normotensive men and women. *Journal of the American Medical Association, 252,* 487–490.

Bolig, E., Borkowski, J., & Brandenberger, J. (1999). Poverty and health across the life span. In T. Whitman (Ed.), *Life-span perspectives on health and illness.* Mahwah, NJ: Lawrence Erlbaum Assoc.

Bond, B., Aiken, L., & Somerville, S. (1992). The health belief model and adolescents with insulin-dependent diabetes mellitus. *Health Psychology, 11,* 190–198.

Botvin, G., & Epstein, J. (1999). Preventing cigarette smoking among children and adolescents. In D. Seidman & L. Covey (Eds.), *Helping the hard-core smoker* (pp. 51–71). Mahwah, NJ: Lawrence Erlbaum.

Briere, J., & Runtz, M. (1988). Symptomatology associated with childhood sexual victimization in a nonclinical adult sample. *Child Abuse and Neglect, 12*(1), 51–59.

Brody, J. (1999, December 28). Paying the price for cheating on sleep. *The New York Times,* p. F7.

Brown, J., & Pollitt, E. (1996). Malnutrition, poverty and intellectual development. *Scientific American, 274,* 38–43.

Brown, B., Zhao, X-Q., Sacco, D., & Albers, J. (1993). Lipid lowering and plaque regression. New insights into prevention of plaque disruption and clinical events in coronary disease. *Circulation, 87,* 1781–1791.

Brownell, K., & Cohen, L. (1995a). Adherence to dietary regimens 1: An overview of research. *Behavioral Medicine, 20,* 149–154.

Brownell, K., & Cohen, L. (1995b). Adherence to dietary regimens 2: Components of effective interventions. *Behavioral Medicine, 20,* 155–164.

Bruhn, J., Scurry, M., & Bunce, H. (1988). Caring for the terminally ill: Attitudes of the house staff. In S. C. Klagsbrun, I. K. Goldberg, & M. M. Rawnsley (Eds.), *Psychiatric aspects of terminal illness.* Philadelphia: The Charles Press Publishers.

Bryan, A., Aiken, L., & West, S. (1996). Increasing condom use: Evaluation of a theory-based intervention to prevent sexually transmitted diseases in young women. *Health Psychology, 15*(5), 371–382.

Buckman, R. (1984). Breaking bad news: Why is it still so difficult? *British Medical Journal, 288,* 1597–1599.

Campo, J. V., & Fritsch, S. L. (1994). Somatization in children and adolescents. *Journal of the American Academy of Child and Adolescent Psychiatry, 33*(9), 1223–1235.

Campo, J. V., Jansen-McWilliams, L., Comer, D. M., & Kelleher, K. J. (1999). Somatization in pediatric primary care: Association with psychopathology, functional impairment, and use of services. *Journal of the American Academy of Child and Adolescent Psychiatry, 38*(9), 1093–1101.

Caplan, G. (1974). *Support systems and community mental health: Lectures on concept development.* New York: Behavioral Publications.

Carmel, S. (1996). Behavior, attitudes, and expectations regarding the use of life-sustaining treatments among physicians in Israel: An exploratory study. *Social Science and Medicine, 43*(6), 955–965.

Cartmill, A., & Betts, T. (1992). Seizure behaviour in a patient with post-traumatic stress disorder following a rape. Notes on the aetiology of pseudo-seizures. *Seizure, 1,* 33–36.

Catania, J., Coates, T., Stall, R., Turner, H., Peterson, J., Hearst, N., et al. (1992). Prevalence of AIDS-related risk factors and condom use in the United States. *Science, 258,* 1101–1106.

Centers for Disease Control (CDC). (1997). *Screening young children for lead poisoning: Guidance for state and local public health officials.* Atlanta: Author.

Cheang, A., & Cooper, C. L. (1985). Psychosocial factors in breast cancer. *Stress Medicine, 1,* 61–66.

Cherpitel, C. (1991). Drinking patterns and problems among primary care patients: A comparison with the general population. *Alcohol and Alcoholism, 26*(5–6), 627–633.

Children's Defense Fund. (1993). *Decade of indifference: Maternal and child health trends 1980–1990.* Washington DC: Author.

Childress, J. (1982). *Who should decide? Paternalism in health care.* New York: Oxford University Press.

Choi, K., & Coates, T. (1994). Prevention of HIV infection. *AIDS, 8,* 1371–1389.

Cobb, S. (1976). Social support as a moderator of life stress. *Psychosomatic Medicine, 38,* 300–314.

Cohen, S., & Hoberman, H. (1983). Positive events and social supports as buffers of life change stress. *Journal of Applied Social Psychology, 13,* 99–125.

Cooper, C., & Faragher, E. (1993). Psychosocial stress and breast cancer: The inter-relationship between stress events, coping strategies and personality. *Psychological Medicine, 23,* 653–662.

Council on Scientific Affairs. (1989). Harmful effects of ultraviolet radiation. *Journal of the American Medical Association, 262*(3), 380–384.

Cross, P., & Gurland. (1986). The epidemiology of dementing disorders. Contract report prepared for the Office of Technology Assessment, U.S. Congress.

Curry, S., & Emmons, K. (1994). Theoretical models for predicting and improving compliance with breast screening. *Annals of Behavioral Medicine, 16*(4), 302–316.

Deber, R. (1994). Physicians in health care management: 8. The patient-physician partnership: Decision making, problem solving, and the desire to participate [see comments]. *Canadian Medical Association Journal, 151,* 423–427.

Deber, R., Kraetschmer, N., & Irvine, J. (1996). What role do patients wish to play in treatment decision making? *Archives of Internal Medicine, 156*(13), 1414–1420.

Delunas, L. (1996). Beyond Type A: Hostility and coronary heart disease-implications for research and practice. *Rehabilitation Nursing, 21*(4), 196–201.

Dembroski, T. , MacDougall, J., Herd, J., & Shields, J. (1979). Effect of level of challenge on pressor and heart rate responses in Type A and Type B subjects. *Journal of Applied Social Psychology, 9,* 209–225.

Desguin, B., Holt, I., & McCarthy, S. (1994). Comprehensive care of the child with a chronic condition. Part 1. Understanding chronic conditions in childhood. *Current Problems in Pediatrics, 24,* 199–218.

DiClemente, C. (1993). Changing addictive behaviors: A process perspective. *Current Directions in Psychological Science, 2,* 101–106.

Diet and health: Implications for reducing chronic disease risk. (1989). Washington, DC: National Academy Press.

DiMatteo, M., & DiNicola, D. (1982). *Achieving patient compliance.* Oxford: Permagon.

Dorgan, J. (1998). Physical activity and breast cancer: Is there a link? *Journal of the National Cancer Institute, 90*(15), 1155–1160.

Draper, G. (1942). Emotional component of ulcer susceptible constitution. *Annals of Internal Medicine, 16,* 633–658.

Dunbar, F. (1946). *Emotions and bodily changes: A survey of the literature on psychosomatic interrelationships.* New York: Columbia University Press.

Dwyer, J., Clarke, L., & Miller, M. (1990). The effect of religious concentration and affiliation on county cancer mortality rates. *Journal of Health & Social Behavior, 31*(2), 185–202.

Ekstrand, M. (1992). Safer sex maintenance among gay men: Are we making any progress? *AIDS, 6,* 875–877.

Emanuel, E., & Emanuel, L. (1992). Four models of the physician-patient relationship. *Journal of the American Medical Association, 267,* 2221–2226.

Ende, J., Kazis, L., Ash, A., & Moskowitz, M. (1989). Measuring patients' desire for autonomy: Decision-making and information-seeking preferences among medical patients. *Journal of General Internal Medicine, 4,* 23–30.

Engel, G. (1959). Psychogenic pain and the pain-prone patient. *American Journal of Medicine, 26,* 899–918.

Engel, G. (1977). The need for a new medical model: A challenge for biomedicine. *Science, 196,* 129–136.

Escobar, J., Swartz, M., Rubio-Stipec, M., & Manu, P. (1991). Medically unexplained symptoms: Distribution, risk factors and comorbidity. In L. J. Kirmayer & J. M. Robbins (Eds.), *Current concepts of somatization: Research and clinical perspectives.* Washington DC: American Psychiatric Press.

Evans, E. (1926). *A psychological study of cancer.* New York: Dodd, Mead & Co.

Eysenck, H. J., & Eysenck, S. B. G. (1975). *Manual for the Eysenck Personality Questionnaire.* London: Hodder and Stoughton.

Expert Panel on Detection, Evaluation, and Treatment of High Blood Cholesterol in Adults. (1990). Summary of the Second Report of the National Cholesterol Education Program (NCEP) Expert Panel on Detection, Evaluation, and Treatment of High Blood Cholesterol in Adults (Adult Treatment Panel II). *Journal of the American Medical Association, 269,* 3015–3023.

Faragher, E., & Cooper, C. (1990). Type A stress prone behaviour and breast cancer. *Psychological Medicine, 20,* 663–670.

Feldman, H., Ploof, D., & Cohen, W. (1999). Physician-family partnerships: The adaptive practice model. *Journal of Developmental and Behavioral Pediatrics, 20*(2), 111–116.

Fins, J., Miller, F., Acres, C., Bacchetta, M., Huzzard, L., & Rapkin, B. (1999). End-of-life decision-making in the hospital: Current practice and future prospects. *Journal of Pain and Symptom Management, 17*(1), 6–15.

Fisher, J., & Fisher, W. (1992). Changing AIDS-risk behavior. *Psychological Bulletin, 111,* 455–474.

Fisher, J., Fisher, W., Misovich, S., Kimble, D., & Malloy, T. (1996). Changing AIDS risk behavior: Effects of an intervention emphasizing AIDS reduction information, motivation, and behavioral skills in a college student population. *Health Psychology, 15*(2), 114–123.

Fleishman, S., & Lesko, L. (1989). Delirium and dementia. In J. Holland & J. Rowland (Eds.), *Handbook of psychooncology: Psychological care of the patient with cancer.* New York: Oxford University Press.

Fletcher, G., Balady, G., Blair, S., Blumenthal, J., Casperson, C., Chaitman, B., et al. (1996). Statement on exercise. Benefits and recommendations for physical activity programs for all Americans. A statement for health professionals by the Committee on Exercise and Cardiac Rehabilitation of the Council on Clinical Cardiology, American Heart Association. *Circulation, 94,* 857–862.

Francis, D., & Chin, J. (1987). The prevention of acquired immunodeficiency syndrome in the United States. An objective strategy for medicine, public health, business, and the community. *Journal of the American Medical Association, 257*(10), 1357–1366.

Frasure-Smith, N., Lesperance, F., Juneau, M., Talajic, M., & Bourassa, M. (1999). Gender, depression, and one-year prognosis after myocardial infarction. *Psychosomatic Medicine, 61,* 26–37.

Frasure-Smith, N., Lesperance, F., & Talajic, M. (1993). Depression following myocardial infarction. Impact on 6-month survival. *Journal of the American Medical Association, 270*(15), 1819–1825.

Freud, S. (1955). *Collected works: Vol. 2. Studies of hysteria.* New York: Hogarth Press.

Friedman, H. (1990). Personality and disease: Overview, review, and preview. In H. Friedman (Ed.), *Personality and disease* (pp. 3–13). New York: John Wiley and Sons.

Friedman, M., & Rosenman, R. (1974). *Type A behavior and your heart.* New York: Knopf.

Fritz, G., Fritsch. S., & Hagino, O. (1997). Somatoform disorders in children and adolescents: A review of the past 10 years. *Journal of the American Academy of Child and Adolescent Psychiatry, 36*(10), 1329–1338.

Fry, R. (1993). Adult physical illness and childhood sexual abuse. *Journal of Psychosomatic Research, 37*(2), 89–193.

Gainesborough, H., & Slater, E. (1946). A study of peptic ulcer. *British Medical Journal, 2,* 253–258.

Garber, J., Walker, L. S., & Zeman, J. (1991). Somatization symptoms in a community sample of children and adolescents: Further validation of the children's somatization inventory. *Psychological Assessment: A Journal of Consulting and Clinical Psychology, 3,* 588–595.

Gatchel, R., Baum, A., & Krantz, D. (1989). An introduction to health psychology (2nd ed.). New York: Newbery Award Records.

Gilligan, J. (1996). *Violence: Our deadly epidemic and its causes.* New York: Putnam.

Golay, A., & Bobbioni, E. (1997). The role of dietary fat in obesity. *International Journal of Obesity and Related Metabolic Disorders, 21*(Suppl. 3), S2–S11.

Goold, S. & Lipkin Jr., M. (1999). The doctor-patient relationship: Challenges, opportunities, and strategies. *Journal of General Internal Medicine, 14*(Suppl. 1), S26–S33.

Gorney, M. (1999). The role of communication in the physician's office. *Medical-Legal Issues in Plastic Surgery, 26*(1), 133–140.

Graham, J. R. (1981). *The Minnesota Multiphasic Personality Inventory (MMPI): A practical guide.* New York: Oxford University Press.

Grant, K. (1992). Informed consent: Medical-legal update for the practitioner on recent judicial opinions applying state laws. *American Surgeon, 58,* 146–152.

Greenfield, S., Kaplan, H., & Ware Jr., J. (1985). Expanding patient involvement in care: Effects on patients' outcomes. *Annals of Internal Medicine, 102,* 520–528.

Greer, S., & Morris, T. (1975). Psychological attributes of women who develop breast cancer: A controlled study. *Journal of Psychosomatic Research, 19,* 147–153.

Grinker, R., & Robbins, F. (1953). *Psychosomatic case book.* New York: Blakiston.

Hagberg, M. (1996). Neck and arm disorders: ABC of work related disorders. *British Medical Journal, 313,* 419–422.

Hamburg, D., Elliott, G., & Parron, D. (1982). *Health and behavior: Frontiers of research in the biobehavioral sciences.* Washington, DC: National Academy Press.

Hanisch, U., & Quirion, R. (1996). Interleukin-2 as a neuroregulatory cytokine. *Brain Research Reviews, 21,* 246–284.

Hardy, M., & Hazelrigg, L. (1993). The gender of poverty in an aging population. *Research on Aging, 15,* 243–278.

Harrison, H. (1993). The principle of family centered neonatal care. *Pediatrics, 92*(5), 643–650.

Hausberg, M., Mark, A., Winniford, M., Brown, R., & Somers, V. (1997). Sympathetic and vascular effects of short-term passive smoke exposure in healthy nonsmokers. *Circulation, 96*(1), 282–287.

Haynes, R., Taylor, D., & Sackett, D. (1979). *Compliance in health care.* London: The Johns Hopkins Press.

Herman, J. (1992). *Trauma and recovery.* New York: Basic Books.

Hersh, D., Kranzler, H., & Meyer, R. (1997). Persistent delirium following cessation of heavy alcohol consumption: Diagnostic and treatment implications. *American Journal of Psychiatry, 154*(6), 846–851.

Herzog, T., Abrams, D., Emmons, K., Linnan, L., & Shadel, W. (1999). Do processes of change predict smoking stage movements? A prospective analysis of the transtheoretical model. *Health Psychology, 18*(4), 369–375.

Hill, A., Weaver, C., & Blundell, J. (1991). Food craving, dietary restraint and mood. *Appetite, 17*(3), 187–197.

Hockey, R. (1973). Changes in information-selection patterns in multisource monitoring as a function of induced arousal shifts. *Journal of Experimental Psychology, 101,* 35–42.

Hoerauf, K., Wiesner, G., Schroegendorfer, K., Jobst, B., Spacek, A., Harth, M., et al. (1999). Waste anaesthetic gases induce sister chromatid exchanges in lymphocytes of operating room personnel. *British Journal of Anaesthesia, 82*(5), 764–766.

Holmes, O. W. (1883). The young practitioner. In *Medical Essays* (p. 338). Boston, MA: Houghton Mifflin.

House, J. (1981). *Work stress and social support.* Reading, MA: Addison-Wesley.

Hubbard, P., Muhlenkamp, A., & Brown, N. (1984). The relationship between social support and self-care practices. *Nursing Research, 33,* 266–170.

Hughes, J. (1988). Clonidine, depression, and smoking cessation. *Journal of the American Medical Association, 259,* 2901–2902.

Hussey, L., & Gilliland, K. (1989). Compliance, low literacy and locus of control. *Nursing Clinics of North America, 24*(3), 605–611.

Institute of Medicine. (1995). *Weighing the options: Criteria for evaluating weight management programs.* Washington, DC: National Academy Press.

Jenkins, C. (1976). Recent evidence supporting psychological and social risk factors for coronary disease: Second of two parts. *New England Journal of Medicine, 294,* 1033–1038.

Johnson, C., & Slaninka, S. (1999). Barriers to accessing hospice services before a later terminal stage. *Death Studies, 23*(3), 225–238.

Kanter, V. B., & Hazelton, J. E. (1964). An attempt to measure some aspects of personality in young men with duodenal ulcer by means of questionnaires and a projective test. *Journal of Psychosomatic Research, 8,* 297–309.

Kaplan, S., Gandek, B., Greenfield, S., Rogers, W., & Ware, J. (1995). Patient and visit characteristics related to physicians' participatory decision-making style. Results from the medical outcomes study. *Medical Care, 33,* 1176–1187.

Kassel, J. (1997). Smoking and attention: A review and reformulation of the stimulus-filter hypothesis. *Clinical Psychology Reviews, 17*(5), 451–478.

Katon, W. (1996). The impact of major depression on chronic medical illness. *General Hospital Psychiatry, 18,* 215–219.

Katon, W., & Walker, E. (1998). Medically unexplained symptoms in primary care. *Journal of Clinical Psychiatry, 59*(suppl 20), 15–21.

Katz, R., & Jernigan, S. (1991). Brief report: An empirically derived educational program for detecting and preventing skin cancer. *Journal of Behavioral Medicine, 14,* 421–427.

Kelner, M., & Bourgeault, I. (1993). Patient control over dying: Responses of health care professionals. *Social Science and Medicine, 36,* 757.

Kernberg, O. (1984). Severe personality disorders: Psychotherapeutic strategies. New Haven: Yale University Press.

King, A., Haskell, W., Young, D., Oka, R., & Stefanick, M. (1995). Long-term effects of varying intensities and formats of physical activity on participation rates, fitness, and lipoproteins in men and women aged 50 to 65 years. *Circulation, 91,* 2596–2604.

Kirmayer, L. J., & Robbins, J. M. (1991). Introduction: Concepts of somatization. In L. J. Kirmayer & J. M. Robbins (Eds.), *Current concepts of somatization: Research and clinical perspectives* (Vol. 31, pp. 1–20). Washington, DC: American Psychiatric Press.

Klerman, L. (1996). Child health: What public policies can improve it? In E. Zigler, S. Kagan, & N. Hall (Eds.), *Children, families and government: Preparing for the 21st century* (2nd ed., pp. 188–206). New York: Cambridge University Press.

Klesges, R, Cigrang, J., & Glasgow, R. (1989). Worksite smoking modification programs: A state-of -the-art review and directions for future research. In M. Johnston & T. Marteau (Eds.), *Applications in health psychology.* New Brunswick, NJ: Transaction.

Kobasa, S. C. O. (1990). Lessons from history: How to find the person in health psychology. In H. S. Friedman (Ed.), *Personality and Disease* (pp. 14–37). New York: John Wiley and Sons.

Koenig, H., & Larson, D. (1998). Use of hospital services, religious attendance, and religious affiliation. *Southern Medical Journal, 91*(10), 925–932.

Koniak-Griffin, D., Nyamathi, A., Vasquez, R., & Russo, A. (1994). Risk-taking behaviors and AIDS knowledge: Experiences and beliefs of minority adolescent mothers. *Health Education Research, 9*, 449–463.

Kozol, J. (1995). *Amazing grace*. New York: Crown.

Kripke, D., Simons, R., Garfinkel, L., & Hammond, E. (1979). Short and long sleep and sleeping pills. Is increased mortality associated? *Archives of General Psychiatry, 36*(1), 103–116.

Kroenke, K., & Mangelsdorff, D. (1989). Common symptoms in ambulatory care: Incidence, evaluation, therapy, and outcome. *American Journal of Medicine, 86*, 262–266.

Kroenke, K., Spitzer, R.L., deGruy, F., Hahn, S. R., Linzer, M., Williams, J. B., et al. (1997). Multisomatoform disorder: An alternative to undifferentiated somatoform disorder for the somatizing patient in primary care. *Archives of General Psychiatry, 54*, 352–358.

Kubler-Ross, E. (1969). *On death and dying*. New York: Macmillan.

Lagerlov, P., Leseth, A., & Matheson, I. (1998). The doctor-patient relationship and the management of asthma. *Social Science and Medicine, 47*(1), 85–91.

Laine, C., & Davidoff, F. (1996). Patient-centered medicine: A professional evolution. *Journal of the American Medical Association, 275*(2), 152–156.

Lavigne, J., Binns, H., Arend, R., Rosenbaum, D., Christoffel, K., Hayford, J., et al. (1998). Psychopathology and health care use among preschool children: A retrospective analysis. *Journal of the American Academy of Child and Adolescent Psychiatry, 37*(3), 262–270.

Law, M., Wald, N., & Thompson, S. (1994). By how much and how quickly does reduction in serum cholesterol concentration lower risk of ischemic heart disease? *British Medical Journal, 308*, 367–372.

Lee, I., Hsieh, C., & Paffenbarger Jr., R. (1995). Exercise intensity and longevity in men. The Harvard Alumni Health Study. *Journal of the American Medical Association, 273*, 1179–1184.

Lerner, D., Stoudemire, A., & Rosenstein, D. (1999). Neuropsychiatric toxicity associated with cytokines. *Psychosomatics, 40*(5), 428–435.

Levenstein, S., Prantera, C., Varvo, V., Scribano, M., Berto, E., Spinella, S., et al. (1995). Patterns of biologic and psychologic risk factors in duodenal ulcer patients. *Journal of Clinical Gastroenterology, 21*(2), 110–117.

Levine, P., Silberfarb, P., & Lipowski, Z. (1978). Mental disorders in cancer patients: A study of 100 psychiatric referrals. *Cancer, 42*, 1385–1391.

Levy, N. (1988). Fatal illness: What should the patient be told? In S. C. Klagsbrun, I. K. Goldberg, & M. M. Rawnsley (Eds.), *Psychiatric aspects of terminal illness*. Philadelphia: The Charles Press.

Levy, S., & Heiden, L. (1990). Personality and social factors in cancer outcome. In H. Friedman (Ed.), *Personality and disease* (pp. 3–13). New York: John Wiley and Sons.

Linde, L., Edland, A., & Bergstrom, M. (1999). Auditory attention and multiattribute decision-making during a 33-hr sleep-deprivation period: Mean performance and between-subject dispersions. *Ergonomics, 42*(5), 696–713.

Lusardi, P., Zoppi, A., Preti, P., Pesce, R., Piazza, E., & Fogari, R. (1999). Effects of insufficient sleep on blood pressure in hypertensive patients: A 24-h study. *American Journal of Hypertension, 12*(1Pt 1), 63–68.

Lynch, J., Helmrich, S., Lakka, T., Kaplan, G. A., Cohen, R. D., Salonen, R., et al. (1996). Moderately intense physical activities and high levels of cardiorespiratory fitness reduce the risk of non insulin-dependent diabetes mellitus in middle-aged men. *Archives of Internal Medicine, 156,* 130–131.

Mai, F. & Merskey, H. (1980). Briquet's *Treatise on Hysteria. Archives of General Psychiatry, 37*(12), 1401–1405.

Maloney, T., & Paul, B. (1991). The consumer movement takes hold in health care. *Health Affairs (Project Hope), 4,* 268–279.

Massie, M., Holland, J., & Glass, E. (1983). Delirium in terminally ill cancer patients. *American Journal of Psychiatry, 140,* 1048–1050.

Masters, W., Johnson, V., & Kolodny, R. (1992). *Human sexuality* (4th ed.). New York: HarperCollins.

Matthews, K., Rosenman, R., Dembroski, T., MacDougall, J., & Harris, E. (1984). Familial resemblance in components of the Type A behavior pattern: A reanalysis of the California Type A twin study. *Psychosomatic Medicine, 46,* 512–522.

McDougall, J. (1989). *Theaters of the body: A psychoanalytic approach to psychosomatic illness.* New York:: W. W. Norton.

McIntosh, J. H., Nasiry, R.W., Frydman, M., Waller, S., & Piper, D. (1983). The personality pattern of patients with chronic peptic ulcer: A case-control study. *Scandinavian Journal of Gastroenterology, 18,* 945–950.

McKenna, M., Zevon, M., Corn, B., & Rounds, J. (1999). Psychosocial factors and the development of breast cancer: A meta-analysis. *Health Psychology, 18*(5), 520–532.

Meichenbaum, D., & Turk, D. (1987). *Facilitating treatment adherence: A practitioner's guide.* New York: Plenum Press.

Mekarski, J. (1999). Stages of adjustment to a medical diagnosis of a serious medical condition. *European Psychiatry, 14,* 49–51.

Melmed, R., & Gelpin, Y. (1996). Duodenal ulcer: The helicobacterization of a psychosomatic disease? *Israeli Journal of Medical Science, 32,* 211–216.

Merrick, N. (1995). Adolescent childbearing as career "choice:" Perspective from an ecological context. *Journal of Counseling and Development, 73,* 288–295.

Milberger, S., Biederman, J., Faraone, S., Chen, L., & Jones, J. (1997). Further evidence of an association between attention-deficit/hyperactivity disorder and cigarette smoking: Findings from a high-risk sample of siblings. *American Journal of Addiction, 6*(3), 205–217.

Miller, F. (1994). Protracted alcohol withdrawal delirium. *Journal of Substance Abuse Treatment, 11,* 127–130.

Miller, T., Balady, G., & Fletcher, G. (1997). Exercise and its role in the prevention and rehabilitation of cardiovascular disease. *Annals of Behavioral Medicine, 19*(3), 220–229.

Morrison, J. (1989). Childhood sexual histories of women with somatization disorder. *American Journal of Psychiatry, 146*(2), 239–241.

Muggleton, J., Allen, R., & Chappell, P. (1999). Hand and arm injuries associated with repetitive manual work in industry: A review of disorders, risk factors and preventive measures. *Ergonomics, 42*(5), 714–739.

Murphy, J., Olivier, D., Monson, R., Sobol, A., Federman, E., & Leighton, A. (1991). Depression and anxiety in relation to social status: A prospective epidemiological study. *Archives of General Psychiatry, 48*(3), 223–229.

Negri, E., LaVecchia, C., Franceschi, S., D'Avanzo, B., Talamini, R., et al. (1996). Intake of selected micronutrients and the risk of breast cancer. *International Journal of Cancer, 65*(2), 140–144.

Nemiah, J. & Sifneos, P. (1970). Affect and fantasy in patients with psychosomatic disorders. In O. Hill (Ed.), *Modern trends in psychosomatic medicine.* London: Butterworth.

Nordevang, E., Azavedo, E., Svane, G., Nilsson, B., & Holm, L. (1993). Dietary habits and mammographic patterns in patients with breast cancer. *Breast Cancer Research and Treatment, 26*(3), 207–215.

North, C. (1996). Alcoholism in women. More common-and serious- than you might think. *Postgraduate Medicine, 100*(4), 221–224, 230, 232–233.

Novack, D., Plumer. R., Smith, R., Ochtill, H., Morrow, G., & Bennet, J. (1979). Changes in physicians' attitudes towards telling the cancer patient. *Journal of the American Medical Association, 241,* 897–900.

Oberg, C., Bryant, M., & Bach, M. (1995). A portrait of America's children: The impact of poverty and a call to action. *Journal of Social Distress and the Homeless, 4,* 43–56.

O'Connor, G., Buring, J., Yusuf, S., et al. (1989). An overview of randomized trials of rehabilitation with exercise after myocardial infarction. *Circulation, 80,* 234–244.

Oken, D. (1961). What to tell cancer patients. *Journal of the American Medical Association, 175,* 1120–1128.

Oldridge, N., Guyatt, G., Fischer, M., & Rimm, A. (1988). Cardiac rehabilitation after myocardial infarction. Combined experience of randomized clinical trials. *Journal of the American Medical Association, 260,* 945–950.

Ornish, D., Brown, S., Scherwitz, L., et al. (1990). Can lifestyle changes reverse coronary heart disease? The Lifestyle Heart Trial. *Lancet, 336,* 129–133.

Paffenbarger Jr., R., Hyde, R., Wing, A., et al. (1993). The association of changes in physical activity level and other lifestyle characteristics with mortality among men. *New England Journal of Medicine, 328,* 538–545.

Paffenbarger Jr., R., Hyde, R., Wing, A., & Hsieh, C. (1986). Physical activity, all-cause mortality, and longevity of college alumni. *New England Journal of Medicine, 314,* 615–613.

Partinen, M., Putkonen, P., Kaprio, J., Koskenvuo, M., & Hilakivi, I. (1982). Sleep disorders in relation to coronary heart disease. *Acta Medica Scandinavica-Supplementum, 660,* 69–83.

Pate, R., Pratt, M., Blair, S., et al. (1995). Physical activity and public health. A recommendation from the Centers for Disease Control and Prevention and the American College of Sports Medicine. *Journal of the American Medical Association, 273,* 402–407.

Persky, V., Kempethorne-Rawson, J., & Shekelle, R. (1987). Personality and risk of cancer: Twenty-year follow-up of the Western Electric Study. *Psychosomatic Medicine, 49,* 435–449.

Perz, C., DiClemente, C., & Carbonari, J. (1996). Doing the right thing at the right time? The interaction of stages and processes of change in successful smoking cessation. *Health Psychology, 15*(6), 462–468.

Piccinelli, M., Rucci, P., Ustun, B., & Simon, G. (1999). Typologies of anxiety, depression and somatization symptoms among primary care attenders with no formal mental disorder. *Psychological Medicine, 29,* 677–688.

Piper, D., McIntosh, J., Ariotti, D., Calogiuri, J., Brown, R., & Shy, C. (1981). Life events and chronic duodenal ulcer: A case control study. *Gut, 22,* 1011–1017.

Pollak, C. P., Perlick, D., Linsner, J. P., Wenston, J., & Hsieh, F. (1990). Sleep problems in the community elderly as predictors of death and nursing home placement. *Journal of Community Health, 15*(2), 123–135.

Powell, K., Thompson, P., Caspersen, C., & Kendrick, J. (1987). Physical activity and the incidence of coronary heart disease. *Annual Review of Public Health, 8,* 253–287.

Prochaska, J., & DiClemente, C. (1983). Stages and processes of self-change in smoking: Toward an integrative model of change. *Journal of Consulting and Clinical Psychology, 51,* 390–395.

Prochaska, J., DiClemente, C., & Norcross, J. (1992). In search of how people change. *American Psychologist, 47,* 1102–1114.

Prochaska, J., Velicer, W., DiClemente, C., & Fava, J. (1988). Measuring processes of change: Applications to the cessation of smoking. *Journal of Consulting and Clinical Psychology, 56,* 520–528.

Rakowski, W., Ehrich, B., Dube, C., Pearlman, D., Goldstein, M., Peterson, K., et al. (1996). Screening mammography and constructs from the transtheoretical "model:" Associations using two definitions of the stages-of-adoption. *Annals of Behavioral Medicine, 18*(2), 91–100.

Reilly, J., Baker, G., Rhodes, J., & Salmon, P. (1999). The association of sexual and physical abuse with somatization: Characteristics of patients presenting with irritable bowel syndrome and non-epileptic attack disorder. *Psychological Medicine, 29,* 399–406.

Renaud, S., de Lorgeril, M., Delaye, J., et al. (1995). Cretan Mediterranean diet for prevention of coronary heart disease. *American Journal of Clinical Nutrition, 61*(Suppl), 1360S–1367S.

Report of the National Commission on Sleep Disorders Research, U.S. Department of Health and Human Services, Vol. 2. P 84 (Washington DC, 1994).

Review Panel on Coronary-Prone Behaviors and Coronary Heart Disease. (1981). Coronary prone behavior and coronary heart disease: A critical review. *Circulation, 63,* 1199–1215.

Ricci Bitti, P., Gremigni, P., Bertolotti, G., & Zotti, A. (1995). Dimensions of anger and hostility in cardiac patients, hypertensive patients and controls. *Psychotherapy and Psychosomatics, 64,* 162–172.

Riether, A., & Libb, J. (1991). Heart and liver transplantation. In A. Stoudemire & B. Fogel (Eds.), *Medical psychiatric practice: Volume I* (pp. 309–346). Washington DC: American Psychiatric Press.

Robinson, L., Klesges, R., Zbikowski, S., & Glaser, R. (1997). Predictors of risk for different stages of adolescent smoking in a biracial sample. *Journal of Consulting and Clinical Psychology, 65*(4), 653–662.

Rook, K. (1984). The negative side of social interaction: Impact on psychological well-being. *Journal of Personality and Social Psychology, 46,* 1097–1108.

Rooney, B., & Murray, D. (1996). A meta-analysis of smoking prevention programs after adjustment for errors in the unit of analysis. *Health Education Quarterly, 23*(1), 48–64.

Roscoe, R., Gittleman, J., Deddens, J., Petersen, M., & Halperin, W. (1999). Blood levels among children of lead exposed workers: A meta-analysis. *American Journal of Industrial Medicine, 36*(4), 475–481.

Rosenbaum, S. (1992). Child health and poor children. *American Behavioral Scientist, 35,* 275–289.

Rosenman, R., Brand, R., Jenkins, C., Friedman, M., Strauss, R., & Wurm, M. (1975). Coronary heart disease in the Western Collaborative Group Study: Final follow-up experience of 8-1/2 years. *Journal of the American Medical Association, 233,* 872–877.

Rosenstock, I. (1966). Why people use health services. *Millband Memorial Fund Quarterly, 44,* 94–127.

Roter, D., Stewart, M., Putnam, S., Lipkin Jr., M., Stiles, W., & Inui, T. (1997). The patient-physician relationship: Communication patterns of primary care physicians. *Journal of the American Medical Association, 277,* 350–356.

Rotter, J. B. (1954). *Social learning and clinical psychology.* New York: Prentice-Hall.

Rotter, J., Sones, J., Samloff, I., Richardson, C., Gursky, J., Walsh, J., et al. (1979). Duodenal ulcer disease associated with elevated serum pepsinogen: An inherited autosomal dominant disorder. *New England Journal of Medicine, 300,* 491–498.

Rowland, A., Baird, D., Shore, D., Weinberg, C., Savitz, D., & Wilcox, A. (1995). Nitrous oxide and spontaneous abortion in female dental assistants. *American Journal of Epidemiology, 141*(6), 531–538.

Russo, J., Katon, W., Sullivan, M., et al. (1994). Severity of somatization and its relationship to psychiatric disorders and personality. *Psychosomatics, 35,* 546–556.

Salisbury, S. (1990). *Outcome in chronic pain: Effects of affect symbolization and capacity for Relatedness.* Unpublished Ph.D. dissertation, California School of Professional Psychology. Alhambra, CA.

Scheidt, S. (1996). A whirlwind tour of cardiology for the mental health professional. In R. Allen & S. Scheidt (Eds.), *Heart and mind: The practice of cardiac psychology* (pp. 15-62). Washington, DC: American Psychological Association.

Schorr, L. B. (1989). *Within our reach: Breaking the cycle of disadvantage.* New York: Anchor Books.

Schulberg, H., Magruder, K., & deGruy, F. (1996). Major depression in primary medical care practice: Research trends and future priorities. *General Hospital Psychiatry, 18,* 395–406.

Searight, H. (1999). *Behavioral medicine: A primary care approach.* Philadelphia: Brunner/Mazel.

Seeland, I. (1988). The importance of discussing death with the dying. In S. C. Klagsbrun, I. K. Goldberg, & M. M. Rawnsley (Eds), *Psychiatric Aspects of Terminal Illness.* Philadelphia, PA: The Charles Press.

Shekelle, R., Gale, M., Ostfeld, A., & Paul, O. (1983). Hostility, risk of coronary disease, and mortality. *Psychosomatic Medicine, 245,* 219–228.

Sherman, A. (1994). *Wasting America's future: The Children's Defense Fund report on the costs of child poverty.* Boston: Beacon Press.

Shorter, E. (1992). *From paralysis to fatigue: A History of psychosomatic illness in the modern era.* Toronto: The Free Press (MacMillan).

Sloan, R., Bagiella, E., Powell, T. (1999). Religion, spirituality, and medicine. *The Lancet, 353,* 664–667.

Sloan, R., Shapiro, P., Bagiella, E., Myers, M., & Gorman, J. (1999). Cardiac autonomic control buffers blood pressure variability responses to challenge: A psychophysiologic model of coronary artery disease. *Psychosomatic Medicine, 61,* 58–68.

Sloan, R., Shapiro, P., Bigger Jr., T., Bagiella, E., Steinman, R., & Gorman, J. (1994). Cardiac autonomic control and hostility in healthy subjects. *American Journal of Cardiology, 74,* 298–300.

Smith, C., Fernengel, K., Holcroft, C., Gerald, K., & Marien, L. (1994). Meta-analysis of the associations between social support and health outcomes. *Annals of Behavioral Medicine, 16*(4), 352–362.

Smith, T. (1992). Hostility and health: Current status of a psychosomatic hypothesis. *Health Psychology, 11,* 139–150.

Spitzer, R., Williams, J., Kroenke, K., et al. (1994). Utility of a new procedure for diagnosing mental disorders in primary care: The Prime-MD 1000 study. *Journal of the American Medical Association, 272,* 1749–1755.

Steptoe, A., Wardle, J., Vinck, J., Tuomisto, M., Holte, A., & Wickstrom, L. (1994). Personality and attitudinal correlates of healthy and unhealthy lifestyles in young adults. *Psychology and Health, 9,* 331–343.

Stern, R., Weinstein, M., & Baker, S. (1986). Risk reduction for nonmelanoma skin cancer with childhood sunscreen use. *Archives of Dermatology, 122*(5), 537–545.

Sternfeld, B. (1992). Cancer and the protective effect of physical activity: The epidemiological evidence. *Medical Science Sports Medicine, 24,* 1195–1209.

Stewart, W., Shechter, A., & Liberman, J. (1992). Physician consultation for headache pain and history of panic from a population-based study. *American Journal of Medicine, 92*(suppl A), 353–405.

Stoudemire, A. (1996). Epidemiology and psychopharmacology of anxiety in medical patients. *Journal of Clinical Psychiatry, 57*(Suppl. 7), 64–72, 73–75.

Strull, W., Lo, B., & Charles, G. (1984). Do patients want to participate in medical decision making? *Journal of the American Medical Association, 252,* 2990–2994.

Stukas, A. Jr., Dew, M., Switzer, G., DiMartini, A., Kormos, R., & Griffith, B. (1999). PTSD in heart transplant recipients and their primary family caregivers. *Psychosomatics, 40*(3), 212–221.

Suls, J., & Rittenhouse, J. D. (1990). Models of linkages between personality and disease. In H. Friedman (Ed.), *Personality and disease* (pp. 38–64). New York: John Wiley and Sons.

Surbonne, A. (1992). Truth telling to the patient. *Journal of the American Medical Association, 268,* 1661–1662.

Szasz, T., & Hollender, M. (1956). A contribution to the philosophy of medicine. *AMA Archives of Internal Medicine, 97,* 582–592.

Tarlau, M., & Smalheiser, I. (1951). Personality patterns in patients with malignant tumours of the breast and cervix. *Annual Review of Microbiology, 13,* 117–121.

Tarnowski, K., & Rohrbeck, C. (1993). Disadvantaged children and families. In T. H. Ollendick & R. J. Prinz (Eds.), *Advances in clinical child psychology* (Vol. 15, pp. 41–79). New York: Plenum Press.

Taylor, C., Houston-Miller, N., Ahn, D., Haskell, W., & DeBusk, R. (1986). The effects of exercise training programs on psychosocial improvement in uncomplicated post myocardial infarction patients. *Journal of Psychosomatic Research, 30,* 581–587.

Taylor, G. (1987). *Psychosomatic medicine and contemporary psychoanalysis* (Monograph 3). Madison, CT: International Universities Press.

Temoshok, L. (1990). On attempting to articulate the biopsychosocial model: Psychological-psychophysiological homeostasis. In H. Friedman (Ed.), *Personality and disease* (pp. 203–225). New York: John Wiley and Sons.

Temoshok, L., Heller, B., Sagebiel, R., Blois, M., Sweet, D., DiClemente, R., et al. (1985). The relationship of psychosocial factors to pronostic indicators in cutaneous malignant melanoma. *Journal of Psychosomatic Research, 29,* 139–154.

Tennant, C., Goulston, K., & Langeluddecke, P. (1986). Psychological correlates of gastric and duodenal ulcer disease. *Psychological Medicine, 16,* 365–371.

Terre, L. & Ghiselli, W. (1997). A developmental perspective on family risk factors in somatization. *Journal of Psychosomatic Research, 42*(2), 197–208.

Thomas, J., Greig, M., & Piper, D. (1980). Chronic gastric ulcer and life events. *Gastroenterology, 78,* 905–911.

Tochikubo, O., Ikeda, A., Miyajima, E., & Ishii, M. (1996). Effects of insufficient sleep on blood pressure monitored by a new multibiomedical recorder. *Hypertension, 27*(6), 1318–1324.

Tran, Z., & Weltman, A. (1985). Differential effects of exercise on serum lipid and lipoprotein levels seen with changes in body weight. A meta-analysis. *Journal of the American Medical Association, 254,* 919–924.

Trzepacz, P. (1996). Delirium: Advances in diagnosis, pathophysiology, and treatment. *Psychiatric Clinics of North America, 19,* 429–448.

U.S. Department of Health and Human Services. (1994). *Youth and tobacco: Preventing tobacco use among young people.* Atlanta, GA: Public Health Service, Centers for Disease Control, U.S. Department of Education.

Van Horn, L. & Kavey, R. (1997). Diet and cardiovascular disease prevention: What works? *Annals of Behavioral Medicine, 19*(3), 197–212.

Vanichseni, S., Des Jarlais, D., Choopanya, K., Friedman, P., Wenston, J., Sonchai, W., et al. (1993). Condom use with primary partners among injecting drug users in Bangkok, Thailand and New York City, United States. *AIDS, 7,* 887–891.

Ventres, W., Nichter, M., Reed, R., & Frankel, R. (1992). Do-not-resuscitate discussions: A qualitative analysis. *Family Practice Research Journal, 12*(2), 157–169.

Viinamaki, H., Niskanen, L., & Koskela, K. (1997). Factors predicting health behavior. *Nordic Journal of Psychiatry, 51*(6), 431–438.

Walden, C., Retzlaff, B., Buck, B., McCann, B., & Knopp, R. (1997). Lipoprotein lipid response to the National Cholesterol Education Program Step II diet by hypercholesterolemic and combined hyperlipidemic women and men. *Arteriosclerosis, Thrombosis, and Vascular Biology, 17,* 375–382.

Walker, E., Katon, W., & Jemelka, R., (1993). Psychiatric disorders and medical care utilization among people in the general population who report fatigue. *Journal of Internal Medicine, 8,* 436–440.

Wallston, K., & Smith, M. (1994). Issues of control and health: The action is in the interaction. In G. Penny, P. Bennett, & M. Herbert (Eds.), *Health psychology: A lifespan perspective.* London: Harwood.

Wallston, K., Wallston, B., & DeVellis, R. (1978). Development of the Multidimensional Health Locus of Control (MHLC) scales. *Health Education Monographs, 6*(2), 160–170.

Ward, M. (1993). A different disease: HIV/AIDS and health care for women in poverty. *Culture, Medicine, and Psychiatry, 17,* 413–430.

Watts, G., Lewis, B., Brunt, J., et al. (1992). Effects on coronary artery disease of lipid lowering diet, or diet plus cholestyramine, in the St. Thomas' Atherosclerosis Regression Study (STARS). *The Lancet, 339,* 563–569.

Webb, W. L. (1983). Chronic pain. *Psychosomatics, 24*(12), 1053–1063.

Weinberg, D. (1996). *Press briefing on 1995 income, poverty, and health insurance estimates.* U.S. Bureau of the Census [Online].Available: http://www.census.gov/ftp/pub/hhes/income/income95/prs96asc.

Weiss G. & Larsen, D. (1990). Health value, health locus of control, and the prediction of health protective behaviors. *Social Behavior and Personality, 18,* 121–136.

Wenger, N., Froelicher, E., Smith, L., et al. (October 1995). *Cardiac Rehabilitation. Clinical Practice Guideline No. 17,* ACHCPR Publication NO. 96-0672. Rockville, MD: U.S. Department of Health and Human Services, Public Health Service, Agency for Health Care Policy and Research and the National Heart, Lung, and Blood Institute.

Whitehouse, P., Lerner, A., & Hedera, P. (1993). Dementia. In K. Heilman & E. Valenstein (Eds.), *Clinical neuropsychology* (3rd ed., pp. 603–635). New York: Oxford University Press.

Williams, R. (1987). Refining the Type A hypothesis: Emergence of the hostility complex. *American Journal of Cardiology, 60*(27), 27J–32J.

Williams, R., Barefoot, J., Haney, T., Harrell, F., Blumenthal, J., Pryor, D., & Peterson, B. (1988). Type A behavior and angiographically documented atherosclerosis in a sample of 2,289 patients. *Psychosomatic Medicine, 50,* 139–152

Wing, R. (1995). Changing diet and exercise behaviors in individuals at risk for weight gain. *Obesity Research, 3*(Suppl. 2), S277–282.

Wingard, D. L., & Berkman, L. F. (1983). Mortality risk associated with sleeping patterns among adults. *Sleep, 6*(2), 102–107.

Wingard, D., Berkman, L., & Brand, R. (1982). A multivariate analysis of health related practices: Nine years mortality follow-up of the Alameda County study. *American Journal of Epidemiology, 116,* 765–775.

Wirsching, M., Hoffman, F., Stierlin, H., Weber, G., & Wirsching, B. (1985). Prebioptic psychological characteristics of breast cancer patients. *Psychotherapy and Psychosomatics, 43,* 69–76.

Wrezesniewski, K., Wonicki, J., & Turlejski, J. (1988). Type A behavior pattern and illness other than coronary heart disease. *Social Science Medicine, 27,* 623–626.

Wulsin, L., Vaillant, G., & Wells, V. (1999). A systematic review of the mortality of depression. *Psychosomatic Medicine, 61,* 6–17.

Zuckerman, B. (1993). Developmental considerations for drug- and AIDS-affected infants. In R. P. Barth,, J. Pietrzak, & M. Ramler (Eds.), *Families living with drugs and HIV: Intervention and treatment strategies* (pp. 37–58). New York: Guilford.

Zuckerman, C. (1997). Issues concerning end-of-life care. *Journal of Long Term Home Health Care, 16*(2), 26–34.

Medical Conditions

3

Psychosocial Sequelae of Cancer Diagnosis and Treatment

MICHAEL A. ANDRYKOWSKI
JANET S. CARPENTER
RITA K. MUNN

Each year in the United States, over one million new cases of cancer are diagnosed and more than 500,000 people die of cancer (American Cancer Society, 2002). Malignant disease is the second most common cause of death in America; only heart disease takes more lives. However, the picture is not completely grim. The number and percentage of cancer survivors in the U.S. increases annually, and is estimated to be about 8 million (American Cancer Society, 2002). Many of these individuals can be considered cured of their disease. In other words, cancer is no longer present and their disease is not expected to recur. Even if not cured, the length of time between diagnosis and death has been extended for many people with cancer. The combination of high incidence, high mortality, and large numbers of individuals living with cancer for an extended period of time has increased the attention that must be paid to the psychological and social ramifications of malignant disease.

This chapter will review and examine the psychosocial impact and sequelae associated with the diagnosis and treatment of cancer. To begin, however, we will provide a brief overview of cancer as well as current cancer treatment.

CANCER: BASIC MEDICAL CONSIDERATIONS

While cancer may strike individuals at any time in life, it is primarily a disease of aging. The typical age at which cancer is initially diagnosed is in the 50s and 60s for the most common cancers. The natural history of one type of cancer may vary widely from another type, but all malignancies share abnormalities in growth characteristics. Malignant cells must be evaluated with regard to two separate but often linked properties: (1) the speed and ability to grow locally in an unregulated manner; and (2) the ability to invade adjacent tissues and other organs. The mortality rate of some cancers results primarily from uncontrolled growth at the site of cancer development (e.g., pancreatic cancer). Others (e.g., colon cancer and breast cancer) may be localized at initial diagnosis but have the potential to metastasize to other sites in the body and become fatal with time. Still other cancers are systemic and often widespread at the time of diagnosis (e.g., leukemias and lymphomas).

When cancer is suspected, a sample of the abnormal tissue is obtained using one of several biopsy techniques (see Table 3.1). In general, the least invasive method is used. This general principle results in the use of different diagnostic tests in different malignancies. Different diagnostic tests are also used in patients with the same malignancy who show varying signs and symptoms.

The tissue obtained in the biopsy is then carefully evaluated by a trained pathologist to ensure that the correct diagnosis is made and that the disease is correctly staged. Staging involves classification of a malignancy with regard to its size and extent of local, regional, and distal (or metastatic) spread. Local disease refers to tumors that are usually small and have not spread beyond the original organ involved. Regional disease refers to tumors that have spread beyond the initial organ site into adjoining tissue or nearby lymph nodes. Distal (or metastatic) disease refers to tumors that have spread beyond the initial organ site into not only adjoining tissue or regional lymph nodes, but to other more distant body or organ sites as well. Staging information is critical to determine which therapy will be most effective, as well as the patient's likely prognosis.

TABLE 3.1. Techniques Used to Diagnose Malignancy

Biopsy Technique	Invasive
Endoscopic	
Bronchoscopy	No
Colonoscopy	No
Laparoscopy	Minimally
Video assisted thoracoscopy	Minimally
Fine needle aspiration*	No
Core needle aspiration*	No
Bone marrow	No
Incisional	Yes
Excisional	Yes
Surgery	Yes

*May be performed on palpable lesions or nonpalpable lesions with X-ray (CT scan, mammogram) guidance.

A variety of modalities are used in treating cancer, each with their own acute and chronic side effects (see Table 3.2). In general, cancer treatment involves a combination of surgery, chemotherapy, and radiotherapy. Additionally, hormonal therapy may be used for cancers of the breast or prostate. In selecting a therapy, the age and general health of the patient are considered. In considering the patient's general health, the patient's Karnofsky Performance Status score is important. The Karnofsky Performance Status score rates a patient's ability to perform routine daily activities, such as walking, lifting, or feeding and clothing himself or herself. The Karnofsky score can predict how well cancer therapy will be tolerated as well as its efficacy (Schag, Heinrich, & Ganz, 1984).

TABLE 3.2. Cancer Treatment Modalities

Treatment	Effective site	Side Effects	
		Acute	Chronic
Surgery	Local	Tissue-dependent anesthesia, pain, wound healing	May include organ loss (breast, limb); rehab important
Radiosurgery			
Gamma knife	Highly localized (brain)	Minimal	Memory loss, balance abnormal
Radiation	Local	Tissue-dependent, skin erythema, nausea, fatigue, if head or neck—mucositis, difficulty swallowing	Some sites prone to fistula formation (cervix), gland dysfunction (salivary gland)
Brachytherapy	Highly localized	Tissue-dependent	Cervix-vaginal scarring, sexual dysfunction
Hormonal	Systemic	Few	Symptoms of hormone deprivation, weight gain, hot flashes, decreased libido
Chemotherapy	Systemic	Nausea, vomiting, fatigue, low blood counts, mucositis, diarrhea	Infertility, increased risk of second malignancy, ototoxicity, neuropathy, renal dysfunction
Multimodality*	Variable	Side effects often greater than with single modality; therapies planned to prevent overlapping toxicities whenever possible	

*May be any combination of above therapies.

A diagnosis of cancer can be emotionally devastating. Psychological and emotional sequelae must be anticipated by the multidisciplinary health care team and managed appropriately. The team must be prepared to treat the cancer patient for pain, dehydration, depression, and other psychological and social sequelae. The team must also educate the patient, the family, and other caregivers about these problems. The health care team must share with the patient and his or her family the goals of therapy. Patients diagnosed with incurable malignancy may obtain relief from symptoms and have prolonged survival with therapy. However, the side effects of therapy must be weighed against the benefits. Patients with a curable malignancy may be willing to tolerate greater short-term side effects to achieve the benefits of a longer life.

Cancer is a very broad term that covers over 100 different diseases. Despite this diversity, all cancers involve a defect in the normal biological mechanisms that control the growth and differentiation of normal human cells. This section will provide a brief medical overview of some of the more common malignancies, with information provided regarding the nature and course of the disease, major diagnostic procedures, staging, and major forms of treatment. Readers desiring more information are referred to a comprehensive handbook edited by DeVita and colleagues (DeVita, Hellman, & Rosenberg, 1997). Tables 3.3 and 3.4 present basic epidemiological information regarding some of the more common cancers we will review. Table 3.3 presents information regarding incidence and mortality. Table 3.4 presents information regarding the proportion of patients surviving five or more years following a cancer diagnosis.

Lung Cancer

Lung cancer is the third most common type of cancer but it is the most common cause of cancer death in the United States. Lung cancer constitutes approximately 13% of all cancers diagnosed in the United States. In 2002, there were 169,400 new cases of lung cancer diagnosed in the United States, with 154,900 individuals dying of the disease (American Cancer Society, 2002). Carcinoma of the lung originates in epithelial cells lining the bronchia. There are no proven methods to screen for the disease. Lung cancer patients typically present with cough, often with traces of blood in the sputum, shortness of breath, chest pain or weight loss, but the cancer is usually advanced by that time. Occasionally, when the disease is in an advanced stage, a chest X-ray obtained for an unrelated reason will show a mass, leading to the subsequent diagnosis of lung cancer.

Tissue may be obtained for diagnosis in a number of ways—bronchoscopy, needle biopsy, or surgery. Microscopic exam of the tissue allows the pathologist to determine if the histologic type is squamous cell, adenocarcinoma, large-cell, or small-cell type. Patients diagnosed with small cell-lung carcinoma must be treated systemically (i.e., with chemotherapy) as this type of lung cancer spreads through the blood stream. Therapeutic decisions for patients with other types of lung cancer will be made based on the stage of disease when found. Patients

TABLE 3.3. Estimated Incidence and Mortality Associated With Specific Cancer Diagnoses in 2002 (in Thousands)

Diagnosis	2002 New cases			2002 Deaths		
	Total	Male	Female	Total	Male	Female
All diagnoses	1284.9	637.5	647.4	555.5	288.2	267.3
Lung	169.4	90.2	79.2	154.91	89.2	65.7
Head and neck						
Oral cavity and pharynx	28.9	18.9	10.0	7.4	4.9	2.5
Larynx	8.9	6.9	2.0	3.7	2.9	.8
Hematologic						
Leukemias	30.8	17.6	13.2	21.7	12.1	9.6
Lymphomas	60.9	31.9	29.0	25.8	13.5	12.3
Gastrointestinal						
Colorectal	148.3	72.6	75.7	56.6	27.8	28.8
Pancreas	30.3	14.7	15.6	29.7	14.5	15.2
Stomach	21.6	13.3	8.3	12.4	7.2	5.2
Gynecologic						
Cervix	13.0	—	13.0	4.1	—	4.1
Ovary	23.3	—	23.3	13.9	—	13.9
Endometrium	39.3	—	39.3	6.6	—	6.6
Genitourinary						
Prostate	189.0	189.0	—	30.2	30.2	—
Testis	7.5	7.5	—	0.4	0.4	—
Bladder	56.5	41.5	15.0	12.6	8.6	4.0
Kidney	31.8	19.1	12.7	11.6	7.2	4.4
Melanoma	53.6	30.1	23.5	7.4	4.7	2.7
Sarcomas						
Bone/joint	2.4	1.3	1.1	1.3	0.7	0.6
Soft tissue	8.3	4.4	3.9	3.9	2.0	1.9
Breast	205.0	1.5	203.5	40.0	.4	39.6

Note: Data is estimated new cases and deaths in 2002 from American Cancer Society (2002).
Source: From the American Cancer Society's Cancer Facts and Figures, 2002. Reprinted with permission.

with local disease, confined to the bronchia or directly adjacent lymph nodes, are evaluated for local therapies (i.e., surgery and radiation). Patients must also be evaluated for metastasis to nonadjacent lymph nodes, bone, liver, and brain. Patients with disease at these sites may be offered systemic therapy (i.e., chemotherapy) combined with local treatments such as surgery and/or radiation.

Recent statistics suggest that only 15% of all individuals diagnosed with lung cancer survive at least five years following diagnosis (American Cancer Society, 2002). The likelihood of surviving five years after a diagnosis of lung cancer is effected by disease stage, the presence of other medical conditions such as chronic obstructive airway disease, and the effectiveness of therapy. Patients di-

TABLE 3.4. Percentage of Individuals Surviving at Least Five Years Following Diagnosis of Various Cancers By Stage at Diagnosis (American Cancer Society, 2002).

Diagnosis	All stages	Local	Regional	Distant
Lung	15	48	21	3
Head and neck				
Oral cavity	56	82	46	21
Larynx	65	83	50	38
Gastrointestinal				
Colon	61	90	64	8
Pancreas	4	16	7	2
Stomach	22	59	22	2
Gynecologic				
Cervix	70	92	49	15
Ovary	52	95	81	29
Endometrium	84	96	63	26
Melanoma	89	96	61	12
Breast (female only)	86	96	76	21
Genitourinary				
Prostate	96	100	*	34
Testis	95	99	95	76
Kidney	62	89	61	9

Note: Percentages are adjusted for normal life expectancy. *The rate for local stages of prostrate cancer represents local and regional stages combined.

Source: From the American Cancer Society's Cancer Facts and Figures, 2002. Reprinted with Permission.

agnosed with early (stage I) disease are often cured of their disease with surgery. Patients diagnosed with advanced (stage IV) disease have a median survival of 8 to 12 months even when treated systemically with chemotherapy.

Head and Neck Cancers

Cancers of the head and neck constitute approximately 3.4% of all cancers diagnosed in the United States. In 2002, 37,800 new cases of head and neck cancer were diagnosed in the United States with 11,100 individuals dying of this cancer (American Cancer Society, 2002). Head and neck cancers include those of the oral cavity, pharynx, sinuses, larynx, salivary glands, or skin of the face and neck. Presenting symptoms vary with site of disease and range from a skin lesion to hoarseness. Staging involves evaluation by a physician specialized in examination of the aerodigestive tract (e.g., otolaryngologist or ENT specialist). Patients with head and neck cancer may have multiple primary tumors (Vokes, Weichselbaum, Lippman, & Hong, 1993). Hence, surgery and radiotherapy are the optimal treatments. Surgical cure may require sacrifice of tissues crucial to speech and nutrition. Accordingly, a multidisciplinary team including a plastic surgeon, speech therapist, nutritionist, and oral surgeon may be required to construct a prosthesis and to support physical and emotional recovery. Control of local or regional disease is especially challenging in head and neck cancers as the risk of relapse is high. In general, risk of local relapse after aggressive therapy is related to the size of the primary tumor and the extent of lymph node involvement. Chemotherapy is generally reserved for patients when surgery and radiotherapy has failed to control their disease.

Recent statistics indicate that the percentage of patients who live for five years following diagnosis of cancer of the larynx or oral cavity is 65% and 56%, respectively (American Cancer Society, 2002). Again, however, five-year survival is highly dependent upon the stage of disease at diagnosis. Five-year survival for both types of cancers for patients with local disease at diagnosis exceeds 80%. In contrast, five-year survival for patients with distal (i.e., metastatic) disease at diagnosis is 38% for cancer of the larynx and only 21% for cancers of the oral cavity.

Hematologic Cancers

Hematologic malignancies include acute and chronic leukemias as well as both Hodgkin's and non-Hodgkin's lymphomas. Patients with these diseases are typically categorized together as these diseases involve the bone marrow and lymphatic system. Hematologic malignancies comprise 7.4% of all cancers diagnosed in the United States. In 2002, 91,700 new cases of leukemia and lymphoma will be diagnosed in the United States with 47,500 individuals dying of these cancers (American Cancer Society, 2002). Hematologic malignancies are often curable even in advanced stages.

Patients with hematologic cancers typically present with symptoms of fever, night sweats, weight loss, reduced appetite, and abnormalities in the complete blood count. Leukemia originates in the bone marrow and therefore is always a systemic disease. The diagnosis of leukemia may be made by demonstration of premature or very young cells (blasts) in the peripheral blood or bone marrow. Leukemia is associated with abnormalities in white blood cells, red blood cells, and platelets, resulting in increased risk of infection, anemia, and bleeding. Patients with acute leukemia present with dramatic evidence of these abnormalities such as nosebleeds, bleeding from the mouth or gums, or life-threatening infection. These patients have only a short history of illness. Individuals with acute leukemia require immediate support with blood products, antibiotics, and chemotherapy. Patients with chronic leukemia may present with less dramatic symptoms and often have a history of a long period of fatigue. Those with chronic disease may be observed without treatment for some time before therapy is required. The untreated natural history of acute leukemia is a short, severe, life-threatening illness; however, the disease is cured in approximately 50% of patients. The natural history of chronic leukemia is more lengthy and less symptomatic. Patients may live for many years after their diagnosis. Their disease is often responsive to chemotherapy initially but becomes more resistant over time. Most patients with chronic leukemia will eventually die of their disease. Young patients in good general health with either acute or chronic leukemia may be candidates for high-dose chemotherapy followed by bone marrow transplantation.

Lymphoma may be of the Hodgkin's or non-Hodgkin's type. Patients may present with the same symptoms as those with leukemia. Lymphoma may involve an isolated lymph node site, multiple lymph node sites, or the bone marrow. The diagnosis is made by microscopic examination of an involved lymph node—noting the type of malignant cell in the node and the pattern of its involvement. Careful staging is required to determine the optimal therapy. Patients with stage I or II Hodgkin's disease may be cured with radiation therapy. Patients with advanced disease (stage III or IV) may be cured with chemotherapy or combined chemotherapy and radiation therapy. Non-Hodgkin's lymphoma must be subclassified into aggressive, intermediate, and indolent subtypes. Treatment for patients with aggressive disease is designed to produce a cure and is similar to that provided for patients with acute leukemia. Patients with intermediate subtypes of non-Hodgkin's lymphoma may be candidates for aggressive therapy if they are young and in good general health. The natural history and treatment response of individuals with indolent lymphomas often mirrors that of patients with chronic leukemia.

Colorectal and Other Gastrointestinal Cancers

Colorectal cancer (i.e., cancer of the colon and rectum) is the most common gastrointestinal cancer and is the second leading cause of cancer death within the United States. The presenting signs and symptoms of colorectal cancer include prolonged constipation or diarrhea, rectal bleeding or blood in the stools, abdominal pain, and weight loss. Some colorectal cancers may cause bowel obstruction which can cause nausea, vomiting, and abdominal pain.

Cancers of the stomach, esophagus, pancreas, gallbladder, small intestine, and other digestive organs comprise the rest of the malignancies of the gastrointestinal tract. Together, these cancers comprise about 16% of all cancers diagnosed in the United States. In 2002, 250,600 cases of gastrointestinal cancer will be diagnosed in the United States, with 132,300 individuals dying of gastrointestinal malignancies; 56,600 of those deaths will be from colorectal cancer (American Cancer Society, 2002).

The most effective diagnostic tool for colorectal cancer is colonoscopy. By using a fiber-optic tube, the physician is able to view the entire length of the colon in motion, projected onto a television screen. Through the same tube, tissue samples can be taken and some polyps can be removed. Tissue samples are essential to staging the disease. Prognosis and treatment are dependent upon the stage of the cancer at diagnosis. The five-year survival rate for patients diagnosed with local colorectal or stomach cancer exceeds 60%. In contrast, five-year survival for those diagnosed with distal disease is less than 10%.

If staging X-rays reveal no evidence of distant spread to the liver or lungs, the treatment is typically surgery. Patients with rectal cancer may be given radiation and chemotherapy prior to surgery to improve the chance of complete removal of the tumor and sparing of the rectum. At the time of surgery, the regional lymph nodes are examined. Patients with lymph node involvement may be offered combination chemotherapy to minimize their risk of disease recurrence at a distant site. Patients with disease that has spread to distant sites cannot be cured. For these patients, chemotherapy and radiotherapy may be palliative and can result in prolonged survival. However, the side effects of these treatments, such as nausea, vomiting, and fatigue can be aversive and must be monitored carefully.

Individuals with inflammatory bowel disease or a strong family history of colorectal cancer are at increased risk for this type of cancer. Screening by digital rectal exam, fecal occult blood testing, and flexible sigmoidoscopy for colorectal cancer are recommended and improve survival by detecting disease either at a premalignant or early stage (Levin & Murphy, 1992). These exams can be done between colonoscopies, which require more preparation and are usually recommended every two years, and even more frequently for patients at highest risk.

Genitourinary Cancers

Genitourinary cancers include testis, bladder, renal, and prostate cancers. The incidence, presenting symptoms, and prognoses for these cancers vary widely. Testis cancer is rare but curable in all stages. Approximately 7,500 cases of testis cancer will be diagnosed in the U.S. in 2002 with only 400 men dying of the disease (American Cancer Society, 2002). There are few early symptoms of testis cancer. Men typically present with a testicular mass as their first symptom. Staging includes assessment of regional lymph nodes and measurement of certain biochemical markers in the blood. Patients with no evidence of spread to the regional lymph nodes may be cured with surgery (i.e., orchiectomy). Those with more advanced stage II or III disease are likely to be given additional chemotherapy or radiation. Tumor markers measured in the blood are often elevated in testis cancer and may be sensitive measures of therapy effectiveness. Patients with testis cancer are often diagnosed at a young age and may be partially or completely infertile by the time of diagnosis. These men should be counseled that chemotherapy will further decrease their ability to father children. Sperm banking may be possible for some patients who are still at least partially fertile at diagnosis.

Prostate Cancer

Prostate cancer is the most common cancer in the United States, comprising approximately 15% of all cancers diagnosed in the United States. In 2002, 189,000 new diagnoses of prostate cancer will be made and 30,200 men will die of the disease (American Cancer Society, 2002). Incidence increases with age, with a median age of diagnosis of 70. While most men are asymptomatic at diagnosis, urinary hesitancy and bladder outlet obstruction may be presenting symptoms. Those with advanced disease typically have bone pain, as the disease commonly metastasizes to bone. The diagnosis of prostate cancer is typically made by a needle biopsy procedure which follows either an abnormal physical exam or detection of an elevated prostate-specific antigen (PSA) level in the blood. If there is no evidence that the disease has spread to bone or regional lymph nodes, surgery may be the treatment of choice. Improved surgical techniques for prostate cancer have reduced the risk of subsequent problems with incontinence and impotence. Since many prostate cancers are slow-growing and relatively benign, "watchful waiting" may be chosen in lieu of surgery. In watchful waiting, the growth of the patient's cancer is monitored by periodic physical examination and measurement of PSA levels in the blood. Surgery and other additional treatments may be implemented later, if deemed necessary. Patients with regionally advanced disease may be treated with radiation. Men with advanced prostate cancer may be treated with hormonal therapy—involving either removal of the testicles or an androgen blockade (i.e., medication to reduce androgen levels). While hormonal therapy can improve life expectancy, it is not curative. Hormonal therapy eventually fails to control the spread of prostate cancer and patients with advanced stage IV disease will eventually succumb to their cancer. Given the potential aversive side effects of hormonal therapy, including reduced libido, impotence, breast enlargement, weight gain, and hot flashes, the decision to employ hormonal therapy must be carefully considered for each individual patient.

Early detection of prostate cancer is critical in determining long-term prognosis since prostate cancer is curable only when it is detected in its earliest stages. The proportion of men living at least five years following diagnosis of local or regional prostate cancer is 100% and 94%, respectively. Five-year survival following diagnosis with distal disease is only 34% (American Cancer Society, 2002). Screening with digital rectal exam and PSA have increased the likelihood that men will be diagnosed at an early stage, with potentially curable disease (Catalona et al., 1991; Jewett, Bridge, Gray, & Shelley, 1968).

Gynecologic Cancers

Cervical, endometrial, and ovarian cancer comprise the bulk of gynecologic cancers. These three cancers comprise approximately 6% of all cancers diagnosed in the U.S. In 2002, 75,600 women in the U.S. were diagnosed with one of these three cancers, and 24,600 women will die of these forms of the disease (American Cancer Society, 2002). The lifetime risk of developing cervical cancer has declined over the last decade, primarily due to treatment of precancerous growths detected by Pap smear. Patients with disease involving the uterus but without spread to the pelvic wall have a 50% likelihood of cure with surgery. Those with larger tumors and those which spread to the pelvic lymph nodes may also receive radiation and chemotherapy. However, these women are still likely to have a very poor prognosis. Five-year survival for women with distal cervical cancer is only 15% (American Cancer Society, 2002).

Endometrial cancer is primarily a disease of postmenopausal women. Those with local disease may be cured with total abdominal hysterectomy and removal of both ovaries. Five-year survival for women diagnosed with local endometrial cancer is 96% (American Cancer Society, 2002). Those with more advanced disease may be treated with radiation, chemotherapy, and/or hormonal therapy. However, prognosis is poorer than those with local disease. Five-year survival for women diagnosed with regional and distal disease is 63% and 26%, respectively (American Cancer Society, 2002).

While ovarian cancer is less frequent than cervical cancer, ovarian cancer causes more deaths than any other gynecologic cancer. In part, this is because ovarian cancer is often a "silent" cancer, with few symptoms or signs occurring in early stages of the disease. The common symptoms associated with ovarian cancer, including abdominal pain, abdominal swelling, bloating, or pelvic pressure, are often evident only with advanced disease.

Ovarian cancer is curable if detected at an early stage. The five-year survival rate for women with local disease at diagnosis is 95%. In contrast, five-year survival rates for regional or distal disease at diagnosis are 81% and 29%, respectively (American Cancer Society, 2002). Unfortunately, the majority of women with ovarian cancer are diagnosed with advanced disease.

Additional information on the screening, diagnosis, and treatment of gynecological cancers is available in chapter 9.

Melanoma and Skin Cancer

Nearly one million new cases of squamous and basal cell carcinomas of the skin are diagnosed each year in the U.S. (American Cancer Society, 2002). Few deaths result from these relatively benign skin cancers. Skin cancers are typically cured by surgical removal. Recurrence of a surgically removed basal cell or squamous cell carcinoma is rare unless the lesion has been neglected. In this case, recurrence is typically local.

Melanomas comprise only 4.2% of all cancer diagnosed in the United States. In 2002, 53,600 new cases of melanoma will be diagnosed and 7,400 individuals will die of the disease (American Cancer Society, 2002). Melanomas usually first appear as pigmented lesions with irregular borders, color variation, and a variable diameter. Treatment involves surgical removal of the lesion. Risk of regional or distal spread of the disease via the lymphatic or circulatory system is directly related to overall thickness of the lesion and extent to which it has penetrated through layers of the skin. Patients with advanced disease or at high risk for disease spread may be offered chemotherapy with the usual attendant side effects of nausea, vomiting, and fatigue. Melanoma may recur years after its initial diagnosis. Patients may relapse with disease in the brain, lung, liver, or lymph nodes.

Early detection of melanoma is critical to survival. The five-year survival rate for patients diagnosed with local disease is 95%. Five-year survival rates for those diagnosed with local or distal disease are 61% and 16%, respectively. Sun exposure is a significant risk factor for melanoma as well as squamous and basal cell carcinomas. Individuals with a fair complexion are also at higher risk for all forms of skin cancer.

Sarcomas

Sarcomas are a diverse group of cancers which involve soft tissue or bone. Soft tissue sarcomas most commonly occur in the arms and legs, and less often in the abdomen and trunk of the body. Surgical removal is the mainstay of therapy for soft tissue sarcomas. Soft tissue sarcomas generally do not respond to chemotherapy or radiotherapy. Amputation may be required for individuals with large tumors in an extremity. The trauma of amputation cannot be overstated. Prosthetics and rehabilitation will permit many of these patients to resume active lives. Individuals with large primary tumors or disease spread to regional lymph nodes at diagnosis are at risk for developing local recurrence or lung metastasis. While chemotherapy may be used in such instances, the treatment is basically palliative and may result in a spectrum of toxicities including hair loss, nausea, vomiting, weight loss, fatigue, and increased risk of infection. Sarcomas of the bone (i.e., osteosarcomas), including Ewing's sarcoma, are most common in individuals less than 25 years of age. These sarcomas require treatment by a multidisciplinary team of physicians including an orthopedic surgeon, pathologist, and medical oncologist. Symptoms at initial diagnosis typically involve pain and swelling. Many patients with sarcomas of bone originating in an extremity may be treated with surgery without the need for amputation and loss of the affected limb. Additional treatment with chemotherapy has resulted in improved survival and the need for less disfiguring surgery. However, chemotherapy treatment for sarcomas of the bone generally involves multiple drugs and a prolonged course of therapy. In addition to the usual side effects of nausea, vomiting, and fatigue, the risk of infertility is increased and additional delayed complication may appear even in patients cured of their disease.

Breast Cancer

Breast cancer is the most common cancer in women and is second to lung cancer as a cause of cancer mortality in women. Breast cancer comprises nearly 15% of all cancers diagnosed in the U.S. and nearly 30% of all cancers diagnosed in women. Early diagnosis of breast cancer is critical to prognosis. The five-year survival rate for those with local disease at diagnosis is 96%. Five-year survival rates for those with regional or distal disease at diagnosis drop to 76% and 21%, respectively. Physical examination of the breasts by a trained clinician and regular mammography examinations are effective screening tools and have been shown to decrease mortality and morbidity associated with breast cancer.

Additional information on the screening, diagnosis, and treatment of breast cancer is available in chapter 9.

PSYCHOSOCIAL CONSIDERATIONS

Expectable Responses to Cancer Diagnosis

Response of the Patient

A cancer diagnosis is a traumatic event for most individuals and their loved ones. Despite some recent improvements in cancer survival rates, cancer remains a life-threatening disease and many individuals continue to equate the word "cancer" with death. A diagnosis of cancer can awaken feelings of personal vulnerability and heighten awareness of personal mortality. Weisman and Worden (1976) coined the phrase "existential plight" to refer to the first 100 days following the initial diagnosis. During this time, a patient's reaction to the diagnosis revolves around life and death issues. The initial concerns are typically, "Will I die?" and "How long might I live?"

Immediate reactions to the diagnosis may include disbelief, denial, anger, depression, anxiety, and confusion. Patients may question the accuracy of their diagnosis and attempt to distance or numb themselves from thoughts and feelings about cancer. Disbelief and denial can accentuate the patient's distress. Patients may have difficulty sleeping or eating and experience large mood swings, but are not necessarily depressed. All of these early reactions to diagnosis can be considered normal since cancer is a life-threatening disease. The distress that is experienced during this time period is generally acute and transient. If initial reactions of sadness and anxiety persist beyond the initial phase of diagnosis or become severe enough to interfere with functioning, a diagnosis of adjustment disorder with either anxious or depressed mood may be warranted. It is estimated that nearly 50% of cancer patients experience transitory feelings of anxiety and depression in response to their diagnosis, while an additional 30% of cancer patients experience adjustment disorders with depressed or anxious mood. Major depression and other serious psychiatric disorders are uncommon reactions to a diagnosis of cancer (Derogatis et al., 1983).

Response of Life Partner and Family

Cancer is a disease that affects the entire family unit. As one would expect, reactions to a cancer diagnosis are not limited to the patient alone. The spouse, partner, or children may experience similar feelings of disbelief, depression, anxiety, and guilt as they begin to cope with the implications of the cancer diagnosis. Such psychological reactions are generally acute and time-limited and rarely develop into serious psychiatric disorders. Difficulties are likely to arise when there is a mismatch between patient and family members' reactions to the diagnosis. For example, a breast cancer patient may wish to discuss thoughts and feelings regarding her own mortality in an effort to cope with feelings of depression or anxiety. Her spouse or partner, on the other hand, may respond with disbelief or denial and refuse to discuss the possibility of death. In this type of situation, patients may feel unsupported, misunderstood, or alienated from their significant other. This can impede their adjustment to the diagnosis, which can then negatively affect family adaptation, including parent-parent and parent-child relationships (Lewis, Hammond, & Woods, 1993).

Tumor Markers and Psychological Sequelae. Tumor markers, the genetic or biochemical changes that can be associated with neoplastic deviations, are among technological advances that are affecting the diagnostic process. Markers now exist that can be used in roughly four categories: determining genetic risk, where certain cancers are known to be associated with other family members; screening for "occult" presence of disease in seemingly healthy patients; determining the prognosis in patients who are newly diagnosed; and attempting to calculate the likelihood of cancer recurrence (Fertig & Hayes, 1998). Patients may be greatly relieved to learn that their prospects are better than they would have known without using tumor markers. They also benefit by earlier or more aggressive treatment where indicated. But there may also be the burden, especially among those who are screened because of disease (e.g., ovarian cancer) in close relatives, of discovering that although they are healthy now, they do carry the genetic markers indicating that susceptibility to the particular cancer.

Expectable Responses to Cancer Treatment

Physical and Cognitive Side Effects of Cancer Treatment

Cancer treatment is associated with a number of physical and cognitive side effects, including nausea, pain, fatigue, sleep disorders, sexual dysfunction, and cognitive dysfunction. Each of these symptoms can vary from individual to individual in frequency, severity, and duration. While some individuals may experience relatively mild symptoms related to cancer treatment, other individuals may experience frequent or severe symptoms. For these latter individuals, physical side effects of treatment may be psychologically distressing and may lead to impaired physical or social functioning.

In this section, we will briefly describe the scope, onset, duration, and treatment for five classes of common side effects of cancer treatment These "on treatment" side effects will include nausea and vomiting, pain, fatigue, sexual dysfunction, and cognitive dysfunction. In some instances, these side effects may persist, or initially emerge, long after the conclusion of treatment. Such "off treatment" side effects will be examined in a later section.

Nausea and Vomiting. Nausea may occur with or without vomiting and may be related to the cancer itself or to cancer treatments, typically radiation and chemotherapy. Nausea may be relatively mild, with little or no vomiting, and cause little interference with eating or other activities. On the other hand, nausea and vomiting may be severe, potentially requiring hospitalization for dehydration and nutritional support. The extent to which patients experience nausea is dependent on cancer type and the dose and type of radiation or chemotherapy received. Certain cancers, such as gastrointestinal or brain tumors, are more likely to be associated with nausea either because of their location within the gastrointestinal tract or their proximity to brain centers which control nausea and vomiting. Other cancers, such as lung cancer and lymphoma, may cause nausea because they are likely to cause electrolyte and other physiologic disruptions (Groenwald, Frogge, Goodman, & Yarbro, 1996).

Radiation-induced nausea depends on the site and size of the area treated and the dose of radiation received. Radiation to the gastrointestinal tract, not only in gastrointestinal cancers but also uterine, bladder, ovarian cancers or other cancers, is more likely to cause nausea or vomiting than radiation to areas away from the gastrointestinal tract. In one study, 60–70% of patients receiving abdominal or pelvic radiation experienced vomiting, compared with 21% of patients receiving chest radiation (King & Makale, 1991). In addition, nausea is more likely to be experienced by patients receiving larger doses of radiation or having larger amounts of tissue irradiated (e.g., total body irradiation for some hematologic malignancies). Nausea can begin within hours of radiation therapy and often lasts throughout the duration of therapy. Since radiation therapy for many malignancies may require almost daily radiation doses over a period of several weeks, the potential impact of radiation-induced nausea and vomiting upon physical and psychosocial status is considerable.

Chemotherapy-induced nausea typically varies with the drug and dosage received. Drugs such as cisplatin and dacarbazine are more likely to cause nausea and vomiting than busulfan and bleomycin (Tenenbaum, 1989). In addition, higher dosages of chemotherapy, such as those received prior to bone marrow transplantation, are associated with more nausea, as are regimens containing multiple chemotherapy drugs. Nausea related to chemotherapy may be acute, delayed or even anticipatory. Acute nausea is experienced within the first 24 h of chemotherapy, typically beginning within the first 1 to 2 h postinfusion. Delayed-onset nausea occurs 1 to 4 days postchemotherapy and is especially common with cisplatin. Anticipatory nausea is experienced prior to a chemotherapy treatment. Stimuli (e.g., sights, sounds, smells, tastes, etc.) associated with nausea during prior chemotherapy infusions may invoke nausea prior to the actual administration of subsequent dosages of the drug. Between 25% and 50% of patients may develop some anticipatory nausea at least occasionally (Redd &

Andrykowski, 1982). Consistent with a classical learning theory explanation for the development of anticipatory nausea, the severity of postchemotherapy nausea is positively associated with a risk for developing anticipatory nausea (Andrykowski, Redd, & Hatfield, 1985).

Treatment of nausea involves administration of single or combination antiemetic agents prior to and during cancer treatment. The goal is to prevent nausea and vomiting. Agents included in antiemetic regimens are prescribed based on their potential to relieve nausea and the underlying cause and pattern of the nausea being experienced (Groenwald et al., 1996). Although no agent is 100% effective, recent pharmacological advances, development of combination antiemetic regimes, and use of cognitive-behavioral strategies, such as guided imagery and relaxation, have been shown effective in decreasing treatment-induced nausea and vomiting.

Pain. Pain is often a major concern for cancer patients. Their concerns are not unwarranted. Nearly 75% of cancer patients in the U.S. with advanced cancer experience pain (Breitbart & Payne, 1998). However, the incidence and severity of pain are highly variable. Cancer pain varies with the location, size, and stage of the tumor, the types of diagnostic and treatment procedures employed, and the type and severity of treatment complications, such as infection or muscle atrophy (Management of Cancer Pain Guideline Panel, 1994).

Cancer pain may be acute or chronic. Acute pain usually has a well-defined onset and course and is typically associated with objective autonomic (e.g., increased heart rate and respiratory rate) and behavioral signs (e.g., limping). With chronic pain, physiologic adaptation occurs and signs of physiologic arousal are generally absent (Foley, 1985). Chronic pain affects about one-third of all cancer patients and as many as 90% of patients with advanced cancer (Portenoy, 1992). Both acute and chronic pain may cause significant psychological distress, such as depression and anxiety, and significantly interfere with a person's quality of life. While the distinction between acute and chronic pain is important, patients may experience both types of pain throughout the course of their treatment.

Although up to 90% of cancer pain can be relieved, many patients do not receive adequate pain relief (Cherny & Portenoy, 1994; Management of Cancer Pain Guideline Panel, 1994). Factors contributing to inadequate pain relief include patients' unwillingness to report pain and fears of analgesic side effects. Additionally, clinicians too often fail to appropriately assess and treat pain due to unwarranted fears of addiction or inadequate training in pain management techniques (Wallace, Reed, Pasero, & Olsson, 1995; Ward et al., 1993). Careful pain assessment, including eliciting patients' subjective reports of pain location, intensity, and pattern, combined with appropriate pain treatment are crucial for minimizing psychological distress and long-term functional limitations. Appropriate pain treatment can involve a combination of pharmacologic and nonpharmacologic therapies. Pharmacologic therapies include the use of narcotics and nonnarcotics to manage pain as well as the use of additional agents to manage analgesic side effects. Nonpharmacologic management includes noninvasive physical (i.e., exercise, immobilization, heat, or cold) and psychological modalities (i.e., relaxation, imagery, or other cognitive-behavioral interventions) as well as more invasive modalities such as nerve blocks or surgery.

Pain management is integral to the emotional well-being of the cancer patient at every stage of disease. Among the challenges of pain management is the fact that there is a subjective element to all pain. This applies even to acute pain, which usually can be observed through autonomic signs, such as those indicated earlier, and other "objective" symptoms, such as limping, also mentioned above.

Further complicating adequate pain management are studies which have shown emotional disturbance to be a predictor of patients' perception of pain. However, inadequately treated pain can lead to depression, anxiety, hopelessness, a sense of helplessness, and suicidal ideation. Effective treatment of pain often results in the disappearance of transient psychiatric disorders (Breitbart & Payne, 1998).

Assessment of pain must be repeated over the course of treatment, since pain levels change throughout the course of the disease. Moreover, patients' tolerance for pain may diminish even as the pain caused by advanced cancer increases. End-stage cancer patients may experience their pain more intensely if they strongly associate their pain with spread of the disease and the imminence of death.

Under-utilization of pain medication causes 25% of cancer patients to die in severe pain, despite the fact that current treatment methods could substantially reduce the number of patients suffering severe pain.

Among the most prevalent fears associated with cancer in the general population is painful death. The sense of helplessness inherent in being diagnosed with a disease defined by uncontrolled cell division is easily compounded by inadequately addressed pain. Cancer patients are approximately twice as likely to commit suicide as the general population. Among those who do, multiple studies have shown that the patients at greatest risk have end-stage disease combined with inadequately controlled pain.

Fatigue. Fatigue is the most common symptom experienced during cancer treatment (Rhodes, Watson, & Hanson, 1988; Winningham et al., 1994), and may stem from many sources including the disease itself or the treatment. In addition, psychological distress or other physical symptoms, such as nausea and pain, may lead to sleep disturbance and subsequent fatigue. Fatigue can have both physical and cognitive components. Physically, patients may report feeling tired, exhausted, or worn out, whereas cognitively patients may experience concentration and memory difficulties (Cimprich, 1992, 1993). Fatigue can significantly interfere with daily functioning and lead to psychological distress and disrupted quality of life. Individuals may curtail work and leisure activities, limit social interactions, and alter family role functioning in response to fatigue.

The incidence of fatigue in persons with cancer varies with cancer type, stage, and extent of treatment received. In general, more severe fatigue is believed to be associated with higher dosages or more extensive therapy. For example, women with breast cancer receiving combination therapy (i.e., chemotherapy and radiation therapy) experienced more severe fatigue than women receiving only radiation therapy (Woo, Dibble, Piper, Keating, & Weiss, 1998).

Despite being recognized as a clinically significant problem, treatments for cancer-related fatigue are limited. Persons undergoing cancer treatment may benefit from modifying their behavior to decrease activities and allow for adequate rest periods. Exercise may also be an effective means of reducing treatment-related fatigue. Women with breast cancer enrolled in a moderate walking exercise program while receiving radiation therapy reported significantly less fatigue than those who did not participate in the program (Mock et al., 1997).

Sexual Dysfunction. Impaired sexual functioning can be a significant problem for persons with cancer (Andersen, 1985; Auchincloss, 1989; Ganz, Rowland, Desmond, Meyerowitz, & Wyatt, 1998). Cancer-related sexual dysfunction encompasses a wide variety of problems for both males and females, including dyspareunia (i.e., painful intercourse), infertility, impotency, and altered body image. Sexual dysfunction is not limited to patients with cancers of the genitourinary system (i.e., testicular, ovarian, prostate cancers). Prevalence varies widely by cancer site and treatment, leading to widely varying estimates of the proportion of cancer patients that experience some type of sexual function at some time (Andersen, 1985). Cancer-related sexual dysfunction may not have a single definitive cause, and may stem from either the physical or psychosocial effects of cancer and cancer treatment.

Physically, sexual dysfunction may result from direct damage to reproductive organs. For example, tumors or surgery may inhibit blood or nerve supplies to reproductive organs, leading to infertility or erectile dysfunction. Surgery may involve removal of organs involved in the sexual response, such as ovaries or testes. Chemotherapy-induced menopause and subsequent estrogen deprivation in breast or ovarian cancer patients can cause vaginal atrophy and subsequent pain during intercourse (Ganz et al., 1998; Thranov & Klee, 1994). In addition, treatment side effects such as pain, nausea, and fatigue may interfere with sexual desire and performance.

Psychosocial effects of cancer and cancer treatment can also play a role in sexual dysfunction. Physical changes resulting from surgery (e.g., mastectomy) or side effects of radiation and chemotherapy, such as temporary hair loss, can interfere with feelings of sexual desirability and attractiveness. Anxiety and depression, either in the patient or their partner, can hinder sexual desire and performance. Finally, unfounded fears of transmitting cancer through sexual intercourse may also interfere with sexuality (Krumm & Lamberti, 1993).

When sexual dysfunction is reported, it is important to recognize the factors that reduce sexual satisfaction and their impact upon specific stages of the sexual response cycle: desire, arousal, orgasm, and resolution (Andersen, Andersen, & DeProsse, 1989). For example, anxiety and depression might reduce sexual desire or inhibit sexual arousal or orgasm. Physical disabilities or symptoms might leave sexual desire unaltered yet interfere with excitement and orgasm. The key to treatment is recognition that sexual dysfunction encompasses a variety of specific problems such as inhibited sexual desire, painful intercourse, or erectile dysfunction. Treatment will vary depending on the type, extent, and duration of the problem. Medical interventions, such as hormone replacement therapy or reconstructive surgery, may be beneficial in helping to restore sexual function and confidence in one's sexuality. In addition, patients and their partners may benefit from psychological or behavioral interventions, including education and psychotherapy.

Cognitive Dysfunction. Cognitive functioning refers to the ability to acquire, process, store, and retrieve information and thus encompasses activities such as awareness, attention, memory, perception, orientation, comprehension, and abstraction. These changes may occur in cancer patients of all ages, evidenced by changes in memory, concentration, reasoning, and judgement, as well as confusion and disorientation. Symptoms of cognitive dysfunction may include interrupted sleep patterns, irritability, and inappropriate behavior. Two broad categories of cognitive dysfunction include delirium and dementia (Fleischman & Lesko, 1989). Delirium is generally acute and transitory, whereas dementia is insidious and irreversible. Delirium includes periods of disorientation, memory loss, impaired attention span, and possibly delusions and hallucinations. Episodes of delirium, often brief, may occur in cancer patients, particularly the elderly, hospitalized, and terminally ill (Breitbart & Cohen, 1998; Fleischman & Lesko, 1989; Pereira, Hanson, & Bruera, 1997). Dementia is characterized by memory loss and personality changes, such as apathy and withdrawal. The latter, of course, can be associated with depression, making careful diagnosis important. Dementia is a relatively rare complication of cancer diagnosis and treatment but may be seen in patients with lung cancer or brain tumors receiving treatments which are toxic to the central nervous system (e.g., brain radiation) (Fleishman & Lesko, 1989).

While both delirium and dementia can be caused by a variety of factors, the underlying cause can be broadly classified as either systemic (i.e., disease-related) or iatrogenic (i.e., treatment-related) in origin. Systemic etiologies include primary tumors of the brain or central nervous system, brain metastases, metabolic encephalopathy, and central nervous system infection. Iatrogenic causes include radiation and chemotherapy and medications used to diminish the side effects of cancer treatment. The latter include medications that affect pain, nausea, and sleep (Breura, Macmillan, Hanson, & Macdonald, 1989; Silberfarb, 1983), while the former include cranial and total body irradiation as well as a host of specific chemotherapeutic drugs.

Although most chemotherapy drugs are not directly toxic to the central nervous system, some drugs, such as cytarabine, are capable of crossing the blood/brain barrier and causing cognitive dysfunction (Winkelman & Hines, 1983). Other drugs, such as methotrexate, can lead to cognitive dysfunction, when administered intrathecally (i.e., directly into the central nervous system) during treatment for leukemia or brain metastases (Breitbart & Cohen, 1998). In general, delirium is viewed as reversible, provided the underlying organic cause is identified and addressed.

Cognitive dysfunction in cancer patients can be distressing for both patients and their families. Patients may be particularly distressed if periods of delirium alternate with periods of normal cognition, resulting in their temporary or occasional awareness of memory lapses, confusion, or inappropriate behavior. In addition, cognitive dysfunction can interfere with patients' abilities to make decisions about their health care. Memory lapses may also interfere with patient-education efforts or patients' ability to self-monitor for side effects and complications of treatment. Irritability and inappropriate behavior may interfere with patients' abilities to participate in their long-term treatment program.

COPING WITH CANCER DIAGNOSIS AND TREATMENT

Regardless of disease site, every cancer patient confronts a reasonably predictable sequence of stressors as the course of the illness unfolds. These stressors are physical and psychological in nature. Successful adaptation to cancer results from effective coping with the challenges posed by each succeeding stressor confronted during the course of the disease. In this section, we will describe the sequence of stressors confronted by cancer patients, identify the primary coping tasks posed by each, the potential resources for coping with these stressors, and review some of the theoretical and empirical literature germane to coping with cancer diagnosis and treatment.

Specific Stressors Associated with Cancer Diagnosis and Treatment

The course of a patient's illness begins with the initial diagnosis of malignant disease. As indicated earlier, the initial diagnosis typically triggers a range of psychological reactions including shock, anger, denial, depression, and anxiety. The primary coping task confronting the patient at this time is to maintain cognitive and emotional equilibrium. This equilibrium will be necessary for the patient to effectively confront the next major stressor in the course of the illness: the need to make decisions about treatment. Effective decision-making at this time is dependent upon the patient's ability to remain emotionally and cognitively engaged with the health care team and to form an effective alliance. This alliance is necessary for the proper flow of information in both directions. The health care team must effectively communicate information about treatment options and the associated risks and benefits. The patient must communicate his or her treatment preferences as well as the value placed upon potential treatment outcomes. For example, in choosing between mastectomy or lumpectomy as treatment for breast cancer, it is important to understand the value a woman places upon personal appearance. Alternatively, in deciding between "watchful waiting" or surgical or hormonal treatments for prostate cancer, it is important to understand the value a man places upon preservation of sexual function.

Once a course of treatment has been selected and embarked upon, the patient must be prepared to cope with side effects such as pain, nausea, and fatigue. Additionally, patients may need to cope with temporary or permanent cosmetic changes, such as hair loss induced by chemotherapy or radiation or loss of a limb or breast as a result of surgery. Many of these prospects cause stress prior to surgery, as the patient anticipates, often with great trepidation, relationship changes that will come as a result of alterations in appearance or sexual functioning. The patient may fear abandonment by a spouse or partner, and be unable to speak about it with that very person. In all instances, the primary coping task for the patient is to minimize the experience of such side effects and/or minimize the impact of such side effects upon performance of routine, daily activities and social roles. In doing so, the patient is more likely to maintain the morale and motivation essential to successful completion of their treatment course.

While completion of chemotherapy and radiation is often viewed by the health care team and the patient's family as a cause for celebration, completion of cancer treatment can be surprisingly stressful for many patients. Despite the side effects associated with treatment, many patients derive comfort from knowing that action is being taken to combat their disease. Thus, completion of treatment can trigger anxiety about recurrence. Furthermore, completion of treatment often means a profound shift in the patient's network of social support, a shift which can itself be highly stressful. Specifically, during chemotherapy and radiation treatment, patients visit their health care facility and are seen by staff on a very frequent basis, perhaps weekly or even daily. Close, supportive relationships are often formed between patients and the health care team during this time. Completion of treatment means some separation of the patient from this supportive social network.

Additionally, completion of cancer treatment may be viewed by family and friends as the appropriate time for a cancer patient to "get on with his or her life." At this time, friends and loved ones who were highly supportive during the period of diagnosis and active treatment might become less tolerant of continuing physical or psychological frailties in the patient. Even when subtle, such shifts in the patient's supportive milieu can be a source of resentment and interpersonal conflict. In light of this, the primary coping task confronting the patient at the time of treatment completion is to cope with shifts in social support which

might occur. This might mean gradually adjusting to lower, perhaps more typical levels of social support, or actively seeking additional support such as that
provided by participation in a cancer support group.

As indicated earlier, completion of cancer treatment signals a shift from
the acute phase of diagnosis and treatment to a phase of "watchful waiting."
During the months and years following completion of treatment, routine visits
to the oncology clinic for medical follow-up may serve as periodic stressors. In
addition to arousing nagging fears that a cancer recurrence will be found, re-
exposure to the clinic environment can trigger classically conditioned reactions
of anxiety or nausea in some patients (Redd & Andrykowski, 1982). This may
occur years after completion of active treatment (Cella, Pratt, & Holland, 1986).
In addition, recent research suggests that some cancer patients may develop cancer-related posttraumatic stress disorder (PTSD) (Alter et al., 1996;
Andrykowski, Cordova, Studts, & Miller, 1998). One of the hallmarks of PTSD
is avoidance of trauma reminders and distress upon exposure to such reminders. Follow-up clinic visits might then be particularly stressful for patients exhibiting symptoms of cancer-related PTSD. Thus, a primary coping task for
patients is to manage any anxieties they might have in order to maintain a good
quality of life as well as remain compliant with recommendations for routine
clinic follow-up.

The sequence of stressors just described is applicable to most cancer patients. In some patients, however, cancer will recur and these patients must again
confront the issue of their mortality. Additionally, decisions regarding treatment
must again be made, the side effects of any subsequent treatment must be endured, and the conclusion of treatment and initiation of another period of
"watchful waiting" will also likely be faced. While the familiarity of this sequence
of stressors might be stress-reducing for some, for many patients the thought of
going through this process again exacerbates their distress. The primary coping
task confronting patients at the time of a cancer recurrence is the maintenance
of their emotional equilibrium in order to maintain a reasonable quality of life,
participate effectively in decisions about further treatment, and maintain motivation to adhere to whatever course of action is selected.

Coping Resources

According to the Transactional Model of Stress and Coping (Lazarus & Folkman,
1984), coping is based upon an individual's primary and secondary appraisal of
a potential stressor. Primary appraisal refers to an individual's decision regarding whether or not a potential stressor poses a threat to either his or her current
or future well-being. An individual may decide that a potential stressor does not
pose a threat. In that case, no coping behavior is likely to be initiated since the
object or event has been deemed nonthreatening (i.e., not a stressor). Secondary
appraisal refers to an individual's evaluation of potential courses of action; the
resources available for enacting those options, and the likely consequences of

those actions on current or future well-being. Interestingly, awareness that one possesses adequate coping resources in itself reduces the threat generated by the potential stressor. In short, perception of the availability of adequate coping resources can reduce the number and magnitude of potential stressors. Additionally, possession of adequate coping resources increases the likelihood that effective action will be taken to reduce or eliminate the potential threat to an individual's well-being posed by any stressor.

Coping resources can be viewed as either personal or interpersonal in nature. Personal resources include psychological or behavioral characteristics such as personality or coping style as well as more tangible resources such as education or income. Interpersonal resources include what is commonly referred to as social support. Evidence suggests that adequate personal and interpersonal resources are essential to effectively cope with the stresses posed by cancer diagnosis and treatment (Helgeson, Cohen, & Fritz, 1998; Rowland, 1989a; 1989b)

Coping Resources: Personal

Psychological adjustment in cancer patients is often found to be positively associated with variables like education, income, or socioeconomic status. Several explanations for this relationship have been suggested. For example, greater income and education might be related to better awareness and access to community resources, such as support groups, personal counseling, or information about cancer and cancer treatment. Similarly, patients of higher socioeconomic status might be better able to access existing sources of social support, including support from physicians or medical staff. Finally, less educated patients may be more likely to respond to diagnosis with fear and helplessness, or may cognitively "process" their experience less effectively. Effective processing of a traumatic event is associated with enhanced physical and psychological outcomes (Esterling, Antoni, Fletcher, Margulies, & Schneiderman, 1994; Pennebaker, 1993), as is the ability to derive "meaning" from one's experience with cancer (Taylor, 1983).

Personality and coping style have also been linked to psychological adjustment in cancer patients. Coping style refers to the relatively enduring or characteristic ways in which an individual responds to stressful situations (Lipowski, 1970). Two coping styles have received a fair amount of attention in the literature and are relevant to cancer: optimism and informational coping style. Optimism refers to the tendency to expect positive outcomes in the future (Scheier & Carver, 1985). When confronted by stress, such as that posed by cancer diagnosis and treatment, optimistic individuals are likely to respond with engagement. That is, by active coping and by continuing to pursue normal life goals and activities as far as possible. In contrast, pessimistic individuals, those with a tendency to anticipate negative future outcomes, are likely to respond to stress by disengaging—suspending or limiting coping efforts, becoming depressed, and withdrawing from pursuit of normal life goals and activities (Scheier & Bridges, 1995).

Informational coping style refers to an individual's tendency to seek or avoid potentially stressful information about a threatening medical condition, such as cancer (Miller, 1995). Two such coping styles have been identified: *monitoring* and *blunting*. Monitoring refers to the extent to which an individual is alert for and sensitized to the negative, potentially painful, or dangerous aspects of information and experience. Such individuals actively seek information about their cancer and its treatment, particularly those aspects which might be threatening or aversive. Blunting refers to the extent to which individuals avoid or distract themselves from such information. Significantly, research has demonstrated that "monitors" experience greater treatment side effects, are more knowledgeable about their medical situation, are less satisfied with and more demanding regarding psychosocial aspects of their care, more adherent to medical recommendations, and display greater distress in response to cancer-related threats (Miller, 1995). In general, monitors do better (psychologically, behaviorally, and physiologically) when provided with more information while those with a blunting style do better with less information (Miller, 1995). Clearly this distinction has significant implications for managing each type of patient.

Coping Resources: Interpersonal

The quality and quantity of social support available to an individual constitutes a significant resource for coping with stress. While various definitions of social support have been advanced, here social support will refer to the comfort, assistance, and/or information received through informal and formal contacts with individuals or groups (Wallston, Alagna, DeVellis, & DeVellis, 1983). This definition emphasizes that social support may come in different forms. In general, two broad types of social support are identified. *Instrumental* social support refers to assistance with tangible needs such as food, finances, information, and transportation, to name a few. *Affective* social support refers to assistance in the form of affiliation or provision of emotional support or comfort. Social support should be distinguished from the social network. The latter refers to the size and nature of an individual's social contacts—which may or may not serve to provide social support (Berkman & Syme, 1979).

The extent of social support available to cancer patients can profoundly effect their psychological, if not their clinical, status. There is strong correlational data suggesting that greater social support, particularly affective support, is associated with better psychological adjustment in cancer patients (Bloom, 1982; Helgeson et al., 1998; Peters-Golden, 1982; Rowland, 1989b). While the specific type of supportive intervention provided has varied across studies, better psychological adjustment in patients receiving supportive intervention has been a consistent finding. A small number of studies favorably compared the survival rates of cancer patients randomly assigned to supportive group intervention to those in a control group receiving no such treatment (Spiegel, Bloom, & Yalom, 1981). Other studies also linked better social support to lengthier survival following cancer diagnosis (Ell, Nishimoto, Mediansky, Mantell, & Hamovitch, 1992; Funch & Marshall, 1983; Stavraky, Donner, Kincade, & Stewart, 1988). Further reinforcing these results were studies linking supportive intervention with both lengthier postdiagnosis survival (Fawzy et al., 1993; Spiegel, Bloom, Kraemer, & Gottheil, 1989) and lengthier time before cancer recurrence (Fawzy et al., 1993). But these results have not been confirmed in recently reported studies of women with metastatic breast cancer. Survival was *not* longer for women who received group intervention (Cunningham et al., 1998; Edelman, Bell, & Kidman, 1999; Goodwin, Leszcz, & Ennis, 2001). This does not mean there were no benefits from the group intervention. Goodwin et al. found that women who were more distressed did experience an improvement in their mood and in their perception of pain. This confirms previous results of the beneficial effects of psychosocial group intervention (Edelman et al., 1999; Fukui et al., 2000) and supportive-expressive group therapy (Spiegel et al., 1981; Classen et al., 2001).

Some cancer patients are the beneficiaries of more than adequate social support throughout the course of their disease. This occurs either because their social network is adept at offering support or because they themselves are skilled at generating and accessing sources of support. Other cancer patients receive inadequate levels of social support, either because their social network is inherently small and/or unsupportive, or because they lack the communication or interpersonal skills necessary to engage their existing social network. It is important to distinguish between these sources of inadequate social support because they suggest different routes to remediation. It is also critical to recognize that while cancer patients will differ in the quantity and quality of social support available to them, they will also differ with regard to their perceived need for such support. In certain respects, the degree to which available social support is congruent with the perceived need for support is more important than simply the amount and type of social support available. Obviously, efforts by friends or medical staff to provide social support for individuals who do not perceive a need for social support would constitute a waste of time at best and, at worst, might generate anger and interpersonal conflict.

Coping Strategies

In contrast to coping style, coping strategy refers to specific behavior patterns that emerge in the face of stress and that are intended to minimize threat and reduce distress. Coping strategies can be grouped into two broad categories: problem-focused and emotion-focused (Lazarus & Folkman, 1984). Both types of coping strategies succeed through their impact upon primary or secondary appraisal of a potential stressor. Problem-focused strategies are intended to directly eliminate a stressor or, at minimum, reduce its impact. Problem-resolution or reduction is the general aim. In the context of cancer, seeking information or advice about potential courses of treatment, enrolling in a support group, or learning how to use relaxation techniques for controlling pain or nausea would be examples of problem-focused coping strategies. Emotion-focused strategies are behaviors which are intended to minimize distress while leaving the fundamental problem unresolved. Regulation of affect is the aim. In the context of cancer, using drugs or alcohol to relieve anxiety or depression, avoiding discussion of one's cancer with family, friends, or acquaintances, or redefining cancer as a challenge or opportunity for personal growth are all examples of emotion-focused strategies. It is important to note that neither type of coping strategy is inherently adaptive or maladaptive. In general, problem-focused coping is most adaptive when something objective can be done about a stressful situation. Emotion-focused coping is likely more adaptive when a stressful situation must be endured. Thus, persistent problem-focused coping efforts in the face of an immutable stressor are likely maladaptive, as is withdrawal or avoidance when a stressor can be effectively managed. As a result, flexible coping strategies are critical to the well-being of cancer patients.

Studies suggest that coping strategies adopted by cancer patients can be related not only to psychological adjustment, but clinical outcomes as well (Watson & Greer, 1998). In particular, recently diagnosed cancer patients can be categorized with regard to the predominant coping strategy they evidence with regard to their disease and treatment. General coping strategies include: (1) *fighting spirit*, characterized by full acceptance of the diagnosis, an optimistic attitude, determination to combat the disease, and a desire to participate in treatment decisions; (2) *avoidance*, characterized by rejecting or minimizing the seriousness of the cancer diagnosis as well as avoidance of thinking about or discussing their disease; (3) *stoic acceptance* (or fatalism), characterized by acceptance of the diagnosis but adoption of a resigned, fatalistic stance toward the disease; (4) *anxious preoccupation*, characterized by constant rumination about cancer, fears that physical aches or pains signal disease spread or recurrence, and a continual need for reassurance; and (5) *helplessness/hopelessness*, characterized by pessimism, a sense of being overwhelmed and engulfed by the cancer diagnosis, a desire to give up, and minimal active coping efforts. While not completely distinct from one another, those familiar with the care of cancer patients will readily recognize these coping strategies. Importantly, stoic acceptance, anxious preoccupation, and helplessness/hopelessness have been linked to worse disease outcomes (i.e., increased tumor growth, increased risk of recurrence, and death) in some cancer patients (Andrykowski, Brady, & Henslee-Downey, 1994; Greer, Morris, Pettingale, & Haybittle, 1990; Morris, Pettingale, & Haybittle, 1992).

Determinants of Coping

The particular coping strategies employed by a cancer patient are affected by many factors. As indicated above, these can include coping style, the type and extent of social support available, and the extent of tangible personal resources available (e.g., money). Additional factors that influence the cancer patient's coping strategies include personal religious values and beliefs, developmental stage, prior personal experiences with cancer, and site and stage of their disease (Rowland, 1989b). With regard to the latter, it is readily apparent that prognosis and treatment course can differ dramatically from patient to patient. A woman diagnosed with localized, early-stage breast cancer faces a much more favorable prognosis and a less intensive course of treatment than a woman diagnosed with advanced, metastatic breast cancer. In effect, the nature of the stressor confronted by each woman is significantly different, with the result being that different coping behaviors are likely. Prior personal experiences with cancer can also affect coping. The newly diagnosed cancer patient who has witnessed a number of close relatives or friends die from the disease is likely to appraise his or her situation far differently than a newly diagnosed patient with limited personal experience with the disease or who has witnessed more favorable outcomes in relatives or friends. Again, different appraisals of the stressor, in this case cancer, are likely to result in different coping strategies.

The point in the patient's life at which cancer occurs is also a significant determinant of coping. At each point in life, the individual is faced with accomplishing certain developmental tasks. These tasks include creating an independent and autonomous self during adolescence, developing the capacity for intimate relationships during adolescence and young adulthood, marriage and child-rearing during young or middle adulthood, and establishing a career or life's work during middle or later adulthood. Cancer's impact on individuals often depends upon their developmental stage. For example, diagnosis of lymphoma in a man in his early 20s may raise serious concerns regarding how the illness and its treatment will affect his ability to ultimately accomplish developmental tasks appropriate for his age group: forming intimate relationships, marrying, and having children. A similar diagnosis in a man in his mid 50's is unlikely to raise these same concerns. As a result, the nature of the threat posed by cancer differs, likely resulting in differential coping.

Finally, personal religious values and beliefs are also likely to influence coping. Evidence suggests that strong personal religious beliefs are associated with greater health and well-being in the general population (Levin & Schiller, 1988) and with positive coping and adjustment in cancer patients (Jenkins & Pargament, 1995; Mickley, Soeken, & Belcher, 1992). Several explanations have been advanced for why this might be so (Musick, Koenig, Larson, & Matthews, 1998). Religious beliefs might allow cancer patients to cope by relinquishing control of the situation to God, thus relieving themselves of the burden of personal agency. Religious beliefs might also allow the cancer patient to attach a positive, less stressful meaning to illness, pain, and suffering. Participation in a religious community can increase opportunities for accessing social support and perhaps can enable the cancer patient to confront critical existential issues with equanimity rather than fear.

Compliance with Medical Treatment

Compliance or adherence to treatment is an especially important consideration for oncology patients for three reasons. First, treatment often involves a highly complex regimen of scheduled clinic visits and/or hospitalizations as well as use of oral and intravenous medications to treat the cancer and side effects of cancer treatment. Second, cancer treatment continues past the end of therapy to include long-term follow-up appointments for laboratory tests, screening procedures, and physical examinations. Finally, compliance with treatment can directly influence long-term survival (Richardson, Shelton, Krailo, & Levine, 1990). Despite the importance of compliance, and in contrast to the wealth of information concerning compliance in other medical populations, information on compliance in cancer patients is limited. Attention has tended to focus on compliance with cancer prevention and cancer screening recommendations in healthy populations rather than on persons already diagnosed with the disease.

Compliance rates vary as a function of both type of cancer treatment and personal characteristics of the patient, such as self-esteem or general tendencies toward anxiety (i.e., trait anxiety). In general, compliance with standard intravenous chemotherapy protocols is typically high (Taylor, Lichtman, & Wood, 1984), while compliance with oral medications, including oral chemotherapy (e.g., cyclophosphamide, allopurinol, prednisone) is often much lower (Lebovits et al., 1990; Levine et al., 1987; Smith, Rosen, Trueworthy, & Lowman, 1979). In general, treatment regimens that require the patient to take personal responsibility and for which monitoring by the health care team is minimal are more likely to have lower rates of compliance. Additionally, patients with high levels of trait anxiety or with high levels of self-esteem appear to be most likely to comply with cancer treatment regimens, including clinic appointments, laboratory tests, and medication (Itano et al., 1983). On the other hand, patients with many competing demands or fewer resources (e.g., financial) may be less compliant. For example, only 16% of Latina cervical cancer patients were fully compliant with their prescribed course of radiation therapy, with lack of compliance largely due to increased stressors associated with work, child care, and transportation (Formenti et al., 1995).

Strategies for increasing treatment compliance in cancer patients include education, home psychological support, and training in pill taking (Levine et al., 1987). Education combined with either home visits, training, or both were equally effective in improving compliance with oral chemotherapeutic regimens. These strategies have proven effective in improving compliance in a variety of chronically ill populations (Meichenbaum & Turk, 1987).

CANCER RECURRENCE

Persons diagnosed with cancer live with the continual threat of recurrence. Fear, anxiety, and uncertainty about the future are not uncommon reactions (Mast,

1998). Because individuals may develop a subjective interpretation of their risk for recurrence, the actual levels of psychological distress that are experienced may not correspond to their medical risk. In other words, fears of recurrence are not limited to those patients who are at highest risk for recurrence (e.g., those treated for more advanced disease). In addition to causing distress, the ongoing threat of recurrence may lead to behavioral changes. Some cancer survivors may alter their lifestyles and adopt more healthy activity and nutritional patterns in the hope of avoiding a recurrence. Other survivors may avoid medical follow-up altogether to avoid confronting the prospect of recurrence.

A cancer recurrence may be associated with the same psychological reactions that were present at the initial cancer diagnosis, including shock, anger, denial, depression, and anxiety. Some individuals will report feeling more distress than they did at their initial diagnosis (Mahon, Cella, & Donovan, 1990). Heightened awareness of mortality and concerns regarding immediate and long term survival may increase feelings of anxiety and depression. Physical health, functional status, psychological distress, social functioning, and marital and sexual adjustment may all be negatively affected by cancer recurrence (Dorval, Maunsell, Deschenes, Brisson, & Masse, 1998). Patients may express anxiety and fears concerning potential long-term physical disability and role limitations, even in the absence of such limitations at the time of recurrence (Mahon et al., 1990). While the personal meaning of a recurrence varies, recurrence inevitably means cancer treatment is needed again. In addition to the anxiety and discomfort of additional medical tests, individuals must face decisions about the type and extent of treatment they are willing to undergo. While patients' prior experience with cancer treatment makes them more knowledgeable regarding surgery, radiation, and chemotherapy, this knowledge may hinder rather than help treatment decision making at the time of recurrence. For example, prior experience of significant or severe treatment-related side effects may increase patients' anxieties and make it difficult to accept certain treatment options at recurrence. In addition, patients may question treatment decisions made at the time of initial cancer diagnosis (Mahon et al., 1990). Since recurrence suggests that initial treatment "failed," patients may blame themselves for not choosing the "correct" treatment course at time of diagnosis. For example, a woman with recurrent breast cancer might regret her initial choice of lumpectomy rather than mastectomy, believing that recurrence might have been prevented had mastectomy been chosen initially. Such thinking increases anxiety and uncertainty, making treatment decisions at the time of recurrence more difficult.

Even as the stress of recurrence and symptoms associated with subsequent treatment subside, patients may become increasingly pessimistic concerning their lives and futures (Schulz et al., 1995). Recurrence and its aftermath can bring fear, anxiety, and uncertainty. After a recurrence the will to resume normal life activities may be weakened. The patient may ask, "Will I rebuild my life only to find more cancer lurking?" Because the threat of recurrence is present to some degree for all cancer survivors, uncertainty is built into every cancer diagnosis.

SUICIDE

Although the vast majority of cancer patients neither commit suicide nor attempt it, and there is evidence suggesting that the majority of those who do had pre-existing psychiatric disorders, the suicide rate among cancer patients is nonetheless at least twice that of the general population. Strikingly, suicidal ideation without actual intent is reported by clinicians treating cancer patients as almost universal, once a safe and trusting relationship between patient and doctor has been established. Thoughts of suicide may provide the patient with a sense of control, representing "a way out" if things get too bad, and thus may give the patient the resilience to endure difficulties ahead (Breitbart & Krivo, 1998).

The actual suicide rate in cancer patients is unknowable, due to "passive suicide" in a variety of forms, including nonreporting of symptoms (new or recurring) and noncompliance. To the degree that these "passive" methods represent deliberate decisions to end life, the true suicide rate among cancer patients is underestimated.

A constellation of factors is associated with heightened suicide risk in oncology patients. These include advanced disease with poor prognosis, depression and hopelessness; a sense of helplessness; augmented by pain (often not controlled to the degree it could be, therefore contributing to many more cancer suicides than necessary), and fatigue in the form of exhaustion of physical, emotional, financial, familial, and other resources (Breitbart & Krivo, 1998). In addition, men are more likely to commit suicide than women, and men in their sixth or seventh decades are at even greater risk.

Finally, in ordinary circumstances, suicidal ideation is a symptom of psychiatric disturbance. But particularly in late-stage cancer, suicide is understood by many people in our society to be a not unreasonable option to consider, or even self-imposed euthenasia. The ultimate goal is preserving the patient's human dignity.

ISSUES WITH SPECIAL POPULATIONS OF CANCER PATIENTS

Children and Adolescents

Pediatric oncology has undergone a dramatic shift during the last 25 years as treatment advances have led to markedly improved survival rates. Focus on clinical outcomes such as decreasing morbidity and mortality has been augmented by important work on quality of life issues important to children and their families (Bradlyn et al., 1996; Lauria, Hockenberry-Eaton, Pawletko, & Mauer, 1996). In particular, two areas have received attention: (1) psychosocial adjustment of patients and their families, and (2) long-term physical effects of cancer treatment.

Although pediatric cancer patients experience a trajectory of diagnosis, treatment, and long-term follow-up similar to their adult counterparts, these events may be experienced quite differently depending on the age and developmental stage of the child (Last & Van Veldhuizen, 1992; MacLean, Foley, Ruccione, & Sklar, 1996). For example, hospitalization can be associated with significant separation anxiety in young children, but not in older children or adolescents. Adolescents, however, may be more distressed by hair loss and other outward changes associated with cancer treatment. In addition, anger, depression, anxiety, and other normal reactions to diagnosis and treatment may be manifested as behavioral problems in children and adolescents. Feelings of helplessness, uncertainty, and the lack of control of the cancer experience may lead to regressive behavior, acting out, or periods of hyperactivity or lethargy.

Diagnosis and treatment of childhood cancer is stressful and anxiety-provoking for parents and siblings as well. Siblings may resent the extra attention afforded their ill sibling or may experience guilt over their sibling's illness. The heightened stress in the household may trigger misbehavior or withdrawal. Parents have the burden of balancing work and family life with the increased demands of the child with cancer. Transporting the child with cancer for frequent clinic visits, staying overnight with the child during hospitalizations, and helping the child manage side effects of treatment can be exhausting responsibilities. These added responsibilities can disrupt the normal family routine, strain the marital relationship, and interfere with parental work responsibilities. While research suggests the majority of parents cope well with their child's illness, mothers and fathers appear to cope differently (Larson, Wittrock, & Sandgren, 1994). Mothers may use more engaged coping styles, more depression, and more social support than fathers.

One particular source of distress for children and parents is the numerous, invasive medical procedures children must undergo in the course of their cancer treatment. Procedures such as venipunctures for chemotherapy and bone marrow aspirations in leukemic patients can be painful and frightening for pediatric patients. Behavioral distress (e.g., crying, screaming, and writhing) is common in children and anxiety-provoking for parents who may be asked by staff to help physically restrain their child (Jacobsen et al., 1990; Manne et al., 1990). However, behavioral interventions such as attentional distraction, positive motivation, and positive reinforcement can be effective in reducing child distress and parental anxiety (Manne et al., 1990; Redd, 1989).

Childhood cancer is associated with long-term side effects, such as infertility, growth impairment, and neurological damage (Groenwald, Frogge, Goodman, & Yarbro, 1997). Both radiotherapy and chemotherapy can damage testes and ovaries in growing children and lead to infertility. Cranial radiation can damage the hypothalamus, causing growth hormone deficiency and subsequent short stature in children. Cranial radiation and intrathecal chemotherapy for treatment of leukemia and brain tumors can lead to decrements in intellectual functioning, attention deficits, and changes in visual and motor skills. Currently unknown long-term side effects of cancer treatment may become better known as survivors of childhood cancer increase.

The Elderly

Two demographic phenomena are of particular importance to the field of geriatric oncology. First, by the year 2030, more than 20% of Americans will be 65 years of age and older (Yancik, 1997). Second, over 60% of new cancer cases occur in individuals aged 65 and older (Kennedy, 1997). Thus, the number of older persons affected by cancer is rapidly increasing. Furthermore, older persons with cancer are likely to have more advanced cancers at diagnosis, in part because symptoms of other chronic conditions, such as arthritis pain, may be difficult for patients and clinicians to differentiate from cancer symptoms (Yancik, 1997). They are also more likely to receive less aggressive treatment than younger patients, due in part to the increased frequency of other pre-existing conditions (Kennedy, 1997; Muss, 1995; Reuben, 1997). Furthermore, while older individuals are able to tolerate cancer treatment when comorbid conditions are absent (Lipschitz, 1995), such conditions may interfere with patients' ability to tolerate certain types or large doses of chemotherapy (Hainsworth, 1995; Wei, 1995). In addition, functional limitations due to other pre-existing conditions may affect long-term recovery from surgery, radiation, or chemotherapy. Sensory and cognitive limitations can interfere with educational efforts, treatment-related decision making, and compliance with treatment.

Social conditions of the elderly can also interfere with cancer diagnosis and treatment (Reuben, 1997). Widowed elderly, or those who have outlived their close friends and immediate relatives, may lack the social support they need to help them cope with the psychological and physical challenges of cancer. Psychological reactions, management of side effects and complications of treatment, and transportation to and from clinic visits can all be compromised by lack of a supportive network. In addition, the high costs of medical care can be particularly troublesome for elderly cancer patients living on fixed incomes.

Racial and Ethnic Groups

Cancer is a disease that crosses all racial and ethnic groups. However, the incidence of cancer is not evenly distributed across these groups. Cancer incidence rates, in general, are higher among African Americans than among Caucasians (American Cancer Society, 2002; Parker, Davis, Wingo, Ries, & Heath, 1998). Specifically, in 1994 the incidence of cancer in African Americans was 454 per 100,000 individuals, while that of Caucasians was 394 per 100,000 individuals. The incidence rates for a number of cancers, including cancers of the cervix, esophagus, prostate, stomach, pancreas, and liver are at least 50% higher in African Americans than Caucasians. This higher incidence may reflect genetic differences in cancer physiology or may be related to behavioral factors such as nutrition, smoking, or participation in cancer prevention programs (Meyerowitz, Richardson, Hudson, & Leedham, 1998; Parker et al., 1998).

African Americans also possess higher cancer mortality rates than other racial or ethnic groups. African Americans are approximately 30% more likely to die of cancer than Caucasians (American Cancer Society, 2002). Cancer mortality rates in 1992 to 1998 for African Americans was 218 per 100,000 individuals, while the comparable mortality rate for Caucasians was 164.5 per 100,000 individuals. African Americans are at least 50% more likely to die of cancers of the esophagus, cervix, larynx, prostate, stomach oral cavity, endometrium, liver, and pancreas than Caucasian Americans (American Cancer Society, 2002). Additionally, the percentage of African Americans surviving more than five years following a cancer diagnosis is lower than in Caucasians For individuals diagnosed between 1992 and 1997, five-year survival among African Americans was 52% while that of Caucasians was 63%. While differences in mortality rates may reflect racial differences in the biology of the disease, much of this difference in five-year survival is due to the tendency for African Americans to be initially diagnosed at a later stage of disease. Along these lines, it should be acknowledged that economic factors may also play a critical role in the higher mortality and poorer survival rates observed in African Americans. Inadequate medical insurance or access to health care providers may result in longer delay in diagnosing an existing cancer or in receipt of less than optimal medical care.

Culture influences all aspects of the cancer experience. Health beliefs and practices of ethnic groups can interfere with cancer screening behaviors and subsequent early diagnosis and treatment of cancer. Differences in role expectations and family relationships can affect treatment decision making. In addition, cultural differences in expressing psychological and symptom-related distress may prevent the clinician from recognizing severe pain, depression, and anxiety. Complicating matters, research in psychosocial and behavioral oncology has tended to focus on Caucasians, rather than persons of color (Meyerowitz et al., 1998).

Female Breast Cancer Patients

Each type of cancer has psychosocial sequelae unique to it. However, breast cancer is the most common cancer in women in the U.S., second to lung cancer in female cancer mortality, and it effects a part of the female body associated with a sense of "womanliness" and, depending upon the time of life, fertility. Moreover, despite many new treatment options, radical mastectomy is often still necessary due to late detection and is still chosen by some women even when lumpectomy is a viable option. Radical mastectomy is amputation, which is always highly traumatic, and carries special self-esteem challenges for women who are losing something integral to female identity.

Today's breast cancer patient, especially if her cancer is caught at an early stage, but even when it is caught later, has an unusual variety of treatments from which to choose. There are three basic treatment modalities for breast cancer patients: (1) lumpectomy followed by radiation; (2) modified mastectomy; and (3) radical mastectomy, which may include immediate reconstructive surgery (or reconstruction may be done later). Some women choose not to have reconstructive surgery, either due to personal beliefs, insurance limitations, or the lack of a plastic surgeon in whom the patient has confidence.

This variety of choices has obvious advantages that did not exist as recently as 10 years ago. It is now well-established, for instance, that when breast cancer is caught while still localized, it can be treated with lumpectomy and radiation rather than mastectomy, with the same five-year survival rates. However, the psychosocial sequelae of deciding which treatment is best for herself must be considered as the patient goes through the decision-making process. Valanis and Rumpler noted that personal and demographic characteristics, as well as her network of family and friends, influence the patient's treatment choice (Rowland & Massie, 1998) in addition to her choice of physician (who is also likely to be a reflection of her demographic position). The possible downside of this is that the patient may be tempted to make her treatment choices to please her spouse, partner, or friends, rather than herself. For instance, in both localized and regionalized breast cancer, she will be offered the choice of lumpectomy followed by several weeks of radiation, or a modified mastectomy. The patient may be eager to remove the entire effected breast, to alleviate anxiety or avoid the severely fatiguing daily radiation therapy which follows lumpectomy. But she may be afraid of alienating her spouse or partner.

Another example of a new treatment option and its psychological sequelae is immediate reconstruction at the time of the mastectomy. This may seem ideal, and although Schain and colleagues have shown that immediate reconstruction does not interfere with the "mourning process" associated with loss of a breast or breasts, or the threat to life (Rowland & Massie, 1998), other clinicians have reported this as a problem in long-term follow-ups of these patients. This choice should also be examined for its fostering or reinforcement of denial in the patient.

Women may be unaware of the implications of their choices. Lumpectomy and radiation, for instance, can, in the event of recurrence requiring mastectomy later, make breast reconstruction more problematic. The number of new choices present many excellent options for breast cancer patients, but also can be overwhelming rather than advantageous as they were intended to be.

CANCER SURVIVAL

It is estimated that 60% of those diagnosed with cancer in 2001 will be alive five years after diagnosis (American Cancer Society, 2002), when adjusted for normal life expectancy. Approximately 8.9 million Americans with a history of cancer were alive in 1997 (American Cancer Society, 2002). Many of these individuals can be considered cured and might expect to achieve a normal lifespan. Others are alive with some evidence of their disease or are still at high risk for recurrence. Still, many individuals live for an extended period of time following cancer diagnosis and treatment, and the number continues to grow. This has critical implications. In addition to recognizing the immediate impact that cancer diagnosis and treatment has on a person's physical and psychosocial functioning, it is important to recognize cancer's long-term impact as well. Accordingly, in evaluating cancer therapies clinicians should consider both *quantity* and *quality* of life. In this section, we will examine some of the long-term sequelae, or "late effects" associated with cancer diagnosis and treatment. These sequelae will be grouped into two categories: physical and cognitive, and psychosocial.

LONG-TERM PSYCHOSOCIAL SEQUELAE OF CANCER

Cognitive Dysfunction

As noted earlier, cognitive functioning may be impaired during cancer treatment as a result of both systemic or treatment-related factors. Both delirium and, more rarely, dementia may be observed. While delirium and dementia represent profound disturbances in cognitive functioning, the majority of research examining long-term cognitive sequelae of cancer has focused upon the presence of more subtle cognitive impairments in cancer survivors. Initially, attention was limited to the long-term effects of cancer treatment on cognitive function in individuals treated during childhood or adolescence (Walch, Ahles, & Saykin, 1998). Those with brain tumors and leukemia were the primary focus of study because of the potential for neurological complications from these cancers as well as the neurotoxicity of the methods employed in treating these cancers. In particular, cranial radiation is used in the treatment of both types of malignancy, and chemotherapy is often administered directly into the central nervous system (i.e., intrathecally) in the treatment of leukemia. While many of the studies in this area suffer from one or more methodological weaknesses, some generalizations can be drawn. Specifically, children and adolescents treated for brain malignancies are likely to subsequently perform below their healthy peers on standard tests of intellectual development. Fortunately, the magnitude of impairment is generally not large. Mean IQ scores of brain tumor survivors are generally around 90, compared to a mean of 100 in the general population. Higher doses of cranial radiation and treatment at a younger age are risk factors for greater intellectual impairment. Finally, tumor location and extent of surgery are generally unrelated to the extent of cognitive impairment (Mulhern, Hancock, Fairclough, & Kun, 1992). The extent of intellectual impairment observed following treatment for leukemia is generally less with younger age at treatment. This is particularly true for individuals receiving cranial radiation as treatment for leukemia (Walch et al., 1998).

Recently, some attention has shifted to examining the possibility that cranial radiation and certain types of systemic chemotherapy might produce long-term cognitive impairment even when treatment occurs during adulthood (e.g., Ahles, Tope, Furstenberg, Hann, & Mills, 1996; Ahles et al., 1998; Andrykowski et al., 1992; van Dam et al., 1998). While individuals with lung cancer treated with systemic chemotherapy and cranial radiation have been the major focus of the adult literature (e.g., Ahles et al., 1998), some evidence for long-term cognitive impairment has also been obtained in women receiving adjuvant chemotherapy for breast cancer (Brezden, Phillips, Abdolell, Bunston, & Tannock, 2000; van Dam et al., 1998); in candidates for bone marrow transplantation previously treated for leukemias and lymphomas (Andrykowski et al., 1992); and in adults treated with autologous bone marrow transplantation (Ahles, Tupe, Furstenberg, Han, & Mills, 1996). In particular, memory, attention, and higher order cognitive processing appear to be most strongly affected. Deficits, if present, are typically subtle, but nevertheless can adversely affect compliance with medical recommendations, work performance, social and leisure activities, and overall quality of life. Additionally, such symptoms, even when mild, can be profoundly upsetting to the patient and the family. Coupled with the adverse impact upon daily activities, such symptoms can result in anxiety or depressive reactions.

Fatigue

As indicated earlier, fatigue is commonly reported during the course of cancer treatment. Increasingly recognized, however, is the fact that some patients continue to report fatigue long after conclusion of cancer treatment; in some instances, several years or more following completion of treatment. For example, Devlen, Maguire, Philips, Crowther, and Chambers (1987) found that reports of "loss of energy" and "feeling tired" were common in disease-free lymphoma patients one year postdiagnosis. Fobair et al. (1986) reported that over one third of 403 Hodgkin's disease survivors a median of nine years post-treatment indicated their energy level had not "returned to normal." These individuals were more likely to have received combined modality therapy and to have been older and had more advanced disease at diagnosis. Andrykowski et al. (1995, 1997) assessed fatigue and diminished energy level problems in a large sample of survivors of bone marrow transplantation for a malignant disease, primarily leukemias and lymphomas. Almost two thirds indicated their current energy level was lower than prior to their cancer diagnosis. While most problems were mild, 15–20% of bone marrow transplant recipients showed moderate to severe problems with corresponding decrements in quality of life.

The most persuasive evidence supporting the existence of "off-treatment" fatigue is provided by studies that have included comparisons of cancer survivors with healthy individuals who have no history of cancer. Andrykowski and colleagues (Andrykowski, Curran, & Lightner, 1998) examined fatigue in 88 breast cancer patients (mean of 28 months post-treatment) as well as age-matched women with benign breast problems but without a history of cancer. Breast cancer patients reported more fatigue and weakness, and less vitality. For breast cancer patients, fatigue was unrelated to either time since treatment completion or type of treatment received. Broekel, Jacobsen, Horton, Balducci, and Lyman (1998) examined fatigue in 61 breast cancer patients 3 to 29 months after completion of adjuvant chemotherapy. Relative to women with no history of cancer, breast cancer patients reported both more fatigue and greater impact of fatigue on quality of life. Greater fatigue in breast cancer patients was associated with poorer sleep quality, more menopausal symptoms, and presence of a mood, anxiety, or adjustment disorder. Hann et al. (1997) examined off-treatment fatigue in breast cancer patients 3 to 62 months following bone marrow transplantation. Transplant recipients reported more fatigue and greater impact of fatigue on quality of life relative to healthy women. More severe fatigue in the bone marrow transplant group was associated with greater sleep disturbance and more symptoms of anxiety and depression. Finally, Hann, Jacobsen, Martin, Azzarello, and Greenberg (1998) assessed off-treatment fatigue in breast cancer patients 5 to 88 months after completion of adjuvant radiotherapy. None of the women received adjuvant chemotherapy. In contrast to the studies cited above, the breast cancer and healthy comparison groups did not differ in reported fatigue.

In sum, evidence is accumulating that cancer patients may display elevated levels of fatigue, with consequent decrements in quality of life, for some time after the conclusion of cancer therapy. The mechanisms underlying this off-treatment fatigue are not understood, and additional research in this area is clearly warranted both from an etiological as well as a management standpoint. Treatment-induced hypothyroidism or pulmonary function problems resulting in respiration difficulties upon exercise should be considered (Greenberg, 1998). While the data is certainly not definitive, more heavily treated patients, particularly those receiving adjuvant or high-dose chemotherapy, appear to be most at risk for long-term fatigue. Older patients and females might be at higher risk as well, with some evidence linking fatigue to menopausal symptoms. Finally, links between off-treatment fatigue, sleep disturbance, and mood or adjustment disorders have been reported. The overlap among these problems needs to be considered in planning how to manage complaints of fatigue or lack of energy.

Sleep Dysfunction

Clinical observation and subjective reports suggest that sleep difficulties, such as insomnia or frequent waking during the night, are a common problem in cancer patients (Savard, Savard, & Morin, 2001). Consistent with this observation, hypnotics have been found to be the most frequently prescribed psychotropic medication among cancer patients (Derogatis et al., 1979). However, little research has explicitly examined sleep difficulties in cancer patients. Information regarding the nature and extent of sleep difficulties in cancer survivors has generally been obtained as part of larger assessments of symptom experience or quality of life. Thus, the specific data obtained regarding sleep difficulties is often quite limited, crude, and difficult to interpret.

A study that compared the sleep of breast and lung cancer survivors to healthy normal-sleeping individuals and otherwise healthy insomniacs found that lung cancer survivors slept as poorly as insomniacs while breast cancer survivors slept similarly to normal-sleeping healthy individuals (Silberfarb, Hauri, Oxman, & Schnurr, 1993). Forty-three percent of a sample of 125 adult long-term bone marrow transplant (BMT) survivors 6–18 years post-transplant reported "sleep disturbance" to be a current problem (Bush, Haberman, Donaldson, & Sullivan, 1995). In two other studies approximately 25% of BMT survivors reported "poor" or "variable" sleep habits (Chao et al., 1992; Schmidt et al., 1993). Syrjala, Chapko, Vitaliano, Cummings, and Sullivan (1993) reported that 27% of patients one year post-BMT scored in the impaired range on a standardized self-report measure of sleep function. Finally, Andrykowski et al. (1997) assessed sleep problems in 172 adult survivors of BMT for a malignant disease. Based upon interview data, 51% of individuals studied were classified as reporting sleep problems. However, the majority of these problems were rated as mild. Only 8% of the entire sample was rated as reporting a "severe" sleep problem. These results were mirrored in questionnaire data obtained from these same patients. About half (47%) of study participants indicated their current sleep quality was worse than prior to their cancer diagnosis and 52% reported a current "sleep problem," mostly in the mild to moderate range. Current sleep problems were most common in females and those who had received total body irradiation prior to bone marrow transplant.

The nature and extent of sleep dysfunction in adult long-term cancer survivors is an area which merits focused investigation. Good sleep contributes to a satisfactory quality of life and promotes good health through tissue restoration, maintenance of immune function, and adequate cognitive functioning. Poor sleep is associated with increased fatigability, decreased tolerance for pain, and can cause or contribute to depression (Sheely, 1996). Investigations utilizing appropriate control groups and addressing the etiology of sleep difficulties in cancer survivors are needed. While research has demonstrated that cancer survivors often do not differ from other clinical groups without malignant disease with regard to sleep difficulties (Lamb, 1982; Shapiro, 1980), the basic question of whether cancer survivors are at greater risk for sleep difficulties than the general population has not yet been adequately addressed. There are many reasons why cancer patients might evidence sleep difficulties, including pain, psychological problems such as anxiety or depression, fatigue, or menopausal symptoms (e.g., hot flashes). Additionally, the possibility that the disease or its treatment contributes to chronic disruption of normal circadian patterns has been raised (Andrykowski et al., 1997). Few if any studies have been explicitly designed to investigate these potential sources of sleep difficulties in cancer patients or survivors.

Sexual Dysfunction

As noted earlier, sexual functioning is often negatively affected during the time when patients are recovering from surgery or when patients are undergoing chemotherapy or radiation. Problems in sexual functioning may persist, or even emerge for the first time, long after conclusion of the acute phase of diagnosis and treatment. One of the reasons that sexual problems might not emerge until several months or more following diagnosis is that sexual activity may be suspended during the acute phase of diagnosis and treatment. This may be particularly likely following surgery for breast, gynecologic, or prostate malignancies. Thus, only when treatment is concluded and attempts to resume sexual behaviors are initiated do sexual problems emerge (Andersen, 1987). As with sexual dysfunction experienced during the active treatment phase, the origins of sexual dysfunction in cancer survivors are multifactorial.

There is clear evidence that the specific nature and extent of sexual dysfunction in cancer survivors varies by disease site (Andersen, 1985; Kornblith, 1998). Considering sexual dysfunction as decreased sexual interest and activity as well as poorer sexual functioning when sexual activity is attempted, Kornblith (1998) found prevalence rates for sexual dysfunction of 31–40% for testis cancer and 22–36% for breast cancer. In a study of women with early-stage gynecologic cancers (i.e., cervix, ovary, vulva, endometrium), 30% were diagnosed with a sexual dysfunction (Andersen et al., 1989). Several recent studies of men treated with surgery or external beam radiotherapy for prostate cancer suggest sexual dysfunction may be present in the majority of men, particularly those over the age of 65 (Bieri, Miralbell, Rohner, & Kurtz, 1996; Litwin et al., 1995; Talcott et al., 1998).

Sexual dysfunction is not limited to survivors of cancer of the genitals, breast, or pelvis. Kornblith (1998) found prevalence rates of 18–25% in Hodgkin's disease and 21–29% in leukemia. Significant rates of sexual dysfunction in colon, rectal, and bladder cancers also exist (Andersen, 1985). While inhibited sexual desire may be experienced by all groups of cancer patients, problems with painful intercourse might be prevalent in women undergoing radical pelvic surgery for gynecologic malignancies or receiving chemotherapy which produces symptoms of early menopause, such as vaginal dryness. Difficulties with erections and ejaculations are most common in men undergoing surgery for prostate or testis cancer.

As with all of the long-term problems associated with cancer survival, identification of "at risk" individuals is key to effective prevention and treatment. In this respect, the limited data suggest that younger or partnerless cancer survivors might be at elevated risk, as are those with a prior history of sexual dysfunction. In addition, previous sexual behavior and attitudes can affect risk for sexual dysfunction (Andersen, 1985; Andersen & Cyranowski, 1994). Those with a more limited repertoire of sexual behavior and/or a lower frequency of intercourse prior to cancer diagnosis are at greater risk for sexual dysfunction following cancer diagnosis and treatment.

Infertility

Infertility, or impaired fertility, is common in cancer patients of both sexes (Kornblith, 1998; Meirow & Schenker, 1995). In contrast to sexual dysfunction, fertility problems are almost always a direct consequence of cancer treatment or of the disease itself. Obviously, surgical removal of the ovaries or womb in ovarian or other gynecologic cancers will create permanent infertility. Similarly, surgical removal of the affected testicle will produce azoospermia (i.e., lack of sperm) or significant oligospermia (i.e., deficient sperm count) in about 30% of men with testis cancer (Kornblith, 1998). Radiotherapy and chemotherapy can also cause either temporary or permanent fertility problems. In men, infertility can result from exposure of the testes to direct radiation or to scatter radiation directed at male reproductive organs.

The risk for infertility is not uniform for all chemotherapy drugs or drug combinations. Certain drugs or combinations of drugs are more harmful to fertility than others. Alkykating agents are considered to be most gonadotoxic. For example, cyclophosphamide is often implicated in the ovarian dysfunction and consequent fertility problems evidenced in breast cancer patients treated with this drug. In a recent study, nearly two thirds of premenopausal breast cancer patients receiving a regimen including cyclophosphamide experienced amenorrhea (Bines, Oleske, & Cobleigh, 1996). Similarly, men and women with Hodgkin's disease treated with chemotherapy regimens for Hodgkin's disease are at high risk for decreased fertility. In a summary of 20 years experience in treating Hodgkin's disease with standard chemotherapy regimens, it was reported that nearly all men were rendered permanently infertile and nearly 80% of women over the age of 25 underwent premature menopause, with 41% becoming permanently amenhorreic (Longo et al., 1986; Urba & Longo, 1992). Finally, BMT survivors of both sexes evidence high rates of infertility due to the use of high-dose chemotherapy, often in combination with total body irradiation, prior to the transplant (Sanders & the Seattle Marrow Transplant Team, 1991).

Not all infertility problems are a consequence of cytotoxic treatment. Rather, fertility may be impaired as a consequence of the disease itself. For example, 30–50% of males with Hodgkin's disease have reduced fertility at the time of diagnosis (Bookman & Longo, 1986). Similarly, 10–15% of men with testicular cancer may be permanently infertile at the time of diagnosis (Einhorn, Richie, & Shipley, 1993). Some fertility problems are temporary and some patients who are completely or partially infertile at the conclusion of cancer treatment may eventually recover complete or partial gonadal function. In general, patients who have received higher doses of treatment, who are older, or who evidenced poorer gonadal function (e.g., low sperm count) prior to treatment are more likely to experience fertility problems as a result of treatment. They are also less likely to recover gonadal function when treatment is concluded (Meirow & Schenker, 1995). The impact of fertility problems upon the psychosocial functioning of the patient is highly dependent upon the age or developmental stage of the patient. Individuals of childbearing years who have not yet completed their families are likely to be profoundly affected. Unmarried individuals may find it difficult to establish intimate relationships, while married individuals may find their relationship greatly stressed by problems relating to reduced fertility.

Negative Psychosocial Sequelae

As discussed previously, the many varied stressors potentially confronted by cancer patients over the course of their illness provide ample opportunity for the development of a variety of psychosocial difficulties. Anxiety and depressive reactions are fairly common during the initial phases of the disease when the shock of the diagnosis and the hardships imposed by treatment are most acutely experienced. As time passes, treatment is completed, and the individual begins the process of cognitively integrating his experience and returning to a normal, precancer lifestyle. At this point distress is likely to diminish. Research suggests the large majority of cancer patients who remain disease free adapt very well to their experience and show good adjustment within one or two years of their diagnosis (Andersen, 1994). A recent meta-analysis concluded that cancer survivors did not significantly differ from the normal population with regard to measures of anxiety and psychological distress (Van't Spijker, Trijsburg, & Duivenvoorden, 1997).

In light of the above and research suggesting the prevalence of major psychiatric disorder in cancer patients does not exceed that of the general population (Derogatis et al., 1983), it is reasonable to conclude that the psychological adjustment of cancer survivors is comparable, on the whole, to that in the normal population. Of course, such a general statement does not mean that some cancer survivors do not experience difficulties in psychological adjustment, if not a formal psychiatric disorder. In the meta-analysis cited above (Van't Spijker et al., 1997), the authors noted that prevalence rates for psychological or psychiatric problems varied across the studies they reviewed (0–46% for depression, 0.9–49% for anxiety, and 5–50% for general psychological distress). Other reviews suggest that up to 20% of cancer survivors experience significant psychological adjustment difficulties (Dobkin & Morrow, 1985). Identification of those most at risk is paramount to effective clinical management. To this end, Andersen (1994) has proposed a model for identifying cancer survivors at greatest risk for psychologic adjustment difficulties. Cancer survivors most at risk for psychological adjustment difficulties are those with: (a) a current or prior history of psychiatric problems; (b) comorbid medical problems; (c) poor social support; (d) lower socioeconomic status; (e) more advanced disease at diagnosis and more aggressive treatment; and (f) new health problems stemming from cancer treatment. In addition, differences in personality or coping style, such as dispositional optimism, self-esteem, conscientiousness, or sexual schema, can also affect psychological adjustment.

Finally, it is noteworthy that Van't Spijker et al. (1997) found that, compared to the normal population, the amount of depression, anxiety, and psychological distress reported by cancer patients was significantly less in studies published after 1987. Thus, there appears to be a historical trend toward better overall psychological adjustment in cancer patients and cancer survivors. Van't Spijker et al. (1997) speculated that this might be due to improved patient education or to improved medical treatment and earlier diagnosis, leading to better overall prognoses. It is also possible that the experience of cancer has been somewhat "detoxified" or made less stressful by historical changes in the social and health care milieu within which cancer occurs. Advances in supportive care along with increased public knowledge and awareness of cancer may have created a climate that minimizes the distress associated with the disease, promotes positive adaptation to the disease (see below), and normalizes the cancer experience so that psychological and social "cures" are attainable in addition to biological cure (van Eys, 1987).

Positive Psychosocial Sequelae

As indicated in the previous section, the diagnosis and treatment of cancer can produce a range of long-term negative sequelae including decreased self-esteem, dysphoric mood, distressing ruminations, anxiety and depressive disorders, and disrupted interpersonal relationships. However, studies which have compared psychosocial adjustment in cancer survivors to benign disease or healthy, "normal" control groups have often found few, and typically small, differences on measures of psychological distress and adjustment between cancer and noncancer samples (e.g., Andrykowski, Brady, & Hunt, 1993; Andrykowski et al., 1996; Cella & Tross, 1986; Danoff, Kramer, Irwin, & Gottlieb, 1983; Van't Spijker et al., 1997; Vinokur, Threatt, Caplan, & Zimmerman, 1989). Given the physical and psychosocial stresses associated with cancer and its treatment, the failure to find such differences might be surprising. However, the lack of differences makes sense given increasing recognition of the possibility that cancer diagnosis may also trigger a host of positive psychosocial sequelae, including increased self-esteem, heightened spirituality, improved outlook on life, and enhanced interpersonal relationships (Andrykowski et al., 1993, 1996). Simply put, such positive psychosocial sequelae may counterbalance some or all of the negative psychosocial sequelae associated with cancer and its treatment. As a result, comparison of individuals with and without cancer may show few, or only small, differences using measures of psychological adjustment.

How can cancer produce positive psychosocial sequelae? Rather than viewing a cancer diagnosis and treatment as a stressful or traumatic event which possesses only the ability to produce negative outcomes, or neutral outcomes at best, cancer might be more broadly viewed as a "transitional" event (Andrykowski et al., 1993). A transitional event is a stressful or traumatic event which has the potential to serve as a turning point in an individual's life. Such events involve major changes that are lasting in their effects and which alter the set of assumptions an individual previously held about the world. Transitional events require individuals to restructure their worldview as well as their future plans. Most importantly, transitional events can produce a wide spectrum of outcomes. In some instances their impact can be positive and life-enhancing, whereas in other instances their impact can be negative and detrimental. Both positive and negative outcomes can also occur, either simultaneously or sequentially, in the same individual (Andrykowski et al., 1993).

While the media have frequently highlighted cancer patients who have coped well with their disease and who profess to an improved outlook on life, enhanced self-esteem, heightened spirituality, and/or enhanced interpersonal relationships, such positive sequelae, have received little attention in the research literature. Most studies of long-term psychosocial adjustment in cancer survivors have focused their assessment upon negative outcomes, typically with scant or no attention paid to assessment of potential positive outcomes. Only a limited number of studies have made concerted efforts to assess positive psychosocial sequelae. The cancer survivors studied have been diverse and have included BMT survivors (Curbow, Legro, Baker, Wingard, & Somerfield, 1993; Curbow, Somerfield, Baker, Wingard, & Legro, 1993; Ferrell et al., 1992; Fromm, Andrykowski, & Hunt, 1996), individuals primarily treated for leukemias and lymphomas (Andrykowski et al., 1993), breast cancer (Andrykowski et al., 1996; Cordova, Cunningham, Carlson, & Andrykowski, 2001; Coward, 1991; Moch, 1990; Zemore, Rinholm, Shepel, & Richards, 1989), testicular cancer (Rieker, Edbril, & Garnick, 1985), and a mixture of cancer diagnoses (Collins, Taylor, & Skokan, 1990). In general, this research has established that many cancer survivors report their cancer experience has had a positive impact in one or more areas of their life, for example, by enhancing interpersonal relationships, raising self-esteem, creating a better appreciation for life, or deepening spiritual or religious convictions. In some studies, nearly three quarters or more of survivors studied reported one or more areas of positive impact (Collins et al., 1990; Zemore et al., 1989). Beyond this general statement, however, few other conclusions can be drawn. Not enough is yet known regarding either which cancer survivors are most likely to evidence positive sequelae or the temporal course over which such sequelae emerge and perhaps ultimately disappear.

The fact that cancer can have a profoundly positive impact upon the lives of some patients is of more than academic interest. From a clinical standpoint, this observation challenges professionals to rethink what constitutes successful psychosocial adjustment in these individuals. At present, a return to, or maintenance of, the premorbid status quo with regard to psychosocial adjustment is the implied goal. In contrast, recognition that cancer can create a milieu in which positive psychological, behavioral, and interpersonal changes are possible suggests a more ambitious goal would be valuable. Specifically, professionals working with cancer patients might focus upon attainment of the twin goals of both minimizing the patient's distress as well as maximizing the potential for growth and positive life change that the cancer experience can provide, in spite of or because of the challenges it poses.

REFERENCES

Ahles, T. A., Silberfarb, P. M., Herndon, II, J., Maurer, L. H., Kornblith, A. B., Aisner, J., et al. (1998). Psychologic and neuropsychologic functioning of patients treated with chemotherapy and radiation therapy with or without warfarin: A study by the Cancer and Leukemia Group B. *Journal of Clinical Oncology, 16,* 1954–1960.

Ahles, T. A., Tope, D. M., Furstenberg, C., Hann, D., & Mills, L. (1996). Psychologic and neuropsychologic impact of autologous bone marrow transplantation. *Journal of Clinical Oncology, 14,* 1457–1462.

Alter, C. L., Pelcovitz, D., Axelrod, A., Goldenberg, B., Harris, H., Meyers, B., et al. (1996). Identification of PTSD in cancer survivors. *Psychosomatics, 37,* 137–143.

American Cancer Society. (2002). *Cancer facts and figures–2002.* Atlanta: Author.

Andersen, B. L. (1985). Sexual functioning morbidity among cancer survivors. *Cancer, 55,* 1835–1842.

Andersen, B. L. (1987). Sexual functioning complications in women with gynecologic cancer: Outcomes and directions for prevention. *Cancer, 60,* 2123–2128.

Andersen, B. L. (1994). Surviving cancer. *Cancer, 74*(Suppl.), 1484–1495.

Andersen, B. L., Andersen, B., & de Prosse, C. (1989). Controlled prospective longitudinal study of women with cancer: I. Sexual functioning outcomes. *Journal of Consulting and Clinical Psychology, 57,* 683–691.

Andersen, B. L., & Cyranowski, J. M. (1994). Women's sexual self-schema. *Journal of Personality and Social Psychology, 67,* 1079–1100.

Andrykowski, M. A., Brady, M. J., & Henslee-Downey, P. J. (1994). Psychosocial factors predictive of survival following allogeneic bone marrow transplantation for leukemia. *Psychosomatic Medicine, 56,* 432–439.

Andrykowski, M. A., Brady, M. J., & Hunt, J. W. (1993). Positive psychosocial adjustment in potential bone marrow transplant recipients. Cancer as a psychosocial transition. *Psychooncology, 2,* 261–276.

Andrykowski, M. A., Carpenter, J. S., Greiner, C. B., Altmaier, E. M., Burish, T. G., Antin, J. H., et al. (1997). Energy level and sleep quality following bone marrow transplantation. *Bone Marrow Transplantation, 20,* 669–679.

Andrykowski, M. A., Cordova, M. J., Studts, J. L., & Miller, T. W. (1998). Diagnosis of posttraumatic stress disorder following treatment for breast cancer. *Journal of Consulting and Clinical Psychology, 66,* 586–90.

Andrykowski, M. A., Curran, S. L., & Lightner, R. (1998). Off-treatment fatigue in breast cancer survivors: A controlled comparison. *Journal of Behavioral Medicine, 21,* 1–18.

Andrykowski, M. A., Curran, S. L., Studts, J. L., Cunningham, L., Carpenter, J. S., McGrath, P., et al. (1996). Quality of life in women with breast cancer and benign breast problems: A controlled comparison. *Journal of Clinical Epidemiology, 49,* 827–834.

Andrykowski, M. A., Greiner, C. B., Altmaier, E. M., Burish, T. G., Antin, J. H., Gingrich, R., et al. (1995). Quality of life following bone marrow transplantation: Findings from a multicentre study. *British Journal of Cancer, 71*, 1322–1329.

Andrykowski, M. A., Redd, W. H., & Hatfield, A. K. (1985). Development of anticipatory nausea: A prospective analysis. *Journal of Consulting and Clinical Psychology, 53*, 447–454.

Andrykowski, M. A., Schmitt, F. A., Gregg, M. E., Brady, M. J., Lamb, D. G., & Henslee-Downey, P. J. (1992). Neuropsychologic impairment in adult bone marrow transplant candidates. *Cancer, 70*, 2288–2297.

Auchincloss, S. S. (1989). Sexual dysfunction in cancer patients: Issues in evaluation and treatment. In J. C. Holland & J. H. Rowland (Eds.), *Handbook of psycho-oncology* (pp. 383–413). Oxford: Oxford University Press.

Berkman, L. F., & Syme, S. L. (1979). Social networks, host resistance, and mortality: A nine year follow-up study of Alameda County residents. *American Journal of Epidemiology, 109*, 186–204.

Bieri, S., Miralbell, R., Rohner, S., & Kurtz, J. (1996). Influence of transurethral resection on sexual dysfunction in patients with prostrate cancer. *British Journal of Urology, 78*, 537–541.

Bines, J., Oleske, D. M., & Cobleigh, M. A. (1996). Ovarian function in premenopausal women treated with adjuvant chemotherapy for breast cancer. *Journal of Clinical Oncology, 14*, 1718–1729.

Bloom, J. R. (1982). Social support, accommodation to stress and adjustment to breast cancer. *Social Science and Medicine, 16*, 1329–1338.

Bookman, M. A., & Longo, D. L. (1986). Concomitant illness in patients treated for Hodgkin's disease. *Cancer Treatment Reviews, 13*, 77–111.

Bradlyn, A. S., Ritchey, A. K., Harris, C. V., Moore, I. M., O'Brien, R. T., Parsons, S. K., et al. (1996). Quality of life research in pediatric oncology: Research methods and barriers. *Cancer, 78*, 1333–1339.

Breitbart, W., & Cohen, K. R. (1998). Delirium. In J. C. Holland (Ed.), *Psycho-oncology* (pp. 564–575). New York: Oxford University Press.

Breitbart, W., & Krivo, S. (1998). Suicide. In J. C. Holland (Ed.), *Psycho-oncology* (pp. 541–547). New York: Oxford University Press.

Breitbart, W., & Payne, D. K. (1998). Pain. In J. C. Holland (Ed.), *Psycho-oncology* (pp. 450–467). New York: Oxford University Press.

Brezden, C. B., Phillips, K. A., Abdolell, M., Bunston, T., & Tannock, I. F. (2000). Cognitive function in breast cancer patients receiving adjunct chemotherapy. *Journal of Clinical Oncology, 18*, 2696–2701.

Broeckel, J. A. Jacobsen, P. B., Horton, J., Balducci, L., & Lyman, G. H. (1998). Characteristics and correlates of fatigue following adjuvant chemotherapy for breast cancer. *Journal of Clinical Oncology, 16*, 1689–1696.

Bruera, E., Macmillan, K. Hanson, J., & Macdonald, R. N. (1989). The cognitive effects of the administration of narcotic analgesics in patients with cancer pain. *Pain, 39*, 13–16.

Bush, N. E., Haberman, M., Donaldson, G., & Sullivan, K. M. (1995). Quality of life of 125 adults surviving 6-18 years after bone marrow transplantation. *Social Science and Medicine, 40*, 479–490.

Catalona, W. J., Smith, D. S., Ratliff, T. L., Dodds, K. M., Coplen, D. E., Yuan, J. J. J., et al. (1991). Measurement of prostate-specific antigen in serum as a screening test for prostate cancer. *New England Journal of Medicine, 324,* 1156–1161.

Cella, D. F., Pratt, A., & Holland, J. C. (1986). Persistent anticipatory nausea, vomiting, and anxiety in cured Hodgkin's Disease patients after completion of chemotherapy. *American Journal of Psychiatry, 143,* 641–643.

Cella, D. F., & Tross, S. (1986). Psychological adjustment to survival from Hodgkin's disease. *Journal of Consulting and Clinical Psychology, 54,* 616–622.

Chao, N. J., Tierney, D. K., Bloom, J. R., Long, G. D., Barr, T. A., Stallbaum, B. A., et al. (1992). Dynamic assessment of quality of life after autologous bone marrow transplantation. *Blood, 80,* 825–830.

Cherny, N. I., & Portenoy, R. K. (1994). The management of cancer pain. *CA: A Cancer Journal for Clinicians, 44,* 262–303.

Cimprich, B. (1992). Attentional fatigue following breast cancer surgery. *Research in Nursing and Health, 15,* 199–207.

Cimprich, B. (1993). Development of an intervention to restore attention in cancer patients. *Cancer Nursing, 16,* 83–92.

Classen, C., Butler, L. D., Koopman, C., Miller, E., DiMicelli, S., Giese-Davis, J., et al. (2001). Supportive-expressive group therapy and distress in patients with metastatic breast cancer: a randomized clinical intervention trial. *Archives of General Psychiatry, 58,* 494–501.

Collins, R. L., Taylor, S. E., & Skokan, L. A. (1990). A better world or a shattered vision? Changes in life perspectives following victimization. *Social Cognition, 8,* 263–285.

Cordova, M. J., Cunningham, L. L. C., Carlson, C. R., & Andrykowski, M. A. (2001). Posttraumatic growth following breast cancer: A controlled comparison study. *Health Psychology, 20,* 176–185.

Coward, D. D. (1991). Self-transcendence and emotional well-being in women with advanced breast cancer. *Oncology Nursing Forum, 18,* 857–863.

Cunningham, A. J., Edmonds, C. V., Jenkins, G. P., Pollack, H., Lockwood, G. A., & Warr, D. A. (1998). A randomized controlled trial of the effects of group psychotherapy on survival of women with metastatic breast cancer. *Psychooncology, 7,* 508–517.

Curbow, B., Legro, M. W., Baker, F., Wingard, J. R., & Somerfield, M. R. (1993). Loss and recovery themes of long-term survivors of bone marrow transplants. *Journal of Psychosocial Oncology, 10,* 1–20.

Curbow, B., Somerfield, M., Baker, F., Wingard, J., & Legro, M. (1993). Personal changes, dispositional optimism and psychological adjustment to an aggressive cancer treatment. *Journal of Behavioral Medicine, 16,* 423–443.

Danoff, B., Kramer, S., Irwin, P., & Gottlieb, A. (1983). Assessment of the quality of life in long-term survivors after definitive radiotherapy. *American Journal of Clinical Oncology, 6,* 339–345.

Derogatis, L. R., Feldstein, Morrow, G., Schmale, A., Schmitt, M., Gates, C., et al. (1979). A survey of psychotropic drug prescriptions in an oncology population. *Cancer, 44,* 1919–1929.

Derogatis, L. R., Morrow, G. R., Fetting, J., Penman, D., Piasetsky, S., Schmale, A. M., et al. (1983). The prevalence of psychiatric disorders among cancer patients. *Journal of the American Medical Association, 249,* 751–757.

DeVita, V. T., Hellman, S., & Rosenberg, S. A. (Eds.). (1997). *Cancer: Principles & practice of oncology* (5th ed.). Philadelphia: Lippincott-Raven.

Devlen, J., Maguire, P., Philips, P., Crowther, D., & Chambers, H. (1987). Psychological problems associated with diagnosis and treatment of lymphomas. 1. restrospective; 2. prospective. *British Medical Journal, 295,* 953–957.

Dobkin, P. L., & Morrow, G. R. (1985). Long-term side effects in patients who have been treated successfully for cancer. *Journal of Psychosocial Oncology, 3*(4), 23–51.

Dorval, M., Maunsell, E., Deschenes, L., Brisson, J., & Masse, B. (1998). Long-term quality of life after breast cancer: Comparison of 8-year survivors with population controls. *Journal of Clinical Oncology, 16,* 487–494.

Edelman, S., Bell, D. R., Kidman, A. D. (1999). A group cognitive behavior therapy programme with metastatic breast cancer patients. *Psychooncology, 8,* 295–305.

Einhorn, L. H., Richie, J. P., & Shipley, W. U. (1993). Cancer of the testis. In V. T. Devita, Jr., S. Hellman, & S. A. Rosenberg (Eds.), *Cancer: Principles and practice of oncology* (4th ed. (pp. 1126–1151). Philadelphia: J. B. Lippincott.

Ell, K., Nishimoto, R., Mediansky, L., Mantell, J., & Hamovitch, M. (1992). Social relations, social support, and survival among patients with cancer. *Journal of Psychosomatic Research, 36,* 531–541.

Esterling, B. A., Antoni, M., Fletcher, M., Margulies, S., & Schneiderman, N. (1994). Emotional disclosure through writing or speaking modulates latent Epstein-Barr virus reactivation. *Journal of Consulting and Clinical Psychology, 62,* 130–140.

Fawzy, F. I ., Fawzy, N. W., Hyun, C. S., Elashoff, R., Gutherie, D., Fahey, J. L., et al. (1993). Effects of an early structured psychiatric intervention, coping, and affective state on recurrence and survival 6 years later. *Archives of General Psychiatry, 50,* 681–689.

Ferrell, B., Grant, M., Schmidt, G. M., Rhiner, M., Whitehead, C., Fonbeuena, P., et al. (1992). The meaning of quality of life for bone marrow transplant survivors. Part 1. The impact of bone marrow transplant on quality of life. *Cancer Nursing, 15,* 153–160.

Fertig, D. L., & Hayes, D. F. (1998). Psychological responses to tumor markers. In J. C. Holland (Ed.), *Psycho-oncology* (pp. 147–160). New York: Oxford University Press.

Fleishman, S., & Lesko, L. M. (1989). Delirium and dementia. In J. C. Holland & J. H. Rowland (Eds.), *Handbook of psycho-oncology* (pp. 342–355). Oxford: Oxford University Press.

Fobair, P., Hoppe, R. T., Bloom, J., Cox, R., Varghese, A., & Spiegel, D. (1986). Psychosocial problems among survivors of Hodgkin's disease. *Journal of Clinical Oncology, 4,* 805–814.

Foley, K. M. (1985). The treatment of chronic pain. *The New England Journal of Medicine, 313,* 84–95.

Formenti, S. C., Meyerowitz, B. E., Ell, K., Muderspach, L., Groshen, S., Leedham, B., et al. (1995). Inadequate adherence to radiotherapy in Latina immigrants with carcinoma of the cervix. *Cancer, 75,* 1135–1140.

Fromm, K., Andrykowski, M. A., & Hunt, J. (1996). Positive and negative psychosocial sequelae of bone marrow transplantation: Implications for quality of life assessment. *Journal of Behavioral Medicine, 19,* 221–240.

Funch, D. P., & Marshall, J. (1983). The role of stress, social support and age in survival from breast cancer. *Journal of Psychosomatic Research, 27,* 77–83.

Fukui, S., Kugaya, A., Okamura, H., Kamiya, M., Koike, M., Nakanishi, T., et al. (2000). A psychological group intervention for Japanese women with primary breast carcinoma. *Cancer, 89,* 1026–1036.

Ganz, P. A., Rowland, J. H., Desmond, K., Meyerowitz, B. E., & Wyatt, G. E. (1998). Life after breast cancer: Understanding women's health-related quality of life and sexual functioning. *Journal of Clinical Oncology, 16,* 501–514.

Goodwin, P. J., Leszcz, M., Ennis, M., Koopman, J., Vincent, L., Guther, M., et al. (2001). The effect of group psychosocial support on survival in metastatic breast cancer. *The New England Journal of Medicine, 24,* 1719–1726.

Greenberg, D. B. (1998). Fatigue. In J. C. Holland (Ed.) *Psycho-oncology* (pp. 485–493). New York: Oxford University Press.

Greer, S., Morris, T., Pettingale, K. W., & Haybittle, J. L. (1990). Psychological response to breast cancer and 15 year outcome. *Lancet, 1,* 49–50.

Groenwald, S. L., Frogge, M. H., Goodman, M., & Yarbro, C. H. (1996). *Cancer symptom management.* Boston: Jones and Bartlett.

Groenwald, S. L., Frogge, M. H., Goodman, M. & Yarbro, C. H. (1997). *Cancer nursing: Principles and practice* (4th Ed.). Boston: Jones and Bartlett.

Hainsworth, J. D. (1995). The use of mitoxantrone in the treatment of breast cancer. *Seminars in Oncology, 22*(Suppl. 1), 17–20.

Hann, D. M. Jacobsen, P. B., Martin, S. C., Azzarello, L. M., & Greenberg, H. (1998). Fatigue and quality of life following radiotherapy for breast cancer: A comparative study. *Journal of Clinical Psychology in Medical Settings, 5,* 19–33.

Hann, D. M., Jacobsen, P. B., Martin, S. C., Kronish, L. E., Azzarello, L. M., & Fields, K. M. (1997). Fatigue in women treated with bone marrow transplantation: A comparison with women with no history of cancer. *Supportive Care in Cancer, 5,* 44–52.

Helgeson, V. S., Cohen, S., & Fritz, H. L. (1998). Social ties and cancer. In J. C. Holland (Ed.), *Psycho-oncology* (pp. 99–109). New York: Oxford University Press.

Itano, J., Tanabe, P., Lum, J. L., Lamkin, L., Rizzo, E., Wieland, M., & Sato, P. (1983). Compliance of cancer patients to therapy. *Western Journal of Nursing Research, 5,* 5–16.

Jacobsen, P. B., Manne, S. L., Gorfinkle, K., Schorr, O., Rapkin, B., & Redd, W. H. (1990). Analysis of child and parent behavior during painful medical procedures. *Health Psychology, 9,* 559–576.

Jenkins, R. A., & Pargament, K. I. (1995). Religion and spirituality as resources for coping with cancer. *Journal of Psychosocial Oncology, 13* (½), 51–74.

Jewett, H. J., Bridge, R. W., Gray, G. F., & Shelley, W. M. (1968). The palpable nodule of prostatic cancer: Results 15 years after radical excision. *Journal of the American Medical Association, 203,* 403–406.

Kennedy, B. J. (1997). Aging and cancer: Geriatric oncology—keynote address: Integrating geriatrics into oncology education. *Cancer, 80,* 1270–1272.

King, G. L., & Makale, M. T. (1991). Postirradiation emesis. In J. Kucharczyk, D. J. Stewart, & A. D. Miller (Eds.). *Nausea and vomiting: Recent research and clinical advances* (pp.103–142). Boca Raton, FL: CRC Press.

Kornblith, A. B. (1998). Psychosocial adaption of cancer survivors. In J .C. Holland (Ed.), *Psycho-oncology* (pp. 223–254). New York: Oxford University Press.

Krumm, S., & Lamberti, J. (1993). Changes in sexual behavior following radiation therapy for cervical cancer. *Journal of Psychosomatic Obstetrics and Gynaecology, 14,* 51–63.

Lamb, M. (1982). The sleeping patterns of patients with malignant and non-malignant diseases. *Cancer Nursing, 5,* 389–396.

Larson, L. S., Wittrock, D. A., Sandgren, A. K. (1994). When a child is diagnosed with cancer: I. Sex differences in parental adjustment. *Journal of Psychosocial Oncology,* *12,* 123–142.

Last, B. F., & Van Veldhuizen, A. M. (Eds.). (1992). *Developments in pediatric psychosocial oncology.* Amsterdam: Swets & Zeitlinger.

Lauria, M. M., Hockenberry-Eaton, M., Pawletko, T. M., & Mauer, A. M. (1996). Psychosocial protocol for childhood cancer: A conceptual model. *Cancer, 78,* 1345–1356.

Lazarus, R. S., & Folkman, S. (1984). *Stress, appraisal, and coping.* New York: Springer.

Lebovits, A. H., Strain, J. J., Schleifer, S. J., Tanaka, J. S., Bhardwaj, S., & Messe, M. R. (1990). Patient noncompliance with self-administered chemotherapy. *Cancer, 65,* 17–22.

Levin, B., & Murphy, G. P. (1992). Revision in American Cancer Society recommendations for the early detection of colorectal cancer. *CA: A Cancer Journal for Clinicians, 42,* 296–299.

Levin, J. S., & Schiller, P. L. (1988). Is there a religious factor in health? *Journal of Religion and Health, 26,* 9–36.

Levine, A. M., Richardson, J. L., Marks, G., Chan, K., Graham, J., Selser, J. N., et al. (1987). Compliance with oral drug therapy in patients with hematologic malignancy. *Journal of Clinical Oncology, 5,* 1469–1476.

Lewis, F. M., Hammond, M. A., & Woods, N. F. (1993). The family's functioning with newly diagnosed breast cancer in the mother: The development of an explanatory model. *Journal of Behavioral Medicine, 16,* 351–370.

Lipowski, Z. J. (1970). Physical illness, the individual and the coping process. *Psychiatry in Medicine, 1,* 91–102.

Lipschitz, D. A. (1995). Age-related declines in hematopoietic reserve capacity. *Seminars in Oncology, 22* (Suppl. 1), 3–5.

Litwin, M. S., Hays, R. D., Fink, A., Ganz, P. A., Leake, B., Leach, G. E., et al. (1995). Quality-of-life outcomes in men treated for localized prostrate cancer. *Journal of the American Medical Association, 273,* 129–135.

Longo, D. L., Young, R. C., Wesley, M., Hubbard, S. M., Duffey, P. K., Jaffe, E. S., et al. (1986). Twenty years of MOPP therapy for Hodgkin's disease. *Journal of Clinical Oncology, 4,* 1295–1306.

MacLean, W. E., Foley, G. V., Ruccione, K., & Sklar, C. (1996). Transitions in the care of adolescent and young adult survivors of childhood cancer. *Cancer, 78,* 1340–1344.

Mahon, S. M., Cella, D. F., & Donovan, M. I. (1990). Psychosocial adjustment to recurrent cancer. *Oncology Nursing Forum, 17,* 47–54.

Management of Cancer Pain Guideline Panel. (1994). *Management of Cancer Pain. Clinical Practice Guideline No. 9.* (AHCPR Publication No. 94-0592). Rockville, MD: Agency for Health Care Policy and Research, U.S. Department of Health and Human Services, Public Health Service.

Manne, S. L., Redd, W. H., Jacobsen, P. B., Gorfinkle, K., Schorr, O., & Rapkin, B. (1990). Behavioral intervention to reduce child and parent distress during venipuncture. *Journal of Consulting and Clinical Psychology, 58,* 565–572.

Mast, M. E. (1998). Survivors of breast cancer: Illness uncertainty, positive reappraisal, and emotional distress. *Oncology Nursing Forum, 25,* 555–562.

Meichenbaum, D., & Turk, D. C. (1987). *Facilitating treatment adherence: A practitioner's guidebook.* New York: Plenum Press.

Meirow, D., & Schenker, J. G. (1995). Cancer and male infertility. *Human Reproduction,* *10,* 2017–2022.

Meyerowitz, B. E., Richardson, J., Hudson, S., & Leedham, B. (1998). Ethnicity and cancer outcomes: Behavioral and psychosocial considerations. *Psychological Bulletin, 123,* 47–70.

Mickley, J. R., Soeken, K., & Belcher, A. (1992). Spiritual well-being, religiousness and hope among women with breast cancer. *Image, 24,* 267–272.

Miller, S. M. (1995). Monitoring versus blunting styles of coping with cancer influence the information patients want and need about their disease: Implications for cancer screening and management. *Cancer, 76,* 167–177.

Moch, S. D. (1990). Health within the experience of breast cancer. *Journal of Advanced Nursing, 15,* 1426–1435.

Mock, V., Dow, K. H., Meares, C. J., Grimm, P. M., Dienemann, J. A., Haisfield-Wolfe, M. E., et al. (1997). Effects of exercise on fatigue, physical functioning, and emotional distress during radiation therapy for breast cancer. *Oncology Nursing Forum, 24,* 991–1000.

Morris, T., Pettingale, K. W., & Haybittle, J. (1992). Psychological response to cancer diagnosis and disease outcome in patients with breast cancer and lymphoma. *Psychooncology, 1,* 105–114.

Mulhern, R. K., Hancock, J., Fairclough, D., & Kun, L. (1992). Neuropsychological status of children treated for brain tumors: A critical review and integrative analysis. *Medical and Pediatric Oncology, 20,* 181–191.

Musick, M. A., Koenig, H. G., Larson, D. B., & Matthews, D. (1998). Religion and spiritual beliefs. In J. C. Holland (Ed.), *Psycho-oncology* (pp. 780–789). New York: Oxford University Press.

Muss, H. B. (1995). Chemotherapy of breast cancer in the older patient. *Seminars in Oncology, 22* (Suppl. 1), 14–16.

Parker, S. L., Davis, K. J., Wingo, P. A., Ries, L. A., & Heath, C. W. (1998). Cancer statistics by race and ethnicity. *CA: A Cancer Journal for Clinicians, 48,* 31–48.

Pennebaker, J. W. (1993). Putting stress into words: Health, linguistic, and therapeutic implications. *Behaviour Research and Therapy, 31,* 539–548.

Pereira, J., Hanson, J., & Bruera, E. (1997). The frequency and clinical course of cognitive impairment in patients with terminal cancer. *Cancer, 69,* 835–841.

Peters-Golden, H. (1982). Breast cancer: Varied perceptions of social support in the illness experience. *Social Science and Medicine, 16,* 483–491.

Portenoy, R. K. (1992). Cancer pain: Pathophysiology and syndromes. *Lancet, 339,* 1026–1031.

Redd, W. (1989). Behavioral interventions to reduce child distress. In J. C. Holland & J. H. Rowland (Eds.), *Handbook of psychooncology* (pp. 573–581). New York: Oxford University Press.

Redd, W. H., & Andrykowski, M. A. (1982). Behavioral intervention in cancer treatment: Controlling aversion reactions to chemotherapy. *Journal of Consulting and Clinical Psychology, 50,* 1018–1029.

Reuben, D. B. (1997). Geriatric assessment in oncology. *Cancer, 80,* 1311–1316.

Rhodes, V., Watson, P., & Hanson, B. (1988). Patients' descriptions of the influence of tiredness and weakness on self-care abilities. *Cancer Nursing, 11,* 186–194.

Richardson, J. L., Shelton, D. R., Krailo, M., & Levine, A. M. (1990). The effect of compliance with treatment on survival among patients with hematologic malignancies. *Journal of Clinical Oncology, 8,* 356–364.

Rieker, P. P., Edbril, S. D., & Garnick, M. B. (1985). Curative testis cancer therapy: Psychosocial sequelae. *Journal of Clinical Oncology, 3,* 1117–1126.

Rowland, J. H. (1989a). Intrapersonal resources: Coping. In J. C. Holland & J. H. Rowland (Eds.), *Handbook of psycho-oncology: Psychological care of the patient with cancer* (pp. 44–57). New York: Oxford University Press.

Rowland, J. H. (1989b). Interpersonal resources: Social support. In J. C. Holland & J. H. Rowland (Eds.), *Handbook of psycho-oncology: Psychological care of the patient with cancer* (pp. 58–71). New York: Oxford University Press.

Rowland, J. H., & Massie, M. J. (1998). Breast cancer. In J. C. Holland (Ed.), *Psycho-oncology* (pp. 380–401). New York: Oxford University Press.

Sanders, J. E ., & the Seattle Marrow Transplant Team (1991). The impact of marrow transplant preparative regimens on subsequent growth and development. *Seminars in Hematology, 28,* 244–249.

Savard, J., Savard, J., & Morin, C. M. (2001). Insomnia in the context of cancer: A review of a neglected problem. *Journal of Clinical Oncology, 19,* 895–908.

Schag, C. C., Heinrich, R. L., & Ganz, P. A. (1984). Karnofsky performance status revisited: Reliability, validity, & guidelines. *Journal of Clinical Oncology, 2,* 187–193.

Scheier, M. F., & Bridges, M. W. (1995). Person variables and health: Personality predispositions and acute psychological states as shared determinants for disease. *Psychosomatic Medicine, 57,* 255–268.

Scheier, M. F., & Carver, C. S. (1985). Optimism, coping, and health: Assessment and implications of generalized outcome expectancies. *Health Psychology, 4,* 219–247.

Schmidt, G. M., Niland, J. C., Forman, S. J., Fonbeuena, P. P., Dagis, A. C., Grant, M. M., et al. (1993). Extended follow-up in 212 long-term allogeneic bone marrow transplant survivors: Issues of quality of life. *Transplantation, 55,* 551–557.

Schulz, R., Williamson, G. M., Knapp, J. E., Bookwala, J., Lave, J., & Fello, M. (1995). The psychological, social and economic impact of illness among patients with recurrent cancer. *Journal of Psychosocial Oncology, 13*(3), 21–45.

Shapiro, W. (1980). Sleep behavior among narcoleptics and cancer patients. *Behavioral Medicine, 7,* 14–21.

Sheely, L. C. (1996). Sleep disturbances in hospitalized patients with cancer. *Oncology Nursing Forum, 23,* 109–111.

Silberfarb, P. M. (1983). Chemotherapy and cognitive defects in cancer patients. *Annual Review of Medicine, 34,* 35–46.

Silberfarb, P. M., Hauri, P. J., Oxman, T. E., & Schnurr, P. (1993). Assessment of sleep in patients with lung cancer and breast cancer. *Journal of Clinical Oncology, 11,* 997–1004.

Smith, S. D., Rosen, D., Trueworthy, R. C., & Lowman, J. T. (1979). A reliable method for evaluating drug compliance in children with cancer. *Cancer, 43,* 169–173.

Spiegel, D., Bloom, J. R., Kraemer, H. C., & Gottheil, E. (1989). Effect of psychosocial treatment on survival of patients with metastatic breast cancer. *Lancet, 2,* 888–891.

Spiegel, D., Bloom, J. R., & Yalom, I. (1981). Group support for patients with metastatic cancer: A randomized prospective outcome study. *Archives of General Psychiatry, 38,* 527–533.

Stavraky, K. M., Donner, A. P., Kincade, J. E., & Stewart, M. A. (1988). The effect of psychosocial factors on lung cancer mortality at one year. *Journal of Clinical Epidemiology, 41,* 75–82.

Syrjala, K. L., Chapko, M. K., Vitaliano, P. P., Cummings, C., & Sullivan, K. M. (1993). Recovery after allogeneic marrow transplantation: Prospective study of predictors of long-term physical and psychosocial functioning. *Bone Marrow Transplantation, 11*, 319–327.

Talcott, J. A., Rieker, P., Clark, J. A., Propert, K. J., Weeks, J. C., Beard, C. J., et al. (1998). Patient-reported symptoms after primary therapy for early prostate cancer: Results of a prospective cohort study. *Journal of Clinical Oncology, 16*, 275–283.

Taylor, S. E. (1983). Adjustment to threatening events: A theory of cognitive adaptation. *American Psychologist, 38*, 1161–1173.

Taylor, S. E., Lichtman, R. R., & Wood, J. V. (1984). Compliance with chemotherapy among breast cancer patients. *Health Psychology, 3*, 553–562.

Tenenbaum, L. (1989). *Cancer chemotherapy: A reference guide.* Philadelphia: W. B. Saunders.

Thranov, I., & Klee, M. (1994). Sexuality among gynecologic cancer patients—a cross-sectional study. *Gynecologic Oncology, 52*, 14–19.

Urba, W. J., & Longo, D. L. (1992). Hodgkin's disease. *New England Journal of Medicine, 326*, 678–687.

van Dam, F. S. A. M., & Schagen, S. B., Muller, M. J., Boogerd, W., Wall, E. V. D., Droogleever Fortuyn, M. E., & Rodenhuis, S. (1998). Impairment of cognitive function in women receiving adjuvant treatment for high-risk breast cancer: High-dose versus standard-dose chemotherapy. *Journal of the National Cancer Institute, 90*, 210–218.

van Eys, J. (1987). Living beyond cure: Transcending survival. *The American Journal of Pediatric Hematology/Oncology, 9*, 114–118.

Van't Spijker, A., Trijsburg, R. W., & Duivenvoorden, H. J. (1997). Psychological sequelae of cancer diagnosis: A meta-analytical review of 58 studies after 1980. *Psychosomatic Medicine, 59*, 280–293.

Vinokur, A. D., Threatt, B. A., Caplan, R. D., & Zimmerman, B. L. (1989). Physical and psychosocial functioning and adjustment to breast cancer: Long term follow-up of a screening population. *Cancer, 63*, 394–405.

Vokes, E. E., Weichselbaum, R. R., Lippman, S. M., & Hong, W. K. (1993). Head and neck cancer. *New England Journal of Medicine, 328*, 184–194.

Walch, S. E., Ahles, T. A., & Saykin, A. J., (1998). Cognitive sequelae of treatment in children. In J. C. Holland (Ed.), *Psycho-oncology* (pp. 940–945). New York: Oxford University Press.

Wallace, K. G., Reed, B. A., Pasero, C., & Olsson, G. L. (1995). Staff nurses' perceptions of barriers to effective pain management. *Journal of Pain and Symptom Management, 10*, 204–213.

Wallston, B. S., Alagna, S. W., DeVellis, B. M., & DeVellis, R. F. (1983). Social support and physical health. *Health Psychology, 2*, 367–391.

Ward, S. E., Goldberg, N., Miller-McCauley, V., Mueller, C., Nolan, A., Pawlik-Plank, D., et al. (1993). Patient-related barriers to management of cancer pain. *Pain, 52*, 319–324.

Watson, M., & Greer, S. (1998). Personality and coping. In J. C. Holland (Ed.), *Psycho-Oncology* (pp. 91–98). New York: Oxford University Press.

Wei, J. Y. (1995). Cardiovascular comorbidity in the older cancer patient. *Seminars in Oncology, 22* (Suppl. 1), 9–10.

Weisman, A. D., & Worden, J. W. (1976). The existential plight in cancer: Significance of the first 100 days. *International Journal of Psychiatry in Medicine, 7,* 1–15.

Winkelman, M. D., & Hines, J. D. (1983). Cerebellar degeneration caused by high-dose cytosine arabinoside: A clinicopathological study. *Annals of Neurology, 14,* 520–527.

Winningham, M. L., Nail, L. M., Burke, M. B., Brophy, L., Cimprich, B., Jones, L. S., et al. (1994). Fatigue and the cancer experience: The state of the knowledge. *Oncology Nursing Forum, 21,* 23–36.

Woo, B., Dibble, S. L., Piper, B. F., Keating, S. B., & Weiss, M. C. (1998). Differences in fatigue by treatment methods in women with breast cancer. *Oncology Nursing Forum, 25,* 915–920.

Yancik, R. (1997). Cancer burden in the aged: An epidemiologic and demographic overview. *Cancer, 80,* 1273–1283.

Zemore, R., Rinholm, J., Shepel, L., & Richards, M. (1989). Some social and emotional consequences of breast cancer and mastectomy: A content analysis of 87 interviews. *Journal of Psychosocial Oncology, 7,* 33–45.

4

Psychosocial Considerations in Essential Hypertension, Coronary Heart Disease, and End-Stage Renal Disease

TIMOTHY W. SMITH
PAUL N. HOPKINS

INTRODUCTION

The emergence and rapid expansion of behavioral medicine and clinical health psychology during the past 30 years has been influenced by a major historical shift in patterns of health and illness. Infectious diseases that were once leading causes of morbidity and mortality in industrialized nations have been brought under substantial control through advances in public health and medicine, such as vaccines, antibiotics, and improved sanitation. Chronic diseases have become the leading causes of death, as well as the primary source of health care expenditure. Many such diseases are caused or at least affected by behavior.

Management of chronic diseases often requires patients to become integral members of the health care team, responsible for adherence to prescribed regimens and even more complex aspects of their care. The modern treatment of chronic disease may extend life, but it often disrupts the patient's quality of life. The development of a clinical psychological science of chronic physical illness is therefore an essential innovation in medical care. The role of behavior in physical health generally, and chronic disease in particular, is formally acknowledged in the current psychiatric nomenclature (see Table 4.1). The potential emotional impact of serious illness is acknowledged elsewhere in the current psychiatric nosology, as in the case of mental or adjustment disorders due to medical conditions.

TABLE 4.1. *DSM-IV* Criteria for Psychological Factors Affecting a Medical Condition

---

A. The presence of a general medical condition (coded on Axis III).
B. Psychological factors affect the general medical condition in at least one of the following ways:
    1. the factors have influenced the course of the medical condition as shown by a close temporal association between the development, exacerbation, or delayed recovery from general medical condition
    2. the factors interfere with treatment of the general medical condition
    3. the factors constitute additional health risks for the individual
    4. stress-related physiological responses precipitate or exacerbate symptoms of a general medical condition.

Reprinted with permission from the *Diagnostic and Statistical Manual of Mental Disorders* (4th ed.). Text Revision. Copyright 2000 American Psychiatric Association.

The three conditions discussed in this chapter are essential hypertension, coronary heart disease, and end-stage renal disease. These three conditions provide clear examples of both the general clinical psychological science of chronic illness and the specific mechanisms identified in current diagnostic criteria. The conditions are related in several ways. For example, essential hypertension is often a contributing factor in both coronary heart disease and end-stage renal disease. Moreover, the three conditions have overlapping modifiable risk factors, such as obesity, diabetes, and smoking. However, their greatest similarity lies in the fact that a variety of psychological considerations are necessary for comprehensive patient care.

ESSENTIAL HYPERTENSION

Essential hypertension is the designation given to persistently elevated blood pressure without a known secondary cause such as renal vascular disease, kidney failure, or excessive aldosterone production from an adrenal tumor. This typically symptomless condition is a major contributing factor in a variety of life-threatening illnesses, including coronary heart disease, stroke, and end-stage renal disease (Foster & Pearson, 1996; U.S. Renal Data System, 2002). Because of increased awareness among the public and medical professionals, dedicated public health efforts, and improvements in medical care, the prevalence of essential hypertension in the United States has decreased over the past decades (American Heart Association [AHA], 2000). However, this improvement in the public's cardiovascular health has slowed in recent years. Estimates suggest that as many as 50 million Americans have essential hypertension (Burt, Whelton, & Roccella, 1995), yet only about two thirds are aware of this condition. Approximately 50% of those affected receive treatment for the condition, and less than a third of individuals receiving treatment have their blood pressure medically controlled to desired levels (Joint National Committee [JNC] on Prevention, Detection, Evaluation, and Treatment of High Blood Pressure, 1997). The serious impact of this condition is evident in the fact that coronary heart disease and stroke are the first and third most common causes of death, respectively, in the United States. They account for more than $250 billion dollars in health care expenditures and lost productivity each year (JNC, 1997). Essential hypertension is also responsible for about 25% of cases of end-stage renal disease, a condition responsible for almost $18 billion in annual treatment expenditures (National Institutes of Health, 1993).

Definition and Epidemiology of Hypertension

Determinants of Blood Pressure and Definition of Hypertension

Blood pressure reflects the force exerted by circulating blood against the arterial wall. Systolic blood pressure (SBP) is the force associated with the contraction of the heart; diastolic blood pressure (DBP) refers to the force between contractions. Although the physiological determinants of blood pressure are complex, for simplicity they can be considered to involve three factors: cardiac output, peripheral resistance, and blood volume. Cardiac output refers to the volume of blood ejected from the left ventricle of the heart into the aorta per minute, which increases with more rapid and vigorous contraction of the heart muscle. When other influences on blood pressure are held constant, increased cardiac output increases blood pressure. Peripheral resistance refers to the force against which blood moves during circulation. Peripheral resistance increases when the major vascular beds (e.g., muscles, skin, digestive organs, etc.) constrict, also producing a rise in blood pressure. Changes in the resistance to blood flow may be transitory, such as during exercise or after eating, or they may be long-term, as in the case of arteriosclerosis or hardening of the arteries. Cardiac output is in part determined by blood volume, as the heart increases the force of contraction in proportion to the amount of blood returned to it by the venous circulation. Retention of excess fluid in the blood, as is seen in some forms of kidney disease, increases blood volume and can produce increased blood pressure through this mechanism. These simple influences on blood pressure are useful in understanding the mechanisms of action of drug treatments for hypertension as well as the way behavioral factors may influence blood pressure.

Table 4.2 presents the current criteria for the diagnosis of essential hypertension (JNC, 1997). The risk of coronary heart disease, stroke, end-stage renal disease, and other serious medical conditions increases across the full range of blood pressure (National High Blood Pressure Education Program Working Group, 1994; Neaton & Wentworth, 1992). Hence, although reducing high blood pressure within the more severe classifications is a pressing medical priority, there are health benefits to reductions at all levels above normal.

TABLE 4.2. Joint National Committee Classification of Blood
Pressure for Adults Aged 18 and Over

Category	Blood pressure, mmHg		
	Systolic		Diastolic
Optimal	< 120	and	< 80
Normal	< 130	and	< 85
High-normal	130–139	or	85–89
Hypertension			
Stage 1	140–159	or	90– 99
Stage 2	160–179	or	100–109
Stage 3	180	or	110

Source: National Heart, Lung and Blood Institute.

Assessment of Blood Pressure

Blood pressure is quite variable across both time and assessment settings. Therefore, diagnosis of the presence and severity of hypertension requires repeated measurements by trained medical personnel with approved devices. The standard recommendations are that the patient be seated in a firm-backed chair with the arms supported at heart level. Measurement of both SBP and DBP should be taken following 5 min of rest, without talking, and by at least two readings separated by 2 min, which should be averaged (JNC, 1997). Readings below 130/85mmHg suggest that no further assessment is necessary. Progressively shorter intervals to a second assessment are recommended when higher blood pressures are obtained at the initial assessment. For example, levels of 140/90 should be reassessed within two months, whereas levels of 180/110 or higher should be referred for possible treatment immediately (JNC, 1997).

Blood pressures measured in a doctor's office or other clinical setting are often uncharacteristically high (Mancia, Saga, Milesi, Cesana, & Zanchetti, 1997). This phenomenon is sometimes called "white coat hypertension," referring to anxiety evoked by the clinical setting, which may evoke a brief, substantial, but artificial, rise in blood pressure (Myers & Reeves, 1991; Siegel, Blumenthal, & Divine, 1990). Multiple assessment occasions are warranted in such cases, and ambulatory assessment may be indicated. Ambulatory blood pressure assessments involve a standard occluding cuff attached to a small computerized recording device. The apparatus is worn for a period of a day or more, with measurements taken at varying intervals. Ambulatory assessments can provide a more accurate measurement of the patient's "true" blood pressure, and not surprisingly have been found to have more prognostic value than traditional clinic-based assessments (Appel & Stason, 1993; Verdecchia, Porcellati, & Schillaci, 1994).

Epidemiology and Risk Factors

Regardless of how it is assessed, essential hypertension is not randomly distributed in the population. Blood pressure increases with age, such that high blood pressure of all severity grades is more common in older individuals. Hypertension runs in families, most likely reflecting shared lifestyle risk factors, genetics, or the combination of these influences (Ward, 1990). The specific mechanisms of genetic influences on hypertension are not clearly established and are likely to involve a variety of influences in the multifactorial physiologic regulation of blood pressure (Hunt, Hopkins, & Williams, 1996; Lander & Schork, 1994). Essential hypertension is more common among African Americans than among any other ethnic group in the United States (Horan & Mockrin, 1992). It is also much more common among industrialized cultures than among "primitive" cultures, in part because of related differences in body weight, diet, physical activity levels, and stress (Stamler, Stamler, & Neaton, 1993).

Statistical associations between modifiable risk factors and incidence of essential hypertension provide the rationale for behavioral approaches to the disorder. Obesity and physical inactivity are well-established risk factors for high blood pressure, and there is evidence that excessive consumption of salt and alcohol are also important (Stamler et al., 1993). As a result, modification of these "lifestyle" risk factors constitute the core of nonpharmacological approaches.

Evidence from a variety of human and animal research suggests that psychological stress and related emotional factors can contribute to the development of hypertension (Harshfield & Grim, 1997; Lovallo, 1997; Pickering, 1997). For example, chronic job stress is associated with increases in blood pressure (Schnall, Schwartz, Landsbergis, Warren, & Pickering, 1998), as well as the development of hypertensive end-organ damage (e.g., left ventricular hypertrophy) (Schnall, Pieper, & Schwartz, 1990). The tendency to experience anger and respond to it in maladaptive ways (e.g., suppressing or responding aggressively) also increases the risk of developing hypertension (Everson et al., 1998). The specific effects of stress on the etiology of high blood pressure may differ across the natural history of the condition. In early stages, particularly large transitory increases in blood pressure and heart rate (i.e., heightened cardiac output) in response to environmental stressors may be involved (Manuck, 1994). In later stages of the condition, changes in the peripheral vasculature (i.e., increased resistance) and renal function (i.e., increased sodium and fluid retention in response to stress) may mediate the effects of stress on sustained high blood pressure (Lovallo & Wilson, 1992). However, evidence of the role of stress in the development of essential hypertension is not as compelling as the role of other "lifestyle" risk factors, such as obesity, though it is sufficient to warrant consideration in the management of the condition.

Medical Evaluation and the Stepped-Care Approach to Management

After a reliable assessment of persistent high blood pressure, medical evaluation is directed toward the known secondary causes of high blood pressure, assessment of the presence and extent of end-organ damage, and the identification of other cardiovascular risk factors and conditions that may influence prognosis and guide treatment (JNC, 1997). A variety of medical disorders can produce elevations in blood pressure (e.g., kidney disease), and most are treatable. However, these conditions probably account for less than 5% of persons found to have high blood pressure. The assessment of end-organ damage primarily involves evaluation of possible coronary heart disease, cerebrovascular disease, left ventricular hypertrophy, nephropathy, retinopathy, and peripheral artery disease. The potential risk factors evaluated include smoking, blood lipids, diabetes, family history of cardiovascular disease, age, and sex. Risk groupings are made on the basis of the severity of hypertension and the presence of risk factors and end-organ damage. The aggressiveness of treatment is determined by this risk stratification process. For example, with mild hypertension and no other risk factors, lifestyle modification would likely be the sole element of an initial treatment approach. With more severe hypertension or the presence of diabetes or cardiovascular disease, drug therapies would be included in the initial treatment approach (JNC, 1997).

Once a diagnosis of essential hypertension is made and the level of risk classified, the clinical approach to the condition is one of sequential implementation of graded interventions. The first step may include the lifestyle modifications of weight loss, increased physical activity, smoking cessation, and reductions in sodium and alcohol intake. The success of these interventions is assessed over the ensuing months and may be adequate to achieve blood pressures within the desired range. If not, then medication is typically introduced. Common classes of medications include: diuretics (e.g., hydrochlorothiazide), which reduce blood pressure by reducing blood volume; beta-blockers (e.g., propranolol hydrochloride, "Inderol"), which have multiple mechanisms of action including reducing cardiac output; ACE inhibitors (e.g., catopril); and calcium blockers (e.g., diltiazem), which dilate the vasculature. The general pharmacological approach is to begin with low dosages of one agent and increase the dosage until acceptable control is achieved. If the response to the initial drug is not adequate, then a different drug may be prescribed. Alternatively, low doses of a second drug of a different class may be added to the first and increased until control is achieved. Combination therapy involving low doses of two drugs often has an additional benefit of reducing the severity of undesirable side effects. A growing variety of medications are available, each with specific indications. This variety provides physicians with the opportunity to make tailored selections, providing many alternatives to a patient's limited response to initial treatment.

Behavioral Interventions

Many cases of cardiovascular disease occur in individuals whose blood pressure is above the desirable range of 120/80 mmHg but below the level required for the diagnosis of essential hypertension. As a result, "lifestyle" or behavioral interventions described here are potentially useful as general principles of public health rather than specific treatments only for hypertension (Kannel, 1996; Stamler, 1991). For a comprehensive, recent review of behavioral approaches to hypertension, see Blumenthal, Sherwood, Gullette, Georgiades, and Tweedy (2002).

Diet and Weight Loss

Dietary interventions have been shown to reduce blood pressure among individuals with high normal blood pressure and those with other hypertension risk factors (e.g., obesity). For example, the DASH diet (Dietary Approaches to Stop Hypertension) consists of a balanced combination of high levels of fruits, vegetables, grains, and minerals (i.e., potassium, calcium, magnesium) with low levels of saturated fat, and it produces sustained reductions in blood pressure among persons with high normal blood pressure (Appel, Moore, & Obarznek, 1997). Several large clinical trials have indicated that interventions specifically designed to reduce blood pressure through restricting dietary intake of sodium have produced some benefits (Midgley, Matthew, Greenwood, & Logan, 1996), though somewhat less substantial than those observed with weight loss (Dubbert, 1995). It is possible that a subset of hypertensive patients may be responsive to the effects of salt, and as a result this group may benefit substantially from sodium restriction.

Several well-controlled clinical trials indicate that weight loss interventions can produce clinically significant reductions in blood pressure among patients with essential hypertension (Dubbert, 1995; JNC, 1997). A loss of as little as ten pounds can have beneficial effects (Trials of Hypertension Prevention Collaborative Research Group, 1997). Further, weight loss may also increase the effectiveness of antihypertensive medication (Neaton et al., 1993).

The benefits of weight loss must be balanced by a realistic view of the degree and stability of weight loss in most intervention programs. Regrettably, obesity has proven to be difficult to treat, especially when sustained rather than initial weight loss is considered as the outcome. Whether patients are treated by professional, self-help, or commercial approaches to weight reduction, an initial loss of 10–20% of body weight is typical. The specific components of weight loss interventions are not a critical consideration, as the standard practice includes multicomponent treatments: reduced calorie and fat intake; self-monitoring; stimulus control techniques to reduce exposure to cues that evoke the urge to over-eat; instruction to change eating behavior (e.g., eating more slowly);

and moderate exercise (Friedman & Brownell, 1996; Clark & Goldstein, 1995). For a recent review of behavioral approaches to weight loss and the management of obesity, see Wadden, Brownell, and Foster (2002).

Despite initial effectiveness, the majority of patients regain most of the weight lost within one year of treatment (Foreyt & Goodrick, 1994; Wilson, 1994; Wing & Klem, 1997). The initial weight loss is sufficient to reduce blood pressure to acceptable levels, or at least enough to reduce the risk of most of the serious medical consequences of hypertension. The challenge of this behavioral approach to treating high blood pressure is the maintenance of weight loss. Several approaches to maintenance hold promise, such as relapse prevention training (Brownell, Marlatt, Lichtenstein, & Wilson, 1986; Collier & Marlatt, 1995; Marlatt & Gordon, 1985) during the initial treatment phase, cultivation of social support for weight loss, and home-based or lifestyle interventions to increase physical activity levels (Wing & Jeffery, 1999; Andersen et al., 1999; Perri, Martin, Leemakers, Sears, & Notelovitz, 1997). It may be that some of the difficulty in the maintenance of initial weight loss stems from the fact that patients fail to achieve ideal weights or body sizes (Brownell & Rodin, 1994; Foster, Wadden, Vogt, & Brewer, 1997), resulting in discouragement. However, reductions in weight far smaller than those needed to achieve ideal body size have important effects on blood pressure. Hence, weight loss in the context of treating hypertension should emphasize this fact in developing the patient's commitment to maintenance.

Physical Activity

It is well established that a sedentary lifestyle is associated with increased risk of essential hypertension (Paffenbarger, Jung, Leung, & Hyde, 1991). Although some well-controlled studies suggest little or no beneficial effects of exercise training on blood pressure (e.g., Blumenthal, Siegel, & Appelbaum, 1991), recent quantitative and qualitative reviews of available studies suggest that regular aerobic exercise reduces blood pressure by 5–7mmHg (Arroll & Beaglehole, 1992; Kelly & McClellan, 1994; Miller, Balady, & Fletcher, 1997). Current treatment guidelines (JNC, 1997) include exercise as a recommended behavioral approach. Initial increases in exercise have been obtained with a variety of approaches, including behavioral contracting and goal-setting, self-monitoring, and training in distraction during exercise (Dubbert, 2002; Dubbert & Stetson, 1995).

As with weight loss, interventions to increase physical activity suggest that the long-term maintenance of the behavior is difficult (Sallis et al., 1990). Consideration of the patient's readiness for increased exercise levels, and tailoring of interventions to this "stage of change" (Prochaska & DiClemente, 1984), have been found to improve outcomes (Calfas et al., 1996). Patients often complain that lack of time, disruptions in routine, and limited access to exercise facilities are common barriers to maintaining such regimens. Therefore, home-based

(King, Haskell, Young, Oka, & Stefanick, 1995) and lifestyle approaches (Dunn et al., 1999) have been developed as alternatives to traditional intervention programs. In contrast to the typical approach, home and lifestyle approaches focus on increasing activity levels in the course of daily routines, leisure and recreational activities, and other elements of an otherwise sedentary individual's typical schedule.

Stress Management

Despite the apparent role of stress in the development and outcome of essential hypertension, stress-reducing interventions have generally not been effective in the management of high blood pressure (Dubbert, 1995; JNC, 1997). Relaxation training, biofeedback, stress management training, and related techniques have all been evaluated in controlled studies, and many individual reports have found beneficial effects. However, quantitative and qualitative reviews of the literature have not supported the efficacy of these interventions. This contrasts sharply with the apparent benefits of similar techniques in managing coronary heart disease, as reviewed later in this chapter.

Comprehensive or Multicomponent Lifestyle Approaches

Several well-controlled clinical trials have found that interventions addressing several lifestyle risk factors simultaneously have beneficial effects on essential hypertension (e.g., Stamler et al., 1987; 1989). Interventions targeted toward weight loss, dietary changes, and exercise and physical activity levels have many common intervention foci and may be combined in a potentially effective manner. One such example is the Multiple Risk Factor Intervention Trial (MRFIT, 1985). This multicenter controlled trial of over 12,000 men with high levels of cardiovascular risk factors evaluated a multicomponent intervention consisting of smoking cessation, stepped care for hypertension, dietary change, and physical activity. Although the intervention did not have a statistically significant benefit on mortality in the entire sample when compared to an appropriate control group, there were beneficial effects on total mortality and cardiovascular death rates among the subsample of men with essential hypertension (MRFIT, 1990).

Pharmacological Interventions

There is now clear and compelling evidence that pharmacological treatments are not only effective in reducing blood pressure among patients with essential hypertension but also in reducing the negative health outcomes associated with this condition, such as left ventricular hypertrophy, coronary heart disease, stroke, and death from cardiovascular causes (Moser & Helbart, 1996; Psaty,

Smith, & Siscovick, 1997). These benefits are even more apparent among elderly, high-risk patients (MacMahon & Rodgers, 1993). The most recent treatment guidelines (JNC, 1997) are based on clear evidence of this effectiveness, and more recent controlled trials provide further support (Hannson, Zanchetti, & Carruthers, 1998;Hannson, Lindholm, & Niskman, 1999). Indeed, it appears that though there are specific indications for individual drugs and combinations, the lowering of blood pressure, regardless of agent, is more important than the type of drug used in reducing morbidity and mortality (Moser, 1999).

The Problem of Adherence

Despite the obvious benefits of antihypertensive medication, many patients do not adhere to their prescribed regimen. Estimates of nonadherence range from 25–50%, depending on whether patient self-reports or pill counts are used as a criterion (Burke, Dunbar-Jacob, & Hill, 1997; Dunbar-Jacob, Burke, & Puczynski, 1995). This obviously poses a critical challenge in clinical care. A variety of approaches are beneficial, including additional patient education, external reminders, self-monitoring, telephone prompts, and efforts to increase appointment keeping (Burke et al., 1997). Further, the improvements in adherence resulting from these interventions have beneficial effects on cardiovascular disease morbidity and mortality (Pearson & Feinberg, 1997).

Particularly important to treatment adherence is the patient's conceptualization and experience of the condition (Leventhal, Diefenbach, & Leventhal, 1992), since essential hypertension has few, if any, reliable symptoms. The initial diagnosis of high blood pressure is often made during routine checkups or health care visits for other purposes. The patient is rarely *seeking* an evaluation because of a concern about possibly having high blood pressure. As a result, reactions to receiving this initial diagnosis can range from appropriate concern to confusion over the importance and meaning of information. Because they do not feel ill, some patients may even discount the seriousness of the diagnosis. In the absence of any subjective evidence that they are sick, patients may not be motivated to make difficult changes in lifestyle or adhere to drug regimens that produce unpleasant side effects.

Some patients can identify changes in their blood pressure to a greater degree than expected by chance (Brondolo, Rosen, Kasbis, & Schwartz, 1999). However, many patients cannot and those who can are quite limited in this ability. Nonetheless, more report the belief that they can detect changes in blood pressure, and may make decisions about medication adherence based on this very imperfect information (Baumann & Leventhal, 1985; Meyer, Leventhal, & Gutmann, 1985). In contrast to the symptomless nature of high blood pressure, antihypertensive regimens often have unpleasant side effects, such as the fatigue associated with beta-blockers and decreased sexual response which can occur with most classes of antihypertensive medication. Hence, patients' informal theories about their blood pressure can often lead to the "detection" of reasons to skip a prescribed dose. Lifestyle interventions can reduce the dosage of or even need for antihypertensive medication. Further, newer drugs or drug combinations can reduce side effects. Nonetheless, problematic levels of nonadherence are common. Clinical attention to the problem of nonadherence and consideration of the patient's construing of the condition and the associated treatment regimen are important components of comprehensive clinical care for essential hypertension. It is also the case that even in the absence of clinical signs of cerebrovascular disease, many patients with hypertension display mild cognitive impairments on neuropsychological examinations, presumably reflecting mild but detectable impairment in brain function (Waldstein, 1995; Waldstein et al., 1996). Hence, poor adherence attributed to "forgetfulness" could reflect mild cognitive deficits.

CORONARY HEART DISEASE

As noted above, coronary heart disease is the leading cause of death in the United States and many other industrialized nations (AHA, 2002). Although death rates from coronary heart disease have decreased over the past three decades, this improvement has slowed in recent years. A large body of epidemiological research indicates the importance of behavior in the development of this condition, and the clinical literature in cardiology has long noted the role of psychological factors in the patient's adaptation and survival. As a result, behavioral cardiology or cardiac psychology (Allan & Scheidt, 1996) is one of the most extensively developed sub-fields at the interface of behavioral science and medicine. For recent reviews of the role of psychosocial factors in the development, course, and management of CHD, see Smith and Ruiz (2002).

Anatomy and Pathophysiology

The term coronary heart disease refers to several clinical manifestations of a single underlying disease process (for reviews, see Scheidt, 1996; Smith & Leon, 1992). Coronary atherosclerosis refers to the progressive buildup of cholesterol deposits on the interior walls of the blood vessels that bring blood, oxygen, and other nutrients to the heart muscle (i.e., myocardium). As depicted in Figure 4.1, the first arterial branches from the aorta are the coronary arteries. These vessels travel on the surface of the myocardium, branch apart (i.e., bifurcate), penetrate the heart muscle, and bifurcate repeatedly. Various regions of the myocardium are served by different sections of this arterial system. The earliest atherosclerotic changes in the coronary arteries appear in middle or late childhood (Strong et al., 1999). This condition grows slowly and silently, or asymptomatically, for decades. Current research on the atherosclerotic process suggests that the initiating event is injury to or inflammatory activation of the lining or endothelium of the artery. At the site of this inflammation, monocytes and other white blood

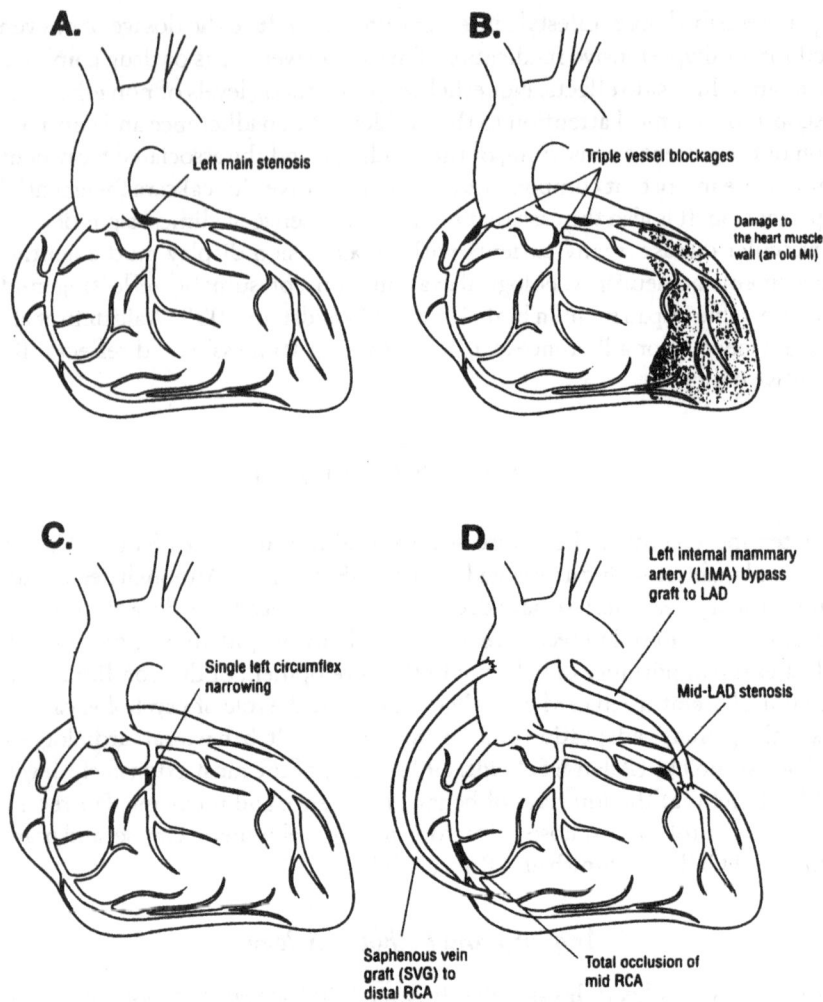

FIGURE 4.1. Diagram of coronary arteries and locations of coronary lesions. From "A Whirlwind Tour of Cardiology for the Mental Health Professional," by S. Scheidt, 1996, in R. Allan and S. Scheidt (Eds.), *Heart and Mind: The Practice of Cardiac Psychology.* Reprinted with permission of the American Psychological Association.

cells are transformed to macrophages. Macrophages, in turn, absorb lipoproteins in an uncontrolled fashion, being thereby transformed to *foam cells*—the hallmark of atherosclerotic lesions. These changes within the arterial wall are accelerated in individuals with high levels of low-density lipoprotein and other atherogenic particles circulating in the blood stream. The growing cholesterol-rich deposit is initially accommodated by an expanding artery wall rather than by encroachment into the opening (i.e., lumen) of the artery. Such encroachment develops later in the disease course, progressively narrowing the opening through which blood can flow. This lesion or plaque is eventually covered with a fibrous, calcified cap. Late in the disease course, the calcified, fibrous cap of the coronary lesions may rupture or fragment. The exposed plaque promotes deposition of blood clots (i.e., thrombi) on the disrupted plaque. These episodes lead to acute coronary events, such as unstable angina or myocardial infarction.

Coronary artery disease is the progressive structural pathology underlying clinical manifestations of coronary heart disease. It contributes to myocardial ischemia, the relative insufficiency of oxygen supply to the heart. Contractions of the heart require oxygen; more rapid and forceful contractions—such as those occurring during physical exertion—require more oxygen. When the heart's demand for oxygen exceeds the supply available, myocardial ischemia results. Advanced coronary artery disease makes this more likely because less blood can flow through narrowed arteries. Also, at the site of coronary artery lesions, transient muscular constriction of the artery (i.e., "spasm") can occur, further reducing blood flow. Ischemia can be severe during a thrombolytic event, because of the drastically restricted blood flow.

Angina pectoris is the chest pain and related discomfort associated with myocardial ischemia. It is a transient symptom, often brought on by activities that provoke ischemia through increased myocardial demand for oxygen (e.g., climbing stairs). Ambulatory monitoring of signs of ischemia in ECG recording has revealed that many episodes of ischemia are not accompanied by pain, discomfort, or other symptoms (e.g., shortness of breath). This phenomenon is called silent ischemia.

Myocardial infarction refers to the death of heart muscle due to severe and prolonged ischemia. This is commonly the result of thrombosis. The location of the infarction is determined by the location of the underlying coronary artery lesion. Heart muscle otherwise nourished by this portion of the arterial circulation is vulnerable to infarction if the occlusion and resulting ischemia are sufficiently severe and prolonged. The medical implications of a myocardial infarction are determined by its location and size. For example, death of a small portion of the right side of the heart can be relatively inconsequential, because the right atrium (i.e., upper chamber) fills the right ventricle, which in turn circulates blood at low pressure through the lungs. In contrast, the left ventricle must generate much higher pressure, sufficient for the systemic circulation. Hence, damage to the left side of the heart can severely impair the heart's capacity to respond to metabolic demands of even routine activities. Some infarcts can disrupt the heart's ability to propagate the electrical impulse necessary for coordinated contraction of the myocardium. The result is disturbances in heart rhythm (i.e., arrhythmias), discussed below. A severely damaged heart muscle resulting in severe restriction of pumping effectiveness is a common cause of congestive heart failure. The term "failure" simply refers to the very poor pump performance, and "congestive" refers to a buildup of excess fluid in the lungs as pressure from the failing left ventricle backs up into the lungs.

The third major clinical manifestation of coronary heart disease is sudden coronary death, defined as death within 1 h of symptom onset in a person not expected to die. On autopsy, such patients are typically found to have severe coronary artery disease, often with recent thrombus formation but no signs of recent myocardial infarction (though they may have old infarcts). Among patients who are resuscitated during an unfolding sudden cardiac death, some (but not most) develop myocardial infarction in the hospital. Hence, the mechanism underlying sudden cardiac death is not infarction. Rather, it is a catastrophic deterioration in heart rhythm. The heart normally contracts via the orderly propagation of an electrical impulse across the myocardium, producing the coordinated, two-step contraction (i.e., "lub-dub") necessary for the filling of the ventricles by the atria, and then the immediately following discharge of blood from the ventricles into the lungs or rest of the body. Ischemia produces disturbances in this rhythm, the most severe of which is ventricular fibrillation. Rather than the coordinated propagation of electrical impulse and heart contraction, in ventricular fibrillation the ventricle muscle twitches chaotically. The heart then ceases to function as an effective pump; lack of oxygen supply to the brain results in death within 6 min unless successful cardiopulmonary resuscitation (CPR) is initiated immediately. About 300,000 sudden coronary deaths occur each year in the United States. For a third or more of these patients, it was their first indication of cardiovascular disease.

The temporal relationship between coronary artery disease and its symptomatic manifestations are depicted in Figure 4.2. This diagram makes clear that associations between risk factors and the development of coronary heart disease could reflect an influence at any point along this decades-long process. Risk fac-

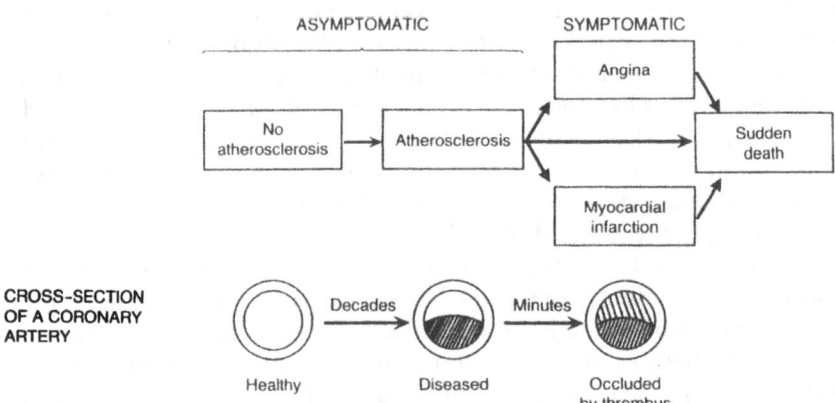

FIGURE 4.2. Relationship of coronary artery disease to manifestations of coronary heart disease. From R. S. Ross, 1975. "Ischemic Heart Disease: An Overview." *American Journal of Cardiology, 36,* 496–505. Copyright 1975 by the American Journal of Cardiology. Adapted with permission.

tors may contribute to the initial endothelial injury or inflammatory activation, deposition of cholesterol at the injury site, plaque rupture, clotting, or thrombosis. Similarly, intervention can be directed toward prevention, slowing, or even reversal of coronary artery disease, or the prevention of ischemia in patients who already have significant coronary artery disease.

There are other types of heart disease, such as valvular heart disease (pathologies of the valves that regulate blood flow into and out of the heart chambers) and cardiomyopathy (diseases of the heart muscle itself). Coronary heart disease is far more common than these conditions and poses much more of a threat to public health. Many of the diagnostic tests, treatment approaches, and psychosocial considerations are similar, but these conditions lie beyond our present scope.

Risk Factors

Several unmodifiable factors confer an increased risk of coronary heart disease; for example, age; male sex, and family history of cardiovascular disease. There are also modifiable risk factors, three of which have the strongest statistical association with coronary disease; such as high cholesterol levels (specifically, low-density lipoprotein), hypertension, and smoking. Moreover, they have a synergistic effect, such that the presence of more than one confers a greater risk than the simple sum of their separate risks. They increase chances for the initial development of coronary disease as well as recurrence. Other modifiable risk factors include obesity, sedentary lifestyle, and diabetes. As with the other modifiable risk factors, these risk factors are associated with both the initial development and the recurrence of disease. Desired levels of these risk factors are presented in Table 4.3.

Psychosocial factors are also associated with increased risk of coronary heart disease (Adler & Matthews, 1994). These include inadequate social support or

TABLE 4.3. Risk Factor Goals

LDL cholesterol	< 100 mg/dl (ideal)
HDL cholesterol	> 40 mg/dl
Triglycerides	< 150
Blood pressure	< 120/80 mmHg (ideal)
Nonsmoking status and no secondary exposure	
Body mass index	18.5–25 kg/m²
Moderate intensity physical activity	> 30 min/day
Vigorous exercise	> 20 min/ 3 times per week
Fasting blood plasma glucose	< 110 mg/dl

Source: Adapted from T. A. Pearson, S. N. Blair, S. R. Daniels, R. H. Eckels, J. M. Fair, S. P. Fortmann, et al. (2002). AHA guidelines for primary prevention of cardiovascular disease and stroke: 2002 update. *Circulation, 106,* 388–391.

social isolation (Berkman, 1995; Uchino et al., 1996), "Type A" behavior (Miller, Turner, Tindale, Posavac, & Dugoni, 1991); anger and hostility (Miller et al., 1996), and depression and anxiety (Frasure-Smith, Lesperance, & Talajic, 1993; Kawachi, Sparrow, Volkonas, & Weiss, 1994; for reviews, see Kubzansky, Kawachi, Weiss, & Sparrow, 1998; Wulsin, Valiant, & Wells, 1999). As noted above, it is not clear whether these psychosocial characteristics influence the development of coronary artery disease itself, precipitate clinical manifestations of coronary heart disease, or both. It is known, however, that stress and related psychosocial factors can promote atherosclerosis, as indicated in experiments with nonhuman primates (Manuck, Marsland, Kaplan, & Williams, 1995).

Stressful environmental circumstances and chronic negative emotions (e.g., anxiety, depression) could promote the initial occurrence of disease through the influence of behaviors such as smoking, poor diet, or physical inactivity. However, statistical control of these behaviors does not eliminate the association of psychosocial risk factors with coronary disease in epidemiological research (Adler & Matthews, 1994; Smith & Gallo, 1994). The prevailing view is that they reflect the cumulative impact of the physiological components of stress. For example, the personality traits of anger and hostility are associated with larger increases in blood pressure, heart rate, and circulating neuroendocrine substances (e.g., catecholamines and cortisol; see Smith & Gallo, 1999). In contrast, social support is associated with smaller physiological stress responses (Uchino et al., 1996). A growing body of research indicates that these responses can initiate and hasten the progression of atherosclerosis (Manuck, 1994; Manuck et al., 1995), and contribute to the precipitation of the clinical manifestations of coronary heart disease (Kamarck & Jennings, 1991; Kop, 1999).

Among patients with established coronary disease, those who are depressed and socially isolated are more likely to have recurrent cardiac events and reduced survival (Berkman, Leo-Summers, & Horowitz., 1992; Carney, Rich, & Freedland, 1988; Frasure-Smith et al., 1993; Ruberman, Weinblatt, Goldberg, & Chadhary, 1984; Williams, Barefoot, & Califf, 1992). Diagnostic techniques used in the clinical evaluation of cardiac disease provide important opportunities to examine psychosocial risk factors as precipitants of myocardial ischemia. For example, the ambulatory electrocardiogram (i.e., Holter monitor) has been used in conjunction with daily diaries to demonstrate that the occurrence of psychological stress during daily activities evokes ischemia—much of it "silent" (Barry et al., 1988; Krantz et al., 1993; Krantz, Hedges, Gabbay, Gottdiener, & Rozanski, 1994). Hostile coronary patients display more episodes of ischemia during daily activities (Helmers et al., 1993). Increased frequency of ischemia during ambulatory monitoring of daily activities is associated with greater risk of angina, cardiac arrhythmias, and sudden cardiac death (Gottlieb et al., 1988).

Laboratory assessment techniques have also been used to demonstrate that emotional stress can precipitate ischemia in coronary patients. For example, Rozanski and his colleagues (1988) measured transient ischemia through the use of radionuclide ventriculography (see below) and found that giving a brief speech about one's personal shortcomings evoked ischemia in patients with coronary artery disease. Ironson and colleagues (1992) found that discussion of an anger-arousing event produced a transient drop in the pumping effectiveness of the left ventricle, a sign of ischemia called left ventricle ejection fraction (i.e., percentage of blood ejected from the left ventricle during myocardial contraction). The effects of anger arousal on ischemia may account for the fact that episodes of anger sometimes precipitate myocardial infarctions (Mittleman et al., 1995). Mental stress can also cause temporary constriction of the coronary arteries at the site of coronary lesions (Yueng et al., 1991) and increase platelet aggregation (the tendency of blood cells to stick together; Kop, 1999). This set of psychophysiological influences on the development of coronary artery disease and precipitation of acute coronary syndromes is depicted in Figure 4.3 (Kop, 1999). Through the mechanism of physiological stress responses, psychosocial risk factors clearly influence coronary heart disease, making stress-reducing interventions a potentially valuable adjunct to traditional medical approaches.

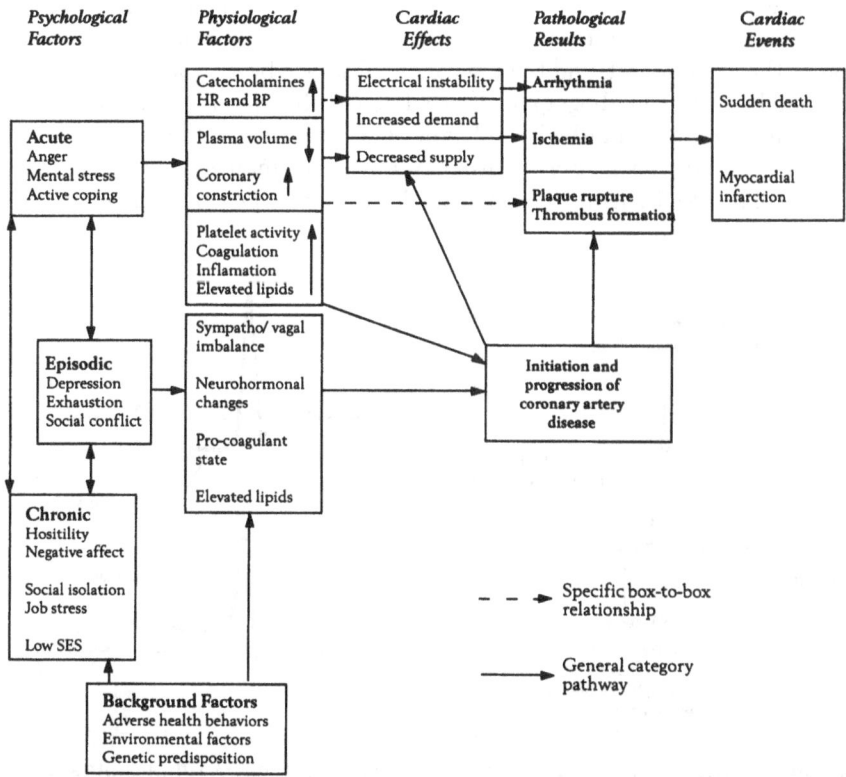

FIGURE 4.3. Psychophysiological influences on coronary artery disease and coronary heart disease. From W. J. Kop, 1999, "Chronic and Acute Psychological Risk Factors for Clinical Manifestations of Coronary Artery Disease." *Psychosomatic Medicine, 61,* 476–487. Reprinted with permission of Lippincott, Williams & Wilkins.

Routine Assessment and Management

Typical care of the coronary patient differs depending whether it is in the context of stable coronary symptoms or an acute coronary crisis. In nonemergent care, patients reporting symptoms of possible disease (e.g., pain, pressure, or shortness of breath during physical exertion) or those with high levels of risk may undergo a variety of tests. The stress ECG (often known as the "stress test") involves recording of the electrocardiogram while progressively increasing physical exertion (e.g., treadmill or bicycle ergometer). In patients with significant coronary artery disease, myocardial demand for oxygen during exercise outstrips the compromised supply, producing ischemia. As depicted in Figure 4.4, this produces a well-established change in the ECG, known as S-T segment depression. S-T segment depression and other ECG anomalies can also be detected by ambulatory ECG monitoring (i.e., Holter monitoring). Both techniques are useful in determining the existence of coronary disease, as well as detecting silent myocardial ischemia.

The stress "thallium scan" is a more sensitive refinement of the exercise ECG. Radioactive thallium is administered intravenously just prior to termination of the exercise test, and the uptake of substance by myocardial tissues is detected by a special radiographic device. Because thallium is carried by blood cells, this uptake is diminished in ischemic or necrotic parts of the heart. Hence, regions that show poor uptake during exercise, but improve after exercise is stopped, indicated ischemic sections of the heart muscle. Regions of poor uptake

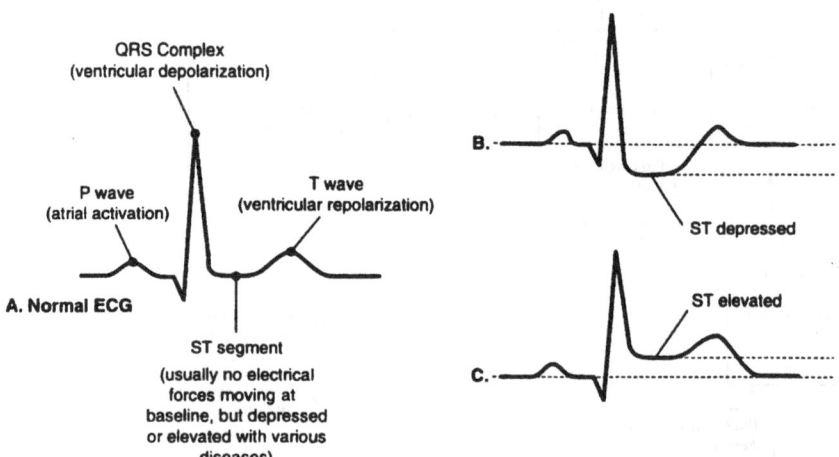

FIGURE 4.4. Normal and Ischemic ECG. From S. Scheidt, 1996, "A Whirlwind Tour of Cardiology for the Mental Health Professional," in R. Allen and S. Scheidt (Eds.), *Heart and Mind: The Practice of Cardiac Psychology* (pp. 15–62). Washington, DC: American Psychological Association. Reprinted with permission of the American Psychological Association.

that do not improve after exercise is stopped reflect the location of prior myocardial infarctions.

Blood pool imaging (i.e., radionuclide ventriculography) and stress echocardiography (i.e., ultrasound techniques) are additional ways of detecting ischemia. They are also used to assess the extent of damage to the left ventricle, as they are used to quantify the ejection fraction and the presence and severity of the ventricular wall motion abnormalities, which are indicators of transient ischemia or prior myocardial damage. (For a review of these techniques and their use in behavioral cardiology, see Rozanski, 1998). These tests produce at most minimal physical discomfort. However, given the seriousness of the diagnostic question, some patients are quite anxious during these procedures.

When one or more of these tests is positive, further testing by cardiac angiography to determine the precise location and extent of coronary artery lesions responsible for ischemia is usually indicated. Because the lesions are on the inside surface of the artery, an invasive test is required—cardiac angiography with coronary arteriography. Precise location and severity must be known in order to select the best approach to medical or surgical management. A small incision is made in either the femoral or brachial artery, and a thin catheter is threaded through the arterial system into the right and then left coronary arteries. A radio-opaque dye is then ejected into the arteries and filmed at high speed. When replayed in slow motion, the locations and severity of coronary lesions or occlusions are revealed as narrowed portions or abrupt ending of the dye path. The procedure is usually safe and well-tolerated, with complications (e.g., injury to the artery or MI) occurring in a small percentage of cases. However, in this 1–2-h hospital-based procedure, the patient must remain awake and comply with simple requests, such as breath holding and lying still during imaging. The physical discomfort involved in the test is only moderate, as the incisions are preceded by a local anesthetic. Some patients report a disconcerting sensation of warmth in the chest when the dye is released from the catheter. Not surprisingly, the procedure is typically experienced as emotionally stressful. The thought of a tube being placed in the heart is anxiety-provoking for most patients, as are the impending test results and implications for future surgical procedures and even life expectancy. Brief psychological preparations, such as provision of sensory and procedural information or rehearsal of coping strategies prior to the procedure, have been found to be effective in reducing patient distress (Kendall et al., 1979).

The results of the cardiac catheterization test influence the choice among three general approaches to management of significant coronary artery disease. In cases of mild disease, the condition may be managed medically with drugs and lifestyle alterations. The most common drugs and their functions are listed in Table 4.4. The effectiveness of these drugs in reducing cardiac morbidity and mortality in patients with coronary artery disease is well documented (Deedwania, 1995; Pearson & Feinberg, 1997; Scandinavian Simvastatin Survival group, 1994; Shepard et al., 1995). However, as in the case of antihypertensive

TABLE 4.4. Protogypes of Drug Classes Used in the Treatment of Coronary Heart Disease

Class	Example	Action
Beta-blockers	Propranolol (Inderol)	Reduces heart rate and strength of contraction
Calcium-blockers	Diltiazem (Cardizem)	Vasodilators in peripheral and coronary arteries
Nitrates	Sublingual nitroglycerin	Coronary and peripheral vasodilation
Lipid-lowering agents	Lovastatin (Mevacor)	Improves lipid profiles
ACE inhibitors	Catopril (Capoten)	Antihypertensive, primary therapy in CHF
Inotropic agents	Digoxin (Lanoxin)	Increases cardiac contraction strength; stabilizes rhythm
Diuretics	Furosemide (Lasix)	Decreases blood volume
Anticoagulants	Warfarin (Coumadin) Aspirin	Reduces blood clotting

therapy, poor adherence decreases their effectiveness. In placebo-controlled trials of drug treatments of coronary disease, poor adherence is associated with subsequent cardiac morbidity and mortality not only among patients taking active drugs but placebos as well (Irvine et al., 1999). That is, better compliance with the medically inert compound was associated with reduced risk of cardiac events and death. Hence, though much of the health threat posed by nonadherence in this population can be attributed to pharmacological effects, psychosocial influences on adherence may themselves impact the course of the disease.

Lifestyle modification in this population involves smoking cessation, regular exercise, weight loss if appropriate, adopting a low-fat diet, and stress management. Recent evidence indicates that lifestyle approaches can reduce cardiac morbidity and mortality, and produce documented evidence (i.e., via angiography or radiographic scan) of regression of coronary artery disease (Gould et al., 1995; Ornish et al., 1990). Though many multicomponent regimens are sufficiently demanding to pose potential adherence problems, these controlled trials do indicate the potential value of aggressive risk reduction in patients with coronary artery disease. As noted previously in the discussion of the treatment of high blood pressure, the patient's understanding of the importance of adherence to medication regimens and lifestyle changes is a key determinant of success in this approach, as the medications and behavior changes are often unpleasant. Patients who understand the importance of these changes may be more successful.

A second medical approach, often used in conjunction with the first, is percutaneous transluminal angioplasty (PCTA). Following a procedure very similar to cardiac catheterization and coronary arteriography, a specialized catheter is inserted into the diseased artery. Once in position, a "balloon" tip on the device is inflated at high pressure, to a precisely determined diameter. This forces an increase in the arterial opening or lumen. Complications during the procedure are rare, higher than the rates observed in coronary arteriography but still acceptable. Restenosis or reocclusion occurs within six months in about one third of patients who undergo this procedure, requiring a second angioplasty or other treatment options. Newer variations on this procedure have been developed primarily to reduce the rate of restenosis (Topol & Serruys, 1998). The most successful of these is insertion of a stent (small metal mesh tube) to mechanically maintain the newly enlarged opening. Controlled trials of angioplasty have indicated success in the reduction of angina, but there is limited evidence of reductions in cardiac events (Gersh, 1994). The patient's experience of this procedure is very similar to that described previously in the discussion of coronary angiography.

Surgical treatment of coronary artery disease typically involves coronary artery bypass graft surgery (CABG). In this procedure, a graft, preferably utilizing the patient's internal mammary artery, but sometimes the saphenous vein from the leg, is attached to the diseased artery, below the site of the lesion. Multiple grafts are often undertaken during a single procedure. The surgery is highly invasive, though fairly routine given the frequency with which it is now performed. The patient is intubated during the 2–4 h procedure a well as for 12–18 h of postsurgical intensive care. The incisions required to open the chest and to remove the graft vein are both painful. Typically after 48 h, the patient is transferred to a postsurgical hospital ward, and discharged within a week to 10 days. The surgery is quite effective in reducing angina, but reductions in cardiac events (i.e., myocardial infarction or sudden coronary death) have been demonstrated only in more severe cases with multivessel disease (Yusuf et al., 1994). Patients are heavily sedated following surgery, and the stress of being intubated and confined can be pronounced. After being weaned from the ventilator, forced coughing to prevent lung infections can be quite unpleasant, given the recently sutured chest incision. In addition to pain and anxiety, some patients experience brief episodes of disorientation. This can be easily managed with low doses of major tranquilizers and is less likely in patients who have undergone preoperative psychological preparation (Smith & Dimsdale, 1989).

Given the stressful nature of the surgery, it is not surprising that brief psychological preparations (e.g., rehearsal of distraction, cognitive restructuring, and other coping skills; supportive therapy; relaxation training) have been found to reduce emotional distress and physical discomfort following CABG (Anderson, 1987; Leserman, Stuart, Mamish, & Benson, 1989). Furthermore, these interventions also reduce the likelihood of medical complications, including postoperative hypertension and the transient cognitive disturbances noted previously (Anderson, 1987; Smith & Dimsdale, 1989). Reduced stress can also hasten the wound healing, diminish related discomfort, and minimize the length of hospitalization (Kiecolt-Glaser et al., 1995, 1998).

Just as individual differences are important in prognosis following diagnosis of coronary artery disease, personality characteristics have been found to predict the outcome of PCTA and CABG. For example, optimistic patients are less likely to experience recurrent coronary events following PCTA (Hegelson & Fritz, 1999) and are less likely to require rehospitalization following CABG (Sheier et al., 1999).

Patients are often referred for structured exercise programs following the decision to pursue medical therapy, after PCTA or CABG, or following release from acute care for myocardial infarction (described below). These programs are the cornerstone of cardiac rehabilitation. The results of many controlled trials indicate that these exercise programs are effective not only in promoting the rapid return to prior levels of functional activity (e.g., work), but also in reducing the risk of future cardiac events, including cardiac death (O'Connor et al., 1989; Oldridge, Guyatt, Fisher, & Rimm, 1988; Haskell et al., 1994). Further, these interventions have been found to be cost effective, reducing cardiac health care costs substantially (Oldridge, Furlong, Feeney, et al., 1993; Ades, Huang, & Weaver, 1992; Bondestam, Briekks, & Hartford, 1995). The degree of improvement in behavioral functioning during cardiac rehabilitation is influenced by psychological factors. For example, patients who tend to display catastrophizing and other negative thoughts about their illness improve less during rehabilitation than do those with a more positive cognitive style (e.g., Christensen et al., 1999).

Management of the Coronary Crisis

Psychosocial influences on the outcome of acute coronary crises such as an unfolding myocardial infarction begin before the patient reaches the hospital. For example, there is a substantial delay between the time when a patient first notices symptoms and the point he realizes he is ill. There are additional delays between the decision that he is ill and the decision that medical care is needed, and between the decision to seek care and the actual initiation of care (Kenyon et al., 1991; Matthews, Siegel, Kuller, Thompson, & Varat, 1983). Given the medical events taking place, the clinical wisdom is that "time equals myocardium." That is, delay increases the likelihood and severity of death of heart tissue. Hence, high risk groups and their families should be trained in the detection and response to coronary crises.

Once hospitalized, the patient undergoes tests to determine if an infarction has taken place (e.g., ECG monitoring, cardiac enzyme testing), and to evaluate the stability of the heart rhythm and pumping effectiveness. Antithrombolitic medications ("clot busters") are an important complement to older medications, such as nitroglycerine, a vasodilator. The patients are often quite distressed on this occasion, as they are understandably afraid of death or disability. In acute care, denial often limits patients' outward displays of emotional distress (Cassem

& Hacket, 1973). Interestingly, denial in patients hospitalized in the coronary care unit is associated with a better short-term prognosis, perhaps because it reduces the physiological arousal associated with emotional upset (Levenson, Kay, Monteperrante, & Herman, 1984;, Levenson et al., 1989; Levine et al., 1987). However, denial is also associated with poor long-term prognosis, perhaps because it interferes with otherwise beneficial lifestyle modifications (Havik & Maeland, 1988; Levine et al., 1987). Brief supportive psychotherapy has been found to promote more rapid medical stabilization among patients hospitalized in the coronary care unit (Gruen, 1975). One of the clinical challenges is supporting adaptive defenses and coping strategies during this critical period without making later behavior changes more difficult. During this phase, the emotional needs of family members may also be acute, and the consulting mental health professional should attend to this issue in patient care, especially given the many benefits of effective social support (Delon, 1996).

When the patient admitted to coronary intensive care becomes stable, the diagnostic procedures described above may be performed, if they were not ordered during the acute phase. The patient then follows one or more of the courses of treatment and rehabilitation that have been described.

The presentation and course of heart disease varies in important ways across demographic groups. For example, women are at reduced risk of developing coronary heart disease, presumably because of the protective effects of estrogen on the cardiovascular system (Mendelsohn & Karas, 1999). As a result, they are often older when they present with coronary heart disease. Further, once they develop coronary heart disease, women are more likely than men to experience complications during hospitalization and to die during the first month after a heart attack (Hochman et al., 1999). Some, but not all of this greater risk during and following hospitalization may be due to the fact that women are, on average, older at the time of their first heart attack. Importantly, in patients with a first heart attack before the age of 50, women are more than twice as likely as men to die during hospitalization (Vaccarino, Parsons, Every, Barron, & Krumholz, 1999). Some of women's greater risk may be due to the fact that they are less likely to be referred for diagnostic angiography than are men, even when presenting similar symptoms and risk factor profiles (Schulman et al., 1999). Thus, women may be at greater risk once they have developed coronary heart disease, because they receive less aggressive diagnostic and treatment procedures at early stages in the course of disease. Similarly, with equivalent levels of cardiac disease, African American patients have a worse prognosis and are likely to die sooner than are white patients (Dries et al., 1999). As with women, some of this additional risk may be due to the fact that African American patients are less likely than white patients to be referred for diagnostic angiography, even when presenting similar symptoms and risk factor profiles (Schulman et al., 1999). Hence, in patients with established coronary heart disease, women and minorities warrant additional attention.

Adjunctive Psychosocial Treatments

As noted earlier, comprehensive behavioral risk-factor reduction interventions hold considerable promise in the treatment of coronary heart disease. Several studies have examined the effectiveness of psychological interventions specifically targeted toward the patient's level of emotional distress. Although there have been some failures (Frasure-Smith et al., 1997), the majority of the evidence indicates that these approaches are successful in reducing rehospitalization, cardiac recurrence, and other measures of disease status as well as functional improvements such as returning to work (Blumenthal et al., 1997; Dusseldorp, van Elderen, Maes, Meulman, & Kraaij, 1999; Friedman et al., 1986; Linden, Stossel, & Maurice, 1996). Further, these interventions produce substantial savings in subsequent medical expenditures (Allison et al., 1995; Black, Allison, Williams, Rummans, & Gau, 1998; Chiles, Lambert, & Hatch, 1999; Lewin, 1997). Pharmacological treatment of emotional distress also has beneficial effects on patient adjustment and medical costs in this population (Thompson et al., 1998). Some potentially beneficial medications, such as tricyclic antidepressants, have been found to have potentially harmful cardiac side-effects (e.g., arrhythmias). However, new classes of medications (e.g., selective seratonin reuptake inhibitors) are safer, and most difficulties with the use of psychopharmacological interventions in the presence of cardiac disease and cardiac medications can be managed effectively (Tabrizi, Littman, Williams, & Scheidt, 1996).

In summary, psychological interventions can be useful in each stage and type of care for the coronary patient. Brief crisis-oriented interventions, such as supportive therapy, relaxation, and rehearsal of coping skills, can be useful in the preparation for stressful diagnostic procedures (e.g., angiography) or cardiac surgery, and during hospitalization for acute infarction. During the rehabilitation stage, these same approaches can be expanded to manage anxiety, anger, depressive symptoms, and general stress, with beneficial effects on physical health and quality of life. This creates the potential for integrated behavioral care. Therapeutic relationships begun during the acute phase and skills introduced in the context of brief interventions, for example, can provide the building blocks for later, more involved approaches to the modification and reduction of psychosocial risk.

END-STAGE RENAL DISEASE

Over 250,000 patients in the United States face the manifold challenges posed by end-stage renal disease (U.S. Renal Data System, 2002). Major causes of this condition, such as diabetes and hypertension, increase with age. Hence, end-stage renal disease is more common among older persons. With an increasing portion of the population being elderly, the prevalence of end-stage renal disease and associated costs will undoubtedly grow in the near future. Deterioration in the kidney's ability to remove waste from the blood and regulate blood volume appropriately poses an immediate and serious threat to life. As recently as 30 years ago, this condition was nearly always fatal, as medical management was limited in effectiveness. The development of artificial renal dialysis was revolutionary in this respect. It created the potential for patients to live many years, assuming that they adhered to strict medical regimens and dietary constraints and avoided the many life-threatening sequelae of the condition. Yet this life-saving treatment entails many severe restrictions and demands on patients, and they are an essential member of their own health care team.

In the decade following the development of renal dialysis, this treatment was not universally available, creating a difficult problem in allocating this expensive health care resource. However, the congressional Medicare End-Stage Renal Disease Act of 1973 mandated access to dialysis for all patients. Although a transforming event in the lives of many patients, this access has also resulted in over 6 billion dollars in annual Medicare expenditures. The development of kidney transplantation and new alternatives to traditional dialysis have further improved the management of this threat to public health. Yet, kidney failure still poses many challenges to patients' adjustment and well-being. All of the treatments involve challenging medical regimens, adherence to which is critical in the success of treatment. For a comprehensive, recent review of these issues, see Christensen and Ehlers (2002).

Pathophysiology and Usual Care

The onset of end-stage renal disease is defined by the total or near-total cessation of kidney function. It is almost always the result of cumulative damage from another medical disorder. The most common of these—accounting for about one third of cases—is diabetes. As with other consequences of diabetes (e.g., retinopathy, coronary artery disease), this endocrine disorder can produce damage to small and large blood vessels. The vascular damage in the kidney results in a progressive loss of renal function. Hypertension is the second major cause of end-stage renal disease. Glomerulonephritis, polycystic kidney disease, and other renal diseases account for most of the remainder. Because renal failure is essentially irreversible, its prevention is one reason why effective treatment of diabetes and essential hypertension is so important. Because it results from cumulative damage from chronic disease, patients are typically aware of the condition and the nature of their likely treatment in advance. This "warning period" provides time for preparation, but also can be the occasion for chronic distress and growing discouragement.

Renal Dialysis

Regardless of the specific underlying cause of renal failure, the critical function of the kidneys in regulating phosphorous, potassium, and blood volume fluid levels must be maintained. The most common form of treatment (i.e., of maintaining kidney function and replacing kidney failure) is renal dialysis, accounting for over 70% of end-stage renal disease cases. There are several forms of dialysis in use, the most common of these being in-center hemodialysis. In this procedure, patients travel to a dialysis center three times each week for a 4-h session. The sessions pose obvious limitations on patients' activities during the week. A trained technician administers treatment by way of a vascular connection between the patients' circulation and the external artificial kidney machine or dialyzer. This connection typically takes the form of an arteriovenus fistula permanently placed in the patient's forearm. Blood is circulated through the machine during the procedure, and the dialyzer removes waste products. The patient typically relaxes, reads, or engages in other activities that can be accomplished while sitting or reclining. Hence, in this component of the treatment, the patient is a passive recipient of the intervention. In a very small minority of patients, hemodialysis may be performed at home, with the assistance of a technician or caregiver. Although the device used to cleanse the blood is similar, the patient is typically more actively involved at home than with in-center dialysis.

An increasingly common approach to management of end-stage renal disease is continuous ambulatory peritoneal dialysis (CAPD). Nationally, about 15% of patients employ this approach. Rather than passive reliance on a mechanical device, the patient is very actively involved. A permanent catheter is surgically implanted in the patient's abdomen. In the procedure, the patient carefully connects the catheter to a bag of sterile dialysis solution via a sterile tube. The bag is raised, allowing the solution to flow into the peritoneal cavity. The bag is then secured under the patient's clothing for a period of 4–8 h, depending on the patient's activity. Blood filters through the peritoneal membrane during this period, and waste products otherwise removed by a healthy kidney are left behind in the solution. After this "dwell time," the fluid is drained back into the attached bag and discarded, and the procedure begins again. It is usually repeated four times daily. Given the delicate nature of this critical procedure, and the associated potential for complications and inadequate performance, the patient's role is crucial in successful treatment. Although CAPD would appear to have many advantages over hemodialysis for patients' quality of life (Symister & Friend, 1996), it is experienced as very demanding and the heightened responsibility for care can be burdensome (Geiser, Van Dyke, East, & Weiner, 1984).

The Role of Adherence

These two approaches to the management of end-stage renal disease pose very different challenges and demands on the patient. As we discussed below, it is not surprising that there are clear individual differences in patient adaptation to these distinct modalities. However, they also have common features, the most important being the critical role of patient adherence to medication, diet, and fluid intake guidelines. Patients undergoing hemodialysis and CAPD must take regular doses of phosphate-binding medication and modify their diet to restrict the intake of phosphates, because of the body's inability to eliminate this metabolite. This medication often produces unpleasant gastrointestinal side-effects, leading to problems with adherence. Poor compliance produces rising serum phosphorous levels, with resulting increases in risk of decreases in calcium, and subsequent bone demineralization (Wright, 1981). Patients are also required to limit intake of potassium-rich foods, because of their inability to regulate serum potassium. Failure to do so can produce dangerous complications of elevations in serum potassium, such as cardiac arrhythmias (Wright, 1981). Serum levels of phosphorous and potassium are typically monitored each month in standard care, with established guidelines for the identification of problematic treatment adherence (Wolcott, Maida, Diamond, & Nissenson, 1986).

For patients undergoing hemodialysis, there are also severe limits on fluid intake because of the intermittent nature of fluid elimination. Prolonged fluid overload can be life threatening in these patients, primarily through the hypertensive effects of increased blood volume and congestive heart failure. Restrictions in fluid intake are perhaps the most common and troubling aspect of patient adherence, and among the most stressful and difficult challenges experienced by hemodialysis patients (Baldree, Murphy, & Powers, 1982; Rosenbaum & Ben-Ari Smira, 1986). The degree of weight gain between dialysis sessions (i.e., interdialytic weight gain) is commonly used to assess degree of adherence to fluid intake restrictions. Increases of 2.5 kg (or 4% of the patient's body weight) or more indicate poor adherence (Manley & Sweeney, 1986).

The health consequences of poor adherence in end-stage renal disease are alarming. The cause of death in about half of all end-stage renal disease-related mortality can be linked to poor adherence to one or more components of the treatment protocol (Abram et al., 1971; Plough & Salem, 1982). Despite this critical importance, rates of nonadherence range from 30% to 50% of patients, and it is somewhat more common for fluid intake than medication and dietary guidelines (Bame, Petersen, & Wray, 1993; Christensen, Benotsch, & Smith, 1997; Schneider, Friend, Whitaker, & Wadhwa, 1991; Wolcott et al., 1986).

Renal Transplantation

Given the burdensome nature of hemodialysis and CAPD, kidney transplant is a desirable alternative in the management of end-stage renal disease. If successful, renal transplant can essentially be considered a cure for the condition, though not an uncomplicated one. Adherence to immunosuppressive medication regimens, for example, is essential. Successful renal transplant typically produces a higher quality of life than observed among patients undergoing hemodialysis or CAPD (Christensen, Holman, Turner, & Slaughter, 1989; Christenson, Holman, Turner, Smith, & Grant, 1991; Levenson & Glocheski, 1991; Symister & Friend, 1996). For example, it provides the greatest amount of independence and the least degree of intrusion of the illness into the patient's normal activities (Devins,

Mandin, et al., 1990; Devins, 1994). However, there are very serious limitations in access to donor organs, and the rejection of transplanted organs is not uncommon. Sometimes, the transplanted organs are donated by family members, potentially creating emotional conflicts for the recipient and complicating the emotional impact of transplant rejection. Transplant surgery itself is no more unpleasant or disruptive than other major surgeries. However, the immunosuppressant treatment can leave the recipient vulnerable to infectious illness, creating the need for heightened precautions against infection. Further, some immunosuppressant medication protocols can have unpleasant side effects, such as weight gain and agitation. The probability of failure of a transplanted kidney remains as high as 50%, even after seven years of successful functioning of the graft (McGee & Bradley, 1994). Many patients on dialysis have returned to dialysis following a failed transplant. Hence, dialysis in its various forms remains the primary treatment for the overwhelming majority of patients with end-stage renal disease (U.S. Renal System, 2002).

Psychosocial Impact of the Disease and Treatment

Even when treatment is going well, hemodialysis, CAPD, and the associated regimens are demanding and unpleasant. Minor complications are common, such as nausea, sleeplessness, and cramping. More serious complications are not unusual and require frequent hospital admissions, as in the case of burst access sites, peritonitis, and hepititis (Devins, Mandin, et al., 1990; Kutner, Brogan, & Kutner, 1986; Wolcott, Nissenson, & Landsverk, 1988). As a result, end-stage renal disease patients report a variety of disruptions and limitations in work, family functioning, social activities, and other dimensions of quality of life (Devins, 1994; Devins, Beanlands, et al., 1997; Devins, Hunsley, et al., 1997; Shulman et al., 1987; Wolcott et al., 1988). Differences in the quality of life, especially in employment and other "objective" indicators are greatest between successful transplant recipients and those patients undergoing the other treatments; differences among types of dialysis are much less pronounced (Symister & Friend, 1996). Mild cognitive impairment has been observed in patients with end-stage renal disease, and this cognitive impairment may, in turn, account for some of the limitations in employment observed in these patients (Bremer, Wert, Durica, & Weaver, 1997). It is not clear whether the cognitive deficits result from metabolic effects of the disease, the presence of cerebrovascular disease, or other medical factors. However, neuropsychological screening of these patients is potentially quite valuable, as it could point to related disability and functional impairment. Cognitive limitations could also play a role in the critical issue of adherence (discussed below).

Given this degree of disruption, it is not surprising that emotional disturbance is common among this group of patients. The prevalence of psychiatric disturbance among renal patients ranges from 25–50%, the most common form being depression (Hinrichsen, Lieberman, Pollack, & Steinberg, 1989; Kalman,

Wilson, & Kalman, 1983; O'Donnell & Chung, 1997). Further, some research indicates that depression is associated with decreased longevity in this population (Burton, Kline, Lindsay, & Heidenheim, 1986; Friend, Singletary, Mendell, & Nurse, 1986; Kimmel, Weihs, & Peterson, 1993; Peterson et al., 1991), though other studies have not supported this conclusion (Christensen, Wiebe, Smith, & Turner, 1994; Devins, Mann, et al., 1990). Distress is more common among patients who perceive the illness and the related treatment as a greater intrusion in their lives (Devins, 1994). The patient's experiences and treatment modalities appear to interact with individual differences to influence adjustment. For example, among patients on dialysis following a failed renal transplant, a belief in their ability to control their health (i.e., internal health locus of control) is associated with *increased* levels of depression. For dialysis patients without this history, belief in their ability to control their own health is associated with *lower* depression levels (Christensen, Turner, et al., 1991). Transplant failure may constitute a powerful disconfirmation of control beliefs, leaving the patient emotionally vulnerable. Similarly, among patients undergoing CAPD, the tendency to blame others for health problems is associated with an increasing level of emotional distress over time, whereas blaming others is associated with better adjustment over time among patients undergoing in-center hemodialysis (Rich, Smith, & Christensen, 1999). When blaming others is a plausible explanation for difficulties (e.g., when receiving treatment from a dialysis center personnel), it may be adaptive. When self-care is paramount and blaming others for difficulties is not plausible, it may represent a maladaptive coping response. Interestingly, a cognitive style consisting of acceptance of responsibility for problems with health, without harsh or punitive self-blame, is associated with improved adjustment over time regardless of treatment modality (Rich et al., 1999). Finally, among patients undergoing CAPD, severity of illness is positively related to the severity of depressive symptoms, but not among in-center hemodialysis patients (Eitel, Hatchett, Friend, Griffin, & Wadhwa, 1995). It is possible that among those with primary responsibility for their own care, worsening disease evokes self-blame and feelings of helplessness, factors known to be associated with depression in this population (Devins et al., 1981; 1982; Rich et al., 1999). Though treatment is likely to be unpleasant, demanding, and limiting for all patients with renal failure, the degree of resulting emotional distress seems to depend on the specific combination of treatment, experience with the illness, and personality characteristics.

The patient's social functioning is also an important adaptational outcome, as well as a determinant of emotional adjustment. Spouses and other family members often experience the illness and its treatment as a source of significant stress (Maurin & Schenkel, 1975; Mlott & Vale, 1982). Spouses often find their necessary involvement with home hemodialysis to be demanding, even if they are pleased to be able to provide valuable instrumental assistance (Brunier & McKeever, 1993; Streltzer, Finkelstein, Feignbaum, Kisten, & Cohn, 1976). Marital adjustment is impacted, often negatively, by the couple's interlocking and possibly conflicting approaches to the condition (Chowanec & Binik, 1982). The degree of disruption in marital functioning increases when the patient and spouse perceive the illness and its treatment as disruptive of their daily lives (Binik, Chowenec, & Devins, 1990). One potential source of marital conflict stems from the fact that relative to their spouses' views of the impact of the disease, patients often underestimate the negative impact of the disease on family life (Kaye, Bray, Gracely, & Levinson, 1989). Women with end-stage renal disease may be particularly vulnerable to decreases in family support (Devins, Hunsley, et al., 1997; Soskolne & De-Nour, 1989), perhaps because affected women are not able to maintain their role caring for others in the family. In contrast, even though it is demanding, their role as the patient's spouse does not conflict with women's general role in family relations (Devins, Hunsley, et al., 1997).

The success of the process of family adaptation is an important influence on the patient's emotional adjustment and physical health. For example, supportive family relationships appear to buffer the patient from the negative effects of illness severity on emotional adjustment (e.g., Christensen, Turner, et al., 1989). In other studies, family support has been associated with increased longevity among end-stage renal disease patients (Christensen, Wiebe, et al., 1994), though other studies have not found this pattern (Peterson et al., 1991).

There is also evidence that other aspects of the patient's social network are important influences on health. Problematic social relationships between patients and the dialysis center staff have been linked to reduced longevity (Foster, Cohn, & McKegney, 1973). Participation in patient-run support groups has been associated with prolonged survival (Friend et al., 1986). It is important to note that these findings come from observational studies and hence could reflect a variety of influences on health other than social relations with staff and other patients. Nonetheless, the broader social context should be examined as a potential influence on adaptation to the condition.

Determinants of Adherence

Given the essential role of patient self-care and adherence in end-stage renal disease and the severe health consequences when adherence lapses, it is not surprising that much of the psychosocial research on this condition reflects attempts to identify high-risk subgroups and potentially modifiable determinants of these critical behaviors (Christensen et al., 1997). Broad demographic variables (e.g., gender, education, ethnicity, etc.) have proven to be inconsistent predictors of patient compliance (Brady et al., 1997; Christensen, Benotsch, & Smith, 1997). However, this is not true for age. Younger patients are typically less adherent than are older patients (Bame et al., 1993; Boyer, Friend, Chlouverakis, & Kaloyanides, 1990; Christensen & Smith, 1995).

Family support (Christensen et al., 1992), individual differences in self-control (Rosenbaum & Ben-Ari Smira, 1986), health beliefs (Friend, Hatchett,

Schneider, & Wadhwa, 1997), and conscientiousness (Christensen & Smith, 1995) have been found to predict adherence in end-stage renal disease patients. However, rather than this "main effects" approach, adherence among end-stage renal disease patients seems to be jointly influenced by treatment modality and individual differences. As in the discussion of adjustment to treatment above, patients seemingly ill-suited for the specific treatment they are undergoing have the worst adherence. Among patients undergoing the more staff-directed, in-center hemodialysis, patients with a strong preference for behavioral involvement in their own health care have worse dietary adherence than those who did not prefer such involvement. In contrast, among patients undergoing home hemo-dialysis where patient involvement and control are much greater, patients who preferred being involved in their own care show better dietary adherence (Christensen, Smith, Turner, Holman, & Gregory, 1990). Similarly, preference for information about medical care and having an internal locus of control have been found to predict better dietary compliance among patients undergoing CAPD, but worse compliance among those receiving in-center hemodialysis (Christensen, Smith, Turner, & Cundick, 1994). It may be that preference for information and belief in one's control are adaptive when there are opportunities that match this style but not when there are few opportunities for self-care. Similarly, use of planning and problem-solving coping strategies is associated with better adherence when patients confront controllable treatment stressors, whereas use of emotional self-control is associated with better adherence when patients confront a largely uncontrollable treatment stressor (Christensen, Benotsch, Wiebe, & Lawton, 1996). This treatment-matching approach could be used to help evaluate various treatment alternatives and their suitability to individual patients. However, many other factors influence this selection. Nonetheless, this matching approach could be useful in the identification of high-risk cases and the implementation of preventive interventions.

Intervention Approaches

Of the two primary domains of psychosocial research on end-stage renal disease, adaptation and adherence, only the latter has been the focus of several controlled intervention studies (Brantley & Hitchcock, 1995; Symister & Friend, 1996). This is understandable, as adherence is arguably the more critical concern; the patient must adhere to treatment regimens in order to live, and live in order for adjustment to be a relevant concern. Even if depression is associated with re-duced longevity in end-stage renal disease, the consequences for health are likely to emerge much more slowly than the potential emergencies associated with poor adherence. The obvious impact of the disease and its treatment on emotional adjustment and quality of life make the lack of treatment research even more glaring; clinical health psychologists have many potentially useful approaches to offer these patients, but they would do so without guidance from controlled research. The potential benefits of psychosocial interventions on quality of life outcomes are evident in the results of a study on employment. Rasgon et al. (1993), found that a psychoeducational intervention consisting of counseling patients on how to best integrate their work and family lives with the demands of treatment doubled the employment rate of dialysis patients.

A variety of behavioral interventions have been effective in promoting better adherence in this population, including behavioral contracting and positive reinforcement (Barnes, 1976; Hart, 1979; Hegel, Ayllon, Thiel, & Oulton, 1992; Keane, Prue, & Collins, 1981). Also, as in many other medical populations, brief educational and cognitive-behavioral approaches seem to facilitate adherence in end-stage renal disease (Cummings, Becker, Kirscht, Levin, 1981; Hegel et al., 1992). However, many of these studies are small and therefore should be considered suggestive rather than definitive.

In most cases, renal failure develops over time, permitting some degree of warning and preparation. It is quite possible for psychologists or social workers consulting with renal practices to design a program of assessment, risk identification, and individualized interventions for patients and their families. Through such a process, patients could be maximally prepared for the rigors of treating this disease before the problems become severe.

CONCLUDING COMMENTS

The intellectual foundations of current behavioral medicine and clinical health psychology rely heavily on the integration of biological, psychological, and social factors in health and illness. The medical conditions discussed here underscore Engel's (1977) critique of the traditional biomedical model and the value of the biopsychosocial model. Adaptation to end-stage renal disease is a challenge created by new, life-sustaining treatments. Likewise, the current landscape of behavioral cardiology reflects advances in cardiac surgery, medical imaging, and interventional cardiology all developed within the last 30 years. There will be many more such changes in the years to come, as opportunities and challenges continue to evolve, with innovations in medicine and styles of practice.

In providing psychological services to patients with essential hypertension, coronary heart disease, and end-stage renal disease, clinicians must be prepared to depart from traditional mental health practices, or at least be prepared to deliver them in unconventional ways and places. They are entering a context in which responsibility for comprehensive care is distributed among a variety of professionals. The best clinical care is a product not only of collaboration among medical specialists but collaborations across the "old" divisions within the biopsychosocial model. The professional challenge of keeping sufficiently informed about developments in the other participating sciences and professions can be daunting (Belar & Deardorff, 1995). However, as illustrated in the three conditions discussed in this chapter, psychosocial assessments and interventions should be valuable and effective components of standard care.

REFERENCES

Ades, P. A., Huang, D., & Weaver, S. O. (1992). Cardiac rehabilitation participation predicts lower rehospitalization costs. *American Heart Journal, 123*, 916–921.

Adler, N., Boyce, W. T., Chesney, M., Folkman, S., & Syme, S. L. (1993). Socioeconomic inequalities in health. *Journal of the American Medical Association, 269*, 340–3145.

Adler, N., & Matthews, K. (1994). Health psychology: Why do some people get sick and some stay well? *Annual Review of Psychology, 45*, 229–259.

Allan, R., & Scheidt, S. (1996). Empirical basis for cardiac psychology. In R. Allan & S. Scheidt (Eds.), *Heart and mind: The practice of cardiac psychology* (pp. 63–124). Washington, DC: American Psychological Association.

Allison, T. G., Williams, D. E., Miller, T. D., Patten, C. A., Bailey, K. R., Squires, R. W., et al. (1995). Medical and economic costs of psychologic distress in patients with coronary artery disease. *Mayo Clinic Proceedings, 70*, 734–742.

American Heart Association. (2000). *2001 heart and stroke statistical update.* Dallas, TX: American Heart Association.

American Psychiatric Association. (2000). *Diagnostic and statistical manual of mental disorders.* (DSM-IV; 4th ed.). Washington, DC: APA.

Andersen, R. E., Wadden, T. A., Bartlett, S. J., Zemel, B., Verde, T. J., & Franckowiak, S. C. (1999). Effects of lifestyle activity vs. structured aerobic exercise in obese women. *Journal of the American Medical Association, 281*, 335–340.

Anderson, E. A. (1987). Preoperative preparation for cardiac surgery facilitates recovery, reduces psychological distress, and reduces the incidence of acute postoperative hypertension. *Journal of Consulting and Clinical Psychology, 42*, 223–232.

Appel, L. J., Moore, T. J., & Obarznek, E. (1997). A clinical trial of the effects of dietary patterns on blood pressure. *New England Journal of Medicine, 336*, 1117–1124.

Appel, L. J., & Stason, W. B. (1993). Ambulatory blood pressure monitoring and blood pressure self-measurement in the diagnosis and management of hypertension. *Annals of Internal Medicine, 118*, 867–882.

Arroll, B., & Beaglehole, R. (1992). Does physical activity lower blood pressure: A critical review of the clinical trials. *Journal of Clinical Epidemiology, 45*, 439–447.

Baldree, K. S., Murphy, S. P., & Powers, M. J. (1982). Stress identification and coping patterns in patients on hemodialysis. *Nursing Research, 31*, 107–112.

Bame, S. I., Petersen, N., & Wray, N. P. (1993). Variation in hemodialysis patient compliance according to demographic characteristics. *Social Science in Medicine, 37*, 1035–1043.

Barnes, M. R. (1976). Token economy control of fluid overload in patient receiving hemodialysis. *Journal of Behavior Therapy and Experimental Psychiatry, 7*, 305–306.

Barry, J., Selwyn, A. P., Nabel, E. G., Rocco, M. B., Mead, K., Campbell, S. & Rebexxa, G. (1988). Frequency of ST-depression produced by mental stress in stable angina pectoris from coronary artery disease. *American Journal of Cardiology, 61*, 989–993.

Baumann, L., & Leventhal, H. (1985). I can tell when my blood pressure is up, can't I? *Health Psychology, 4*, 203–218.

Belar, C. D., & Deardorff, W. W. (1995). *Clinical health psychology in medical settings.* Washington DC: American Psychological Association.

Berkman, L. F. (1995). The role of social relations in health promotion. *Psychosomatic Medicine, 57*, 245–54.

Berkman, L. F., Leo-Summers, L., & Horowitz, R. I . (1992). Emotional support and survival after myocardial infarction: A prospective, population-based study of the elderly. *Annals of Internal Medicine, 117,* 1003–1009.

Binik, Y. M., Chowanec, G. D., & Devins, G. M. (1990). Marital role strain, illness intrusiveness, and their impact on marital and individual adjustment in end-stage renal disease. *Psychology and Health, 4,* 245–257.

Black, J. L., Allison, T. G., Williams, D. E., Rummans, T. A., & Gau, G. T. (1998). Effect of intervention for psychological distress on rehospitalization rates in cardiac rehabilitation patients. *Psychosomatics, 39,* 134–143.

Blumenthal, J. A., Jiang, W., Babyak, M. A., Krantz, D. S., Frid, D. J., Coleman, R. E., et al. (1997). Stress management and exercise training in cardiac patients with myocardial ischemia. *Archives of Internal Medicine, 157,* 2213–2223.

Blumenthal, J. A., Sherwood, A., Gullette, E. C. D., Georgiades, A., & Tweedy, D. (2002). Biobehavioral approaches to the treatment of essential hypertension. *Journal of Consulting and Clinical Psychology, 70,* in press.

Blumenthal, J. A., Siegel, W. C., & Appelbaum, M. (1991). Failure of exercise to reduce blood pressure in patients with mild hypertension. *Journal of the American Medical Association, 266,* 2098–2104.

Bondestam, E., Breikks, A., & Hartford, M. (1995). Effects of early rehabilitation on consumption of medical care during the first year after acute myocardial infarction in patients ≥ 65 years of age. *American Journal of Cardiology, 75,* 767–771.

Boyer, C. B., Friend, R., Chlouverakis, G., & Kaloyanides, G. (1990). Social support and demographic factors influencing compliance of hemodialysis patients. *Journal of Applied Social Psychology, 20,* 1902–1928.

Brady, B. A., Tucker, C. M., Alfino, P. A., Tarrant, D. G., & Finlayson, G. C. (1997). An investigation of factors associated with fluid adherence among hemodialysis patients: A self-efficacy theory based approach. *Annals of Behavioral Medicine, 19*(4), 339–343.

Brantley, P. J., & Hitchcock, P. B. (1995). Psychological aspects of chronic-maintenance hemodialysis patients. In A. J. Goreczny (Ed.), *Handbook of health and rehabilitation psychology* (pp. 497–511). New York: Plenum Press.

Bray, G. A. (1996). Health hazards of obesity. *Endocrinological and Metabolic Clinics of North America, 25,* 907–919.

Bremer, B. A., Wert, K. M., Durica, A. L., & Weaver, A. (1997) Neuropsychological, physical, and psychosocial functioning of individuals with end-stage renal disease. *Annals of Behavioral Medicine, 19*(4), 348–352.

Brondolo, E., Rosen, R. C., Kostis, J. B., & Schwartz, J. E. (1999). Relationship of physical symptoms and mood to perceived and actual blood pressure in hypertensive men: A repeated-measures design. *Psychosomatic Medicine, 61,* 311–318.

Brownell, K. D., Marlatt, G. A., Lichtenstein, E., & Wilson, G. T. (1986). Understanding and preventing relapse. *American Psychologist, 41,* 765–782.

Brownell, K. D., & Rodin, J. (1994). The dieting maelstrom: Is it possible and advisable to lose weight? *American Psychologist, 49,* 781–791.

Brunier, G. M., & McKeever, P. T. (1993). The impact of home dialysis on the family: Literature review. *American Nephrology Nurses Association Journal, 20,* 653–659.

Buchner, D. M., Beresford, S. A. A., Larson, E. B., Lacroix, A. Z., & Wagner, E. H. (1992). Effects of physical activity on health status in older adults. *Annual Review of Public Health, 13,* 469–488.

Burke, L. E., Dunbar-Jacob, J. M., & Hill, M. N. (1997). Compliance with cardiovascular disease prevention strategies: A review of the research. *Annals of Behavioral Medicine, 19,* 239–263.

Burt, V. L., Whelton, P., & Roccella, E. J. (1995). Prevalence of hypertension in the U.S. adult population: Results from the third National Health and Nutrition Examination Survey. *Hypertension, 25,* 305–313.

Burton, H. J., Kline, S. A., Lindsay, R. M., & Heidenheim, A. P. (1986). The relationship of depression to survival in chronic renal failure. *Psychosomatic Medicine, 48,* 261–269.

Calfas, K. J., Long, B. J., Sallis, J. F., Wooten, W. J., Pratt, M., & Patrick, K. (1996). A controlled trial of physician counseling to promote the adoption of physical activity. *Preventive Medicine, 25,* 225–233.

Carney, R. M. J., Rich, M. W., & Freedland, K. E. (1988). Major depressive disorder predicts cardiac events in patients with coronary artery disease. *Psychosomatic Medicine, 50,* 627–633.

Cassem, N. H., & Hackett, T. P. (1973). Psychological rehabilitation of myocardial infarction patients in the acute phase. *Heart and Lung, 2,* 382–388.

Chiles, J. A., Lambert, M. J., & Hatch, A. L. (1999). The impact of psychological intervention on medical cost offset: An analytic review. *Clinical Psychology: Science & Practice, 6,* 204–220.

Chowanec, G. D., & Binik, Y. M. (1982). End-stage renal disease (ESRD) and the marital dyad: A literature review and critique. *Social Science and Medicine, 16,* 1551–1558.

Christensen, A. J., Benotsch, E. G., & Smith, T. W. (1997). Determinants of regimen adherence in renal dialysis. In D. S. Gochman (Ed.), *Handbook of health behavior research II: Provider determinants* (pp. 231–244). New York: Plenum Press.

Christensen, A. J., Benotsch, E. G., Wiebe, J., & Lawton, W. J. (1996). Coping with illness-related stress: Effects on adherence among hemodialysis patients. *Journal of Consulting and Clinical Psychology, 63,* 454–459.

Christensen, A. J., Edwards, D. L., Moran, P. J., Burke, R., Lounsbury, P., & Gordon, E. E. I. (1999). Cognitive distortion and functional impairment in patients undergoing cardiac rehabilitation. *Cognitive Therapy and Research, 23,* 159–168.

Christensen, A. J., & Ehlers, S. L. (2002). Psychological factors in end-stage renal disease: An emerging context for behavioral medicine research. *Journal of Consulting and Clinical Psychology, 70,* 712–724.

Christensen, A. J., Holman, J. M., Turner, C. W., & Slaughter, J. R. (1989). Quality of life in end-stage renal disease: Influence of renal transplantation. *Clinical Transplantation, 3,* 46–53.

Christensen, A. J., Holman, J. M., Turner, C. W., Smith, T. W., & Grant, M. K. (1991). A prospective examination of quality of life in end-stage renal disease. *Clinical Transplantation, 5,* 46–53.

Christensen, A. J., & Smith, T. W. (1995). Personality and patient adherence: Correlates of the five-factor model in renal dialysis. *Journal of Behavioral Medicine, 18,* 305–513.

Christensen, A. J., Smith, T. W., Turner, C. W., & Cundick, K. E. (1994). Patient adjustment and adherence in renal dialysis: A person by treatment interactional approach. *Journal of Behavioral Medicine, 17,* 549–566.

Christensen, A. J., Smith, T. W., Turner, C. W., Holman, J. M., & Gregory, M. C. (1990). Type of hemodialysis and preference for behavioral involvement: Interactive effects on adherence in end-stage renal disease. *Health Psychology, 9*(2), 225–236.

Christensen, A. J., Smith, T. W., Turner, C. W., Holman, J. M., Gregory, M. C., & Rich, M. A. (1992). Family support, physical impairment, and adherence in hemodialysis: An investigation of main and buffering effects. *Journal of Behavioral Medicine, 15*(4), 313–325.

Christensen, A. J., Turner, C. W., Slaughter, J. M., & Holman, J. M. (1989). Perceived family support as a moderator of psychological well-being in end-stage renal disease. *Journal of Behavioral Medicine, 12,* 249–265.

Christensen, A. J., Turner, C. W., Smith, T. W., Holman, J. M., & Gregory, M. C. (1991). Health locus of control and depression in end-stage renal disease. *Journal of Consulting and Clinical Psychology, 59*(3), 419–424.

Christensen, A. J., Wiebe, J. S., Smith, T. W., & Turner, C. W. (1994). Predictors of survival among hemodialysis patients: Effect of perceived support. *Health Psychology, 13,* 521–525.

Clark, M. M., & Goldstein, M. G. (1995). Obesity: A health psychology perspective. In A. J. Goreczny (Ed.), *Handbook of health and rehabilitation psychology.* New York: Plenum.

Collier, C. W., & Marlatt, G. A. (1995). Relapse prevention. In A. J. Goreczny (Ed.), *Handbook of health and rehabilitation psychology. Plenum series in rehabilitation and health* (pp. 307–321). New York: Plenum.

Curry, S. J., & McBride, C. M. (1994). Relapse prevention for smoking cessation: Review and evaluation of concepts and interventions. *Annual Review of Public Health, 15,* 345–366.

Cummings, C. K., Becker, M. H., Kirscht, J. P., & Levin, N. W. (1981). Intervention strategies to improve compliance with medical regimens by ambulatory hemodialysis patients. *Journal of Behavioral Medicine, 4,* 111–127.

Davidson, M. H., Hauptman, J., DiGirolamo, M., Foreyt, J. P., Halsted, C. H., Heber, D., et al. (1999). Weight control and risk factor reduction in obese subjects treated for 2 years with Orlistat: A randomized controlled trial. *Journal of the American Medical Association, 281,* 235–242.

Deedwania, P. C. (1995). Clinical perspectives on primary and secondary prevention of coronary atherosclerosis. *Medical Clinics of North America, 79,* 973–998.

Deffenbacher, J. L. (1994). Anger reduction: Issues, assessment and intervention strategies. In A. W. Sigman & T. W. Smith (Eds.), *Anger, hostility, and the heart* (pp. 239–269). Hillsdale, NJ: Lawrence Erlbaum.

Delon, M. (1996). The patient in the CCU waiting room: In-hospital treatment of the cardiac spouse. In R. Allan & S. Scheidt (Eds.), *Heart and mind: The practice of cardiac psychology* (pp. 421–432). Washington DC: American Psychological Association.

Devins, G. M. (1994). Illness intrusiveness and the psychosocial impact of lifestyle disruptions in chronic life-threatening disease. *Advances in Renal Replacement Therapy, 1,* 251–263.

Devins, G. M., Armstrong, S. J., Mandin, H., Paul, L. C., Hons, R. B., Burgess, E. D., et al. (1990). Recurrent pain, illness intrusiveness, and quality of life in end-stage renal disease. *Pain, 42,* 279–285.

Devins, G. M., Beanlands, H., Mandin, H., & Paul, L. C. (1997). Psychosocial impact of illness intrusiveness moderated by self-concept and age in end-stage renal disease. *Health Psychology, 16,* 529–538.

Devins, G. M., Binik, Y. M., Gorman, P., Dattel, M., McClosky, B., Oscar, G., et al. (1982). Perceived self-efficacy, outcome expectancies, and negative mood states in end-stage renal disease. *Journal of Abnormal Psychology, 91,* 241–244.

Devins, G. M., Binik, Y. M., Hollomby, D. J., Barre, P. E., & Guttman, R. D. (1981). Helplessness and depression in end-stage renal disease. *Journal of Abnormal Psychology, 90,* 531–545.

Devins, G. M., Hunsley, J., Mandin, H., Taub, K. J., & Leendert, C. P. (1997) The marital context of end-stage renal disease: Illness intrusiveness and perceived changes in family environment. *Annals of Behavioral Medicine, 19,* 325–332.

Devins, G. M., Mandin, H., Hons, R. B., Burgess, E. D., Klassen, J., Taub, K., et al. (1990). Illness intrusiveness and quality-of-life in end-stage renal disease: Comparison and stability across treatment modalities. *Health Psychology, 9,* 117–142.

Devins, G. M., Mann, J., Mandin, H., Paul, L. C., Hons, R. B., Burgess, E. D., et al. (1990). Psychosocial predictors of survival in end-stage renal disease. *Journal of Nervous and Mental Disease, 178,* 127–133.

Dries, D. L., Exner, D. V., Gersh, B. J., Cooper, H. A., Carson, P. E., & Domanski, M. J. (1999). Racial differences in the outcome of left ventricular dysfunction. *New England Journal of Medicine, 340,* 609–616.

Dubbert, P. M. (1995). Behavioral (life-style) modification in the prevention and treatment of hypertension. *Clinical Psychology Review, 15,* 187–216.

Dubbert, P. M. (2002). Physical activity and exercise: Recent advances and current challenges. *Journal of Consulting and Clinical Psychology, 70,* in press.

Dubbert, P. M., & Stetson, B. A. (1995). Exercise and physical activity. In A. Goreczny (Ed.), *Handbook of health and rehabilitation psychology* (pp. 255–274). New York: Plenum.

Dunbar-Jacob, J. Burke, L. E., & Puczynski, S. (1995). Clinical assessment and management of adherence to medical regimens. In P. M. Nicassio & T. W. Smith (Eds.), *Managing chronic illness: A biopsychosocial perspective* (pp. 313–350). Washington DC: American Psychological Association.

Dunn, A. L., Marcus, B. H., Kampert, J. B., Garcia, M. E., Kohl III, H. W., & Blair, S. N. (1999). Comparison of lifestyle and structured interventions to increase physical activity and cardiorespiratory fitness: A randomized trial. *Journal of the American Medical Association, 281,* 327–334.

Dusseldorp, E., van Elderen, T., Maes, S., Meulman, J., & Kraaij, V. (1999). A meta-analysis of psychoeducational programs for coronary heart disease patients. *Health Psychology, 18,* 506–519.

Eitel, P., Hatchett, L., Friend, R., Griffin, K. W., & Wadhwa, N. K. (1995). Burden of self-care in seriously ill patients: Impact on adjustment. *Health Psychology, 14,* 457–463.

Emery, C. F., Schein, R. L., Hauck, E. R., MacIntyre, N. R. (1998). Psychological and cognitive outcomes of a randomized trial of exercise among patients with chronic obstructive pulmonary disease. *Health Psychology, 17,* 232–240.

Engel, G. L. (1997). The need for a new medical model: A challenge for biomedicine. *Science, 196,* 129–136.

Everson, S. A., Goldberg, D. E., Kaplan, G. A., Julkunen, J., & Salonen, J. T. (1998). Anger expression and incident hypertension. *Psychosomatic Medicine, 60,* 730–735.

Foreyt, J. P., & Goodrick, G. K. (1994). Impact of behavior therapy on weight loss. *American Journal of Health Promotion, 8,* 466–468.

Foster, F., Cohn, G., & McKegney, R. (1973). Psychobiological factors and individual survival on chronic renal hemodialysis—A two-year follow-up: Part I. *Psychosomatic Medicine, 35,* 64–81.

Foster, G. D., Wadden, T. A., Vogt, R. A., & Brewer, G. (1997). What is a reasonable weight loss? Patient's expectations and evaluations of obesity treatment outcomes. *Journal of Consulting and Clinical Psychology, 65,* 79–85.

Foster, V., & Pearson, T. A. (1996). 27th Bethesda conference: matching the intensity of risk factor management with the hazard for coronary disease events, September 14–15. *Journal of American College Cardiology, 27,* 957–1047.

Frasure-Smith, N., Lesperance, F., Prince, R. H., Verrier, Garber, R. A., Juneau, M., et al. (1997). Randomized trial of home-based psychosocial nursing intervention for patients recovering from myocardial infarction. *Lancet, 350,* 473–479.

Frasure-Smith, N., Lesperance, F., & Talajic, M. (1993). Depression following myocardial infarction. *Journal of the American Medical Association, 270,* 1819–1825.

Friedman, M., & Brownell, K. D. (1996). A comprehensive treatment manual for the management of obesity. In V. B. Van Hasselt & M. Hersen (Eds.), *Sourcebook of psychological treatment manuals for adult disorders.* New York: Plenum Press.

Friedman, M., Thoresen, C. E., Gill, J. J., Ulmer, D., Powell, L. H., Price, V. A., et al. (1986). Alteration of Type-A behavior and its effect on cardiac recurrences in post-myocardial infarction patients: Summary results of the Recurrent Coronary Prevention Project. *American Heart Journal, 112,* 653–665.

Friend, R., Hatchett, L., Schneider, M. S., & Wadhwa, N. K. (1997) A comparison of attributions, health beliefs, and negative emotions as predictors of fluid adherence in renal dialysis patients: A prospective analysis. *Annals of Behavioral Medicine, 19,* 344–347.

Friend, R., Singletary, Y., Mendell, N. R., & Nurse, H. (1986). Group participation and survival among patients with end-stage renal disease. *American Journal of Public Health, 76,* 670–672.

Geiser, M. T., Van Dyke, C., East, R., & Weiner, M. (1984). Psychological reactions to continuous ambulatory peritoneal dialysis. *International Journal of Psychiatry in Medicine, 13,* 299–307.

Gersh, B. J. (1994). Efficacy of percutaneous transluminal coronary angioplasty (PTCA) in coronary artery disease: Why we need clinical trials. In E. J. Topol (Ed.), *Textbook of interventional cardiology* (2nd ed., pp. 251–273). Philadelphia: W.B. Saunders.

Gottlieb, S. O., Gottlieb, S. H., Achuff, S. C., Baumgardner, R., Mellits, E. D., Weisfeldt, M. L. & Gersienblith, G. (1988). Silent ischemia in postinfarction patients. *Journal of the American Medical Association, 259,* 223–232.

Gould, K. L., Ornish, D., Scherwitz, L., Brown, S., Edens, R. P., Hess, M. J., et al. (1995). Changes in myocardial perfusion abnormalities by position emission tomography after long-term, intense risk factor modification. *Journal of the American Medical Association, 274,* 894–901.

Gruen, W. (1975). Effects of brief psychotherapy during the hospitalization period on the recovery process in heart attacks. *Journal of Consulting and Clinical Psychology, 42,* 223–232.

Hannson, L., Lindholm, L. H., & Niskman, K. (1999). Effect of angiotensin-converting-enzyme inhibition compared with conventional therapy on cardiovascular morbidity and mortality in hypertension: The Captopril Prevention Project (CAPPP) randomized trial. *Lancet, 353,* 611–616.

Hannson, L., Zanchetti, A., & Carruthers, S. G. (1998). Effects of intensive blood-pressure lowering and low-dose aspirin in patients with hypertension: Principal results of the Hypertension Optimal Treatment (HOT) randomized trial. *Lancet, 351,* 1755–1762.

Harshfield, G. A., & Grim, C. E. (1997). Stress hypertension: The wrong genes in the wrong environment. *Acta Physiologica Scandanavia, 161* (Suppl. 640), 129–132.

Hart, R. (1979). Utilization of token economy within a chronic dialysis unit. *Journal of Consulting and Clinical Psychology, 47,* 646–648.

Haskell, W. L., Alderman, E. L., Fair, J. M., Maron, D. J., Mackey, S. F., Superdo, H. R., et al. (1994). Effects of intensive multiple risk factor reduction on coronary atherosclerosis and clinical cardiac events in men and women with coronary artery disease: The Stanford Coronary Risk Intervention Project (SCRIP). *Circulation, 89,* 975–990.

Havik, O. E., & Maeland, J. G. (1988). Verbal denial and outcome in myocardial infarction patients. *Journal of Psychosomatic Research, 32,* 145–147.

Hegel, M. T., Ayllon, T., Thiel, G., & Oulton, B. (1992). Improving adherence to fluid-restrictions in male hemodialysis patients: A comparison of cognitive and behavioral approaches. *Health Psychology, 11,* 324–330.

Hegelson, V. S., & Fritz, H. L. (1999). Cognitive adaptation as a predictor of new coronary events after percutaneous transluminal coronary angioplasty. *Psychosomatic Medicine, 61,* 488–495.

Helmers, K. F., Krantz, D. S., Howell, R. H., Klein, J., Bairey, N., & Rozanski, A. (1993). Hostility and myocardial ischemia in coronary artery disease patients: Evaluation by gender and ischemic index. *Psychosomatic Medicine, 55,* 29–36.

Hinrichsen, G. A., Lieberman, J. A., Pollack, S., & Steinberg, H. (1989). Depression in hemodialysis patients. *Psychosomatics, 30,* 284–289.

Hochman, J. S., Tamis, J. E., Thompson, T. D., Weaver, W. D., White, H. D., Van de Werf, F., et al. (1999). Sex, clinical presentation, and outcome in patients with acute coronary syndromes. *The New England Journal of Medicine, 341,* 226–232.

Horan, M. J., & Mockrin, S. C. (1992). Heterogeneity of hypertension. *Journal of Hypertension, 5,* 1108–1135.

House, J. S., Landis, K. R., & Umberson, D. (1988). Social relationships and health. *Science, 241,* 540–545.

Hunt, S. C., Hopkins, P. N., & Williams, R. R. (1996). Hypertension: Genetics and mechanisms. In V. Fuster, R. Ross, & E. Topol (Eds.), *Altherosclerosis and coronary artery disease* (pp. 209–235). Philadelphia: Lippincott-Raven.

Ironson, G., Taylor, C. B., Boltwood, M., Bartzokis, T., Dennis, C., Chesney, et al. (1992). Effects of anger on left ventricular ejection fraction in coronary disease. *American Journal of Cardiology, 70,* 281–285.

Irvine, J., Baker, B., Smith, J., Jandciu, S., Paquette, M., Cairns, J., et al. (1999). Poor adherence to placebo or Amiodaroe therapy predicts mortality: Results for the CAMIAT Study. *Psychosomatic Medicine, 61,* 566–575.

Joint National Committee on Prevention, Detection, Evaluation, and Treatment of High Blood Pressure. (1997). The sixth report of the Joint National Committee on Prevention, Detection, Evaluation, and Treatment of High Blood Pressure. *Archives of Internal Medicine, 157,* 2413–1446,

Kalman, T. P., Wilson, P. G., & Kalman, C. M. (1983). Psychiatric morbidity in long-term renal transplant recipients and patients undergoing hemodialysis: A comparative study. *Journal of the American Medical Association, 250,* 55–58.

Kamarck, T. W., & Jennings, J. J. (1991). Biobehavioral factors in sudden cardiac death. *Psychological Bulletin, 109,* 42–75.

Kannel, W. B. (1996). Blood pressure as a cardiovascular risk factor: prevention and treatment. *Journal of the American Medical Association, 275,* 1575–1576.

Kawachi, I., Sparrow, D., Vokonas, P. S., & Weiss, S. T. (1994). Symptoms of anxiety and risk of coronary heart disease. *Circulation, 90,* 2225–2229.

Kaye, J., Bray, S., Gracely, E. J., & Levinson, S. (1989). Psychosocial adjustment to illness and family environment in dialysis patients. *Family Systems Medicine, 7,* 77–89.

Keane, T. M., Prue, D. M., & Collins, F. L. (1981). Behavioral contracting to improve dietary compliance in chronic renal dialysis patients. *Journal of Behavior Therapy and Experimental Psychiatry, 12,* 63–67.

Kelly, G., & McClellan, P. (1994). Antihypertensive effects of aerobic exercise. A brief meta-analytic review of randomized controlled trials. *American Journal of Hypertension, 7,* 115–119.

Kendall, P. C., Williams, L., Pechacek, T. F., Graham, L. E., Shisslak, C., & Herzoff, N. (1979). Cognitive-behavioral and patient education interventions in cardiac catheterization procedures: The Palo Alto Medical Psychology Project. *Journal of Consulting and Clinical Psychology, 47,* 49–58.

Kenyon, L. W., Ketterer, M. W., Gheorghiade, M., & Goldstein, S. (1991). Psychological factors related to prehospital delay during acute myocardial infarction. *Circulation, 84,* 1969–1976.

Kiecolt-Glaser, J. K., Marucha, P. T., Malarkey, W. B., Mercado, A. M., & Glaser, R. (1995). Slowing of wound healing by psychological stress. *Lancet, 346,* 1194–1196.

Kiecolt-Glaser, J. K., Page, G. G., Marucha, P. T., MacCallum, R. C., & Glaser, R. (1998). Psychological influences on surgical recovery: Perspectives from psychoneuroimmunology. *American Psychologist, 53,* 1209–1218.

Kimmel, P. L., Weihs, K., & Peterson, R. A. (1993). Survival in hemodialysis patients: The role of depression. *Journal of the American Society of Nephrology, 4,* 12–27.

King, A. C., Haskell, W. I., Young, D. R., Oka, R. K., & Stefanick, M. L. (1995). Long-term effects of varying intensities and formats of physical activity on participation rates, fitness, and lipoproteins in men and women aged 50 to 65 years. *Circulation, 91,* 2596–2604.

Kop, W. J. (1999) Chronic and acute psychological risk factors for clinical manifestations of coronary artery disease. *Psychosomatic Medicine, 61,* 476–487.

Krantz, D. S., Gabbay, F. H., Hedges, S. M., Leach, S. G, Gottdiener, J. S., & Rozanski, A. (1993). Mental and physical triggers of silent myocardial ischemia: Ambulatory studies using self-monitoring diary methodology. *Annals of Behavioral Medicine, 15,* 33–40.

Krantz, D. S., Hedges, S. M., Gabbay, F. H., Gottdiener, J. S., & Rozanski, A. (1994). Triggers of angina and ST-segment depression in ambulatory patients with coronary artery disease: evidence for an uncoupling of angina and ischemia. *American Heart Journal, 128,* 703–712.

Kubzansky, L. D., Kawachi, I., Weiss, S. T., & Sparrow, D. (1998). Anxiety and coronary heart disease: A synthesis of epidemiological, psychological, and experimental evidence. *Annals of Behavioral Medicine, 20,* 47–58.

Kutner, N. G., Brogan, D., & Kutner, M. H. (1986). End-stage renal disease treatment modality and patient's quality of life. *American Journal of Nephrology, 6*, 396–402.

Lander, E. S., & Schork, N. J. (1994). Genetic dissection of complex traits. *Science, 265*, 2037–2048.

Leserman, J., Stuart, E. M., Mamish, M. E., & Benson, H., (1989). The efficacy of the relaxation response in preparing for cardiac surgery. *Behavioral Medicine, 2*, 111–117.

Levenson, J. G., & Glocheski, S. (1991). Psychological factors affecting end-stage renal disease: A review. *Psychosomatics, 32*, 382–389.

Levenson, J. L., Kay, R., Monteperrante, J., & Herman, M. V. (1984). Denial predicts favorable outcome in unstable angina pectoris. *Psychosomatic Medicine, 46*, 25–32.

Levenson, J. L., Mishra, A., Hamer, R. M., & Hastillo, A. (1989). Denial and medical outcome in unstable angina. *Psychosomatic Medicine, 51*, 27–35.

Leventhal, H. S., Diefenbach, M., & Leventhal, E. A. (1992). Illness cognition: Using common sense to understand treatment adherence and affect cognitive interactions. *Cognitive Therapy and Research, 16*, 143–163.

Levine, J., Warrenburg, S., Kerns, R., Schwartz, G., Delaney, R., Fontana, A., et al. (1987). The role of denial in recovery from coronary heart disease. *Psychosomatic Medicine, 49*, 109–117.

Lewin, B. (1997). The psychological and behavioral management of angina. *Journal of Psychosomatic Research, 43*, 453–462.

Linden, W., Stossel, C., & Maurice, J. (1996). Psychosocial interventions for patients with coronary artery disease: A meta-analysis. *Archives of Internal Medicine, 156*, 745–752.

Lovallo, W. (1997). *Stress and health*. Thousand Oaks, CA: Sage.

Lovallo, W. R., & Wilson, M. F. (1992). A biobehavioral model of hypertension development. In J. R. Turner, A. Sherwood, & K. C. Light (Eds.), *Individual differences in cardiovascular response to stress* (pp. 265–280). New York: Plenum Press.

MacMahon, S., & Rodgers, A. (1993). The effects of blood pressure education in older patients: an overview of five randomized controlled trials in elderly hypertensives. *Clinical Experimental Hypertension, 15*, 967–978.

Mancia, G., Sega, R., Milesi, C., Cesana, G., & Zanchetti, A. (1997). Blood-pressure control in the hypertensive population. *Lancet, 348*, 455–457.

Manley, M., & Sweeney, J. (1986). Assessment of compliance in hemodialysis adaptation. *Journal of Psychosomatic Research, 30*, 153–161.

Manuck, S. B. (1994). Cardiovascular reactivity in cardiovascular disease: Once more unto the breach. *International Journal of Behavioral Medicine, 1*, 4–31.

Manuck, S. B., Marsland, A. L., Kaplan, J. R., & Williams, J. K. (1995). The pathogenicity of behavior and its neuroendocrine mediation: An example from coronary artery disease. *Psychosomatic Medicine, 57*, 275–283.

Marlatt, G. A., & Gordon, J. J. (1985). *Relapse prevention*. New York: Guilford Press.

Matthews, K. A., Siegel, J. M., Kuller, L. H., Thompson, M., & Varat, M. (1983). Determinants of decisions to seek medical treatment by patients with acute myocardial infarction symptoms. *Journal of Personality and Social Psychology, 44*, 1144–1156.

Maurin, J., & Schenkel, J. (1975). A study of the family unit's response to hemodialysis. *Journal of Psychosomatic Research, 20*, 163–168.

McGee, H., & Bradley, C. (1994). Quality of life following renal failure: An introduction to the issues and challenges. In H. McGee & C. Bradley (Eds.), *Quality of life following renal failure: Psychosocial challenges accompanying high technology medicine* (pp. 1–22). Chur, Switzerland: Harwood Academic.

Mendelsohn, M. E., & Karas, R. H. (1999). The protective effects of estrogen on the cardiovascular system. *The New England Journal of Medicine, 340,* 1801–1811.

Meyer, D., Leventhal, H., & Gutmann, M.. (1985). Common sense models of illness: The example of hypertension. *Health Psychology, 4,* 115–135.

Midgley, J. P., Matthew, A. G., Greenwood, C. M. T., & Logan, A. G. (1996). Effect of reduced dietary sodium on blood pressure: a meta-analysis of randomized controlled trials. *Journal of the American Medical Association, 275,* 1590–1597.

Miller, T. Q., Balady, G. J., & Fletcher, G. F. (1997). Exercise and it's role in the prevention and rehabilitation of cardiovascular disease. *Annals of Behavioral Medicine, 19,* 220–229.

Miller, T. Q., Smith, T. W., Turner, C., Guijarro, M. L., & Hallet, A. J. (1996). A meta-analytic review of research on hostility and physical health. *Psychological Bulletin, 119,* 322–348.

Miller, T. Q., Turner, C. W., Tindale, R. S., Posavac, E. J., & Dugoni, B. L. (1991). Reasons for the trend toward null findings in research on Type-A behavior. *Psychological Bulletin, 110,* 469–485.

Mittleman, M. A., Maclure, M., Sherwood, J. B., Mulry, R. P., Tofler, G. H., Jacobs, S. C., et al. for the Determinants of Myocardial Infarction Onset Study Investigators. (1995). Triggering of acute myocardial infarction onset by episodes of anger. *Circulation, 92,* 1720–1725.

Mlott, S. R., & Vale, W. H. (1982). Hemodialysis: Adjustment difficulties of patient and family. *Southern Medical Journal, 75,* 1366–1368.

Moser, M. (1999). National recommendations for the pharmacological treatment of hypertension: Should they be revised? *Archives of Internal Medicine, 159,* 1403–1406.

Moser, M., & Helbart, P. R. (1996). Prevention of disease progression, left ventricular hypertrophy and congestive heart failure in hypertension treatment trials. *Journal of the American College of Cardiology, 27,* 1214–1218.

Multiple Risk Factor Intervention Trial Research Group. (1985). Exercise electrocardiogram and coronary heart disease mortality in the Multiple Risk Factor Intervention Trial. *American Journal of Cardiology, 55,* 16–24.

Multiple Risk Factor Intervention Trial Research Group. (1990). Mortality after 10 ½ years for hypertensive participants in the Multiple Risk Factor Intervention Trial. *Circulation, 82,* 1616–1628.

Myers, M. G., & Reeves, R. A. (1991). White coat phenomena in patients receiving antihypertensive therapy. *American Journal of Hypertension, 4,* 844–849.

National High Blood Pressure Education Program Working Group (1994). National High Blood Pressure Education Program Working Group report on hypertension in the elderly. *Hypertension, 23,* 275–285.

National Institutes of Health. (1993). Morbidity and mortality of dialysis. *National Institutes of Health Consensus Statement, 11,* 1–33.

Neaton, J. D., Grimm Jr., R. H., Phineas, R. J., Stamler, J., Granoits, G. A., Elmer, P. J., et al. (1993). Treatment of mild hypertension study: Final results. Treatment of mild hypertension study research group. *Journal of the American Medical Association, 270,* 73–74.

Neaton, J. D., & Wentworth, D. (1992). Serum cholesterol, blood pressure, cigarette smoking, and death from coronary heart disease: overall findings and differences by age for 316,099 white men. *Archives of Internal Medicine, 152,* 56–64.

O'Connor, G. T., Buring, J. E., Yusuf, S., Goldhaber, S. Z., Olmstead, B. A., Paffenbarger, R. S., et al. (1989). An overview of randomized trials of rehabilitation with exercise after myocardial infarction. *Circulation, 80,* 234–244.

O'Donnell, K., & Chung, J. Y. (1997). The diagnosis of major depression in end-stage renal disease. *Psychotherapy and Psychosomatics, 66,* 38–43.

Oldridge, N. B., Furlong, W., Feeny, D., Torrance, G., Guyatt, G., Crowe, J., et al. (1993). Economic evaluation of cardiac rehabilitation soon after acute myocardial infarction. *American Journal of Cardiology, 72,* 154–161.

Oldridge, N. B., Guyatt, G. H., Fisher, M. E., & Rimm, A. A. (1988). Cardiac rehabilitation after myocardial infarction. Combined experience of randomized clinical trials. *Journal of the American Medical Association, 260,* 945–950.

Ornish, D., Brown, S. E., Scherwitz, L. W., Billings, J. H., Armstrong, W. T., Ports, T. A., Melanahan, S. M., Kirkeeide, R. L., Brand, R. J. & Gould, K. L. (1990). Can lifestyle changes reverse coronary heart disease? *Lancet, 336,* 129–133.

Paffenbarger, R. S., Jung, D. L., Leung, R. W., & Hyde, R. T. (1991). Physical activity and hypertension: An epidemiological view. *Annals of Medicine, 23,* 319–327.

Pearson, T. A., Blair, S. N., Daniels, S. R., Eckel, R. H., Fair, J. M., Fortmann, S. P., et al. (2002). AHA guidelines for primary prevention of cardiovascular disease and stroke: 2002 up-date. *Circulation, 106,* 388–391.

Pearson, T. A., & Feinberg, W. (1997). Behavioral issues in the efficacy versus effectiveness of pharmacologic agents in the prevention of cardiovascular disease. *Annals of Behavioral Medicine, 19,* 230–238.

Perri, M. G., Martin, A. D., Leemakers, E., Sears, S. F., & Notelovitz, M. (1997). Effects of group-versus home-based exercise in the treatment of obesity. *Journal of Consulting and Clinical Psychology, 65,* 278–285.

Peterson, R. A., Kimmel, P. L., Sacks, C. R., Mesquita, M. L., Simmens, S. J., & Reiss, D. (1991). Depression, perception of illness and mortality in patients with end-stage renal disease. *International Journal of Psychiatry in Medicine, 21,* 343–354.

Pickering, T. G. (1997). The effects of environmental and lifestyle factors on blood pressure and the intermediary role of the sympathetic nervous system. *Journal of Human Hypertension, 11* (Suppl. 1), S9–S18.

Plough, A. L., & Salem, S. (1982). Social and contextual factors in the analyses of mortality in end-stage renal disease: Implications for health policy. *American Journal of Public Health, 72,* 1293–1295.

Prochaska, J. O., & DiClemente, C. C. (1984). *The transtheoretical approach: Crossing traditional boundaries of therapy.* Chicago: Dow Jones/Irwin.

Psaty, B. M., Smith, N. L., & Siscovick, D. S . (1996). Health outcomes associated with antihypertensive therapies used as first-line agents: A systematic review and meta-analysis. *Journal of the American Medical Association, 277,* 739–745.

Rasgon, S., Schwankovsky, L., James-Rogers, A., Widrow, L., Glick, J., & Butts, E. (1993). An intervention for employment maintenance among blue-collar workers with end-stage renal disease. *American Journal of Kidney Diseases, 22,* 403–412.

Rich, M. R., Smith, T. W., & Christensen, A. J. (1999). Attributions and adjustment in end-stage renal disease. *Cognitive Therapy and Research, 23,* 143–158.

Rosenbaum, M., & Ben-Ari Smira, K. (1996). Cognitive and personality factors in the delay of gratification in hemodialysis patients. *American Journal of Personality and Social Psychology, 51,* 357–364.

Ross, R. S. (1975). Ischemic heart disease: An overview. *Journal of Cardiology, 36,* 496–505.

Rozanski, A. (1998). Laboratory techniques for assessing the presence and magnitude of mental stress-induced myocardial ischemia in patients with coronary artery disease. In D. S. Krantz & A. Baum (Eds.), *Technology and methods in behavioral medicine* (pp. 47–67). Mahwah, NJ: Lawrence Erlbaum.

Rozanski, A., Bairey, C. N., Krantz, D. S., Friedman, J., Resser, K. J., Morell, M., et al. (1988). Mental stress and the induction of silent myocardial ischemia in patients with coronary artery disease. *New England Journal of Medicine, 318,* 1005–1012.

Ruberman, W., Weinblatt, E., Goldberg, J., & Chadhary, B. S. (1984). Psychosocial influences on mortality after myocardial infarction. *New England Journal of Medicine, 311,* 552–559.

Sallis, J. F., Hovell, M. F., Hofstetter, C. R., Elder, J. P., Faucher, P., Spry, V. M., et al. (1990). Lifetime history of relapse from exercise. *Addictive Behaviors, 15,* 573–579.

Scandinavian Simvastatin Survival Study Group. (1994). Randomized trial of cholesterol lowering in 4444 patients with coronary heart disease: The Scandinavian Simvastatin Survival Study (4S). *Lancet, 344,* 1383–1389.

Scheidt, S. (1996). A whirlwind tour of cardiology for the mental health professional. In R. Allan & S. Scheidt (Eds.), *Heart and mind: The practice of cardiac psychology* (pp. 15–67). Washington, DC: American Psychological Association.

Scheier, M. F., Matthews, K. A., Owens, J. F., Schulz, R., Bridges, M. W., Magovern, G. J., et al. (1999). Optimism and rehospitalization after coronary artery bypass graft surgery. *Archives of Internal Medicine, 159,* 829–833.

Schnall, P. L., Pieper, C., Schwartz, J. E., Karasek, R. A., Schlussel, Y., Dereveux, R. B., et al. (1990). The relationship between "job strain," workplace diastolic blood pressure, and left ventricular mass index. *Journal of the American Medical Association, 263,* 1929–1935.

Schnall, P. L., Schwartz, J. E., Landsbergis, P. A., Warren, K., & Pickering, T. G. (1998). A longitudinal study of job strain and ambulatory blood pressure: Results from a three-year follow-up. *Psychosomatic Medicine, 60,* 697–706.

Schneider, M. S., Friend, R., Whitaker, P., & Wadhwa, N. K. (1991). Fluid noncompliance and symptomatology in end-stage renal disease: Cognitive and emotional variables. *Health Psychology, 10,* 209–215.

Schulman, K. A., Berlin, J. A., Harless, W., Kerner, J., Sistrunk, S., Gersh, B. J., et al. (1999). The effect of race and sex on physician's recommendations for cardiac catheterization. *New England Journals of Medicine, 340,* 618–626.

Shepherd, J., Cobbe, S. M., Ford, I., Isles, C. G., Lorimer, A. R., Macfarlane, P. W., et al. for the West of Scotland Coronary Prevention Study Group. (1995). Prevention of coronary heart disease with pravastatin in men with hypercholesterolemia.. *New England Journal of Medicine, 333,* 1301–1307.

Shulman, R., Pacey, I., Price, J. D. E., & Spinelli, J. (1987). Self-assessed social functioning on long-term hemodialysis. *Psychosomatics, 28,* 429–433.

Siegel, W. C., Blumenthal, J. A., & Divine, G. W. (1990). Physiological, psychological, and behavioral factors and white hypertension. *Hypertension, 16,* 140–146.

Smith, L. W., & Dimsdale, J. E. (1989). Postcardiotomy delirium: Conclusions after 25 years? *American Journal of Psychiatry, 146,* 452–458.

Smith, T. W., & Gallo, L. C. (1994). Psychological influences on coronary heart disease. *Irish Journal of Psychology, 15,* 8–26.

Smith, T. W., & Gallo, L. C. (1999). Hostility and cardiovascular reactivity during marital interaction. *Psychomatic Medicine, 61,* 436–445.

Smith, T. W., & Leon, A. S. (1992). *Coronary heart disease: A behavioral perspective.* Champaign-Urbana, IL: Research Press.

Smith, T. W., & Ruiz, J. M. (2002a). Psychosocial influences on the development and course of coronary heart disease: Current status and implications for research and practice. *Journal of Consulting and Clinical Psychology, 70,* in press.

Smith, T. W., & Ruiz, J. M. (2002b). Coronary heart disease. In A. J. Christensen & M. Antoni (Eds.), *Chronic physical disorders: Behavioral medicine's perspective.* Oxford: Blackwell.

Soskolne, V., & De-Nour, A. K. (1989). The psychosocial adjustment of patients and spouses to dialysis treatment. *Social Science and Medicine, 29,* 497–502.

Stamler, J. (1991) Blood pressure and high blood pressure: Aspects of risk. *Hypertension, 18* (Suppl.1), l-95–l-107.

Stamler, R., Stamler, J., Gosch, F. C., Civinelli, J., Fishman, J., McKeever, P., et al. (1989). Primary prevention of hypertension by nutritional-hygenic means. *Journal of the American Medical Association, 262,* 1801–1807.

Stamler, R., Stamler, J., Grimm, R., Gosch, F. C., Elmer, P., Dyer, A., et al. (1987). Nutritional therapy for high blood pressure. Final report of a four-year randomized controlled trial-the hypertension control program. *Journal of the American Medical Association, 257,* 1484–1491.

Stamler, J., Stamler, R., & Neaton, J .D. (1993). Blood pressure, systolic and diastolic, and cardiovascular risks. *Archives of Internal Medicine, 153,* 598–615.

Streltzer, J., Finkelstein, F., Feigenbaum, H., Kisten, J., & Cohn, G. L. (1976). The spouse's role in home hemodialysis. *Archives of General Psychiatry, 33,* 35–58.

Strong, J. P., Malcom, G. T., McMahan, C. A., Tracy, R. E., Newman, W. P., Herderick, E. E., Cornhill, J. F., & the Pathobiological Determinants of Atherosclerosis in Youth Research Group (1999). Prevalence and extent of atherosclerosis in adolescents and young adults: Implications for prevention from the pathobiological determinants of atherosclerosis in youth study. *Journal of the American Medical Association, 281,* 727–735.

Symister, P., & Friend, R. (1996). Quality of life and adjustment in renal disease: A health psychology perspective. In R. J. Resnick & R. H. Rozensky (Eds.), *Health psychology through the lifespan: Practice and research opportunities* (pp. 265–287). Washington, DC: American Psychological Association.

Tabrizi, K., Littman, A., Williams, R. B. Jr., & Scheidt, S. (1996). Psychopharmacology and cardiac disease. In R. Allan, & S. Scheidt (Eds.), *Heart and mind* (pp. 397–419). Washington, DC: American Psychological Association.

Thompson, D., Hylan, T. R., McMullen, W., Romeis, M. E., Buesching, D., & Oster, G. (1998). Predictors of a medical offset effect among patients receiving antidepressant therapy. *American Journal of Psychiatry, 155,* 824–827.

Topol, E. J., & Serruys, P. W. (1998). Frontiers in interventional cardiology. *Circulation, 98,* 1802–1820.

Trials of Hypertension Prevention Collaborative Research Group. (1997). Effects of weight loss and sodium reduction intervention on blood pressure and hypertension incidence in overweight people with high-normal blood pressure: The Trials of Hypertension Prevention, phase II. *Archives of Internal Medicine, 157,* 657–667.

Turk, D. C., & Salovey, P. (1995). Cognitive-behavioral treatment of illness behavior. In P. M. Nicassio & T. W. Smith (Eds.), *Managing chronic illness: A biopsychosocial perspective* (pp. 245–284).

Uchino, B. N., Cacioppo, J. R., & Kiecolt-Glaser, J. K. (1996). The relationship between social support and physiological processes: A review with emphasis on underlying mechanisms and implications for health. *Psychological Bulletin, 119,* 488–531.

United States Renal Data System. (1997). *USRDS 1997 Annual Report.* Bethesda, MD: U.S. Department of Health and Human Services, National Institute of Diabetes and Digestive and Kidney Disease.

Vaccarino, V., Parsons, L., Every, N. R., Barron, H. V., & Krumholz, H. M. (1999). Sex-based differences in early mortality after myocardial infarction. *The New England Journal of Medicine, 341,* 217–225.

Verdecchia, P., Porcellati, C., & Schillaci, G. (1994). Ambulatory blood pressure: an independent predictor of prognosis in essential hypertension. *Hypertension, 24,* 793–801.

Wadden, T. A., Brownell, K. D., & Foster, G. D. (2002). Obesity: Responding to the global epidemic. *Journal of Consulting and Clinical Psychology, 70.*

Waldstein, S. R. (1995). Hypertension and neuropsychological function: A lifespan perspective. *Experimental Aging Research, 21,* 321–352.

Waldstein, S. R., Jennings, J. R., Ryan, C. M., Muldoon, M. F., Shapiro, A. P., Polefrone, J. M., et al. (1996). Hypertension and neuropsychological performance in men: Interactive effects of age. *Health Psychology, 15,* 102–109.

Ward, R. (1990). Familial aggregation and genetic epidemiology of blood pressure. In J. H. Laragh & B. M. Brenner (Eds.), *Hypertension: Pathophysiology, diagnosis, and management* (pp. 81–100). New York: Raven Press.

Williams, J. K., Vita, J. A., Manuck, S. B., Selwyn, A. P., & Kaplan, J. R. (1991). Psychosocial factors impair vascular responses of coronary arteries. *Circulation, 84,* 2146–2153.

Williams, R. B., Barefoot, J. C., & Califf, R. M. (1992). Prognostic importance of social and economic resources among medically treated patients with angiographically documented coronary artery disease. *Journal of the American Medical Association, 267,* 520–524.

Wilson, G. T. (1994). Behavioral treatment of obesity: Thirty years and counting. *Advances in Behavioral Research and Therapy, 16,* 31–75.

Wing, R. R., & Jeffery, R. W. (1999). Benefits of recruiting participants with friends and increasing social support for weight loss and maintenance. *Journal of Consulting and Clinical Psychology, 67,* 132–138.

Wing, R. R., & Klem, M. L. (1997). Obesity. In S. L. Gallant, G. P. Keita & Royak-Schaler, R. (Eds.), *Health care for women: Psychological, social, and behavioral influences,* Washington, DC: American Psychological Association.

Wolcott, D. L., Nissenson, A. R., & Landsverk, J. (1988). Quality of life in chronic dialysis patients. *General Hospital Psychiatry, 10,* 267–277.

Wolcott, D. W., Maida, C. A., Diamond, R., & Nissenson, A. R. (1986). Treatment compliance in end-stage renal disease patients on dialysis. *American Journal of Nephrology, 6,* 329–338.

Wright, L. R. (1981). *Maintenance hemodialysis.* Boston: G.K. Hall.

Wulsin, L. R., Valliant, G. E., & Wells, V. E. (1999). A systematic review of the mortality of depression. *Psychosomatic Medicine, 61,* 6–17.

Yeung, A. C., Vekshtein, V. I., Krantz, D. S., Vita, J. A., Ryan, T. J., Ganz, P., et al. (1991). The effect of atherosclerosis on the vasomotor response of coronary arteries to mental stress. *New England Journal of Medicine, 325,* 1551–1556.

Yusuf, S., Zucker, H. D., Peduzzi, P., Fisher, L. D., Takaro, T., Kennedy, J. W., et al. (1994). Effect of coronary artery bypass graft surgery on survival: Overview of 10-year results from randomised trials by the Coronary Artery Bypass Graft Surgery Trialists Collaboration. *Lancet, 344,* 563–570.

5

Psychosocial Dimensions of Gastrointestinal Disorders

KEVIN W. OLDEN
PHILIP R. MUSKIN

INTRODUCTION

The gastrointestinal system has long been associated with the brain and emotions. William Beaumont's experiments with his patient, Alexis St. Martin, whose gastric fistulae demonstrated increased acid secretion in response to stress, is a classic in psychosomatic medicine (Beaumont, 1833). Almy furthered this concept when in 1947, he demonstrated that colonic motility could be altered by acute experimentally induced stress (Almy, 1947, 1949). The relationship between the behavioral sciences and gastroenterology has not always been a smooth one. In the 1940s and 1950s, Alexander investigated the relationship between personality structure and peptic ulcer disease as well as inflammatory bowel disease (Alexander, 1950). These studies, consisting of open-ended interviews with patients with known inflammatory bowel disease, yielded results that were highly examiner-dependent and biased (Olden 1998). Unfortunately this literature, which gained wide acceptance for a time, was also quite stigmatizing and ultimately resulted in an intellectual and cultural breech between gastroenterologists and behavioral scientists. This divergence was further widened when the field of gastroenterology made significant strides in the basic sciences and defined in more precise terms the pathophysiology of various gastrointestinal diseases, including inflammatory bowel disease and peptic ulcer disease. Consequently, many of the psychological hypotheses previously advanced were rendered obsolete. This schism continued into the 1980s.

Since the 1980s, there has been a renaissance of investigative collaboration between gastroenterologists and psychiatrists, psychologists, and other mental health professionals. The adoption of a *biopsychosocial model* and increasing evidence to support this model's usefulness in treating many gastrointestinal disorders has gained increased acceptance (Drossman, 1995a). In addition, the efficacy of psychotherapy and other behavioral interventions in treating gastrointestinal diseases makes this an area ripe for collaborative efforts in both clinical research and in treatment. This chapter will review, by regions of the gut, the literature supporting the importance and efficacy of a biopsychosocial approach in treating gastrointestinal disease, particularly the functional gastrointestinal disorders.

SPECIFIC ANATOMIC REGIONS OF THE GASTROINTESTINAL TRACT: PSYCHOSOCIAL CORRELATES

The Esophagus

The esophagus is often misperceived as a pipe whose only function is to connect the oropharynx and the stomach. Nothing could be further from the truth. The esophagus is an extremely complex structure that is connected by an intricate network of afferent and efferent neuroconnections with the spinal cord and with adjacent organs, including the lungs, the heart, and pericardium. In a highly coordinated manner the esophagus allows for the successful propulsion of food into the stomach, clears acid refluxed from the stomach, and the prevents aspiration of gastric content back into the oropharynx. Indeed, the lower esophageal sphincter is the key apparatus preventing the reflux of gastric contents: specifically, gastric acid is prevented from getting into the esophagus, oropharynx, and lungs. Because the motility of the esophagus is highly coordinated, esophageal dysmotility can be extremely impairing, particularly to a patient's quality of life. The primary motility disorders of the gut are achalasia, nutcracker esophagus (NE), diffuse esophageal spasm (DES), and nonspecific esophageal motility disorders (NSMD). Esophageal motility disorders lead to a wide spectrum of symptoms including chest pain, dysphasia, odynophagia (painful swallowing), and occasionally vomiting (Rao et al., 1996, Brzana & Koch, 1997).

The relationship between psychosocial factors and esophageal motility disorders is fascinating and highly complex. In a seminal article, Clouse and Lustman demonstrated that patients with esophageal motility disorders were much more likely to suffer from a concomitant psychiatric disorder. Using a validated psychiatric interview, patients who presented with esophageal motility disorders were compared to a control group with no esophageal dysmotility. The investigators found that 84% of the patients with esophageal dysmotility also had an Axis I psychiatric diagnosis, particularly depression or an anxiety disorder. The prevalence of psychiatric diagnoses in the patients was significantly higher than in the controls (Clouse & Lustman 1983). The importance of these findings has been demonstrated in two subsequent studies on treatment. Using a double-blind placebo crossover methodology, 29 patients with nonspecific esophageal motility disorders who were complaining of chest pain were treated with the antidepressant trazodone over six weeks. Trazodone was significantly superior to placebo in relieving patients' esophageal symptoms. No changes in the patients' esophageal motility tracings were detected as a result of the treatment with trazodone (Clouse et al., 1987). These findings suggest that trazodone exerted its effect not by changing esophageal motility patterns, but rather through a more complex interaction between the central nervous system and the connections to the esophagus. The finding that patients' overall perceptions of their symptoms improved significantly with trazodone suggests a role for the central nervous system in patients' perception and reporting of their GI symptoms.

Cannon et al. (1994) evaluated 60 patients presenting with chest pain of unclear etiology. These patients were screened using esophageal motility testing, cardiac catheterization to rule out the presence of cardiac disease, and psychiatric consultation that included psychological testing. The psychological testing was designed to detect the presence of psychiatric disorders such as somatization disorder and panic disorder that could present as a complaint of chest pain. After a five-week placebo run, the patients were randomized to either an antidepressant (imipramine 25–50 mg per day), an antihypertensive (clonidine 0.05–0.1 mg twice a day), or placebo for three weeks. The investigators found that imipramine was significantly superior to either clonidine or placebo. They demonstrated that the patients who were treated with imipramine, in addition to experiencing an amelioration of their chest pain symptoms, experienced an improvement in their sense of overall well-being. This finding was independent of the presence of any specific psychiatric diagnosis (Cannon et al. 1994). These studies suggest a complex interaction between psyche and soma, rather than an "either/or" phenomenon. Recognizing that some patients with chest pain and difficulties in swallowing may also have psychological difficulties is important when patients complain of such symptoms during the course of a psychotherapy.

Strategies targeting an end-organ approach support the concept that the symptoms perceived by patients with esophageal dysmotility are related less to actual dysfunction of the esophagus itself but are secondary to the processing of that information by the central nervous system. The distal two-thirds of the esophagus has a smooth muscle plexus that is responsible for generating the peristaltic activity of this part of the organ. This anatomical fact generated research investigating the effect of smooth muscle relaxants to ameliorate symptoms induced by esophageal dysmotility. A review of the literature showed that although many of the patients in these studies had significant improvement in the quality of their esophageal motility as documented by esophageal manometry testing, the patients often experienced no improvement in their chest pain symptoms compared to placebo (Sperling & McQuaid, 1996). Drugs that work on the central nervous system would seem to offer a more effective approach to the patient with symptoms referable to the esophagus, as opposed to attempting to impact esophageal dysmotility itself. However, patients fear they will be told their symptoms are all "in your head." Psychological support, accurate diagnosis and treatment for coexisting psychiatric disorders, and understanding of patients' concerns are necessary to aid them in their recovery.

Gastroesophageal Reflux Disease

Gastroesophageal reflux disease (GERD) occurs most commonly through dysfunction of the lower esophageal sphincter. Lowering the pressure of the lower esophageal sphincter allows for reflux of acid into the esophagus, inducing heartburn (pyrosis) and esophageal dysmotility which in turn can cause chest pain, belching, or dysphagia. The acid reflux can also lead to a host of extraintestinal complications, including exacerbation of asthma and, on a rare occasion, carcinoma of the larynx (Richter, 1999). Gastroesophageal reflux is influenced by factors such as caffeine, high-fat foods, alcohol, and tobacco, which can decrease lower esophageal sphincter pressure. Colloquially, it has been assumed that stress can induce gastreoesophageal reflux that in turn produces symptoms of "heartburn." It is not uncommon for individuals to say, "My job gives me heartburn" or make similar statements about other life stresses. However, the relationship between emotional factors in gastroesophageal reflux disease has been only recently investigated in a systematic manner.

In an extremely well-designed study, Bradley et al. (1995) evaluated a group of patients with known GERD using a 24-h pH monitor. This device allowed the investigators to precisely quantify the amount of acid reflux an individual subject had over a one-day period. Subjects were also evaluated psychologically using the Millon Behavioral Health Index (MBHI). This instrument detects psychological susceptibility to various illness patterns. Specifically, one scale on "GI susceptibility" measures a patient's proclivity to manifest psychological stress as a gastrointestinal symptom. Patients were stratified into two groups, those who had high scores on the GI susceptibility scale of the MBHI, and those with lower MBHI scores. Patients were then exposed to a series of artificial stressors in an attempt to induce reflux and/or reflux symptoms. The results were impressive. Objectively, the presence of artificial stimuli did not induce a significant change in reflux in any of the study subjects. However, patients who scored high on the GI susceptibility scale of the MBHI were much more likely to report symptoms suggestive of reflux, despite the fact that their pH monitor study showed no evidence of reflux. This finding was in contrast to the control subjects who reported no increase in reflux symptoms (Bradley et al., 1993). This study suggests that acute stress does not produce reflux; nevertheless, patients who are psychologically vulnerable are more likely to report reflux symptoms in the presence of acute stress. Identifying a patient's psychological status when the patient complains of any physical symptom can aid in the medical evaluation and eventual diagnosis. Resolution of the psychological factors in psychotherapy may be as important as any other medical treatment for patients with esophageal dysfunction.

Peptic Ulcer Disease

The history of peptic ulcer disease (PUD) speaks powerfully to the concept that all medical knowledge is provisional. Originally considered one of Franz

Alexander's "seven psychosomatic diseases," the psychosomatic status of PUD fell victim to advances in biomedical science. Alexander described patients with PUD as having "repressed help-seeking dependent tendencies" (Alexander, 1950). In Alexander's schema, peptic ulcer disease was presumed to be due to a hypersecretion of acid that was modulated by certain personality traits.

Our understanding of peptic ulcer disease was radically altered in 1985 when it was demonstrated that the bacterium *Helicobacter pylori* (*H. pylori*) could cause both gastric and duodenal ulcers (Marshall & Warren, 1984). Research has unequivocally shown that H. pylori infection is associated with about 70% of gastric ulcers and 30–90% of duodenal ulcers. Eradication of *H. pylori* infection through a combination of antibiotics, acid suppression, and the use of bismuth compounds can cure peptic ulcers and prevent their return (Hunt, 1996). Subsequent research has shown that 11–25% of peptic ulcers are caused by the use of nonsteroidal anti-inflammatory medications (NSAIDS) such as aspirin and ibuprofen (Graham, 1996). There remain approximately 5% of patients with PUD who neither use NSAIDS nor are infected with *H. pylori*. It is this group of patients that deserves further investigation from a psychosocial perspective.

Mental stress can clearly influence acid secretion as demonstrated by Beaumont's work in the nineteenth century. In an investigation of specific personality traits and their influence on acid secretion, Holtmann and colleagues studied four healthy male volunteers who were screened using a standardized personality assessment instrument (Holtmann, Kriehel, & Singr, 1990). They were subjected to artificial stress (performing increasingly difficult arithmetic problems) while undergoing continuous measurement of gastric output. The results of this study were quite dramatic. Individuals with high degrees of impulsivity as part of their personality structure were more likely to have increased gastric acid output during acute periods of mental stress. Patients who scored low on the impulsivity scale had decreased levels of acid secretion in response to the same artificial stress. Holtmann concluded that there was great individual variability in gastric acid response to acute mental stress, and that this variability could be partly attributed to differences in personality traits.

Levenstein and colleagues studied the impact of personality and life events on duodenal ulcer (Levenstein et al., 1992). They investigated 33 patients with duodenal ulcer disease who had symptoms for at least the previous six months and had received no treatment in the previous year. Using the Paykel Interview for Stressful Life Events, the Minnesota Multiphasic Personality Inventory (MMPI) to evaluate personality structure, and the Zung Anxiety and Depression Scales, they found that 65% of their patients with duodenal ulcer disease had abnormal MMPIs. Sixty-one percent evidenced some degree of depression. Sixteen of the patients who had particularly severe stressors prior to the development of their ulcers were found to have more pathological MMPIs than their peers, particularly on the paranoia and dependency scales. These patients were also more depressed than the study group as a whole. They had used NSAIDs significantly less than the patients who had lower levels of pre-existing stress and who subsequently developed duodenal ulcers. The patients with high stress levels were also more likely to be single and of lower socioeconomic status. Anxiety levels did not differ significantly between groups with high pre-existing stress and low stress. The investigators concluded that patients who developed ulcers while experiencing psychosocial stress represented a distinct subgroup. They further concluded that stress might have mediated the use of alcohol and tobacco in these patients, which also might have catalyzed ulcer genesis (Levenstein et al., 1992).

Stress has an impact on the healing of peptic ulcers. Another study by Levenstein investigated 70 patients with duodenal ulcers. The subjects were assessed using the MMPI and queried for their use of tobacco, alcohol, and NSAIDs. In addition to endoscopic diagnosis of their ulcer disease, serum pepsinogen I levels were obtained from each subject at the time of endoscopy. After six weeks of treatment with ranitidine (Zantac) 300 mg per day, the patients underwent repeat endoscopy. Six patients (9%) had persistent ulcers and five patients (7%) had persistently inflamed duodenal mucosa. There were no differences between the patients with healed ulcers and those with nonhealing ulcers in gender, use of tobacco and alcohol, or levels of serum pepsinogen. High levels of anxiety as measured by the MMPI were powerfully associated with both ulcer persistence ($p = 0.03$) and incomplete healing (duodenal mucosa edema; $p = 0.02$). Levenstein concluded that high levels of anxiety have a negative impact on the healing of duodenal ulcers, even in the presence of adequate antisecretory therapy (Levenstein et al. 1996).

The discovery of the importance *H. pylori* in the development of peptic ulcer disease makes it somewhat harder to understand what role stress and personality structure play. A number of key points can help clarify this conundrum. First, *H. pylori* is an extremely common worldwide infection. Despite its wide prevalence, most individuals who are infected with the bacterium never develop ulcers. The same is true for nonsteroidal anti-inflammatory use. Most patients who take these agents never develop ulcers. Finally, there is a population of patients who have never been infected with *H. pylori,* have never taken NSAIDS, but develop peptic ulcer disease (McColl et al., 1993). To help explain this paradox, Levenstein, in an extensive review, suggested that psychological stress, interacting with *H. pylori* infection and/or other risk factors, can potentiate conditions that impair mucosal defense. This ultimately results in ulcer formation (Levenstein, 1998). This hypothesis is important for contemporary psychosomatic medicine. As our scientific knowledge in the behavioral and biological sciences advances, all-or-nothing etiologic theories for the cause of ulcers are passé. The development of ulcer disease results from the interaction of multiple variables which interact in complex ways. This outlook represents the best application of the biopsychosocial model. It can lead to more effective treatments that addresses stress reduction and other behavioral interventions to prevent ulcer disease, in addition to the use of purely medical modalities. In this regard, psychotherapy plays a powerful role in patients who are experiencing distress in life. Alterations of coping skills (see Chapter 10) may enable patients to reduce the physiological impact of stress and thus alter their vulnerability to developing exacerbations of medical disorders.

Inflammatory Bowel Disease

Alexander included both ulcerative colitis and Crohn's disease as two of his "classic" psychosomatic diseases. Alexander's psychoanalytic studies of the 1930s through the 1960s suggested a premorbid personality that first produced a specific immunologic reaction (so-called "specificity theory") and then produced the clinical pattern of inflammatory bowel disease (IBD) (Alexander, 1950). These studies have intrinsic methodologic difficulties and have been thoroughly repudiated by research that demonstrated no relationship between specific personality types and the development of subsequent IBD (Olden, 1992).

Research into the relationship between psychiatric disorders and IBD has been fraught with difficulties. North and colleagues reviewed 138 published studies addressing this topic, analyzing for methodologic flaws, including lack of control subjects, rigorous manner of data collection, and absence of diagnostic criteria (North et al., 1990). Only 7 out of the 138 studies met the investigators' criteria for "valid systematic investigation." In the seven studies, none failed to show an association between psychiatric factors and inflammatory bowel disease. To investigate the applicability of the specificity theory, Helzer et al. (1982) studied 50 patients with ulcerative colitis to determine the lifetime prevalence of psychiatric diagnosis and stressful life events. This group was compared to an age and gender-matched control sample of people with chronic nongastrointestinal medical problems. Helzer et al. (1982) found the frequency of diagnosable psychiatric disorders in ulcerative colitis patients was no greater than the control subjects. Patients with ulcerative colitis and comorbid psychiatric illness did not appear to have more serious gastrointestinal involvement. Likewise, the severity of ulcerative colitis did not predict the frequency, or the seriousness, of any comorbid psychiatric disorder (Helzer et al., 1982).

Helzer conducted another study with patients who had Crohn's disease. Fifty patients with active Crohn's disease were compared to 50 age- and gender-matched controls with nongastrointestinal chronic medical illnesses. Patients with Crohn's disease were significantly more likely to have had a lifetime psychiatric diagnosis. Major depressive disorder and obsessional and phobic symptoms were significantly more common in the Crohn's patients. Helzer was not able to find evidence of an interaction between the Crohn's patients' psychiatric disease and the initial presentation of the Crohn's disease or the ultimate activity of the disease (Helzer et al., 1984).

To further investigate the significance of psychiatric diagnosis in patients with IBD, Walker and colleagues (1988) studied 40 patients with known IBD who were evaluated using the Diagnostic Interview Schedule (DIS) for *DSM-IV.* Patients were screened for functional gastrointestinal symptoms as well as prior episodes of emotional and physical/sexual abuse. A self-reported evaluation of personality and disability was also obtained. Patients with IBD and a concurrent psychiatric diagnosis had a significantly higher average number of lifetime psychiatric diagnoses, a higher rate of physical and sexual abuse, and a greater number of unexplained gastrointestinal and nongastrointestinal complaints. The results of the study show that a higher number of psychiatric diagnoses, symptoms suggestive of a functional gastrointestinal disorder (as opposed to IBD), and elevated levels on the dissociation scale of the DIS, predict lower levels of quality of life and poorer functioning in daily activities. This is independent of a diagnosis of IBD. During the course of the study, eight patients found to have major depressive disorder were treated with antidepressant medications. Their functional disability decreased without any objective change in gastrointestinal severity. Walker concluded that the presence of a psychiatric disorder was not a causal variable for inflammatory bowel disease. Rather, psychiatric disorders, when present, alter patients' perception of their symptoms and disease severity independent of actual disease activity, which, in turn, leads to a worse quality of life (Walker et al., 1996).

To investigate the role of life events in the exacerbation of inflammatory bowel disease, North studied 32 patients with IBD who had at least one relapse in a two-year period prior to entering the study. Life stressors were measured using the Social Readjustment Rating Scale, depression by the Beck Depression Inventory (BDI), and GI symptoms with a symptom inventory. Patients were then followed prospectively for two years. A mean of 2.2 exacerbations per subject was seen during the course of the study. North found that life events were not temporally associated with any changes in intestinal symptoms; however, a significant association was found between the degree of intestinal symptoms and mood levels as measured by the BDI ($p < 0.05$). The study did not demonstrate a directionality in the symptoms, that is, inflammatory bowel disease activity did not trigger depression and vice-versa. North concluded that personal life events or the presence of depressed mood could not be identified as precipitors for IBD exacerbations (North et al., 1991).

The importance of employing a biopsychosocial perspective for inflammatory bowel disease is demonstrated by these findings. The concept of emotional factors "causing" IBD clearly is only of historical interest at this point. Although it is clear that psychological factors are not etiologic, it is also clear that the presence of chronic symptoms of diarrhea, abdominal pain, bloating, arthritis, fatigue, arthralgias, and arthritis associated with chronic IBD in and of themselves can induce significant stress. This comorbid, as opposed to etiologic psychological, distress needs to be acknowledged by the clinician treating these patients (Olden, 1998). However, the misconceptions generated by this flawed theory continue to persist in some circles. This dilemma should not prevent clinicians and investigators from continuing to investigate the interaction between life events and psychiatric diagnosis on disease perception and illness behavior.

Irritable Bowel Syndrome

William Sutton, a British physician, first described irritable bowel syndrome (IBS) in 1818. IBS differs from IBD in that it is a "motility" disorder of the gut as opposed to an "inflammatory" disorder of the gut. Although early investigators referred to IBS using terms such as "colitis" or "interitis," inflammation is not a significant component of IBS. Rather, IBS is a disorder of colonic motility and visceral perception. It is characterized by chronic abdominal pain, alternating constipation and diarrhea of which one or the other is usually more prominent, and an alteration in stool character such as pencil thin stools. The diagnostic criteria for IBS are outlined in Table 5.1. A review of the descriptions of centuries of conditions that are clearly IBS suggests that clinicians perceived a strong emotional component to IBS. Subsequent research has strongly supported this clinical impression. Drossman studied three groups of individuals: patients presenting for treatment for IBS at a tertiary care university-based clinic; individuals sampled from an undergraduate college population who met the Rome diagnostic criteria for IBS but who were not seeking medical care; and normal controls chosen from the hospital medical staff (Drossman et al., 1988). Patients were evaluated for pain behavior by the Magill Pain Inventory and for personality structure by the MMPI. The individuals with IBS who sought medical care were significantly different in their pain scores, personality structure, and adjustment to illness compared to either non-IBS controls or the patients with IBS who choose not to seek medical care. Drossman concluded that psychological factors influenced how patients perceived their symptoms that subsequently led to health care-seeking behavior (Drossman et al., 1988). These findings have been replicated by others (Whitehead, 1991).

A number of psychiatric diagnoses have been associated with IBS. High levels of anxiety disorders, particularly panic disorder, have been found in patients with IBS selected from the Epidemiologic Catchment Area (Lydiard et al., 1994; Fossey & Lydiard, 1990; Walker et al., 1992). Major depressive disorder has also been identified as a common comorbid condition seen in association with IBS (Masand et al., 1995). Somatization disorder is a frequent concomitant of func-

TABLE 5.1. Rome II Diagnostic Criteria for Irritable Bowel Syndrome

---

At least 12 weeks, which need not be consecutive, in the preceding 12 months of abdominal discomfort or pain that has two of three features:

1. relieved with defecation; and/or
2. onset associated with a change in frequency of stool; and/or
3. onset associated with a change in form (appearance) of stool.

From *Rome II: The Functional Gastrointestinal Disorders* (2nd ed.), (2000), edited by Douglas A. Drossman, with Enrico Corazziari, Nicholas Talley, W. Grant Thompson, and William Whitehead. McLean, VA: Degnon. www.romecriteria.org. Used with permission.

tional GI disorders and is associated with a poor outcome in patients with IBS (Whitehead & Crowell, 1991).

TRAUMA AND ABUSE HISTORY

An area of rapidly expanding research in the functional gastrointestinal disorders is the impact of trauma and/or abuse on the subsequent development of a functional gastrointestinal disorder later in life (Leserman et al., 1996). In a study of 239 women who presented to a university-based tertiary care gastroenterology clinic, 66% of patients presented with a history of physical and/or sexual abuse. The patients who were abused were more likely to have a functional as opposed to an organic GI disorder (Leserman et al., 1996).

A positive abuse history is common in patients reporting GI symptoms even outside the medical setting. In a community-based sample of 919 people, 14% of women and 11% of men reported a history of physical or sexual abuse (Talley et al., 1994). This finding resulted in an age/gender adjusted prevalence of 26%. Of the individuals who reported abuse, 14% met Rome criteria for IBS, 23% met criteria for functional dyspepsia, and 12% had frequent heartburn. Talley also demonstrated a statistically significant association between the presence of an IBS diagnosis and a reported history of sexual, emotional, or verbal abuse, either in childhood or adulthood. In addition, both dyspepsia and heartburn were significantly more common in patients who reported an abuse history. The likelihood of visiting a physician was also higher in those individuals reporting an abuse history. Talley concluded that self-reported abuse was common in community populations. People reporting a history of abuse were more likely to have functional GI complaints such as IBS, dyspepsia, or heartburn and were more likely to visit a physician for their symptoms than were patients who had not been abused (Talley et al., 1994).

Other functional gastrointestinal disorders have been associated with abuse. Abraham studied 33 women diagnosed with sphincter of Oddi dysfunction, a functional GI disorder of contractility of the sphincter of Oddi. It is defined as a sphincter of Oddi pressure > 40 mm Hg as measured by endoscopic biliary manometry. These patients were compared to 33 gender- and ethnically-matched controls. Both groups were screened for psychiatric disorders and abuse history. Abraham found a statistically increased prevalence of childhood sexual abuse, but not physical abuse, in women presenting with sphincter of Oddi dysfunction compared to controls ($p < 0.02$). The severity of the abuse correlated strongly with the severity of the patient's gastrointestinal complaint. Abraham also found that severity of childhood abuse correlated with a tendency to develop somatization disorder in adult life (Abraham et al., 1997).

Leserman and colleagues (1992) also studied the tendency for an abuse history to negatively influence disease perception and patient distress. They evaluated 239 patients who presented to a tertiary care GI clinic for functional gastrointestinal complaints. Patients were screened for a history of sexual abuse, severity of abuse, and health status. One hundred twenty-one of the female patients had a history of prior sexual or physical abuse. In those with an abuse history, 24% of their current health status could be explained by serious injury during abuse, victimization by multiple perpetrators, or being raped. Thirty-nine percent of the variance in overall health status was explained in patients who were physically abused, had been raped, or had multiple life-threatening incidents. Using these data, Leserman created an abuse severity index that could be used to evaluate the effect of abuse on a patient's health status. The importance of identifying abuse, particularly in patients who are suffering from particularly poor health status within the context of a given disease, was demonstrated by this study (Leserman et al., 1997).

Individuals with a history of abuse may be vulnerable to a variety of medical disorders (Felitti et al., 1998), and not all patients with IBS report abuse. Many patients with borderline personality disorder report abuse, but not 100% (Herman et al., 1989). We do not yet understand how physical and sexual abuse in childhood influences either medical or psychiatric disorders. An appreciation of the potential consequences of abuse, and sensitive inquiry of these issues, are thus an important part of the interaction with all patients.

PSYCHOTHERAPEUTIC APPROACHES TO FUNCTIONAL GASTROINTESTINAL DISORDERS

Functional gastrointestinal disorders are the most common disorders seen in gastroenterology practice (Drossman et al., 1993; Drossman, 1994). They are characterized by a wide spectrum of severity. Some patients present with minimal symptoms that are amenable to a straightforward modification of diet and lifestyle. However, some patients are extremely distressed and experience more severe symptoms, greater levels of disability, and an impaired quality of life (Camilleri & Choi, 1997; Drossman et al., 1988). Patients who present for treatment of IBS tend to be more emotionally distressed than those who meet the diagnostic criteria for IBS but choose not to seek treatment (Olden, 1997). The reasons for this finding remain unclear. As noted earlier, a history of physical or sexual abuse has been identified as one factor that can be associated with IBS as well as other functional GI symptoms (Drossman et al., 1995, 1999).

The strong association between psychosocial factors and gastrointestinal disorders suggests that behavioral or psychotherapeutic interventions could be useful in the treatment of these patients. The usefulness of psychotherapeutic interventions in the functional GI disorders is supported by research indicating that the efficacy of medical management alone is, at best, mixed (Klein 1988). It is in this context that the usefulness of behavioral interventions in functional GI disorders has been studied.

Psychotherapy has been traditionally used in the treatment of psychiatric disorders. Anxiety disorders, panic disorder, obsessive-compulsive disorder, and phobias have all been shown to be responsive to psychotherapeutic intervention. Depression has also been shown to benefit from a variety of psychotherapeutic approaches. Expanding the applicability of psychotherapy to the treatment of medical disorders has resulted in the use of several modalities of psychotherapy to treat gastrointestinal disorders.

The section below will review the research data that supports the use of various psychotherapeutic techniques for patients with gastrointestinal disorders. Several principles guide the therapist in working with these patients, irrespective of the particular type of psychotherapy. One fear patients have, particularly those with IBS, is that without "objective" findings the illness is not real. The lack of a pathologic finding does not abolish the person's discomfort. The core of working with these patients is to acknowledge but not to focus upon their pain and suffering. Therapists should accept the patient's definition of his/her illness and not seek to challenge the reality of the illness. We must also be mindful that allowing the patient to continue to focus on the diagnostic process (more tests, repeating procedures, finding the "right" doctor) will slow down the process of recovery. This requires an understanding and communication with the physicians who are evaluating and treating the patient's gastrointestinal disorder. Early on in the process the therapist should obtain permission from the patient to be in contact with his/her medical doctors.

Patients may be reluctant to work on what they can do rather than what they feel is not available to them. One strategy is to confront the reluctance to give up the sick role because he or she is not symptom free. At the same time, confronting unrealistic expectations of what the person can do will prevent failures and the development of feeling hopeless and/or helpless. Seeking out meaning in the illness does not imply that the physical symptom is caused by unconscious psychological conflict. This prevents patients from reacting in a negative manner and feeling accused of creating their symptoms. Both the meaning of the symptom itself and the meaning of being ill should be considered in therapies that are insight-oriented.

Cognitive Behavioral Psychotherapy

Cognitive-behavioral psychotherapy (CBT) is predicated on the premise that a patient's feelings and attitudes, and the emotional state resulting from those feelings and attitudes, derive from the patient's "cognition" or intellectual understanding of his/her self-perception and perception of the environment. In the CBT model, patients who are distressed by physical symptoms have a dysfunctional or incorrect perception of their illness. That perception leads to destructive attitudes and maladaptive behavior, including depression, somatization, and loss of social functioning (Whitehead, 1992). CBT involves constructing the *cognitive triad* in which incorrect thoughts lead to dysfunctional attitudes and emotions which result in dysfunctional and/or self-destructive behaviors.

Although originally developed for depression, this technique has been increasingly applied to the treatment of medical conditions. The data arising from studies on the use of CBT-based psychotherapy in IBS patients is quite promising. Blanchard and colleagues (1992) treated 90 patients who were randomized to either CBT delivered in 12 sessions over eight weeks or a regimen of biofeedback and meditation (relaxation therapy). These treatment groups were compared to a symptom-monitoring control group. The results were quite positive. Interestingly, the presence of a psychiatric illness was a negative predictor of response to cognitive behavioral psychotherapy. The authors concluded that the presence of any diagnosable psychiatric disorder would be a poor prognostic indicator for CBT (Blanchard et al., 1992).

To further assess the effectiveness of CBT, Greene and Blanchard (1994) randomized 20 patients with IBS to either individual CBT delivered in 10 sessions over eight weeks or eight weeks of daily symptom monitoring and no treatment. Each group had GI symptoms measured pre- and postintervention. The group who received CBT had significant reduction in GI symptoms between their measurements compared to patients who were randomized to symptom monitoring only ($p = 0.005$). In the post-treatment setting, 80% of the patients who received CBT showed clinically significant reduction in GI symptoms versus only 10% of the symptom-monitored group. The improvement was maintained at the three-month follow-up (Greene & Blanchard, 1994).

To assess the effectiveness of CBT versus self-help support groups, Payne and Blanchard (1995) randomized 34 patients who met the Rome criteria for IBS to one of three treatment options that included individualized CBT, a self-help support group directed by a trained facilitator, and a symptom monitoring group to serve as a control over eight weeks. Patients in both the CBT and self-help support groups received 10 hours of contact time. Patients with diagnosable psychiatric disorders were excluded from the study. Patients treated with CBT showed a significantly better pre- to post-treatment improvement in gastrointestinal symptoms when compared to the self-help support group or the controls. The CBT group also had significant improvement in levels of depression and anxiety as measured on standardized psychological tests when compared to the self-help support group or controls. The study suggests that even without a psychiatric diagnosis, CBT is superior to group social interaction (as typified by the self-help support group arm of the study) for the treatment of functional GI disorders (Payne & Blanchard, 1995).

The ability of the effect of CBT to persist after the initial treatment regimen was addressed by Van Dulmen, Fennis, and Bleijenberg (1996). They treated 45 patients with eight 2-h sessions of CBT lasting over three months, compared this group to 20 patients randomized to a waiting list. At the completion of the eight-week trial the treatment group had significant improvement in abdominal complaints. The study also found that patients who were treated with CBT developed a greater number of successful coping strategies. Patients treated with CBT had less "avoidant behavior," that is, they were less threatened by social situations and were less constrained in their daily activities by their IBS. Both the treatment and control patients were followed for an average of 2.25 years (ranging from six months to four years). At the end of long-term follow-up, the patients treated with CBT showed persistent and significant improvement in the number of abdominal complaints, number of successful coping strategies, and lower avoidance behavior than the patients in the control group. The study is most encouraging because the findings suggest that CBT can produce a persistent improvement over time in patients with chronic functional gastrointestinal complaints (Van Dulmen et al., 1996). The use of cognitive behavioral approaches has been adapted for use in a group setting. Preliminary reports suggest the same effects as for individually based CBT (Toner et al., 1998).

The effectiveness of CBT for patients with gastrointestinal disorders extends beyond IBS. In a study of 100 patients with functional dyspepsia, 50 patients had 10 sessions of CBT, compared to a control group receiving no active psychological treatment. Patients were evaluated for GI symptoms, "target complaints" (issues the patients identified as being most problematic), a specific measure of dyspepsia, and the patient's psychological status. Both groups showed improvement at the four month and one year follow-up assessments in levels of dyspepsia and psychological status. The investigators attributed this improvement in the control group to a nonspecific effect resulting from additional interest and attention shown by the investigators as part of the intake and randomization process. The cognitive psychotherapy group showed greater reduction than the control group in GI symptoms. In addition, the patients who received CBT had significant self-reported improvement in their "target complaints" as compared to controls ($p = 0.001$). These findings suggest that CBT is useful in treating a spectrum of chronic gastrointestinal complaints beyond those associated with IBS alone (Haug et al., 1994).

Psychodynamic Psychotherapy

Psychodynamic psychotherapy is based on the premise that patients' symptoms of depression and anxiety result from the stress of unresolved conflicts. The purpose of psychodynamic psychotherapy is to resolve the nature of the relationships patients have with individuals in their current life as well as experiences in earlier life. Svedlund treated IBS patients with psychodynamic psychotherapy over a period of three months. The patients were significantly improved in somatic symptoms over controls. At a one-year follow-up the psychotherapy patients showed continued improvement while the controls showed deterioration (Svedlund et al., 1983).

Guthrie and Creed randomized 102 patients with IBS to a course of psychodynamic psychotherapy in combination with relaxation techniques and ongoing standard medical treatment, such as, the use of antispasmodics and dietary modifications. The control group consisted of 49 patients randomized to ongoing standard medical treatment. It is important to note that these patients were eligible for entry into the study only if they had been engaged in active medical treatment for at least six months prior to the study and had failed to improve. All patients were assessed psychologically both on entry and completion of the study. Gastrointestinal symptoms were rated both by the patients' treating gastroenterologist who was blinded to the treatment, and by the patients themselves. The treatment group had an initial 2-h psychotherapeutic intake session, six psychotherapy sessions, and relaxation tapes that the patients could use at any time. There was significant improvement in bowel symptoms as rated by the gastroenterologist in the treatment group compared to controls ($p < 0.01$). Patients in the treatment group reported significant improvement in abdominal pain and diarrhea. There was no improvement in symptoms of bloating or consistency of bowel movements between the two groups. Psychiatric assessments were significantly improved in patients in the treatment group compared to controls. It is important to note that 30% of the patients met *DSM-III* criteria for major depressive disorder and 18% met diagnostic criteria for an anxiety disorder. These findings suggest that, for patients with coexisting psychiatric disorders, psychodynamic psychotherapy may be more useful than CBT (Guthrie et al., 1991; Blanchard et al., 1992).

In a similar trial, Guthrie randomized 102 patients to either active psychodynamic psychotherapy or "supportive listening." This latter modality consisted of the same therapist (the investigator) conducting the active psychotherapeutic arm of the study, but spending time with patients by listening to them and not offering comments or active therapeutic intervention. This technique was utilized to mitigate any bias introduced by the personality of the investigator on both experimental and control subjects. Patients randomized to active treatment had significant improvement in abdominal symptoms and psychological status compared to controls, as rated by their treating gastroenterologist and by their own report. The group that received psychodynamic psychotherapy had a 75% reduction in health care utilization in the one year follow-up period after cessation of treatment (Guthrie et al., 1993). This research suggests that a broader psychotherapeutic approach should be a consideration for patients with a variety of GI disorders. Resolution of psychological conflicts may dramatically alter how patients cope with their GI symptoms and thus improve their quality of life.

Other Modalities

Houghton, Heyman, and Whorwell (1996) used hypnotherapy to treat 25 (mostly female) patients with severe IBS. These patients were compared to an age/gender-matched control group of patients with comparable IBS severity. In addition to severity of GI symptoms, the investigators measured quality of life and extraintestinal medical complaints. The hypnotherapy group received 12 30-min sessions during which patients were directed toward "control of gut function" through hypnotic suggestions. GI symptoms improved significantly in the hypnotherapy group. Extraintestinal symptoms such as lethargy, backache, and headache significantly improved in the hypnotherapy group compared to controls. The hypnotherapy group showed significant improvement on a spectrum of quality of life measures including a sense of psychiatric well-being, physical well-being, mood, locus of control, social behavior, and ability to perform and enjoy work ($p < 0.001 - 0.05$). Houghton's study would suggest that innovative behavioral techniques in the hands of skilled clinicians can produce real benefits for patients suffering from functional gastrointestinal disorders (Houghton et al., 1996).

Biofeedback, that is, "multicomponent treatment," involving simultaneous use of multiple behavioral interventions, such as patient education (Blanchard & Schwartz, 1987) and the use of psychodrama (Arn et al., 1989), have all had some investigation. Behavioral treatment research is not easy to perform. Patients who self-select for specific treatments, inclusion criteria, outcome measurements, investigator bias, and the placebo effect can make this area particularly challenging for investigators. Talley highlighted the difficulties associated with this area of research in his review of the literature from 1966 to 1994. In an evaluation of only 14 studies that met rigid methodological criteria (use of a control group and other criteria), Talley found that although 8 of the 14 studies (57%) showed that psychological treatment was superior, only one study exceeded the investigators' standard for a "quality study" as measured by an algorithm that Talley developed (Talley et al., 1996). To improve research in this area, international working teams have undertaken an initiative to devise standard criteria for conducting treatment trials in behavioral research (Veldhuyzan et al., 1999).

CONCLUSIONS

Patients with functional gastrointestinal disorders, particularly those who have failed to respond to medical treatment, are a challenge for any health care professional. It is easy for both parties to become frustrated with the failure of progression in treatment. The evolving area of psychotherapeutic and behavioral interventions in functional gastrointestinal disorders has a small but maturing body of data to support the usefulness of psychotherapeutic intervention, particularly when medical management has failed.

Functional gastrointestinal disorders have repeatedly been shown to be commonly associated with anxiety, mood, and somatoform disorders. The ability to detect and treat comorbid psychiatric disorders has significant implications for improving the quality of life for these patients. Optimal multimodal treatment has yet to be defined for these patients, as many of the studies are methodologically flawed (Talley et al., 1996). However, even with the limitations of past studies, the literature supports the important role for psychiatry and psychology in the treatment of functional gastrointestinal disorders.

REFERENCES

Abraham, H. D., Anderson, C., & Lee, D. E. (1997). Somatization disorder in sphincter of Oddi dysfunction. *Psychosomatic Medicine, 59,* 553–557.

Alexander, F. (1950). *Anonymous psychosomatic medicine: Its principles and applications.* New York: W.W. Norton.

Almy, T. P. (1947). Alterations in colonic function in man under stress. I: Experimental production of changes simulating the "irritable colon." *Gastroenterology, 8,* 616–626.

Almy, T. P., Kern, F., & Tulin, M. (1949). Alterations in colonic function in man under stress. II: Experimental production of sigmoid spasm in healthy persons. *Gastroenterology, 12,* 425–436.

Arn, I., Theorell, T., Uvnas-Moberg, K., & Jonsson, C. (1989). Psychodrama group therapy for patients with functional gastrointestinal disorders—A controlled long-term follow-up study. *Psychotherapy & Psychosomatics, 51,* 113–119.

Beaumont, W. (1833). *Anonymous experiments and observations on the gastric juice and the physiology of digestion.* New York: F. P. Allen.

Blanchard, E. B., Scharff, L., Payne, A., Schwartz, S. P., Suls, J. M., & Malamood, H. (1992). Prediction of outcome from cognitive-behavioral treatment of irritable bowel syndrome. *Behavior Research & Therapy, 30,* 647–650.

Blanchard, E. B., & Schwartz, S. P. (1987). Adaptation of a multi-component treatment program for irritable bowel syndrome to a small group format. *Biofeedback and Self-Regulation, 12,* 63–69.

Bradley, L. A., Richter, J. E., Pulliam, T. J., Haile, J. M., Scarinci, I. C., & Schan, C. A. (1993). The relationship between stress and symptoms of gastroesophageal reflux: The influence of psychological factors. *American Journal of Gastroenterology, 88,* 11–19.

Brzana, R. J., & Koch, K. L. (1997). Gastroesophageal reflux disease presenting with intractable nausea. *Annals of Internal Medicine, 126,* 704–707.

Cannon, R. O., Quyyumi, A. A., Mincemoyer, R., et al. (1994). Imipramine in patients with chest pain despite normal coronary angiograms. *New England Journal of Medicine, 330,* 1411–1417.

Camilleri, M., & Choi, M. G. (1997). Review article: Irritable bowel syndrome. *Alimentary Pharmacology & Therapeutics, 11,* 3–15.

Clouse, R. E., & Lustman, P. (1983). Psychiatric illness and contraction abnormalities of the esophagus. *New England Journal of Medicine, 309,* 1337–1342.

Clouse, R. E., Lustman, P., & Eckert, T. C., Feney, C. M., & Griffith, L. S. (1987). Low-dose trazodone for symptomatic patients with esophageal contraction abnormalities: A double-blind, placebo-controlled trial. *Gastroenterology, 92,* 1027–1036.

Drossman, D. A. (1994). *Functional gastrointestinal disorders: Diagnosis and treatment.* Boston: Little Brown.

Drossman, D. A. (1995). Diagnosing and treating patients with refractory functional gastrointestinal disorders. *Annals of Internal Medicine, 123,* 688–697.

Drossman, D. A., Creed, F. H., Fava, G. A., Olden, K. W. (1995). Psychosocial aspects of the functional gastrointestinal disorders. *Gastroenterology International, 8,* 47–90.

Drossman, D. A., Li, Z., Andruzzi, E. (1993). U.S. householder survey of functional GI disorders: Prevalence, sociodemography and health impact. *Digestive Diseases & Sciences, 13,* 1569.

Drossman, D. A., McKee, D., & Sandler, R. (1988). Psychosocial factors in the irritable bowel syndrome. A multivariate study of patients and nonpatients with irritable bowel syndrome. *Gastroenterology, 95,* 701–708.

Drossman, D. A., Creed, F. H., Olden, K. W., Svedlund, J., Toner, B. B., & Whitehead, W. E. (1999). Psychosocial aspects of the functional gastrointestinal disorders. *Gut, 45,* II25–II30.

Felitti, V. J., Anda, R. F., Nordenberg, D., Williamson, D. F., Spitz, A. M., Edward, V., et al. (1998). Relationship of childhood abuse and household dysfunction to many of the leading causes of death in adults–The Adverse Childhood (ACE) Study. *American Journal of Preventive Medicine, 14*(4), 245–258

Fossey, M. D., & Lydiard, R. B. (1990). Anxiety and the gastrointestinal system. *Psychiatric Medicine, 8,* 175–186.

Graham, D. Y. (1996). Non-steroidal anti-inflammatory drugs, Helicobacter pylori, and ulcers: Where we stand. *American Journal of Gastroenterology, 91,* 2080–2086.

Greene, B., & Blanchard, E. B. (1994). Cognitive therapy for irritable bowel syndrome. *Journal of Consulting Clinical Psychology, 62,* 576–582.

Guthrie, E. A., Creed, F. H., Dawson, D., & Tomenson, B. (1991). A controlled trial of psychological treatment for the irritable bowel syndrome. *Gastroenterology, 100,* 450–457.

Guthrie, E. A., Creed, F. H., Dawson, D., Tomenson, B. (1993). A randomised controlled trial of psychotherapy in patients with refractory irritable bowel syndrome. *British Journal of Psychiatry, 163,* 315–321.

Haug, T. T., Wilhelmsen, I., Svebak, S., Berstad, A., & Ursin, H. (1994). Psychotherapy in functional dyspepsia. *Journal of Psychosomatic Research, 38,* 735–744.

Helzer, J. E., Chammas, S., Norland, C. C., Stillings, W. A., & Alpers, D. M. (1984). A study of the association between Crohn's disease and psychiatric illness. *Gastroenterology, 86,* 324–330.

Helzer, J. E., Stillings, W., Chammas, S., Morland, C. C., & Alpers, D. M. (1982). A controlled study of the association between ulcerative colitis and psychiatric diagnoses. *Digestive Diseases and Sciences, 27,* 513–518.

Herman, J. L. (1989). Childhood trauma and borderline personality disorder. *American Journal of Psychiatry, 146*(4), 490–495.

Holtmann, G., Kriebel, R., & Singer, M. V. (1990). Mental stress and gastric acid secretion: do personality traits influence the response? *Digestive Diseases and Sciences, 35,* 998–1007.

Houghton, L. A., Heyman, D. J., & Whorwell, P. J. (1996). Symptomatology, quality of life and economic features of irritable bowel syndrome–The effect of hypnotherapy. *Alimentary Pharmacology & Therapeutics, 10,* 91–95.

Hunt, R. H. (1996). Eradication of *Helicobacter pylori* infection. *American Journal of Medicine, 100,* 42S–51S.

Klein, K. B. (1988). Controlled treatment trials in the irritable bowel syndrome: A critique. *Gastroenterology, 95,* 232–241.

Leserman, J., Drossman, D. A., Li, Z., Toomey, T. C., Nachman, G., & Glogau, L. (1996). Sexual and physical abuse history in gastroenterology practice: how types of abuse impact health status. *Psychosomatic Medicine, 58,* 4–15.

Leserman, J., Li, Z., Drossman, D. A., Toomey, T. C., Nachman, G., & Glogau, L. (1997). Impact of sexual and physical abuse dimensions on health status: development of an abuse severity measure. *Psychosomatic Medicine, 59,* 152–160.

Levenstein, S. (1998). Stress and peptic ulcer: Life beyond helicobacter. *British Medical Journal, 316,* 538–541.

Levenstein, S., Prantera, C., Varvo, V., Spinella, S., Arca, M., & Bassi, O. (1992). Life events, personality, and physical risk factors in recent-onset duodenal ulcer: A preliminary study. *Journal of Clinicial Gastroenterology, 14,* 203–210.

Levenstein, S., Prantera, C., Scribano, M. L., Scribano, M. L., Berto, E., Spinella, S., et al. (1996). Psychologic predictors of duodenal ulcer healing. *Journal of Clinicial Gastroenterology, 22,* 84–89.

Levenstein, S. (1998). Stress and peptic ulcer: Life beyond helicobacter. *British Medical Journal, 316,* 538–541.

Lydiard, R. B., Greenwald, S., Weissman, M., Johnson, J., Drossman, D. A., & Ballenger, J. C. (1999). Panic disorder and gastrointestinal symptoms: findings from the NIMH epidemiologic catchment area project. *American Journal of Psychiatry, 151,* 64–70.

Marshall, B. J., & Warren, J. R. (1984). Unidentified curved bacilli in the stomach of patients with gastritis and peptic ulceration. *Lancet, 1,* 1311–1315.

Masand, P. S., Kaplan, D. S., Gupta, S., Bhandary, A. N., Nasra, G. S., Kline, M. D., et al. (1995). Major depression and irritable bowel syndrome: is there a relationship? *Journal of Clinical Psychiatry, 56,* 363–367.

McColl, K. E. L., El-Nujumi, A. M., Chittajallu, R. S., Dahill, S. W., Dorrian, C. A., El-Omar, E., et al. (1993). A study of the pathogenesis of Helicobacter pylori negative chronic duodenal ulceration. *Gut, 34,* 762–768.

North, C. S., Clouse, R. E., Sptznagel, E. L., & Alpers, D. H. (1990). The relation of ulcerative colitis to psychiatric factors: a review of findings and methods. *American Journal of Psychiatry, 147,* 974–981.

North, C. S., Alpers, D. H., Helzer, J. E., Spitznagel, E. L, & Clouse, R. E. (1991). Do life events or depression exacerbate inflammatory bowel disease? *Annals of Internal Medicine, 114,* 381–386.

Olden, K. W. (1992). Inflammatory bowel disease: A biopsychosocial perspective. *Psychiatric Annals, 22,* 619–623.

Olden, K. W. (1997). Stress and the GI tract. In J. Hubbard & E. Workman (Eds.), *Handbook of stress medicine: An organ system approach.* Boca Raton, FL: CRC Press.

Olden, K. W. (1998). Inflammatory bowel disease and psychiatry: From causality to comorbidity. *Medical Psychiatry, 1,* 17–21.

Payne, A., & Blanchard, E. B. (1995). A controlled comparison of cognitive therapy and self-help support groups in the treatment of irritable bowel syndrome. *Journal of Consulting and Clinical Psychology, 63,* 779–786.

Rao, S. S. C., Gregersen, H., Hayek, B., Summers, R. W., & Christensen, J. (1996). Unexplained chest pain: The hypersensitive, hyperreactive and poorly compliant esophagus. *Annals of Internal Medicine, 124,* 950–958.

Richter, J. E. (1999). Extraesophageal manifestations of gastroesophageal reflux disease. In L. J. Brandt (Ed.), *Clinical practice of gastroenterology* (pp. 34–43). Philadelphia: Current Medicine, Inc.

Sperling, R. M., & McQuaid, K. R. (1996). Rational medical therapy of functional GI disorders. In K. W. Olden (Ed.), *Handbook of functional gastrointestinal disorders* (pp. 269–328). New York: Marcel Dekker.

Svedlund, J., Sjodin, I., Ottosson, J. O., & Dotevall, G. (1983). Controlled study of psychotherapy in irritable bowel syndrome. *Lancet, ii,* 589–592.

Talley, N. J., Fett, S. L., Zinsmeister, A. R., & Melton, L. J., 3rd. (1994). Gastrointestinal tract symptoms and self-reported abuse: a population-based study. *Gastroenterology, 107,* 1040–1049.

Talley, N. J., Owen, B. K., Boyce, P., & Paterson, K. (1996). Psychological treatment for irritable bowel syndrome: a critique of controlled clinical trials. *American Journal of Gastroenterology, 91,* 277–286.

Toner, B. B., Segal, Z. V., Emmott, S., Myran, D., Ali, A., DiGasbarro, I., et al. (1998). Cognitive-behavioral group therapy for patients with irritable bowel syndrome. *International Journal of Group Psychotherapy, 48,* 215–243.

Van Dulmen, A. M., Fennis, J. F. M., & Bleijenberg, G. (1996). Cognitive-behavioral group therapy for irritable bowel syndrome: Effects and long-term follow-up. *Psychosomatic Medicine, 58,* 508–514.

Veldhuyzen van Zanten, S. J., Talley, N. J., Bytzer, P., Klein, K. B., Whorwell, P. J., & Zinsmeister, A. R. (1999). Design of treatment trials for functional gastrointestinal disorders. *Gut, 45,* II69–II77.

Walker, E. A., Katon, W. J., Jemelka, R. P., et al. (1992). Comorbidity of gastrointestinal complaints, depression and anxiety in the epidemiologic catchment area (ECA) study. *American Journal of Medicine, 92,* 26S–30S.

Walker, E. A., Gelfand, M. D., Gelfand, A. N., Creed, F., & Katon, W. J. (1996). The relationship of current psychiatric disorder to functional disability and distress in patients with inflammatory bowel disease. *General Hospital Psychiatry, 18,* 220–229.

Whitehead, W. E., & Crowell, M. D. (1991). Psychologic considerations in the irritable bowel syndrome. *Gastrointestinal Clinics of North America, 20,* 249–267.

Whitehead, W. E. (1992). Behavioral medicine approaches to gastrointestinal disorders. *Journal of Consulting Clinical Psychology, 60,* 605–612.

CHAPTER

6

Endocrine Disorders

ELBERT F. SHOLAR
SUSAN G. KORNSTEIN
DAVID F. GARDNER

Endocrine and metabolic disorders are among the most frequent medical causes of psychiatric symptoms. These disorders can occur at any age, but are most commonly seen during the third and fourth decades of life, and occur more frequently in women. Cognitive, affective, and behavioral changes were noted in the earliest accounts of endocrine disorders described by Addison (1868), Cushing (1932), Sheehan (1939), and others.

Early in the course of an endocrine disorder, a patient may present primarily with psychiatric symptoms, and may be misdiagnosed as depressed, neurotic, demented, or psychotic. In the elderly, endocrine disorders may be easily overlooked, as the physical symptoms may not be evident and the mental changes mistaken for dementia. As the disease progresses, the psychiatric symptoms will worsen and physical symptoms will emerge, as hormones affect many organ systems.

Screening for endocrine dysfunction should be an essential part of the diagnostic work-up whenever patients present with symptoms that could be caused by underlying endocrine disorders, especially in the elderly and in women. Ideally, such screening would take place whenever a new patient seeks psychotherapy. Persistent insomnia, for instance, prompts many individuals to seek treatment. Some of these patients are actually in need of thyroid medication rather than antianxiety medication. Laboratory tests may include serum electrolytes, fasting blood sugar, thyroid stimulating hormone (TSH), and calcium levels. Psychiatric symptoms will not improve until the underlying endocrine disorder is treated; in fact, they may worsen if the individual is treated with psychotropic medication alone. Psychiatric disorders resulting from an endocrine disease are categorized as "mental disorder due to a general medical condition" in *DSM-IV*, and the medical condition is noted on Axis III (APA, 1994).

There has been little research into the capacity for psychiatric or psychological factors to trigger endocrine disorders. Stressful life events have been thought to play a role in the onset of illness in Graves' and Cushing's diseases. However, research into the effects of psychological factors on endocrine disorders has been limited by methodological deficiencies.

In this chapter, we focus on those endocrine disorders that most often manifest psychiatric syndromes. These include disorders of glucose metabolism, thyroid and adrenal malfunction, disorders of calcium homeostasis, and pituitary irregularities.

OVERVIEW OF THE ENDOCRINE SYSTEM

Endocrinology involves the study of chemical mediators (hormones) that travel from their site of production to other parts of the body, where they influence the function of other tissues. Endocrine disorders result from either too much or too little of a hormone, or from resistance to a hormone's action at the target tissue. Hormone production takes place in the pituitary gland, the hypothalamus, and the major endocrine organs (the adrenal, thyroid, and parathyroid glands; the pancreatic islets; and the ovaries and testes). The hypothalamus produces antidiuretic hormone, which regulates urinary concentration by the kidney, and oxytocin, which is necessary for milk letdown during breastfeeding. Both of these hormones are stored in the posterior pituitary. In addition, the hypothalamus produces several releasing and inhibiting hormones that influence hormone production in the anterior pituitary. These include growth hormone releasing hormone (GHRH) and growth hormone release inhibiting factor (GHRF), which influence production and secretion of growth hormone (GH); and gonadotropin releasing hormone (GnRH), which influences production and secretion of luteinizing hormone (LH) and follicle stimulating hormone (FSH) by the anterior pituitary. Both LH and FSH are necessary for normal gonadal functioning in men and women. Also produced by the hypothalamus are prolactin release inhibiting factor (dopamine) and prolactin releasing hormone (PRH), which influence prolactin (PRL) production by the anterior pituitary, and thus milk production and lactation; thyrotropin releasing hormone (TRH) and corticotropin releasing hormone (CRH), which affect the release of TSH and adrenocorticotropic hormone (ACTH), which control adrenocortical production of glucocorticoids by the anterior pituitary, respectively. The anterior pituitary produces a total of six hormones: TSH, GH, PRL, LH, FSH, and ACTH.

DISORDERS OF GLUCOSE METABOLISM

Diabetes Mellitus

Definition, Epidemiology, and Etiology

Diabetes mellitus is the most common clinical endocrine disorder, with a prevalence rate of 1–2% in the United States. It occurs twice as often in African Americans as in Caucasians. The incidence is nearly equal in men and women. The onset and severity of some complications of diabetes (in particular, nephropathy, retinopathy, and neuropathy) are directly related to the adequacy of control of blood glucose levels.

Diabetes mellitus occurs in two primary forms. In Type 1 (often referred to as insulin-dependent or juvenile-onset diabetes), the destruction of beta cells in the pancreas causes severe insulin deficiency. This results in decreased glucose utilization, increased glucose production, and significant hyperglycemia. It typically begins in childhood or adolescence, and is most common in Caucasians. Etiologic factors include genetic, autoimmune, environmental/toxic, and viral causes. Type 2 (noninsulin-dependent or maturity onset) is most common in adults over age 40 who are obese. It is much more common than Type 1 and is thought to have a different etiology and mechanism. Genetic and environmental/toxic factors are believed to be involved in the development of Type 2 diabetes. Hyperglycemia in Type 2 diabetic patients is related to abnormalities in insulin secretion and insulin action, the latter often referred to as insulin resistance.

Diabetes mellitus represents a group of heterogeneous disorders affecting multiple organ systems. An elevated blood glucose level and a number of potentially disabling complications characterize the disease. These complications include disorders of the small blood vessels (microvascular disease), involvement of larger blood vessels (macrovascular disease), and other complications, such as neuropathy, increased susceptibility to infections, poor wound healing, and high-risk pregnancies. Microvascular disease results in diabetic retinopathy and nephropathy. Macrovascular disease causes accelerated atherosclerosis, resulting in coronary artery disease, cerebrovascular disease (such as strokes), and peripheral vascular disease. For a review of the chronic complications of diabetes and overall management see Brownlee and King (1996) and Hirsch and Riddle (1997).

The central nervous system (CNS) is very sensitive to acute changes in blood glucose levels, as it cannot manufacture glucose and cannot store more than a few minutes' supply of glucose. Plasma glucose levels are normally maintained in a narrow range. Insulin, produced by the pancreas, lowers blood glucose levels by increasing uptake of glucose in peripheral tissues and decreasing glucose production. Glucagon, also produced by the pancreas, acts on the liver to increase the production of glucose from glycogen (a form of sugar stored in the liver), and to increase the production of glucose from amino acids and fatty acids. Epinephrine from the adrenal medulla stimulates the liver to produce and release glucose and decreases the utilization of glucose by peripheral tissues (thus ensuring that the brain receives more glucose). Growth hormone and cortisol antagonize insulin action and, therefore, tend to raise plasma glucose concentrations.

The role of psychosocial factors in diabetes is controversial. The evidence suggesting a role for psychosocial factors in the onset of illness is inconclusive;

however, many studies have shown a relationship between psychosocial factors and control of blood sugar.

Symptoms

The symptoms of hyperglycemia are sometimes initially misdiagnosed as hypochondriasis. Increased urination, appetite, and thirst are typically seen, along with nausea and vomiting, fatigue, blurred vision, and paresthesias ("pins and needles" sensations in the fingers and toes). Fewer than 5% of patients present with delirium due to diabetic ketoacidosis. Cognitive deficits, such as impaired attention, memory problems, and poor problem-solving abilities, may be seen. Infrequently, a patient will present with impotence as his only symptom of hyperglycemia.

Course of Illness

Diabetes may result in a number of acute and chronic complications. Severe hyperglycemia in Type 1 diabetes may be associated with diabetic ketoacidosis, a condition in which the body breaks down fatty acids and proteins to produce keto acids, which provide fuel for the brain. This results in metabolic acidosis, with symptoms of tremendous thirst, severe fatigue, nausea, vomiting, and sometimes coma. In Type 2 diabetes, severe hyperglycemia may result in hyperosmolar nonketotic coma (these patients do not develop ketoacidosis for unknown reasons). Both of these conditions may cause death if not rapidly and appropriately treated. Diabetic neuropathy is common and often presents as a bilateral, symmetric, sensory syndrome characterized by paresthesias and loss of sensation. Painful neuropathies may also occur, typically with burning and shooting pains in the lower extremities. Other potential complications, such as retinopathy and nephropathy, are discussed in the previous section.

Diagnostic Tests

The best screening test for diabetes mellitus is a fasting plasma glucose determination. A level over 125 mg/dl is diagnostic for this disorder. A glucose tolerance test (measuring the reaction to consumption of a large amount of glucose over a several-hour period) may be done if the fasting plasma glucose level is normal but there is still a suspicion that the illness exists. Patients with borderline results should undergo periodic testing of blood glucose levels and follow the recommendations regarding diet, exercise, and weight loss given by their physician. Glycemic control may be monitored in patients with diabetes by measurement of hemoglobin A1c levels, which give an indication of plasma glucose levels over the preceding 8 to 10 weeks. In poorly controlled diabetes, the hemoglobin A1c concentration will be markedly elevated.

Treatment

Type 1 diabetes is treated with dietary management, an exercise program (as fatty tissue increases insulin resistance), and insulin replacement therapy (via injection of insulin into subcutaneous tissue). Type 2 diabetes is treated with dietary management, weight loss in most patients, exercise, oral medication (hypoglycemic agents) to lower blood sugar, and, sometimes, insulin injections. Treatment must be individualized to the patient, and may need frequent adjustment. For example, individuals who exercise frequently require less insulin than those who are more sedentary; and insulin requirements increase during periods of stress and infection. Patients are required to monitor their blood sugar several times a day. The overall goal of treatment is to return plasma glucose concentrations to the "near-normal" range, which has been shown in several studies to reduce the risk of diabetic complications.

Some tricyclic antidepressants (e.g., amitriptyline, nortriptyline, and desipramine) have shown success in treating the painful neuropathies associated with diabetes mellitus. Anticonvulsants (carbamazepine, gabapentin) may be helpful as well.

Psychological Sequelae

As a lifelong illness that requires attention to almost every aspect of daily life, diabetes mellitus may have profound emotional effects on both the patient and those close to him or her. Patients and family members commonly experience denial, anger, depression, anxiety, and feelings of frustration. Mood swings may occur, along with feelings of irritability. Additionally, blood sugar levels may be affected by stress, which in turn will have emotional effects. Psychosocial factors may also influence control of blood sugar by influencing compliance with treatment. Studies suggest that psychosocial factors affect blood sugar both directly (via neuroendocrine effects) and indirectly (via patient compliance) (Helz & Templeton, 1990; Jacobson, 1996).

Initially, the individual and family experience a sense of loss upon learning of the diagnosis of diabetes mellitus. Sometimes, there is a period of bereavement as well (Jacobson, 1996). Intermittent periods of sadness, loneliness, apprehension, irritability, and a longing for health are often seen in children and adolescents (Kovacs et al., 1995). Parents may worry about their child's future and may feel guilty, blaming themselves for their child's illness. Adjustment difficulties are more likely in families with antecedent psychosocial problems (Hauser et al., 1985). Future noncompliance with appointments and control of blood sugar may be predicted by the presence of family problems at the time of diagnosis. Early difficulty in adjustment also predicts the later development of anxiety and depression (Kovacs et al., 1995).

Early treatment of emotional problems and education of the patient and family are important. Initially, the patient and significant others should be given only necessary information and helped through the process of grieving the loss of a "normal" life. The immediate goal is stabilization of blood sugar levels. More complete information is beneficial when the patient has adjusted emotionally and is familiar with the skills needed to live with the illness (i.e., monitoring blood glucose, taking medication, proper technique for insulin injections if necessary, following a diet and exercise program, and monitoring for symptoms and complications of the illness). The patient should develop an understanding that diabetes mellitus is compatible with living a happy and healthy life (Jacobson, 1996).

Patients may fear the daily pain from pricking their finger several times a day to test blood glucose. They may be concerned that insulin will make them fat. They may become frustrated with the dietary restrictions and the need to take medication. Jacobson provides an excellent review of common concerns in patients with diabetes mellitus (Jacobson, 1996). When a patient has an abnormal test result, they may react with anger, anxiety, or depression. The clinician will need to listen to the expressed emotions, explain what the information means, and try to allay the patient's fears. In patients with serious complications, prolonged periods of mourning are common (Jacobson et al., 1994). Patients may feel uncertain about their future; they may be more upset by transient changes than by prolonged periods of more stable (but more severe) complications. Group and individual therapy may help patients to cope with major complications such as visual loss (Bernbaum et al., 1989). Couples may benefit from therapy to help them adjust to sexual problems with impotence due to diabetes (McCulloch et al., 1986).

Various psychological problems may affect compliance with treatment. Psychosocial interventions have been primarily evaluated in children and adolescents. These studies suggest that behavioral interventions based on social learning theory and groups focusing on building coping skills can improve adjustment to illness, adherence to treatment, and control of blood glucose (Padgett et al., 1988).

Women with insulin-dependent diabetes mellitus appear to be at greater risk than the general population for developing eating disorders (Rodin & Daneman, 1992). They may try to lose weight by skipping or reducing their insulin dose. These behaviors are associated with difficulty controlling blood sugar (Polonsky et al., 1994), and they predispose patients to the development of visual problems (Rydall et al., 1994). Cognitive-behavioral treatments may be useful in these patients to address eating disorders.

Major depressive disorder and dysthymia are common in both Type 1 and Type 2 diabetes. The estimated prevalence of major depressive disorder in diabetics is about 33%. Depressive disorders are best treated with SSRI antidepressants, as they have less effect on glucose metabolism, a lower incidence of weight gain and carbohydrate craving, and no anticholinergic or cardiac side effects. The newer antipsychotics are preferred in the treatment of psychosis in patients with diabetes mellitus, as they have lower risks of extrapyramidal side effects (EPS) and therefore minimize the need for anticholinergic agents, which may adversely affect control of blood glucose. However, olanzapine and clozapine may cause weight gain and diabetes in some individuals. Anticonvulsants are preferable in the treatment of bipolar disorder in diabetic individuals, as lithium may have more effects on blood glucose levels. Buspirone and benzodiazepines are useful in treating anxiety, and thereby may improve control of blood glucose (Lustman et al., 1997). Beta-blockers should be used with care, as they may mask the symptoms of hypoglycemia.

Hypoglycemia

Definition and Etiology

Hypoglycemia is a syndrome that may be defined by a triad of clinical findings: (1) appropriate symptoms (as noted below); (2) a plasma glucose level below 50–60 mg per dl; and (3) reversal of symptoms upon administration of glucose. Reactive (postprandial, postabsorptive) hypoglycemia occurs within 5 h after the ingestion of food. Fasting (spontaneous) hypoglycemia occurs more than 5 h after eating.

Fasting hypoglycemia may be seen in a variety of disorders: insulin-secreting tumors of the islet cells of the pancreas, large nonislet cell tumors, severe liver or kidney disease, endocrine deficiency states (e.g., adrenal insufficiency, hypopituitarism), severe starvation, autoimmune disorders with antibodies to insulin or the insulin receptor, and drugs or toxins (Field, 1989). Drugs that most commonly cause fasting hypoglycemia are insulin and oral hypoglycemic agents used to treat diabetes. In many cases, alcohol, aspirin and other salicylates, and propranolol may be the cause. The differential diagnosis of fasting hypoglycemia should always include surreptitious administration of insulin or an oral hypoglycemic agent. In patients suspected of surreptitious ingestion of an oral hypoglycemic, a blood or urine toxicology test should be performed.

Reactive hypoglycemia may be divided into three major categories: (1) alimentary hypoglycemia, usually associated with previous gastric surgery; (2) mild diabetes, characterized by a delayed but excessive insulin response to glucose; and (3) idiopathic ("functional") hypoglycemia (Hofeldt, 1989).

Hypoglycemia is frequently overdiagnosed; for a review of this subject, see Gastineau (1983) and Nelson (1985). This is particularly true for reactive hypoglycemia, which became a fashionable diagnosis to explain a variety of poorly defined psychological and physical ailments, including depression, anxiety, fatigue, sexual difficulties, and overall loss of vitality (Yager & Young, 1974).

Symptoms and Course of Illness

Symptomatic hypoglycemia is marked by the presence of multiple symptoms of autonomic arousal (anxiety, palpitations, sweating, feelings of panic, and lightheadedness). Other symptoms include headache, restlessness, irritability, blurred or double vision, weakness, dizziness, incoordination, slurred speech, and paresthesias. In cases of prolonged hypoglycemia, seizures, personality changes, cognitive problems, coma, and even death may occur.

Diagnostic Tests

Patients should be evaluated with a plasma glucose determination at the time symptoms occur. For patients with reactive hypoglycemia, this measurement should be done following ingestion of a normal meal of mixed carbohydrates, proteins, and fats (Service, 1997). In patients with fasting hypoglycemia, the plasma glucose determination should be done after an overnight fast, although fasting may need to be extended up to 72 h to get diagnostic information.

Treatment

In most patients with reactive hypoglycemia, dietary changes in terms of content and frequency of meals may be sufficient to alleviate symptoms. Therapy in patients with fasting hypoglycemia will vary with the etiology of the underlying disorder. In diabetic patients receiving insulin, modifications of the insulin regimen will be critical to eliminating hypoglycemic symptoms. The inhibition of epinephrine release by maintaining normal blood glucose levels will prevent the development of physiological and psychological symptoms. Alcoholics should be encouraged to abstain from alcohol, and nutritional disturbances should be corrected.

THYROID DISEASE

Disorders of the thyroid are among the most common endocrine conditions, especially in women. There are two types of functional thyroid disorders, hyperthyroidism (thyrotoxicosis) and hypothyroidism. Thyrotoxicosis occurs eight times more frequently in women than men. Hypothyroidism also occurs much more often in women, particularly elderly women.

The thyroid gland produces thyroid hormones, which are necessary for the regulation of the basal metabolic rate and carbohydrate, fat, and protein synthesis and degradation. Triiodothyronine (T3) and thyroxin (T4) are produced from a common precursor, thyroglobulin, which is stored in thyroid follicles. In peripheral tissues, T4 is converted to T3, the metabolically active form of the hormone. The hypothalamus produces TRH, which stimulates the anterior pituitary to release TSH. TSH promotes the synthesis and release of T4 and T3.

Thyrotoxicosis

Etiology

Thyrotoxicosis (hyperthyroidism) is a clinical syndrome with multiple etiologies, all resulting in an increase in circulating thyroid hormone concentrations. The most common cause of thyrotoxicosis is Graves' disease, a systemic autoimmune disorder characterized by diffuse thyroid enlargement and extrathyroidal manifestations involving the eyes and skin. More than 95% of all cases of thyrotoxicosis are caused by Graves' disease, toxic nodular goiter, subacute thyroiditis, or excessive thyroid hormone replacement. Rare causes include thyrotropin-secreting pituitary tumors, trophoblastic tumors, struma ovarii, and iodine-induced thyrotoxicosis.

Symptoms

The typical patient with thyrotoxicosis appears hyperactive and has lost weight. He or she may have rapid and rambling speech, and may appear anxious and apprehensive. Other important signs include rapid heartbeat, warm, smooth, and moist skin, a fine tremor of the hands, hyperreflexia, and an enlarged thyroid (the front of the neck may appear swollen). Eyes may appear enlarged with a characteristic "bug-eyed" stare. Mental changes commonly occur and are often the initial complaint. Most frequently, the patient experiences anxiety, irritability, emotional lability, a feeling of apprehension, difficulty concentrating, and insomnia. He or she may report distractibility and a decrease in short-term memory. Psychosis occurs less commonly and is usually not severe.

Symptoms of thyrotoxicosis are variable, but the following are most often reported: nervousness, increased sweating, heat intolerance, fatigue, shortness of breath, palpitations, weight loss despite increased appetite, eye symptoms, muscle weakness, hair loss, and increased frequency of bowel movements. Menstrual cycle abnormalities may also be observed. Occasionally, a patient will lack many of the classical symptoms, and the diagnosis may be missed. This occurs most often in elderly patients who present with unexplained weight loss, muscle weakness, atrial fibrillation, and heart failure, a condition known as "apathetic thyrotoxicosis."

Thyrotoxicosis is frequently misdiagnosed as an anxiety disorder. Distinguishing features include the cognitive impairment, rapid heartbeat, fatigue, and constant state of anxiety, as well as palms that are warm and dry rather than cool and clammy. Other misdiagnoses may include depression, bipolar disorder, anorexia nervosa, schizophrenia, substance abuse, and cognitive impairment disorders of other etiologies.

Treatment

Treatment consists of normalization of circulating thyroid hormone levels. Initial therapy, however, is often symptomatic, with beta-adrenergic blocking medications (such as propranolol) effectively reversing many signs and symptoms of thyrotoxicosis. Definitive treatment for most patients involves antithyroid drugs or radioactive iodine. The role of surgery is limited. Hypothyroidism often develops during the first one to two years after treatment of thyrotoxicosis with radioactive iodine, although sometimes it does not appear for more than 5 to 10 years. As thyroid function returns to normal, anxiety, affective symptoms, and cognitive difficulties usually improve. Some patients who have severe prolonged thyrotoxicosis may have persistent mental impairment despite treatment of the underlying thyroid disorder.

The newer antidepressants such as the SSRIs, bupropion, and nefazodone appear to be safe in treating affective symptoms associated with thyrotoxicosis. The atypical antipsychotics (risperidone, olanzapine, and quetiapine) are preferred agents for the treatment of related psychosis. Benzodiazepines and buspirone may be useful adjuncts in managing anxiety and agitation.

Hypothyroidism

Hypothyroidism results from inadequate synthesis of thyroid hormone. It may be categorized as overt, with low thyroid hormone levels, elevated TSH, and presence of symptoms; or as subclinical, with normal thyroid hormone levels, elevated TSH, and absence of symptoms. The prevalence of overt hypothyroidism is about 1 percent, but increases with age. It is estimated that up to 15% of elderly women have overt hypothyroidism. Subclinical hypothyroidism occurs in about 3% of men and 7.5% of women; up to 16% of elderly women have subclinical hypothyroidism. About 5–15% of patients with subclinical hypothyroidism progress to overt hypothyroidism each year, and thus are more likely to be diagnosed.

Etiology

The most common cause of hypothyroidism is autoimmune thyroiditis, also known as Hashimoto's disease. This disorder, which occurs with increased frequency in women, is associated with the production of antibodies against thyroid tissue. Other causes include idiopathic atrophy, deficiency of dietary iodine (rare in the United States), hypopituitarism, hypothalamic disease, and iatrogenic hypothyroidism caused by drugs, surgery, or radioactive iodine.

Symptoms

Symptoms and signs of hypothyroidism are numerous and include cold intolerance, constipation, muscle cramps, menstrual disturbances, shortness of breath, dizziness, fainting spells, reduced hearing, poor appetite, abnormal sensations, weight gain, brittle and thinning hair, slow heart rate, enlargement of the heart, and husky voice. Anemia and elevated levels of cholesterol and triglycerides may occur. Psychiatric symptoms include depressed mood, poor memory and concentration, apathy, and slow responses to questions. Some patients develop auditory hallucinations and paranoia, which is called "myxedema madness" (myxedema is an older term for hypothyroidism). Subclinical hypothyroidism may produce symptoms of depression and cognitive difficulties; however, these are generally less severe than in overt hypothyroidism. The latter may increase the risk of developing major depression, and studies have reported reduced efficacy of antidepressant medications in these patients.

Course of Illness

Hypothyroidism usually develops gradually, except when it is the result of surgical or radioactive iodine treatment of hyperthyroidism. Neonates with hypothyroidism may develop permanent physical and mental retardation (cretinism). Children who develop hypothyroidism often exhibit poor school performance and reversible growth retardation. In adults, the physical and mental symptoms are generally reversible with thyroid replacement therapy; however, hypothyroidism of long duration may produce permanent cognitive deficits.

Diagnostic Tests

The serum TSH concentration is the most sensitive test for diagnosing hypothyroidism. Depressed circulating thyroid hormone concentration results in elevated TSH levels in most patients. However, hypothyroidism due to hypothalamic or pituitary disease is associated with inappropriately low TSH levels.

Treatment

Levothyroxine (T4) is the preferred treatment for hypothyroidism. Treatments with L-triiodothyronine (T3) or mixed preparations of T4 and T3 should be avoided. Thyroid hormone should be gradually replaced, with adjustment of dose as indicated by TSH levels. Clinical improvement may not occur for several weeks after the initiation of thyroid hormone replacement therapy. Depression secondary to hypothyroidism usually improves with thyroid replacement therapy alone. Antidepressant therapy may be necessary for more severe cases; however, without treatment of the underlying hypothyroidism, antidepressant therapy is usually insufficient. In patients with severe psychiatric symptoms, such as psychosis or depression with suicidal ideation, urgent treatment with psychotropic medication is necessary. Low starting doses and less-sedating drugs are suggested. The SSRI antidepressants as well as bupropion, nefazodone, venlafaxine, and mirtazapine (used at higher doses to decrease the likelihood of sedation) are recommended. The newer antipsychotics are preferred for the treatment of psychosis. Buspirone may be useful in treating anxiety and agitation in these patients.

ADRENAL DISORDERS

Cushing's Syndrome

Etiology

Cushing's syndrome results from prolonged exposure of tissues to inappropriately elevated levels of plasma glucocorticoids. It may occur spontaneously or in association with chronic administration of glucocorticoids (e.g., cortisone, hydrocortisone, prednisone, methylprednisolone, triamcinolone, and dexamethasone). Spontaneous Cushing's syndrome may result from excessive secretion of ACTH by the pituitary gland, usually due to a pituitary adenoma (Cushing's disease), primary neoplasms of the adrenal cortex, or ectopic production of ACTH by a malignancy (in another tissue of the body).

Symptoms and Course of Illness

Typical clinical manifestations of Cushing's syndrome include truncal obesity, moon faces, hypertension, violaceous striae of the skin (violet lines), muscle weakness (primarily proximal muscles), excessive bruising, facial plethora (a swollen, red complexion), acne, hirsutism, menstrual disturbances (usually absence of menses), and peripheral edema. Metabolic consequences include carbohydrate intolerance (elevated blood sugar), hypokalemic alkalosis, and osteoporosis.

In exogenous Cushing's syndrome, similar physical manifestations are seen; however, myopathy, glucose intolerance, and osteoporosis tend to be more prominent. Cataracts and aseptic necrosis of the head of the femur may also be found. Hypertension is less common, and signs of masculinization and hyperpigmentation do not occur. The diagnosis of exogenous Cushing's syndrome is based on a history of prolonged administration of either ACTH or high doses of glucocorticoids. The duration of therapy and the dose given determines the likelihood of developing clinical features of Cushing's syndrome. Up to 14% of patients receiving high doses of glucocorticoids develop significant psychiatric symptoms. The occurrence of symptoms is clearly related to the dose of drug administered. Patients receiving the equivalent of more than 40 mg per day of prednisone are at greatest risk. Mental changes may be seen at any point, but are most common within the first 5 days of steroid treatment. Alterations in mood are seen most often; euphoria occurs in most cases, with irritability, increased appetite, increased libido, and insomnia.

In spontaneous Cushing's syndrome, psychiatric disturbances occur in over

50% of patients. Mental symptoms may precede physical signs or symptoms. The most frequent psychiatric presentation is depression accompanied by irritability, insomnia, crying spells, low energy, poor concentration and memory, decreased libido, and suicidal ideation. Agitation may alternate with periods of psychomotor retardation. Rapid mood fluctuations with episodic acute anxiety may occur. Occasionally, euphoria and manic excitement are noted, typically prior to the onset of depression. Cognitive impairment with confusion and disorientation may also be seen. However, paranoid states and schizophreniform syndromes rarely occur.

Diagnostic Tests

Patients with Cushing's syndrome may be misdiagnosed as having major depression, mania, bipolar depression, schizophrenia, or a variety of secondary, toxic, or metabolic conditions. However, misdiagnosis can be prevented, and excessive laboratory tests avoided, by the alert clinician. The distinctive physical signs of Cushing's syndrome (moon faces, hirsutism, etc.) should be observed, and an in-depth medical history should always be taken when seeing a new patient. If a patient is taking glucocorticoid medication, the psychotherapist should be aware of this before beginning treatment. Definitive diagnosis requires the demonstration of cortisol overproduction and an abnormality in the suppression of cortisol secretion. Screening tests include the overnight dexamethasone suppression test (DST), and the 24-h urinary free cortisol assay. Any patient with a positive result on either of these tests should be referred to an endocrinologist for further investigation and treatment.

Treatment

Successful treatment of Cushing's syndrome requires an accurate determination of the cause of the hypercortisolism. Removal of an underlying neoplasm is the treatment for patients with primary adrenal tumors or ectopic ACTH syndrome. Inhibitors of cortisol biosynthesis (aminoglutethimide, metapyrone, or ketoconazole) are used in patients when removal of a tumor is not possible. Exogenous (iatrogenic) Cushing's syndrome is treated by discontinuing glucocorticoid therapy. Cushing's syndrome secondary to an ACTH-secreting pituitary tumor (Cushing's disease) is best treated by trans-sphenoidal pituitary surgery.

As cortisol levels are reduced to normal, psychiatric symptoms usually remit. In exogenous Cushing's syndrome, remission of psychiatric and behavioral symptoms occurs over several weeks to months. Reduction of the steroid medication dosage alone may cause symptoms to remit.

Low doses of antipsychotics, SSRI antidepressants, or electroconvulsive therapy may be helpful for the relief of psychiatric symptoms. Antidepressants may precipitate a manic episode, and therefore should not be used unless the depression is severe or persists after cortisol levels are normalized. In steroid psychosis, the newer antipsychotics are preferable because patients tolerate them more easily. ECT has been reported to ameliorate steroid psychosis, whereas tricyclic antidepressants have been reported to cause a worsening of symptoms. Prophylactic treatment with lithium reduced psychiatric complications in one study of patients receiving ACTH for multiple sclerosis; however, this study has not been replicated. A study by Hall et al. (1979) suggests that there is no correlation of previous steroid psychosis to subsequent events. However, still, lithium prophylaxis for patients with a history of steroid psychosis might be considered if steroid treatment is again required (Falk, Mahnke, & Poskanzer, 1979).

Addison's Disease (Adrenocortical Insufficiency)

Definition and Etiology

The adrenal glands produce three major types of steroid hormones: glucocorticoids, mineralocorticoids, and sex steroids. Glucocorticoids are involved in sugar and protein metabolism, maintenance of blood pressure, and response to physical stress, as well as the release of certain pituitary hormones. Mineralocorticoids are involved in maintaining fluid balance in the body. Sex steroids have actions similar to those of the hormones produced by the ovaries and testes. Addison's disease (primary adrenal insufficiency) results from a variety of adrenal gland disorders. Inadequate secretion of ACTH (due to pituitary disease) results in secondary adrenal insufficiency. In the past, tuberculosis was the major cause of Addison's disease. Today, most cases are due to autoimmune destruction of the adrenal gland. Other causes include fungal infection, metastatic tumors, hemorrhage due to anticoagulant therapy, infiltrative disorders (amyloidosis, sarcoidosis, and hemochromatosis), and previous adrenal surgery. The incidence is 5.6 per million per year, and the prevalence is 110 per million in the United States.

Long-term administration of steroid medication may cause atrophy of the adrenal glands and lowered secretion of ACTH (secondary adrenal insufficiency). Recovery may take 6 to 12 months after the cessation of steroid medication.

Symptoms and Course of Illness

Typical symptoms of Addison's disease include generalized weakness and fatigue, weight loss, anorexia, vomiting, hyperpigmentation, abdominal pain, low blood pressure with dizziness on standing, nonspecific muscle and joint pain, and perceptual abnormalities (hallucinations). Common laboratory abnormalities include elevated potassium and low sodium levels, and occasionally an elevated calcium level.

Psychiatric symptoms are seen in 60–90% of patients with Addison's disease. Symptoms develop slowly and often precede the classic physical symptoms. Apathy, social withdrawal, fatigue, irritability, negativism, and poverty of thought are early manifestations. Moderate to severe depression occurs in 30–50% of patients. Memory impairment is often present. Mental changes tend to be episodic and to fluctuate in severity. During Addisonian crisis (acute adrenal failure), delirium may occur. Common misdiagnoses include depression, hypochondriasis, and conversion disorders.

Diagnostic Tests

Adrenal insufficiency is suspected in an individual with a low 8 AM serum cortisol concentration. The rapid ACTH test with synthetic ACTH (Cortrosyn) is the best screening study; a normal result virtually eliminates the diagnosis of primary adrenal insufficiency. An abnormal result requires confirmation, and the individual should be referred to an endocrinologist for further testing and evaluation. A clearly elevated serum ACTH in a patient with an abnormal Cortrosyn test is virtually diagnostic of primary adrenal insufficiency. The diagnosis of secondary adrenal insufficiency due to a hypothalamic or pituitary abnormality is more complex and may require performance of an insulin tolerance test, CRH test, or metyrapone test.

Treatment

Treatment of Addison's disease usually requires replacement of both glucocorticoids and mineralocorticoids. Patients with secondary adrenal insufficiency require only glucocorticoid replacement. Physical and mental symptoms respond rapidly to steroid replacement. The long-term prognosis depends on the underlying cause of the adrenal insufficiency. In chronic adrenal insufficiency, patients have a life-long illness requiring ongoing treatment with steroids. Mood and cognitive disturbances usually respond rapidly when the patient is treated with glucocorticoid and mineralocorticoid replacement. Psychosis may persist for several weeks. Irreversible mental changes rarely occur. Psychotropic medications should only be used with careful monitoring and low initial dosages. Olanzapine and quetiapine are useful in treating psychosis in these patients, as they are less likely to cause extrapyramidal side effects (EPS) and have no anticholinergic side effects. Nefazodone may be preferable in the treatment of depression in Addison's disease, as it has little effect on appetite, no anticholinergic side effects, and may decrease anxiety and agitation. The SSRIs, bupropion, venlafaxine, and mirtazapine should be used cautiously in depression associated with Addison's disease, as their potential side effects of nausea, headache, dizziness, agitation, anxiety, and postural hypotension may worsen some symptoms of the illness. Tricyclics should be reserved for those patients who do not respond to (or do not tolerate) the antidepressants noted above, as they are more likely to cause carbohydrate craving, increased appetite and weight gain, and nausea, headache, dizziness, agitation, anxiety, and postural hypotension.

DISORDERS OF CALCIUM METABOLISM

Hyperparathyroidism

Etiology

Excessive parathyroid hormone (PTH) secretion causes primary hyperparathy-roidism, characterized by an elevated serum calcium concentration. It is the most common cause of hypercalcemia in the ambulatory population. Women are affected more commonly than men; the prevalence in women over 60 may be as high as 1 in 600. In approximately 85% of cases, excessive PTH secretion is due to a single parathyroid adenoma. Fifteen percent of cases are due to parathyroid hyperplasia; hyperparathyroidism is rarely associated with multiple adenomas or a parathyroid carcinoma. In hospitalized patients, malignancy is responsible for a far larger proportion of cases of hypercalcemia. The malignancies most commonly associated with hypercalcemia are lung, breast, prostrate, renal cell, cervix, multiple myeloma, and head and neck cancers. Other causes of hypercalcemia include hyperthyroidism, sarcoidosis, vitamin A and vitamin D intoxication, immobilization, drugs (thiazide diuretics, lithium), Addison's disease, and acute renal failure with rhabdomyolysis.

Symptoms and Course of Illness

Prior to 1970, more than 90% of patients with primary hyperparathyroidism presented with either renal disease (kidney stones and calcium deposits in the kidney) or bone disease. With the advent of screening blood tests as part of the routine medical examination, the clinical presentation of this disorder changed dramatically. Currently, more than 50% of patients with primary hyperparathy-roidism are asymptomatic; 20–30% have vague, nonspecific symptoms; and fewer than 20% present with renal or bone disease. The onset of symptoms is often insidious, and they are often subtle. Patients may complain of nonspecific muscle weakness, fatigue, lethargy, anorexia, nausea, constipation, increased thirst, and vague abdominal and muscle and/or joint pain. More acute symptoms may occur with a kidney stone, peptic ulcer disease, pancreatitis, or a pathologic fracture.

Psychiatric symptoms have been reported in 5–65% of patients with hyperparathyroidism. In general, mental status changes parallel the degree of elevation of serum calcium. With mildly elevated calcium levels personality changes, loss of spontaneity, and lack of initiative are common complaints. With moderate elevation symptoms are primarily those of depression, with dysphoria, anhedonia, apathy, anxiety, irritability, impaired concentration and recent memory, and sometimes suicidal ideation. With severe elevation or a rapid rise in serum calcium, psychotic and cognitive symptoms predominate; these include confusion, disorientation, catatonia, agitation, paranoid ideation, delusions, and auditory and visual hallucinations. With very high levels, stupor and coma are common. Some patients may have significant (but not severe) elevations in serum calcium without observable mental status changes; this is more likely in individuals in which the elevation in serum calcium occurs gradually.

Diagnostic Tests

A serum calcium determination is the single best screening test for primary hyperparathyroidism. The definitive diagnosis of hyperparathyroidism requires the exclusion of other causes of hypercalcemia and demonstration of an elevated serum PTH concentration. The combination of elevated serum calcium and elevated serum PTH is diagnostic in most patients. Patients on chronic lithium therapy may have a clinical picture indistinguishable from that of primary hyperparathyroidism. Discontinuation of lithium treatment should result in the return of serum calcium to normal levels.

Because of its insidious onset and frequent lack of specific symptomatology, the diagnosis of hyperparathyroidism is frequently overlooked and often not screened for. Common misdiagnoses include neuroses, hypochondriasis, mood disorders, schizophrenia, and cognitive impairment disorders of other etiology.

Treatment

Surgery is the definitive treatment for primary hyperparathyroidism, with a cure rate of 90–95%. In elderly patients and those with mildly elevated serum calcium, the indications for surgery are controversial. Two small studies showed improvement in elderly patients with dementia who had successful surgery for hyperparathyroidism. Correction of elevated serum calcium brings about rapid reversal of many of the psychiatric manifestations of hyperparathyroidism (Borer & Bhanot, 1985; Peterson, 1968).

Hypoparathyroidism

Definition and Etiology

Hypoparathyroidism is characterized by a decreased serum calcium concentration in association with an elevated serum phosphate level. It occurs more frequently in women (1.6 times as often as in men). The peak age of onset is in the sixth decade. The most common etiology is accidental damage to or removal of the parathyroid glands during surgery to the thyroid or for head and neck cancer. Other causes include magnesium deficiency (often associated with alcoholism), parathyroid aplasia (DiGeorge's syndrome), neck irradiation, infiltrative disorders (e.g., amyloid, sarcoidosis, hemosiderosis), and autoimmune destruction (usually as part of autoimmune polyglandular deficiency syndrome)

(Eisenbarth & Verge, 1998). Pseudohypoparathyroidism is a rare inherited disorder in which there is impaired end-organ responsiveness to PTH. Other conditions causing hypocalcemia include malabsorption syndrome, acute pancreatitis, multiple blood transfusions, and chronic renal failure.

Symptoms and Course of Illness

Symptoms of hypoparathyroidism are primarily a reflection of low serum calcium, which typically results in increased neuromuscular irritability. Symptoms range in severity from mild paresthesias to tetany, muscle cramps, and spasms of the muscles in the feet and hands. More severe hypocalcemia may result in difficulty breathing (due to spasm of the larynx) and generalized seizures. Physical findings include a positive Chvostek sign (facial twitch in response to tapping of the facial nerve) or Trousseau sign (carpopedal spasm due to nerve compression in the arm when a blood pressure cuff is inflated above systolic pressure for 3 min) (Parfitt, 1989), cataracts, and a Parkinson's-like syndrome (most often seen in patients with basal ganglia calcification associated with low serum calcium concentration of long duration).

Psychiatric symptoms occur in 30–50% of hypoparathyroid patients (Popkin & Mackenzie, 1980). The severity of complaints seems to be related mostly to the rapidity of change in the serum calcium and other electrolytes. Anxiety, depression, irritability, emotional lability, social withdrawal, phobias, and obsessions may be present. In severe cases, delirium with confusion, disorientation, agitation, paranoia, and auditory and visual hallucinations may occur. Intellectual deterioration is seen in one third of patients with primary hypoparathyroidism, a result of a long duration of illness prior to diagnosis and treatment. Cognitive changes are rare in surgically induced illness, as the condition is usually treated promptly. Symptoms may be mistaken for neuroses, hypochondriasis, conversion disorders, anxiety disorders, depression, schizophrenia, dementia, and cognitive impairment disorders of other etiology.

Diagnostic Tests

The finding of a low serum calcium concentration associated with a low serum PTH level confirms the diagnosis of hypoparathyroidism.

Treatment

Oral vitamin D and calcium supplements are used to return the serum calcium level to the low-normal range. Normalization of serum calcium levels typically resolves symptoms. If intellectual impairment is present, residual cognitive deficits often persist. Patients with hypoparathyroidism have shown an increased sensitivity to acute dystonias secondary to treatment with phenothiazine antipsychotics, such as chlorpromazine and fluphenazine (Schaff & Payne, 1966). Given their lower side effect profile, the newer antipsychotics and antidepressants are preferred agents in treating psychiatric symptoms of hypoparathyroidism.

DISORDERS OF PITUITARY FUNCTION

Most clinically significant disorders of pituitary function are the result of benign pituitary tumors. These usually present with neurologic symptoms such as headaches and visual disturbances, evidence of endocrine dysfunction, or both. (Most headaches are not due to pituitary tumors). Less often, cranial nerve abnormalities, hypothalamic dysfunction, and, rarely, hydrocephalus will bring the patient to treatment. Endocrine presentations are divided into those due to pituitary hormone hypersecretion (e.g., acromegaly due to excess growth hormone, Cushing's disease due to excess ACTH, and hyperprolactinemia), and those due to inadequate pituitary hormone secretion (hypopituitarism).

Hyperprolactinemia

Definition and Etiology

Hyperprolactinemia (elevated blood level of prolactin) results from excessive secretion of prolactin. It is the most common hypothalamic-pituitary abnormality found in clinical practice. Its etiology may be divided into five major categories: (1) hypothalamic disorders that interfere with normal inhibition of prolactin secretion by dopaminergic neurons; (2) prolactin-secreting pituitary tumors (prolactinomas); (3) "neurogenic" factors, such as chest wall lesions and nipple stimulation; (4) endocrine causes, such as normal pregnancy and hypothyroidism; and (5) drugs. Drugs associated with hyperprolactinemia include antipsychotic medications (especially phenothiazines, haloperidol, and risperidone), tricyclic antidepressants, antihypertensive agents, and dopamine receptor antagonists (metoclopramide, sulpiride). Other drugs that may cause hyperprolactinemia include verapamil, cimetidine, estrogens, and opiates. Hyperprolactinemia occurs more commonly in women.

Symptoms and Course of Illness

Symptoms of hyperprolactinemia in women are primarily menstrual dysfunction, galactorrhea, and infertility. Sexual dysfunction (decreased libido, painful intercourse) and hirsutism (excessive hair growth) may also be seen (Evans, Carlsen, & Ho, 1990). Psychological symptoms such as anxiety, depression, and hostility have been reported (Fava et al., 1981). Men with hyperprolactinemia usually present with decreased libido and impotence, which may be mistaken for a primary sexual disorder. Men most often present with apathy without dysphoric mood (Cohen, Greenberg, & Murray, 1984). Irritability and impulsive behavior are also seen. Patients with a pituitary tumor may present with headaches and visual symptoms in addition to the endocrine dysfunction.

Diagnostic Tests

A serum prolactin level higher than 200 ng/ml is virtually diagnostic of a prolactinoma. Most nonpituitary causes of hyperprolactinemia are associated with a serum prolactin concentration of less than 100 ng/ml. Some patients with small pituitary tumors may have lower serum prolactin concentrations (30–200 ng/ml), which may overlap with the levels seen in other causes of hyperprolactinemia. A pituitary imaging study (MRI or CT scan) is essential to evaluate the presence of a tumor.

Treatment

Prolactinomas are most often treated with bromocriptine, and less frequently with trans-sphenoidal pituitary surgery. The cure rate with surgery ranges from 70–80% for microadenomas (tumors < 10 mm) and 0–40% with macroadenomas. Hyperprolactinemia has been reported to recur in some cases after apparent surgical cure (Vance & Thorner, 1987). Thus, bromocriptine is the primary treatment. Bromocriptine is generally well tolerated, with the most common side effects being nausea and orthostatic hypotension. Bromocriptine will usually decrease the size of the prolactinoma, resulting in reversal of visual disturbances, headaches, and other neurological symptoms. Radiation therapy is usually reserved for larger tumors that have not responded to bromocriptine and surgery. Symptoms generally remit, with reduction in prolactin levels, with medication, surgery, or radiation therapy. However, medication must be given indefinitely, as hyperprolactinemia and symptoms will recur once medication is stopped. In women, successful therapy results in normal ovulatory menstrual cycles, resolved galactorrhea, and restored fertility, generally. In men, normal sexual function generally returns.

Acromegaly

Definition and Etiology

Acromegaly usually results from the excess secretion of growth hormone by a pituitary tumor in an adult. Rarely, a tumor elsewhere in the body will secrete GHRH, resulting in sustained elevation of circulatory growth hormone levels. The prevalence of acromegaly is about 4 per 100,000.

Symptoms and Course of Illness

Patients with acromegaly typically present with enlargement of the nose, tongue, jaw, and soft tissues of the hands and feet. Internal organs (the liver, heart, and kidneys) may also enlarge. Excessive sweating and pain in the bones/joints may be noted. Headaches and visual problems may occur due to the expansion of the pituitary mass outside the sella turcica, placing pressure on the brain. Frequently, patients will have elevated blood glucose levels.

Psychiatric symptoms may occur in some cases. Personality changes have been reported (apathy, lack of initiative and spontaneity, and mood lability) (Bleuler, 1951). Patients may have psychological reactions to their altered appearance, particularly to the changes in facial structure. Untreated acromegaly may cause serious problems due to the effects on internal organs as well as the circulatory system. Treatment will prevent further symptoms but will not reverse many of the physical changes associated with prolonged growth hormone excess.

Diagnostic Tests

Acromegaly is diagnosed with two tests: (1) failure of the suppression of serum growth hormone levels to less than 1 ng/ml after an oral glucose tolerance test; and (2) an elevated level of somatomedin-C (IGF-1) in the serum. A head CT or MRI scan will usually document the presence of a pituitary tumor.

Treatment

Surgical removal of the pituitary adenoma is the treatment of choice in most cases. Adjunctive radiation treatment may be used in patients not cured by surgery. Octreotide has potent inhibitory effects on GH release in acromegalic patients (O'Dorisio & Redfern, 1990). It is generally reserved for the treatment of patients who do not respond to surgery and radiation treatment.

Psychological Sequelae

Patients may have difficulty adjusting to the changes in their appearance. They may also have trouble adapting to living with a chronic illness.

Hypopituitarism

Definition and Etiologies

Hypopituitarism may result from a number of destructive processes affecting the pituitary and hypothalamus (Vance, 1994). Pituitary tumors, pituitary surgery, irradiation of the pituitary, and serious head injury are some common causes of hypopituitarism. Less common etiologies are tumors of the hypothalamus, hemochromatosis and sarcoidosis, metastatic tumors (commonly of the lung or breast), lymphocytic hypophysitis, and postpartum pituitary infarction (Sheehan's syndrome).

Symptoms and Course of Illness

In adults, the symptoms seen are due to a deficiency of hormone production by the glands targeted by the pituitary hormones (i.e., hypothyroidism, hypoadrenalism, and hypogonadism). Diabetes insipidus may occur if the posterior pituitary and hypothalamus are affected. Because the symptoms are nonspecific and slow to develop, the diagnosis of hypopituitarism may be delayed.

Amotivation, dysphoria, and cognitive impairment are common psychological symptoms. If hypopituitarism develops rapidly (as in pituitary apoplexy), acute confusional states or psychosis may be seen (Khanna et al., 1988).

Diagnostic Tests

Imaging studies (CT scan or MRI) help define abnormal pituitary and hypothalamic anatomy. Screening studies should consist of thyroid function tests, serum testosterone (in males), and measurement of serum cortisol at 8 AM.

Treatment

Replacement of deficient hormones is essential, and is treated as discussed in previous sections covering hypothyroidism and hypoadrenalism. Psychotropic medications should only be considered after the underlying endocrine abnormalities have been corrected.

Psychological Sequelae

Expected reactions to this illness are similar to those seen in other endocrine disorders requiring long-term replacement therapy. Individuals must adjust to having a chronic, incurable but treatable illness.

MISCELLANEOUS ENDOCRINE DISORDERS

Pheochromocytoma

Definition and Etiology

Pheochromocytomas are rare tumors that secrete catecholamines, usually occurring in the adrenal medulla. These tumors occur with equal frequency in men and women. Most patients present with symptoms of the disorder between the ages of 30 and 50.

Symptoms

Patients present with hypertension, which may be sustained or paroxysmal. The blood pressure is often quite labile. Common symptoms include headaches, palpitations, and sweating. Nausea, vomiting, tremor, abdominal pain, and anxiety may also be seen. Patients may have elevated blood sugar and weight loss. In severe cases, death may occur due to abnormal heart rhythms and hypertensive crisis. This disorder may be confused with hyperthyroidism. The most common psychological symptom is anxiety, although one study (Starkman et al., 1985) found minimal overlap with anxiety disorders as defined by *DSM-IV* criteria. Affective lability may be seen in some cases.

Course of Illness

Pheochromocytoma may be fatal if untreated, with death occurring due to cardiac arrhythmia or cerebrovascular accident (from elevated blood pressure).

Diagnostic Tests

The best screening test is measurement of catecholamines and metanephrines in a urine sample collected over a 24-h period. If a patient has normal test results but suspicious symptoms, additional tests such as plasma catecholamine levels or a "clonidine suppression" test (Sheps et al., 1990) should be performed.

Treatment

Surgical removal of the pheochromocytoma is the definitive treatment. Prior to removal, phenoxybenzamine, propranolol, and/or phentolamine are used. Cardiac arrhythmia may be treated with lidocaine or propranolol.

Male Hypogonadism

Definition and Etiologies

Male hypogonadism is the inadequate secretion of testosterone by the testes, insufficient production of sperm, or both. Infertility is the primary symptom of insufficient production of sperm, while the symptoms of inadequate testosterone secretion depend on the stage of sexual development of the individual. In teenage boys, testosterone deficiency results in delayed puberty, while in adult males symptoms include decreased libido and energy, decreased body hair and muscle mass, and sexual dysfunction. See Plymate (1994) for an excellent review of this subject.

Causes of hypogonadism in men are divided into two categories: those associated with diseases of the testes (primary hypogonadism) and those associated with disorders of the hypothalamic-pituitary axis (secondary hypogonadism). Primary hypogonadism is most commonly caused by Klinefelter's syndrome, a genetic disease in which the male has an extra copy of the X chromosome (i.e., chromosomal constitution 47 XXY). Other causes include myotonic dystrophy, mumps orchiitis, testicular trauma or irradiation, cancer chemotherapy, and autoimmune disease. Secondary hypogonadism is due to pathology of the pituitary or hypothalamus. The most common hypothalamic disorder resulting in male hypogonadism is Kallmann's syndrome, characterized by a deficiency of GnRH, which is produced in the hypothalamus. Patients with Kallman's syndrome have minimal development of secondary sexual characteristics and present as prepubertal eunuchs. Pituitary causes of male hypogonadism include prolactinomas, destructive pituitary tumors, hemochromatosis, sarcoidosis, irradiation or surgery of the pituitary, or severe systemic illness.

Symptoms and Course of Illness

As indicated above, untreated male hypogonadism will result in either absence of secondary sexual characteristics in prepubertal boys, delayed puberty, or sexual dysfunction, and often associated loss of muscle mass and decreased energy and libido.

Diagnostic Tests

The initial diagnostic evaluation for male hypogonadism consists of a careful history and physical exam, focusing on the signs and symptoms noted above. Special attention should be paid to the stage of sexual development, size of the testicles, and the presence of any evidence of pituitary dysfunction. Serum testosterone level, prolactin level, and LH and FSH levels should be obtained. If the history and physical exam and blood tests indicate an abnormality of the hypothalamic-pituitary axis, a CT or MRI scan of the pituitary should be performed.

Treatment

Testosterone replacement therapy, in the form of an intramuscular depot preparation or a transdermal testosterone patch, is appropriate for the chronic treatment of testosterone deficiency. If the patient desires fertility, he may be treated with clomiphene, gonadotropin replacement, or pulsatile GnRH infusions.

Psychological Sequelae

Male hypogonadism may cause significant psychological distress and impaired social adjustment. It is common for patients to have low self-esteem and self-confidence, along with feelings of inadequacy. Alienation and isolation from others are frequently seen. Patients with Klinefelter's syndrome may have a range of psychiatric disorders, including mental retardation, personality disorders, depression, bipolar illness, neuroses, alcoholism, sexual deviance, and schizophrenia (Caroff, 1978; Swanson & Stipes, 1969). The most consistently seen psychiatric disorder in individuals with Klinefelter's syndrome is a personality disorder characterized by passivity, dependency, and poor socialization.

In patients with hypogonadism that develops in adulthood, replacement of testosterone should result in return of normal sexuality and prevention of any further psychological difficulties.

Anabolic Steroid Use

Definition and Etiology

Athletes sometimes use anabolic steroids as a means to improve their performance. Surveys suggest as many as 6–11% of high school males have taken anabolic steroids (Merck Manual online, 2002; Sect. 22, Ch. 35). This is up from 7% in the 1980s (Buckley et al., 1988). Studies have consistently shown that college athletes use them at approximately twice the rate of high school athletes (Windsor & Dumitri, 1989). Most athletes obtain these drugs illegally and use both oral and injectible forms. Illicit testosterone administration may result in blood levels of testosterone 10 to 100 times normal.

Symptoms and Course of Illness

Anabolic steroids may be highly toxic. Jaundice, altered blood levels of LDL and HDL cholesterol, acne, breast tissue enlargement, impotence, sleep apnea, decreased glucose tolerance, and low sperm levels may be seen. Psychiatric manifestations include mood disorders (depression or mania), psychoses, and aggressive behavior and irritability (Pope & Katz, 1988). Individuals may become dependent on these drugs and experience withdrawal symptoms such as fatigue, decreased sex drive, depression, insomnia, anorexia, craving for more drugs, and dissatisfaction with body image.

Individuals who become addicted require higher doses, which will produce more physical problems. Liver failure and liver cancer may result from the use of these drugs. Elevations in cholesterol may produce cardiovascular illness over a prolonged period.

Treatment

Abstinence from using steroid drugs is indicated. The individual may need substance abuse treatment to maintain abstinence. Antipsychotic medications and mood-stabilizing agents may be helpful in treating the psychiatric symptoms. Once the individual discontinues the use of steroids, the psychological symptoms should remit.

Hirsutism

Definition and Etiology

Hirsutism is characterized by the excessive growth of coarse, dark hair in women in some or all of the following areas: the upper lip, chin, neck, chest, lower abdomen, and perineum. There are four major categories of causes of hirsutism: (1) ovarian; (2) adrenal; (3) drug-induced; and (4) idiopathic. (See the reviews of Rittmaster & Loriaux, 1987; and Mechanick & Dunaif, 1990, for a detailed discussion of these different etiologies.)

Polycystic ovary syndrome is the most common cause of hirsutism and is usually associated with oligomenorrhea or amenorrhea. Many drugs may cause hirsutism; for a more detailed discussion, see Kornstein, Sholar, and Gardner (2002). A detailed discussion of this disorder is beyond the scope of this chapter.

Symptoms and Course of Illness

The symptoms of hirsutism are as noted above. Mood disturbances are commonly seen in hirsutism of various causes. Patients with hirsutism may socially isolate themselves because of the unwanted changes in their body image. Depression is common and should be treated with appropriate means (medication, psychotherapy).

Diagnostic Tests

Screening tests consist of serum testosterone, dehydroepiandrosterone sulfate, LH, FSH, and prolactin. In patients suspected of having Cushing's syndrome, an overnight dexamethasone suppression test should be done. Further testing should be pursued in consultation with an endocrinologist or gynecologist.

Treatment

The treatment of hirsutism depends on the underlying cause. Hirsutism associated with polycystic ovary syndrome may be treated with androgen antagonists (e.g., spironolactone), birth control pills, and (based on very recent studies) metformin. Weight reduction may also significantly alleviate symptoms. Stopping the medication causing the hirsutism treats drug-induced hirsutism; however, if hirsutism is due to treatment with a steroid, the medication must be carefully tapered to prevent acute adrenal insufficiency.

CONCLUSIONS

Endocrine disorders frequently present with psychiatric symptoms. Certain groups of patients are at high risk of having endocrine disorders and should be carefully evaluated. These include patients with affective symptoms and coexistent cognitive dysfunction; patients with inconsistent or atypical presentations of psychiatric disorders; patients with psychiatric symptoms refractory to standard psychiatric treatments; patients with symptoms of dementia; patients with known pre-existing endocrine abnormalities; and patients with affective symptoms following a closed head injury. Patients with endocrine disorders may have difficulty adjusting to the changes necessary in dealing with a chronic but not necessarily life-threatening illness. Appropriate therapy is helpful in their adaptation to living with their illness. Additionally, it must be remembered that medications used to treat endocrine disorders may produce psychiatric symptoms; such symptoms should be investigated and treated appropriately.

REFERENCES

Addison, T. (1868). On the constitutional and local effects of disease of the suprarenal capsules. In S. Wilkes & E. Daldey (Eds.), *A collection of the unpublished writings of Thomas Addison* (Vol. 36). London: New Sydenham Society.

American Psychiatric Association. (1994). *Diagnostic and statistical manual of mental disorders* (DSM-IV; 4th ed.). Washington, DC: APA.

Bernbaum, M., Albert, S. G., Brusca, S. R., Drimmer, A., Duckro, P. N., Cohen, J. D., et al. (1989). A model clinical program for patients with diabetes and vision impairment. *Diabetes Education, 15,* 325–330.

Bleuler, M. (1951). The psychopathology of acromegaly. *Journal of Nervous and Mental Disease, 113,* 497–511.

Borer, M. S., & Bhantot, V. K. (1985). Hyperparathyroidism: Neuropsychiatric manifestations. *Psychosomatics, 26,* 597–601.

Brownlee, M., & King, G. L. (1996). Chronic complications of diabetes (symposium). *Endocrinology and Metabolism Clinics of North America, 25,* 217–490.

Buckley, W. E., Yescalis, C. E., III, Friedl, K. E., Anderson, W. A., Strett, A. L., & Wright, J. E. (1988). Estimated prevalence of anabolic steroid use among high school seniors. *Journal of the American Medical Association, 160,* 3441–3445.

Caroff, S. N. (1978). Klinefelter's syndrome and bipolar affective illness: A case report. *American Journal of Psychiatry, 135,* 748–749.

Cohen, L. M., Greenberg, D. B., & Murray, G. B. (1984). Neuropsychiatric presentation of men with pituitary tumors (the "four A's"). *Psychosomatics, 25,* 925–928.

Cushing, H. (1932). The basophil adenomas of the pituitary body and their clinical manifestations. *Johns Hopkins Medical Journal, 50,* 137–195.

Eisenbarth, G. S. & Verge, C. F. (1998). Immunoendocrinopathy syndromes. In J. D. Wilson, D. W. Foster, H. M. Kronenberg, & P. R. Larsen (Eds.), *Williams textbook of endocrinology, 9th ed.* (pp. 1651–1662), Philadelphia: W. B. Saunders.

Evans, W. S., Carlsen, E., & Ho, K. Y. (1990). Prolactin and its disorders. In K. L. Becker (Ed.), *Principles and practice of endocrinology and metabolism* (pp. 134–139). Philadelphia: Lippincott.

Falk, W. E., Mahnke, M. W., & Poskanzer, D. C. (1979). Lithium prophylaxis of corticotropin-induced psychosis. *Journal of the American Medical Association, 24,* 1011–1012.

Fava, G. A., Fava, M., Kellner, R., Serafini, E., & Mastrogiacomo (1981). Depression, hostility, and anxiety in hyperprolactinemic amenorrhea. *Psychotherapy Psychosomatics, 36,* 122–128.

Field, J. B. (1989). Hypoglycemia: Definition, clinical presentations, classification, and laboratory tests. *Endocrinology and Metabolism Clinics of North America, 18,* 27–41.

Gastineau, C. F. (1983). Is reactive hypoglycemia a clinical entity? *Mayo Clinic Proceedings, 58,* 545–549.

Hall, C. W., Popkin, M. K., Stickney, S. K., & Gardner, E. R. (1979). Presentation of the steroid psychoses. *The Journal of Nervous and Mental Diseases, 167,* 229–236.

Hauser, S. T., Jacobson, A. M., Wertlieb, D., Brink, S., et al. (1985). The contribution of family environment to perceived competence and illness adjustment in diabetic and acutely ill adolescents. *Family Relations, 34,* 99–108.

Helz, J. W., & Templeton, B. (1990). Evidence for the role of psychosocial factors in diabetes mellitus: A review. *The American Journal of Psychiatry, 147,* 1275–1282.

Hirsch, I. B., & Riddle, M. C. (1997). Current therapies for diabetes (symposium). *Endocrinology and Metabolism Clinics of North America, 26,* 443–701.

Hofeldt, F. D. (1989). Reactive hypoglycemia. *Endocrinology and Metabolism Clinics of North America, 18,* 185–201.

Jacobson, A. M. (1996). The psychological care of patients with insulin-dependent diabetes mellitus. *The New England Journal of Medicine, 334,* 1249–1253.

Jacobson, A. M., Hauser, S. T., Anderson, B. J., & Polonsky, W. (1994). Psychosocial aspects of diabetes. In C. R. Kahn & G. C. Weir (Eds.), *Joslin's diabetes mellitus* (13th ed., pp. 431–450). Philadelphia: Williams & Wilkins.

Khanna, S., Ammini, A., Saxena, S., & Mohan, D. (1988). Hypopituitarianism presenting as delirium. *International Journal of Psychiatry in Medicine, 18,* 89–92.

Kornstein, S. G. Sholar, E. F., & Gardner, D. F. (2000). Endocrine disorders. In A. Stoudemire, B. S. Fogel, & D. B. Greenberg (Eds.), *Psychiatric care of the medical patient, second edition* (pp. 801–819). New York: Oxford University Press.

Kovacs, M., Ho, V., & Pollack, M. H. (1995). Criterion and predictive validity of the diagnosis of adjustment disorder: A prospective study of youths with new-onset insulin-dependent diabetes mellitus. *The American Journal of Psychiatry, 152,* 523–528.

Lustman, P. J., Griffith, L. S., Freedland, K. E., & Clouse, R. E. (1997b). The course of major depression in diabetes. *General Hospital Psychiatry, 19*(2), 138–143.

McCulloch, D. K., Hosking, D. J., & Tobert, A. (1986). A pragmatic approach to sexual dysfunction in diabetic men: Psychosexual counseling. *Diabetic Medicine, 3,* 485–489.

Mechanick, J. I., & Dunaif, A. (1990). Masculinization: A clinical approach to the diagnosis and treatment of hyperandrogenic women. *Advances in Endocrinology and Metabolism, 1,* 129–173.

Nelson, R. L. (1985). Hypoglycemia: Fact or fiction? *Mayo Clinic Proceedings, 60,* 844–850.

O'Dorisio, R. M., & Redfern, J. S. (1990). Somatostatin and somatostatin-like peptides: Clinical research and clinical applications. *Advances in Endocrinology and Metabolism, 1,* 175–230.

Padgett, D., Mumford, E., Hynes, M., & Carter, R. (1988). Meta-analysis of the effects of educational and psychosocial interventions on management of diabetes mellitus. *Journal of Clinical Epidemiology, 41,* 1007–1030.

Parfitt, A. M. (1989). Surgical, idiopathic, and other varieties of parathyroid hormone-deficient hypoparathyroidism. In L. J. Degroot (Ed.), *Endocrinology* (pp. 1049–1064). Philadelphia: WB Saunders.

Peterson, P. (1968). Psychiatric disorders in primary hyperparathyroidism. *Journal of Clinical Endocrinology, 28,* 1491–1495.

Plymate, S. R. (1994). Hypogonadism. *Endocrinology and Metabolism Clinics of North America, 23,* 749–772.

Polonsky, W. H., Anderson, B. J., Lohrer, P. A., Ponte, J. E., Jacobson, A. M., & Cole, C. F. (1994). Insulin omission in women with IDDM. *Diabetes Care, 17,* 1178–1185.

Pope, H. G., Jr., & Katz, D. L. (1988). Affective and psychotic symptoms associated with anabolic steroid use. *American Journal of Psychiatry, 145,* 487–490.

Popkin, M. K., & Mackenzie, T. B. (1980). Psychiatric presentations of endocrine dysfunction. In R. C. W. Hall (Ed.), *Psychiatric presentations of medical illness* (pp. 139–156). New York: Spectrum Publications.

Rittmaster, R. S., & Loriaux, D. L. (1987). Hirsutism. *Annals of Internal Medicine, 30,* 95–107.

Rodin, G. M., & Daneman, D. (1992). Eating Disorders and IDDM: A problematic association. *Diabetes Care, 15,* 1402–1412.

Rydall, A., Rodin, G., Olmsted, M., Daneman, M. B., & Devenyi, M. D. (1994). A four year follow-up study of eating disorders and medical complications in young women with insulin-dependent diabetes mellitus. *Psychosomatic Medicine, 56,* 179.

Schaff, M., & Payne, C. (1966). Dystonic reactions to prochlorperazine in hyperparathyroidism. *New England Journal of Medicine, 275,* 991–994.

Service, F. J. (1997). Hypoglycemia. *Endocrinology and Metabolism Clinics of North America, 26,* 937–955.

Sheehan, H. L. (1939). Simmonds disease due to post partum necrosis of the anterior pituitary. *The Quarterly Journal of Medicine, 8,* 277–307.

Sheps, S. G., Jiang, N. S., Klee, G. G., &Van Heerdan, J. A. (1990). Recent developments in the diagnosis and treatment of pheochromocytoma. *Mayo Clinic Proceedings, 65,* 88–95.

Starkman, M. N., Zelnick, T. C., Nesse, R. M., & Cameron, O. G. (1985). Anxiety in patients with pheochromocytoma. *Archives of Internal Medicine, 145,* 248–252.

Swanson, D. W., & Stipes, A. H. (1969). Psychiatric aspects of Klinefelter's syndrome. *American Journal of Psychiatry, 126,* 82–90.

Vance, M. L. (1994). Hypopituitarism. *New England Journal of Medicine, 330,* 165–166.

Vance, M. L., & Thorner, M. O. (1987). Prolactinomas. *Endocrinology and Metabolism Clinics of North America, 16,* 731–753.

Windsor, R., & Dumitri, D. (1989). Prevalence of anabolic steroid use by male and female adolescents. *Medicine and Science in Sports and Exercise, 21,* 494–497.

Yager, J., & Young, R. T. (1974). Non-hypoglycemia is an epidemic condition. *New England Journal of Medicine, 291,* 907–908.

7

Neurological Illnesses

LAURIE STEVENS
JULIE K. SCHULMAN

INTRODUCTION

Despite our diverse backgrounds in mental health, all mental health professionals agree on one thing about the mind: it rests, physically, in the brain. As a result, diseases of and injuries to the brain can lead to changes, not only in a person's ability to control physical movements, remember things, or use language, but also to changes in a person's ability to experience or regulate emotions, or even to comprehend his or her condition. Because of these factors, patients with neurological disorders are among the most complicated and challenging patients with whom a mental health professional can work.

Given the complexity of the human brain and nervous system, it is not surprising that there is a wide variety of neurological illness about which the mental health practitioner must become familiar. Knowing the location in the brain that an illness affects and the illness' prognosis are critical to understand the physical and cognitive problems that the person will have, and they can also give you important cues about the likely emotional sequelae (Table 7.1).

This chapter will outline the major neurological conditions and discuss some representative illnesses within these categories. Each selection discusses the physical, psychological, and cognitive sequelae of at least one illness in a particular category, as well as the emotional and behavioral consequences that may result. It will also highlight some of the psychological issues that may arise as the patient undergoes common medical tests or procedures, or receives medications. We hope that this chapter will enable the mental health practitioner with a foundation in neuroanatomy to develop a broader understanding of neurological illnesses in general and to identify common scenarios for psychosocial intervention.

TABLE 7.1. Neurological Illnesses

Cerebrovascular Diseases
Ischemia/Infarction: transient ischemic attacks, lacunae style, hypertensive encephalopathy, cerebral vascular accidents
Hemorrhage: cerebral, subarachnoid
Vascular Lesions: arteriovenous malfomations, aneurysms
Arteritis: collagen vascular diseases (i.e., lupus)

Infections
Brain abscess
Creutzfeld-Jacob Disease
Encephalitis: viral, Lyme, protozoa, fungi
HIV
Meningitis
Syphilis
Opportunistic Infections
Sarcoid

Tumors
Gliomas
Meningiomas
Metastatic from a noncerebral site
Pineal
Pituitary
Neuronal or retinal origin

Movement disorders
Parkinson's Disease
Wilson's Disease
Huntington's Disease
Sydenhams
Tardive Dyskinesia
Myoclonus
Essential Tremor
Tourette's Syndrome

Demyelinating
Multiple sclerosis
Progressive multifocal leukoencephalopathy

Seizure Disorders
Epilepsy

Trauma
Concussion
Contusion

Dementias
Alzheimer's
Senile
Multi-infarct

Pain Disorder
Headache: migraine, cluster
Neuralgia
Causalgia

Degenerative
Vitamin deficiency
Metabolic
Post-viral
Amyotrophic Lateral Sclerosis

Disorders of Cerebrospinal Fluid and Brain Fluid
Hydrocephalus

Birth and Developmental Abnormalities
Cerebral Palsy
Mental Retardation
Attention Deficit Disorders
Autism

Spinal Cord Disease
Paraplegia

Ataxias

Neuromuscular Junction Disease
Myasthenia gravis
Genetic Disease
Muscular dystrophy
Neurofibromatosis

Toxins
Alcohol
Heavy metals
Industrial
Medications
Substances of abuse

Other
Dizziness
Sleep Disorders: narcolepsy, sleep apnea
Metabolic Disturbances: fluid/electrolyte, endocrine

CEREBROVASCULAR DISEASE

Diseases of the cerebrovascular system are among the most common neurological disorders, and are the third leading cause, after cardiac disease and cancer, of illness and mortality in the United States. Transient ischemic attacks (TIAs) and cerebrovascular accidents (CVAs) can be caused by thrombosis (blockage) in or by hemorrhage (bleeding) from the cerebral arteries that supply blood to the brain. They may arise in patients who have generalized cardiovascular or cerebrovascular disease, in the setting of pre-existing structural damage to the cerebral arteries such as aneurysms (ballooning of blood vessels caused by weakness in the vessel walls) or arteriovenous malformations (abnormal collections of blood vessels in the brain which are present at birth), or as a result of traumatic brain injury.

Transient Ischemic Attacks

TIAs occur when there is a temporary insufficient supply of blood and oxygen to a part of the brain. TIAs are manifested by focal impairment in neurological function—for example, left-sided weakness or trouble speaking—with a complete resolution of symptoms within 24 h. These symptoms are early warning signs of an impending stroke and signal that a patient should consult with his or her physician to undergo a neurological evaluation and work-up. Though no permanent damage occurs, they can be very frightening to patients.

Cerebrovascular Accident (Stroke)

A CVA occurs when there is an insufficient supply of blood and oxygen to a portion of the brain for a long enough time to damage or destroy brain tissue. Strokes may be hemorrhagic, in which there is bleeding from a damaged blood vessel, or nonhemmorhagic, in which a vessel supplying blood to areas of the brain is blocked by a clot or by an embolus (a piece of another clot or other solid material) that originated in another area of the body, often the carotid arteries. Strokes may occur in any area of the brain, though there are certain areas that are more likely to be affected than others because of the nature of the cerebral arteries. The severity of the injury, the portion of the brain affected, and the age of the individual are all important in predicting the outcome of a stroke.

If the patient comes to an emergency room quickly enough with a nonhemorrhagic stroke, clot-dissolving agents such as t-PA (tissue plasmogen activator) and streptokinase may be recommended. The goal is to avoid progression of the stroke and reverse the damage to the brain by resupplying blood to the area that has been blocked by a clot in the blood vessel. If the patient is unable to make medical decisions, the spouse or family may be called upon to decide whether they want these treatments administered. This decision is extremely difficult to make because, although they are touted as "miracle drugs," the medications have potentially fatal complications. They block the person's ability to produce any clots for several hours, and as a result, the person may develop bleeding in the brain or somewhere else in the body. Whatever the patient or family decides, if the patient's outcome is poor, they may feel tremendous guilt, anger, or grief about the situation.

On the other hand, a patient who delays coming in to the hospital when the symptoms occur may later become depressed when discovering that they could have had this option if they had arrived sooner. A worried spouse may also feel intense anger at a patient who minimized symptoms and delayed getting treatment, believing that the patient is partly responsible for the problems with which the spouse will now also have to cope.

The effects of the stroke are always the worst initially, when there may be edema (swelling) or temporary damage to some neurons that have not died. Over time, the patient can expect to recover some functions that they have lost, and some will recover almost completely, but it is difficult to give a specific prognosis. If the CVA leaves the patient with significant physical and functional impairment, then they will require a period of physical and cognitive rehabilitation. This usually occurs in the inpatient setting and will often include physical therapy, occupational therapy, and psychotherapeutic support (group and individual). Extensive discharge planning is necessary so that the patient and family can start to adapt to changes in the patient's functional capabilities and can make any physical alterations to the home (elevators, special toilet/shower facilities, special beds, wheelchair accessibility, etc.). There can be an enormous impact on the social, emotional, and financial dynamics of the family system.

Regardless of the severity of the stroke, anticoagulant therapy may be recommended as prophylaxis to avoid future strokes. Patients who take these need to get regular blood draws to be sure they are taking the right dosage of medication, and need to be very careful about doing anything that may cause them to bleed—for example, tripping and falling down—because their blood will not clot as easily. Patients may also notice that they bruise more easily than they used to. All of these things can cause fear and anxiety. Plus, patients may need to consider surgical options if significant stenosis (narrowing) is present in the carotid arteries, which are the main source of blood supply to the brain. Such surgery can offer hope of avoiding future strokes but also carries significant risks, especially if a person is elderly and has other medical problems.

Psychological Sequelae and Interventions

It is vital for patients who have had strokes to receive appropriate psychosocial treatment. The neuropsychiatric sequelae of strokes—including emotional problems, behavioral changes, and cognitive or language disorders—have a negative effect not only on the social functioning and overall quality of life of patients (King, 1996), but also on patients' physical recovery from the motor deficits caused by strokes (Clark & Smith, 1997).

Depression and dysthymia occur in 30–50% of patients immediately following stroke (Robinson et al., 1983; Sinyor et al., 1986; Pohjasvaara et al., 1998). The incidence and duration of the depression is related to the anatomical location of the brain injury, as well as to the degree of impairment in daily functioning. The mean duration of major depression following stroke appears to be about nine months, but there are a significant percentage of patients with either severe or mild depression who remain depressed for several years after a stroke (Chemerinski et al., 2000). Patients with depression following a stroke have significant impairment in their activities of daily living (ADLs) when compared with similar poststroke patients without depression.

Poststroke anxiety is another significant problem. One study showed that poststroke anxiety occurs in about 30% of patients (Castillo et al., 1993), and poststroke depression and anxiety often occur comorbidly. A three-year longitudinal study by Astrom (1996) revealed that right hemisphere brain lesions appear to be associated more with generalized anxiety alone, and left hemisphere brain lesions are associated more with comorbid depression and anxiety. Even among patients who have had mild strokes, or who have recovered fully, the impact of a sudden stroke can bring on considerable anxiety about one's susceptibility to illness or death. Poststroke psychosis, on the other hand, is rarely seen. It is usually an indication of a delirium caused by another occult medical problem, or a misdiagnosed fluent aphasia, in which the person speaks in a disorganized or nonsensical manner as the result of damage to the area of the brain controlling language expression.

Assessing a stroke survivor's mental state and mood can be quite challenging if an aphasia (speech and language impairment) is present, or if the stroke itself has caused affective lability (extreme swings of emotion) or apathy. One study showed that depression was not properly diagnosed by nonpsychiatric physicians in 50–80 % of poststroke patients (Schubert et al., 1992). In some cases, the mental health practitioner will have to base his or her diagnosis almost entirely on observations of the patients' behavior or on the family's report.

For significant depression, anxiety, or mood lability, medications can be very helpful. Benzodiazepines are effective for anxiety, but in elderly patients they can impair memory and increase the risk of falls, so they should always be used with caution. Nonbenzodiazepine anxiolytics or antidepressants with anxiolytic properties are often better choices for poststroke patients. If a patient has mood lability, a mood stabilizer, such as lithium or valproate, or a mild antipsychotic medication can be very helpful. Of course, careful consideration always needs to be made of the patient's age and any other medications they may be taking.

Psychosocial interventions need to address both the patient and the patient's family. Speech and language therapists can be very helpful with aphasic or speech-impaired patients by aiding patients in regaining language functions and in developing alternative ways to express their feelings and needs. Physical and occupational therapists also have important roles in helping patients regain better physical functioning, greater independence, and improved self-esteem. Finally, a psychotherapist can help the patient address the issue of grief over the loss of functioning and enable them to develop ways of coping with their new situation.

Educating family and caregivers about such problems as mood lability or poststroke depression or anxiety can be very helpful. Supportive group therapy for caregivers or family members also aids in adjustment to the degree of the patient's disability and their special needs. They should be encouraged to independently seek out information and support from peers through advocacy groups.

DEMENTIAS

Dementia is a general term that refers to the condition of impaired cognitive skills, often associated with impaired emotional regulation, which is acquired after birth. Dementias are caused by a wide variety of illnesses and may be classified in a number of ways. They can be progressive or nonprogressive, cortical or subcortical, reversible (such as induced by B12 deficiency) or nonreversible (such as Alzheimer's). Contrary to popular belief, old age does not cause dementia *per se*.

With the progress in modern society in many areas related to public health, our expected lifespan has increased. As a result, we are now seeing many more individuals with illnesses that tend to occur late in life. Though there are some types of dementias that occur in middle age, the elderly are the ones who are most likely to develop the medical conditions that cause dementia. Individuals with dementia are also living longer due to the advances in medical care, which means that the proportion of those with progressive dementia who reach advanced stages has also increased.

This section reviews the presentation and symptoms of three of the most common types of dementia, with psychological sequelae and interventions common to these dementias discussed at the end.

Alzheimer's Disease

The most common cause of dementia in industrialized societies is Alzheimer's Disease (AD). AD is a progressively degenerative disease that affects 4 million Americans. The disease usually begins in people in their midfifties, and its incidence and prevalence increase with advancing age. In approximately 5–10% of cases, AD is thought to be a hereditary illness (Evans et al., 1989).

The diagnosis of Alzheimer's Disease is usually a clinical one, based on symptoms, as there is no simple medical test that can confirm or rule out Alzheimer's. Magnetic Resonance Imaging (MRI) or computer tompgraphy (CT) may show atrophy and help exclude other possible brain diseases, but the definitive diagnosis of AD can be made only with examination of brain tissue via brain biopsy or at autopsy, which shows the characteristic amyloid plaques and neurofibrillary tangles.

AD usually has an insidious onset, and the intellectual deterioration is slow but relentless. The classic presentation of Alzheimer's is an older person with memory problems—typically with a loss of short-term memory more than long-term memory—and a language or communication impairment. The language deficit may start as a mild decrease in spontaneous speech or word-finding problems, but gradually worsens over time, and the person's verbal communication may become increasingly difficult to comprehend as it is more and more constricted to familiar words and phrases. In advanced stages, the person may be completely mute and there is a loss of verbal comprehension, also.

Along with the language deficits, patients with Alzheimer's develop apraxia—problems with motor skills—which initially is limited to complex or fine motor tasks. As the illness progresses, patients have increasing trouble with dressing, grooming, and using utensils, and in the final stages, even with walking or movement of any kind. They also develop incontinence at some point as the illness progresses. Problems with visuospatial abilities also develop as a part of the illness, so that the patients may have some visual agnosia (the inability to recognize objects) or frequent misperceptions (for example, mistaking a coat rack in the hall for a person).

Neuropsychiatric symptoms that may present in AD include psychotic symptoms especially delusions and hallucinations (primarily visual), personality changes, mood disturbances (dysphoria, depression, irritability, elation, and lability of mood), anxiety symptoms, and behavior changes (apathy and disinhibition, or infantile behavior).

There is no known cure for Alzheimer's disease but there are medications such as anticholinesterase inhibitors that can help in slowing the progression of the disease and the subsequent cognitive deterioration.

Pick's Disease

In Pick's disease, the frontal and anterior temporal lobes of the brain become gradually atrophied, while the parietal lobes are spared. Characteristically, patients develop Pick's disease by the age of 65, and unlike Alzheimer's—in which the risk of disease increases with increased age—the incidence peaks in the late 60's and declines thereafter. However, like Alzheimer's, the disease is progressive and nonreversible.

Because the frontal lobe—which is the part of the brain that controls executive functioning and the inhibition of expression of unwanted behaviors and emotions—is the area most affected by Pick's, patients often develop personality changes and disinhibited behavior in the early stages of the illness, which may even be mistaken for mania. The disease is usually diagnosed by CT scan, which shows the characteristic disproportionate shrinking of the frontal lobes. Over time, the clinical posture becomes more similar to that of Alzheimer's disease, with the exception that visuospatial function, which resides in the parietal lobe, may be spared for a much longer period of time.

Vascular Dementia

Vascular dementia is generally believed to be the second most common cause of dementia after Alzheimer's disease. It is usually caused by multiple infarcts (areas of cell death) in the brain. This may be the result of several major strokes like the ones described earlier, or of a small emboli that block the tiny blood vessels supplying the brain. However, vascular dementia can also be caused by cerebral vasculitis (an inflammation of the blood vessels that supply blood to the brain) due to autoimmune disease or infections.

In some unfortunate cases, vascular dementia can be produced even by a single stroke in a vital area of the brain, which is then associated with a unique constellation of symptoms. For example, patients with a stroke in the angular gyrus develop fluent aphasia, visuospatial disorientation, agraphia, and memory loss. An infarct in the thalamus can also cause memory loss, but with ocular palsies (difficulty with eye movements), apathy, and slowness or drowsiness (Geldmacher & Whitehorse, 1996).

The hallmarks of classic multi-infarct vascular dementia are the sudden onset of cognitive problems, with a "stepwise" progression—discrete episodes of decline in functioning that are the result of new infarcts—in a person with a history of TIAs or strokes. On neurological exam, there are usually focal neurological deficits such as asymmetric motor strengths or reflexes. Unlike Alzheimer's and Pick's diseases, in which cortical areas are injured and the subcortical areas remain relatively intact, in multi-infarct dementia the subcortical areas are more severely affected. Because of this, the cognitive and memory problems are not generally quite as severe as with Pick's or AD, but apathy and slowed thinking are more likely to be prominent.

Unfortunately, unlike AD, there are currently no medications or treatments that have been shown to slow or reverse the course of vascular dementia once it has developed.

Psychological Sequelae

Patients with dementia have varying degrees of memory impairment, and may have associated problems with complex judgments, abstract reasoning, or calculations. Often, patients will appear perfectly fine to their families when they are in familiar environments and talking about events that occurred many years ago, but when tested they have significant problems with recent memory or with following directions with more than one or two steps. Symptoms may become worse or more evident in the presence of a systemic illness (like a respiratory infection) or when the patient is in unfamiliar surroundings (as with hospitalization).

Sleep and appetite disturbances are often present in dementia patients. There is a well-known phenomenon called *sundowning* which occurs in the evening and night hours and is characterized by a sudden loss of orientation and severe agitation. Sundowning is caused by the lessening of sensory stimuli that the patient uses to orient him or herself in space and time, especially if the patient has any visual or hearing impairments. It is also not uncommon for patients with AD or Pick's to develop a reversal in their sleep cycles as the illness progresses. Simple maneuvers like leaving on a light or a radio, placing family photos and a clock on the bed table, and hanging a calendar on the wall can be very reassuring to a demented patient and help them orient themselves at nighttime. Sometimes a low-dose antipsychotic medication can also help to quell agitation, assist with orientation, and aid in helping the person sleep.

The psychopharmacologic treatment of dementia is directed as treating depression, anxiety, and agitation that cannot be managed with behavioral interventions. Agitation can often be treated effectively with low doses of antipsychotic medications or mood stabilizers. Mood and anxiety disorders can be treated with antidepressants or mood stabilizers, as well as beta-blockers or the careful use of bezodiazepines if needed.

Therapeutic interventions include cognitive-behavioral therapy to teach patients who have good insight how to compensate for memory problems, family therapy, supportive therapy, and group therapy, especially for the caregivers. Education should be provided to the family members, and caregivers, and social services should be available to assist with obtaining home health aides, day programs, and eventually with nursing home placement if it becomes necessary. The decision to place a loved one with dementia in a nursing home is often fraught with guilt and sadness for family members. The family may need a great deal of support to make such a decision and go through the laborious process of application and placement. Legal assistance may be necessary to organize health care proxies and powers of attorney for health care decisions and financial planning.

TUMORS

Tumors of the brain come in many different forms (Table 7.2). There are several ways in which cerebral tumors arise. Cerebral tumors may develop from structures outside the brain, including the meninges, pituitary gland, or cranial nerves. These tumors are generally benign in the sense that they do not metastasize and can be cured by surgical resection, but as they grow they will compress the brain within the skull and can be fatal. Tumors may also develop from a type of brain cell, including ependymal cells, glia, and astrocytes. These tumors, which in-

TABLE 7.2. Relative Frequencies of Common Histologic Types
of Brain Tumors

Tumor type	Frequency (%)
Primary	
Giliomas	40–50
Astrocytomas	10–15
Glioblastomas	20–25
Others	10–15
Meningiomas	10–20
Pituitary adenomas	10
Neurilemmomas	5–8
(mainly acoustic neuromas)	
Medulloblastomas and pinealomas	5
Miscellaneous primary tumors	5
Metastatic	15–25

Reprinted from J. B. Lohr and J. L. Cadet, 1987. "Neuropsychiatric Aspects of Brain Tumors," in R. E. Hales & S. C. Yudofsky (Eds.), *The American Psychiatric Press Textbook of Neuropsychiatry* (p. 356). Washington, DC: American Psychiatric Press. www.appi.org. Used with permission.

clude ependymonas, medulloblastomas, gliomas (including astrocytomas), and oligodendrogliomas, can all be—and generally are—malignant. Plus, cerebral tumors may also occur as the result of cancer elsewhere in the body that metastasize to the brain, and these metastases may infiltrate the brain itself (the most common scenario) or they may form in the meninges or attach to the skull wall.

All types of tumors grow and displace the brain within the closed case of the skull. The increase in intracranial pressure can create neurological symptoms and emotional symptoms, and may affect the level of consciousness. Depending on the location and the speed of growth of the tumor, patients may first present with a seizure, headaches, personality changes, or cognitive slowing (all caused by the increased intracranial pressure) rather than focal signs caused by the location of the tumor). A seizure is actually the first symptom in 30–50% of patients, and headaches are also quite common, occurring in approximately one-third of patients (Joseph, 1996).

The diagnostic approaches used to evaluate a brain tumor include CT scan, MRI, electroencephalogram (EEG), and brain biopsy. Once a brain tumor has been diagnosed, the course of treatment needs to be determined. For some patients, this will be surgery to remove the tumor, if it is felt to be resectable without too much injury to healthy brain tissue. Sometimes radiation therapy will be indicated to shrink the size of a brain tumor. Steroids, such as hydrocortisone, are often prescribed to reduce swelling of the brain. After malignant tumors are resected, radiation therapy may be recommended to further shrink the tumor or to try to prevent recurrence of the tumor.

Depending on the aggressivity of the tumor, the clinical course may vary from a slow progression of symptoms to a rapidly downhill process. For example, glioblastoma multiforme, a highly aggressive type of glioma, tends to start in the frontal-temporal region but quickly infiltrates the entire brain and is very resistant to chemoradiation. It is often very widespread before discovery, and it has a one-year survival rate in adults of only 20% (Joseph, 1996). Meningiomas, on the other hand, grow very slowly and do not recur if the surgeon is able to fully resect the tumor.

Psychological Sequelae and Interventions

The level of functional impairment caused by the tumor or the surgery, as well as the prognosis, have a major impact on the patient's and family's adjustment to the illness. If the patient experiences personality or behavioral changes prior to diagnosis, family members may sometimes experience guilt if they had been angry at the patient, not knowing that a tumor was the cause of those changes.

Should significant psychiatric symptoms (depressed mood, anxiety), delirium, or behavioral problems occur in the brain tumor patient, they can be treated pharmacologically with lower dosages of psychiatric medications than are used in functional psychiatric disorders. Psychotherapeutic interventions for patient and family vary widely depending on the particular situation. A patient who has a successful resection and a good prognosis, but who must then adapt to living with a residual disability, will benefit from speech and language therapy if needed, physical and occupational therapy, and supportive individual or group psychotherapy. On the other hand, a patient with an extremely poor prognosis will benefit more from immediate medical and social service planning that anticipates the patient's needs for increasing physical care, and psychotherapeutic support for the patient and the family that focuses on grief and end-of-life issues.

Naturally, all of the various health care providers—including general physicians, neurologists, surgeons, nurses, therapists, psychiatrists, social workers, and psychologists—need to communicate well to provide optimal care to the patient.

MOVEMENT DISORDERS

The complexity of the human nervous system ensures that there are many different neurons involved in the simplest of movements, or in the inhibition of movements. Because of this, a wide variety of neurological disorders exist—degenerative, metabolic, and toxic, just to name a few—that cause problems with movement. These disorders vary considerably in their potential effects on cognition or emotions. For example, amytrophic lateral sclerosis (a progressive loss of lower and upper motor neurons) rarely causes changes in cognition, while other disorders such as Parkinson's disease lead to dementia in up to one in four patients. This section will focus on Parkinson's disease as one example of a movement disorder, but the reader should be aware that each of these disorders has a very distinct presentation and prognosis.

Parkinson's Disease

Parkinson's Disease (PD) is a movement disorder characterized by tremor, rigidity, balance difficulties, flattened facial expression, and bradykinesia (slowed movements). Patients with this disorder have a loss of dopaminergic neurons (nerve cells that contain the neurotransmitter dopamine) in the substantia nigra area of the basal ganglia. It is a progressive disease and there may be a genetic basis for the disorder. Patients with this disease may experience cognitive and intellectual impairment as well as mood changes, notably depressed mood (Doonief et al., 1992; Starkstein et al., 1990), in addition to their neurological symptoms. Such patients may experience sudden "freezing," which is associated with an inability to initiate walking or turning (Giladi et al., 1992). Parkinson's patients can have severe constipation as well as impaired voice, speech, chewing, and swallowing (Hartelius, 1994).

The cognitive deficits in PD include memory impairment, attention deficits, and visual/spatial impairment. Such cognitive impairment can lead affected individuals to be unable to accomplish familiar daily tasks or cause them to feel emotionally overwhelmed in performing these tasks (Marsh, 2000). About 25% of patients with PD will develop a dementia, with features of aphasia (language difficulty), apraxia, and memory deficits (Mohr, Mendis, & Grimes, 1995), and 65% of Parkinson's patients will have an associated dementia by age 85 (Mayeux & Stern, 1983). The combination of social isolation and cognitive disturbance commonly seen in early dementias is often mistaken for depression in this population, and the dementia may be missed. Treating this type of patient with antidepressant medication can be complicated, as medication side effects can worsen the patient's cognitive deficits and even cause delirium.

Medications are used to treat Parkinson's disease, and the pharmacotherapy is continually evolving. Selegiline (Deprenyl) may be used early in the course of the disease in order to delay the need for L-dopa therapy. It acts by preventing the breakdown of dopamine in the brain. Dopamine agonists like bromocriptine, pergolide, pramipexole, and ropinirole are also used for as long as possible until L-Dopa therapy is necessary. These dopamine agonists act by increasing postsynaptic dopamine activity (Marsh, 2000) Tolcapone, a catecholamine transferase inhibitor, can be used to increase dopamine in the synapse. L-Dopa is often recommended as the disease progresses.

The anti-Parkinsonian agents may lose their efficacy over time and can also cause neuropsychiatric side effects, like visual hallucinations, agitation, mood changes, psychosis, and confusion. The side effects and potential of loss of efficacy can be very demoralizing and frustrating for both the patients and their families.

In the most severe cases of PD, experimental surgery involving transplantation of dopaminergic neurons has been performed. Neurosurgical procedures can also be performed to diminish the symptoms of PD. Pallidotomy can be used for treatment-related dyskinesias and motor changes in PD. Thalamotomy, the procedure performed in the well-publicized case of the actor Michael J. Fox, can treat the tremor in PD. Deep brain stimulation (DBS) involves the use of a pacemaker-like device that sends electrical impulses to the thalamus or globus pallidus to reduce tremor. Implantation of fetal brain tissue is still an experimental procedure to treat PD (Olanow, Kardower, & Freeman, 1996).

Psychological Sequelae and Interventions

The very nature of the disease, often with a chronically progressive downhill course, can be very frightening to all involved. The patient and family may envision him/her becoming totally dependent and disabled, even to the point of being unable to chew and swallow food, with uncontrollable shaking. This may bring about depression and fear. Some patients may contemplate suicide when faced with deterioration and loss of independent functioning in association with depression. The family may have to make adjustments in the patient's living space to accommodate the balance problems and shuffling gait. This may not always be possible, creating stress in the family and the potential for nursing home placement.

Approximately 90% of PD patients experience neuropsychiatric disorders. These include mood disorders, adjustment disorders, anxiety disorders, drug-induced psychiatric symptoms, affective lability, dementia, apathy, psychosis, and delirium (Starkstein & Mayberg, 1993). The prevalence of depression is about 40%, with reports ranging from 4–70%. Other mood disorders, such as dysthemia, bipolar disorder, and adjustment disorders with mood alteration may also occur. There appears to be no clear association between depression and age of onset or duration of PD, family history of mood disorders, or past history of depression (Cummings, 1992). It is also difficult to assess whether depression in a PD patient is secondary to the neurochemical changes in the brain from the disease process, a reaction to the disability and motor symptoms, or some combination of the two.

Emotional lability is common. PD patients will have episodes of frequent crying and/or laughing, which are inappropriate, unrelated to emotional events, and not under voluntary control. This may lead to socially embarrassing situations for patients and their families. Anxiety is present in approximately 40% of PD patients and seems to be associated with the dysregulation of the noradrenergic neurotransmitter system (Cash et al., 1987). Psychosis is also present in about 40% of PD patients, and may be the result of the illness itself or—not infrequently—iatrogenically induced by the medications for PD that increase the levels of dopamine in the brain. Psychosis can also be caused by delirium secondary to other medical problems, like an infection or a low sodium level. In some instances, the psychosis is associated with other mood symptoms like depression or mania.

Most pharmacologic treatment for the psychiatric syndromes that occur in PD patients is similar to that of functional psychiatric disorders. However, it must be remembered that patients with brain diseases, especially PD, have an increased risk for side effects and generally require reduced dosages of psychotropic medications. Standard antidepressant medication can be used to treat depression. Psychosis or agitation, however, requires a very careful selection and titration of antipsychotic medications—ideally, atypicals such as olanzapine or quetiapine—so as not to worsen the underlying Parkinson's disease.

Education for the patient and caretakers about the functional changes caused by PD and a program of physical therapy can be immensely beneficial in helping the patient maintain good functioning and keep a sense of dignity as the disease progresses. Supportive psychotherapeutic interventions for the patient and family should also be provided to help them cope with the psychological burden of this illness. It is often helpful to point out that the depression is part of the disease process and not just a reaction to disability. This will often make patients and families more receptive to the intervention of mental health professionals. Support groups are often available for affected individuals and their caregivers, and these groups are a good resource for both information and support.

DEMYELINATING DISEASES

Multiple Sclerosis

Multiple sclerosis (MS) is the most well-known example of a demyelinating disease—a disease that damages the myelin sheath on the axons of neurons, which act like insulation on a wire. Demyelination by MS causes problems with nerve conduction that may present gradually or acutely in a variety of ways—a loss of sight, problems with movement, or changes in sensation. Although there are other causes of demyelination, they are much rarer and tend to have an acute and sometimes fulminant course.

The onset of MS is generally in the third decade of life, with the incidence being highest in the young female population. Because the presentation varies, it is generally not clinically diagnosed until the patient develops at least two neurological symptoms in different parts of the body at different times. Some patients initially have such mild symptoms that they are diagnosed as "hysterical" or psychogenic in origin. The final diagnosis is usually made with an MRI scan and a spinal tap, which shows the presence of oligoclonal bands.

MS can have a rapidly progressive or slowly progressive course, or a relapsing and remitting course. The cause of MS remains an enigma. Physical symptoms depend on the location of the lesions in the brain. Lesions most commonly occur in the long tracts of the spinal cord, the optic nerve, cerebellum, and the brain stem. Patients can have gait (walking) disturbances, tremors, paraparesis (partial paralysis), sensory loss in limbs, spasticity in the extremities, and can have bowel, bladder, and sexual dysfunction. Fatigue is extremely common in MS, affecting as many as 90% of patients, with considerable debate about how it is related to neurological and psychological factors. Neuropsychiatric disorders and impairments in cognition (commonly problems with memory, attention, conceptual reasoning, verbal fluency, and abstraction) can also occur even in the early stages of the disease, before physical disability develops (Brassington & Marsh, 1998).

Symptomatic treatments may be helpful for MS patients. Baclofen can help with spasticity, although the medication may cause sedation and other serious side effects. Patients may need to be instructed in bowel and bladder care in order to prevent urinary retention and constipation. Bowel and bladder accidents may be quite humiliating to patients. Newer immunologic treatments are available like Betaseron and Interferon, which may help in stabilizing the course of the disease.

Psychological Sequelae and Interventions

As this disease usually strikes individuals early on and in the prime of their lives, it can be particularly emotionally devastating. The disease can have an impact on their educational, professional, personal, and social lives.

Early on in the course of the disease, many patients experience significant denial of illness and resist modifying their lifestyles to accommodate their illness and symptoms. Formerly active individuals may find it hard to accept that there are real physical limitations imposed by the MS. For example, MS patients often report a worsening of symptoms when they are overheated or dehydrated, but some patients will refuse to change intense exercise regimens that lead to MS exacerbations. Similarly, though times of high life-stress can also cause a flare-up of MS symptoms, many patients are reluctant initially to change their work schedules or change to less-demanding types of work.

As the disease progresses, the denial tends to break down and the patient may become depressed as he or she comes to recognize the progressive and degenerative nature of the disease. Fear of loss of control of one's body and one's life and fear of abandonment by loved ones are common. Fear of becoming dependent on others is also prominent. Demoralization is common in this population, especially as functional abilities decline. Having to accommodate physical modifications, like using a cane or a wheelchair, is particularly difficult for young people. When ability to be employed or to function in one's usual role (i.e., as a homemaker or parent) is impaired, this can also be quite devastating.

Along with these expectable reactions to the development of serious illness, MS patients are at increased risk for other neuropsychiatric disorders. Bipolar disorder is more prevalent in MS patients than in the general population, even in the absence of any family history, and mania can also be induced by the use of steroids. Depression also affects a very large proportion (27–54%) of patients with MS (Minden & Schiffer, 1990, review) though there is still no clear consensus on how much is neurologically based and how much is explainable by the psychological impact of having a serious and unpredictable illness. Psychosis and organic personality syndromes (Surridge, 1969) may also occur, and even temporal lobe epilepsy secondary to lesions in the temporal lobes. Many of these disorders may be secondary to lesions in the temporal lobes. Many of these disorders may be effectively treated symptomatically with mood stabilizers, antidepressants, or antipsychotics as approriate, though lower doses will often need to be used. It is also important to screen MS patients carefully for impairments in cognition that often go unrecognized but can have significant impact on the patient's functioning.

Certain neuropsychiatric disorders are particular to MS, such as euphoria. Patients with euphoria are not animated or manic, but rather seem to have developed a persistent state of serenity and outward optimistic cheerfulness that is incongruent to their situation (Minden & Schiffer, 1990; Minden, 1992). Euphoria is presumed to be primarily neurologically based, the result of demyelinating lesions in the frontal lobes, basal ganglia, and the limbic system that serve to "disconnect" the emotional areas of the brain. Other patients develop pathological laughing and weeping, which occurs independently of the patient's underlying mood, and seems to be related neuroanatomically to damage in the subcortical forebrain structures. Pathological laughing and weeping has been reported to respond well to low-dose amitriptyline, 25–75 mg qd (Schiffer, Herndon, & Rudick, 1985).

A therapist for an MS patient will wear many hats. Patients may have a variety of needs over time and may present different demands on therapists at different stages of the illness. It is sometimes helpful to actively refocus demoralized, frightened, or somatically preoccupied patients on their assets and what they are able to do to take charge of their lives, so as to take the emphasis for these patients off the deficits and restrictions. At other times, it is important to gently confront denial in overly optimistic patients and emphasize the need to make realistic accommodations for the effects of the disease, while still encouraging the patient to be as active as he or she is able to be. Helping patients with specific suggestions about managing the disease—e.g., by planning their activities to minimize fatigue and stress—is a useful strategy.

Unfortunately, patients often look to the new drugs like Betaseron and Avinex as magical cures. They expect a complete remission of their symptoms and may be gravely disappointed when the only benefit is a slowed progression of their disease. When these medications are prescribed, careful attention should be paid to focusing patients on being as realistic as possible about the potential benefits of the medications. Oftentimes, the most that one can hope for is a slowing in the progression of the disease or a decrease in the frequency of exacerbations or disabling attacks.

Although many good support groups and organizations exist for people with

MS, caution should be exercised when referring patients to support groups. Patients should be steered to participate in groups with others at a similar stage of disease. Some patients in early stages of the disease will become very distressed and frightened if placed in a group too soon with patients at a more advanced stage, who may be wheelchair bound and very functionally impaired. However, these groups can be important sources of comfort and practical information about coping with MS, so that patients should be encouraged to make use of these groups when they are emotionally ready.

SEIZURE DISORDERS

Epilepsy

Epilepsy affects about 40 million people across the globe. More than 2 million Americans are being treated for epilepsy. An epileptic seizure is caused by a temporary abnormal electrical discharge of neurons in the brain (Pedley, Scheur, & Walczak, 1995). There are several types of epilepsy (Table 7.3), including partial seizures (simple and complex), generalized seizures (typical absence, atypical absence), myoclonic seizures, clonic seizures, tonic seizures, tonic-clonic seizures, and atonic seizures.

TABLE 7.3. International League Against Epilepsy Revised Classification of Epileptic Seizures

1. Partial (focal, local) seizures
   A. Simple: motor, somatosensory, autonomic, or psychic
   B. Complex
      1) Impaired consciousness at outset
      2) Simple partial followed by impaired consciousness
   C. Partial seizures evolving to generalized tonic-clonic (GTC)
      1) Simple to GTC
      2) Complex to GTC
2. Generalized seizures (convulsive or nonconvulsive)
   A. 1) Absence seizures
      2) Atypical absences
   B. Myclonic
   C. Clonic
   D. Tonic-clonic
   F. Atonic
   G. Combinations
3. Unclassified epileptic seizures

Adapted from Commission on Classification and Terminology of the International League Against Epilepsy, 1981.

A focal seizure is one that arises from a particular area of the brain, but may spread and become generalized. A generalized seizure arises from the thalamus and hypothalamus and immediately spreads to the cortex of both hemispheres of the brain. Seizures that have motor symptoms are manifested by rhythmic jerking (clonic movements) of an area of the body. These movements may be confined to a segment as small as one finger, although more commonly they involve one side of the body. This period of motor activity can last from several seconds to many minutes. If the whole body becomes involved in the seizure, there may be a loss of bowel and bladder function, a loss of consciousness, as well as jerking movements of all of the voluntary muscle groups. After the motor activity subsides, the person's extremities are often weakened. In the postictal state (after seizure has ended), the patient may seem confused and sleepy. Although we typically associate seizures with motor movements, 60% of epilepsy patients have nonconvulsive seizures with no motor symptoms (Hauser & Rocca, 1996).

Some seizure disorders are associated with an impairment of consciousness; others have focal signs and symptoms (motor, sensory, or visual). Patients may report visual disturbances, such as seeing objects which appear to be too small, too large, or misshapen. Some people may hear voices or musical phrases during a seizure. However, these auditory hallucinations differ from those in functional psychiatric illness in that they are usually the same words or sounds repeated over and over again and the patient is aware that they are not real. If a person is conscious during a seizure, he or she may seem inattentive or apathetic and will perform poorly on tests of intellectual function, especially memory. Other patients may have speech disturbances and stereotypical automatisms (Pedley et al., 1995). These automatisms are simple movements the patient repeatedly performs and might forcefully resist attempts to interrupt. Typical automatisms are continual swallowing or kissing movements, abdominal rubbing, and even quasi-masterbatory movements. Speech may consist of mutterings of a few sounds or phrases. Preservation of speech and simple activities may occur.

Some patients may have "auras" that precede the seizure or continue during the seizure. These are cognitive, affective, perceptual, or sensory experiences. Some may have cognitive auras, like depersonalization or deja vu experiences. Some may have affective auras, like fear or pleasure. Some may have perceptual changes (illusions, hallucinations). Some may have sensory changes (strange smells, like "burning rubber").

EEG is helpful in diagnosing a seizure disorder; however, the EEG may be normal when a patient is not seizing, despite strong clinical evidence of a seizure disorder. Generally seizure disorders are diagnosed by clinical symptoms. Each type of epilepsy has its own natural course and response to a treatment.

The medical therapy of seizure disorders has three goals: (1) to eliminate seizures or reduce their frequency as much as possible, (2) to avoid side effects associated with long-term treatment, and (3) to assist the patient in maintaining or restoring normal psychosocial and vocational functioning (Tucker &

McDavid, 1997). There are many anticonvulsant medications available to treat seizure disorders. However, the most widely-used anticonvulsant medications have significant unpleasant side effects like sedation, weight gain, and acne. Not surprisingly, compliance with treatment can be a major issue for some patients.

Psychological Sequelae and Interventions

The impact of seizures on one's quality of life can be tremendous. Driving may be restricted, independence may be threatened, and workplace discrimination may occur. Patients must learn to avoid circumstances that may precipitate a seizure. Understanding these factors can help a patient to avoid situations, substances, and medications that may encourage generation of a seizure. Table 7.4 shows the factors that may increase the risk of seizures.

A special difficulty for the person with epilepsy is the episodic nature of the illness and the unpredictability of when a seizure may occur. This may lead to social isolation and decreased autonomy. Psychological factors may have a great impact on a patient's clinical course (Tucker & McDavid, 1997). These factors include demoralization and feelings of helplessness, hopelessness, and incompetence (Frank & Frank, 1991). Occupational aspirations may be compromised, and interpersonal and intimate relationships may be affected by this illness.

Psychiatric symptoms are common in individuals with seizure disorders. The incidence of suicidal behavior has been reported by Robertson and Trimble (1983) to be up to 25 times greater than that of the general population, especially in temporal lobe epilepsy. However, there is conflicting evidence whether or not epileptics have a higher incidence of mood disorders (Robertson, 1986). Depression needs to be differentiated from the demoralization that can result from living with epilepsy. Mood disorders in epilepsy can cause substantial morbidity and contribute to a higher risk of mortality (see Schwartz & March, 2000).

Panic attacks in patients with epilepsy have a lifetime prevalence of 21%,

TABLE 7.4. Factors that Lower the Seizure Threshold

Common	Occasional
Sleep deprivation	Barbiturate withdrawal
Alcohol withdrawal	Hyperventilation
Stress	Flashing lights
Dehydration	Diet and missed meals
Drugs and drug interactions	Specific "reflex" triggers
Systemic infection	
Trauma	
Malnutrition	

From T. A. Pedley, M. L. Scheur, & T. S. Walczak (1995). "Epilepsy," in L. P. Rowland (Ed.), *Merritt's Textbook on Neurology* (pp. 845–884). Reprinted with permission of Lippincott, Williams & Wilkins.

compared with the prevalence rate of 1% in the general population (Katerndahl & Realini, 1993). Panic episodes that occur interictally (in between seizure episodes) can be mistaken for seizure activity, and some panic-like symptoms can occur physiologically before or during seizures, making it difficult to properly differentiate between anxiety symptoms and seizure symptoms. Consequently, patients may not receive either the proper antipanic medication or the proper dosage of anticonvulsant medication

The risk of psychosis in patients with epilepsy is greater than the nonepileptic population (McKenna, Kane, & Parish, 1985). A "dyscontrol" syndrome can occur, manifested by uncontrollable rage that occurs with little or no provocation (Elliot 1984). A psychotic-like symptom complex may occur in temporal lobe epilepsy. Seizures have to be distinguished diagnostically from a variety of neurological and psychiatric disorders, like panic disorder (Weilberg, Bear, & Sachs, 1987), hyperventilation, cerebral ischemia, migraine, narcolepsy, malingering and conversion disorder (Tucker & McDavid, 1986).

Pseudoseizures, or "nonepileptic seizures," often occur in patients with real seizure disorders and need to be properly identified and diagnosed as such, even though this may be a difficult task. Pseudoseizures would fit into the category of somatoform disorders. They look like an actual ictal or seizure event, but often are missing some of the salient features of a true seizure, such as urinary incontinence or tongue biting (Peguero et al., 1995). Treatment of pseudoseizures is focused on identifying, with the patients, the emotions and thoughts leading to the events, as well as the secondary gain (extra attention, a sense of protection and safety, etc.) that the patient achieves from having these seizures. Ideally, the patient can then learn to tolerate his or her emotions and develop other ways of expressing his or her wishes. Whether or not a formal mood disorder is present should also be investigated and treated accordingly.

BRAIN AND SPINAL CORD TRAUMA

Traumatic injuries to the brain and spinal cord are monumental health problems in light of their prevalence, financial impact, and dramatic life-changing natures.

Brain Trauma

Each year over 2 million people in the U.S. are victims of traumatic brain injury (TBI). Aside from the impact on the affected individuals, brain trauma has a huge public health and economic impact. It is estimated that $40 billion is spent annually in the U.S. to treat the 400,000 patients with brain injury (Max, McKenzie, & Rice, 1991). When substances of abuse like alcohol are involved at the time of injury, the prognosis regarding morbidity and mortality is worse (Corrigan, 1995).

Just as with strokes or brain tumors, the severity of brain injury and the areas of the brain which are damaged will determine the subsequent neurological and psychiatric problems. Unlike strokes or tumors, however, the damage may not be limited to a single area of the brain, and some of the damage caused by trauma, (such as injury of the brain from hitting the side of the skull, when the head is moving and hits a solid object) may not be as easily visible in brain scans. Post-traumatic seizures may occur in up to 12% of patients in the first five years following head trauma (Annegers et al., 1980)

Even when brain injury is though to be "mild" in severity, i.e., following a concussion, the cognitive impairment may be significant. Such impairment may include confused or clouded thinking, problems with concentration, short-term memory disturbance and word-finding difficulties, among other problems. There may be continued complaints of headache and dizziness for many months after the injury.

Psychological Sequelae and Interventions

Not all brain injury results in serious sequelae. Adults may be more seriously affected than children following brain trauma. The psychological and social consequences that result from brain injury may be lifelong and devastating. After severe brain injury, many patients have difficulties in functioning in all areas of life (occupational, interpersonal, familial, educational, etc.), which bring their own personal and financial costs. The psychological and cognitive problems that result often heavily contribute to the extent of disability and stress on the patient and family following brain injury.

Perhaps one of the most distressing problems that can occur following brain injury is personality change. This may be accompanied by behavioral changes, especially aggressiveness, irritability and inappropriate social behavior. In a study of 40 patients with brain injury, Thomsen (1984) found that 80% had personality changes lasting two to five years and 65% had personality changes lasting greater than 10 years following the injury. Brooks et al. (1986) found that 74% of patients had personality changes five years following brain injury. For the families of TBI patients, these are the most disturbing effects of the brain injury and some families describe the experience as "living with an entirely different person." Compounding this problem is the fact that many TBI patients have little or no insight into their personality and behavioral changes and are more distressed by the cognitive deficits they experience.

Other neuropsychiatric symptoms commonly result from traumatic brain injury. Depression has reported in from 6–77% (Silver, Yudofsky, & Hales, 1991) of patients, sometimes related to the severity of the trauma, and mania, hypomania, and delirium have also been reported. Psychotic symptoms may occur immediately following brain injury or may develop several months later (Silver et al., 1991). Anxiety disorders may very effective in treating these problems as well as irritability or mood lability, but the medications must be carefully chosen so as to relieve the patient's symptoms; medications such as fluoxetine are a better choice for depression than tricyclic antidepressants, which often cause anticholinergic side effects.

Treatment usually involves a multidisciplinary approach, including physical therapy, occupational therapy, psychiatric treatment, neurological treatment, social services, and supportive group therapy for patients and their families. This approach should start early in the recovery phase, usually in the rehabilitation setting. One study (Leach et al., 1994) showed that patients with TBI whose families learned how to implement problem-solving techniques and behavioral coping strategies had a significantly lower risk of developing depression than patients with TBI whose families had not learned these skills.

The patient and family often go through a parallel, but not identical grieving process in response to the loss of brain function and resulting deficits and disabilities in the patient. The accident itself often has great symbolic significance for the patient, and the therapist may need to explore the patient's beliefs about the meaning of the accident itself. On a more concrete level, therapists also need to provide social skills training, teach cognitive strategies for compensating for impaired memory or concentration, and continually reinforce these skills in patients who have impaired insight and poor compliance. While treatment of these patients can be very challenging, some patients with TBI do gain insight and benefit tremendously from treatment, which is an extremely rewarding goal to accomplish.

Spinal Cord Trauma

Basic Medical Facts

Like brain trauma, spinal cord injury is another potentially devastating life event. It often occurs in the younger population, who engage in more risky activities such as sports, horseback riding, driving cars fast, or riding motorcycles. The level at which injury occurs to the spinal cord determines the level of functional disability. Injuries at the lumbosacral level lead to paralysis of the lower extremities and cause both bowel and bladder dysfunction. Injuries at the cervical level can lead to paralysis of the upper and lower extremities and sometimes paralysis of the muscles of respiration, necessitating a tracheotomy and the use of a respirator to preserve life. As with brain injury, the level of functional disability affects the patient's emotional state and ability to be autonomous and independent. Unlike with brain injury, the cerebral functions remain intact.

Psychological Sequelae and Interventions

Depression may occur in this patient population, although the incidence is not as high as one might expect (Howell et al., 1981). A bigger problem is chronic pain, which is reported in about 50% of spinal cord injury patents (Umlauf, 1992). The psychological response to spinal cord injury is similar to the loss of a body part or of a loved one. A grief reaction should be expected, with the emergence of the psychological stages of denial, anger, despair, bargaining, and acceptance. Much of how the spinal cord-injured individual reacts to his injury is related to his preinjury personality and functioning. DeJong, Branch, and Corcoran (1984) found that the factors that predicted the best independent living outcomes were being married, higher education, few transportation barriers, economic advantages and milder severity of disability.

After spinal cord injury, there is usually a period of intensive rehabilitation. The patient's home may need to be modified to accommodate the disabilities and wheelchair-accessibility. A multidisciplinary team usually works with the patient and the family to prepare for living with the disabilities and the physical and/or psychological accommodations that will need to be made. Involving the family is vital to minimizing the patient's feelings of loss, sadness, helplessness, and fears of abandonment.

Family members, especially spouses, may also go through a period of grief. Providing psychological support to the family is very helpful and often necessary to help with the patient's discharge from the hospital and return to daily life. Sexual issues are often hidden unless specifically addressed. For example, patients and their sexual partners can be reassured that sexual relations are still possible and spinal cord patients can continue to derive satisfaction from sexual relations as well as provide that for their partners. However, there may need to be counseling about different sexual techniques and devices which may be necessary to make sexual relations successful for both partners. The treating clinician's openness and willingness to bring up and explore sexual issues is important to allowing patients and partners to communicate about this very important part of life.

PAIN SYNDROMES

Headaches

Headaches can be classified into primary and secondary headaches. Primary headaches include migraine, cluster, and tension headaches. Secondary headaches are those resulting from an underlying problem, like a brain tumor, a metabolic disturbance, or other brain diseases (Table 7.5).

Migraine Headaches

Basic Medical Facts. Migraine headaches have a typical pattern, beginning with a prodromal state, lasting from hours to days prior to the actual headache; the

TABLE 7.5. International Headache Society Classification

1. Migraine
2. Tension-type headache
3. Cluster headache and chronic paroxysmal hemicrania
4. Miscellaneous headaches unassociated with structural lesion
5. Headache associated with head trauma
6. Headache associated with vascular disorders
7. Headache associated with nonvascular disorder
8. Headache associated with substances or their withdrawal
9. Headache associated with noncephalic infection
10. Headache associated with metabolic disorder
11. Headache or facial pain associated with disorder of cranium, neck, eyes, ears, nose, sinuses, teeth, mouth, or other facial or cranial structures
12. Cranial neuralgias, nerve trunk pain, and deafferentation pain
13. Headache not classifiable

From "Classification and Diagnostic Criteria for Headache Disorders, Cranial Neuralgias and Facial Pain." (1998). *Cephalagia, 8,* 1–96. Reprinted with permission of Blackwell Science Ltd.

aura, occurring immediately prior to the headache; the actual headache; the termination of the headache, which occurs as the pain subsides; and the postdromal period, during which patients experience symptoms similar to the prodromal state. Migraine headaches have many variants (typical, classic, and atypical), which may occur with or without an aura.

Migraine headache pain is quite severe and can be very debilitating. Patients will complain of pain so severe that they cannot function even at the most elementary level. They may experience nausea, vomiting, and photophobia (which means that they cannot tolerate light so they have to be an in a darkened room). The headache may last for hours.

There is no consensus as to the cause of migraine headaches. A vascular hypothesis has been offered as well as a neural inflammation hypothesis as to causation. There is often a co-morbidity between migraine headaches and other medical and neuropsychiatric conditions. Migraines may coexist with mood disorders, especially depression, seizure disorders, and stroke.

Treatment involves migraine prophylaxis as well as acute pain management. Drugs that provide prophylaxis act on the 5-HT-2 system. These drugs include methysergide, ergotamines, antidepressants, calcium channel blockers, and anticonvulsants. Medications like sumatriptan (Imitrex), a 5-HT-1D agonist, have revolutionized the acute treatment of migraines. These drugs block the release of serotonin (5-HT) from the neuron. Other agents that may be helpful in the acute treatment include analgesics (pain medications), antiemetics (antinausea medications), anxiolytics, steroids, nonsteroidal anti-inflammatory agents, narcotics, and tranquilizers.

Cluster Headaches

Cluster headaches are headaches that occur in series that last from weeks to months followed by periods of long remissions. There are distinct clinical criteria for diagnosis of cluster headaches (Table 7.6).

Acute treatment includes sumatriptan, ergotamines, dihydroergotamine (HE), and local anesthetics. Oxygen therapy may also be helpful. Prophylactic (preventative) treatment includes ergotamines, methysergide, steroids, calcium channel blockers, lithium carbonate, and divalproex. Although there has been speculation about a comorbidity between psychiatric disorders and cluster headaches, there have been no studies that confirm such an association.

Psychological Sequelae and Interventions. Epidemiological evidence and treatment modalities point to the possibility that headaches and psychiatric disorders may overlap and result from similar neural mechanisms. Therefore, the clinician should be sensitive to this possible linkage and alert to looking for psychiatric illness in the headache patient, especially migraine patients.

Depending on the patient's response to pharmacological intervention and treatments, headache patients experience different levels of interference from the illness in their everyday lives. A good response usually causes little change in daily functioning. However, poor responsiveness can lead to profound alterations in how patients cope with daily life and their usual activities. Aggressive management of the headache and patient education about the illness are important in helping patients cope with the various types of headaches described in this section.

TABLE 7.6. Diagnostic Criteria for Cluster Headache

A. At least five attacks fulfilling B–D
B. Severe unilateral orbital, supraorbital, and/or temporal pain lasting 15–180 min if untreated
C. Headache is associated with at least one of the following signs, which have to be present on the pain side:
  1. Conjunctival injection
  2. Lacrimation
  3. Nasal congestion
  4. Rhinorrhea
  5. Forehead and facial sweating
  6. Miosis
  7. Prosis
  8. Eyelid edema
D. Frequency of attacks: from one every other day to eight per day

From "Classification and Diagnostic Criteria for Headache Disorders, Cranial Neuralgias and Facial Pain." (1998). *Cephalagia, 8,* 1–96. Reprinted with permission of Blackwell Science Ltd.

INFECTIONS

Basic Medical Facts

Encephalitis and meningitis are caused by bacteria, fungi, or viruses. Some types of meningitis, such as meningococcal meningitis, are extremely contagious, and exposed individuals must seek immediate medical attention. Encephalitis and meningitis are especially prevalent in the immunocompromised patient population, such as patients with AIDS or cancer. These disorders usually present with an acute or sudden change in the patient's usual mental state. One may see changes in the person's behavior, level of consciousness, a change in personality, changes in cognitive or thinking ability or even acute psychotic symptoms. Symptoms such as headache, nausea, vomiting, fever, and stiff neck may also be present.

Lyme Disease

Lyme disease, caused by the tick-borne Lyme spirochete, has been recognized to cause a variety of confusing neuropsychiatric and physical symptoms. They may include unusual fatigue, poor concentration, memory loss, emotional lability, sleep disturbances, depression, arthralgias (joint aches), myalgias (muscle aches), and seizures (Shaddick et al., 1994). For more information about this disease, please see Chapter 8.

Psychological Sequelae and Interventions

These patients are usually managed acutely by their internists and neurologists. Mental health practitioners may be consulted to help with the recovery after the initial infection is diagnosed and treated. With successful diagnosis and treatment with antibiotics, the patient often has a complete return to the previous level of functioning.

However, if the infection is of a chronic or more indolent nature, the mental status and neurological changes may not be reversible. Such chronic infections include neurosyphilis (syphilis that affects the central nervous system), viruses like Herpes virus, and fungi-like cryptococcus. In these situations, patients may no longer be able to care for themselves and may need home or nursing care with proper medical supervision and assistance.

In the case of Lyme disease, physiologically based cognitive and mood symptoms may falsely be attributed to functional causes (Fallon & Nields, 1994). Many of these patients are labeled as "crocks" or are thought to have conversion disorders or hysterical reactions. All complaints need to be thoroughly investigated and, if Lyme disease is present, treated with aggressive antibiotic therapy.

Some patients with Lyme disease have little or no change in physical and psychological symptoms after antibiotic therapy is completed. Some of these patients continue to suffer from continuing cognitive disturbances, unusual fatigue, sleep disturbance, and mood swings. This is more often the case in patients in whom there was a delay in diagnosis. There is controversy whether long-term antibiotic treatment is of benefit to this group of patients.

Generally, the mental health practitioner needs to build a solid and trusting alliance with the patient. This will help sort out any secondary gain the patient may experience from continuing physical disability. Group treatment may be helpful, but this can be a double-edged sword. Just like with the chronic fatigue syndrome population, there will be support group members who obtain enormous secondary gain, which actually may encourage the "sick role" instead of promoting healthy psychological adaptation to a physical problem. Patients should be supported to maximize their assets and make suitable accommodations for their disabilities in order to function as well as possible in social and occupational arenas.

DIAGNOSTIC PROCEDURES

The major diagnostic tests used in evaluating neurological disease are listed in Table 7.7.

TABLE 7.7. Diagnostic Procedures Used in Neurological Disorders

Neuroimaging Techniques
    Computerized Tomography (CT)
    Magnetic Resonance Imaging (MRI)
    Single Photon Emission Computerized Tomography (SPECT)
    Positron Emission Tomography (PET)
    Magnetic Resonance Angiography (MRA)

Angiography

Electrodiagnostic Techniques
    Electroencephalogram (EEG)
    Evoked Potentials
    Electromyography (EMG)
    Nerve conduction studies

Noninvasive Cartoid Evaluation
    Doppler Assessment
    Ophthalmodynamometry
    Oculoplethysmography

Muscle and nerve biopsy
    Lumbar Puncture (LP) and cerebrospinal fluid examination
    Neuropsychological testing

Neuroimaging Techniques

Diagnostic imaging techniques can give information about the physical structure and anatomy of the brain or about functional changes in blood flow and activity of neuronal tissue.

Computerized Tomography (CT) Scan

CT scanners are just tunnel-shaped X-ray machines that project X-rays around a 360° axis in order to take cross-sectional pictures ("slices") of any part of the body. Because the information is stored in a computer and can be manipulated, CT scans can even be used in some cases to construct three-dimensional images by putting together information from a series of very thin cross-sectional pictures, also knows as a "spiral CT." CT scans are relatively less expensive than other imaging techniques, have minimal risks to the patient if done without contrast dyes, and are widely available in the United States.

CT scans record variations in tissue density in the brain. They are very good for detecting bone fractures and acute brain hemorrhages and can be done quickly, which is why head CTs are usually ordered first in cases of stroke or head trauma. They are also suitable for detecting general atrophy of the brain and for seeing lacunae, or holes, that are the result of old strokes, which makes head CTs a good choice for evaluating dementia as well. On the other hand, while they are good at detecting calcified lesions (because any calcium, like bone, appears bright white), CT scans can miss even large tumors or aneurysms if there is no swelling or edema, because the density of these may be similar to normal brain tissue. Plus, because of the signal interference caused by large amounts of bone reflecting the X-rays around the temporal lobes, brain stem, and posterior fossa, CT scans are of little use to detect brain lesions in those areas.

The use of intravenous contrast material, both ionic and nonionic agents, enhance the detection of brain lesions, especially when there has been a disruption of the blood-brain barrier (Chan, Khandji, & Hilal, 1995). However, the use of contrast material carries the risk of potentially severe allergic reactions or damage to the kidneys. It is contraindicated in patients who have had a previous major allergic reaction to contrast material or shellfish, and is generally not used in patients who are pregnant, have renal failure, or are in sickle-cell crisis.

Patients having a CT scan may feel closed in or claustrophobic and may experience an anxiety reaction. They should be informed about this possibility in advance and offered antianxiety medication. They should also be informed that if they have an intravenous injection of contrast material, it may cause a "burning" sensation that may be alarming; they can be reassured that this is a normal experience and given forewarning and reassurance should it occur.

Magnetic Resonance Imaging (MRI)

MRI refers to the use of a machine to create a small but very powerful magnetic field, which temporarily reverses the spin of electrons around the nucleus of the hydrogen atom, a major component of water in brain tissue. MRIs are generally less available than CT scans because of the greater expense, but they have superior sensitivity to detect brain pathology, especially small brain tumors (Chan et al., 1995). Intravenous contrast media called gadolinium can enhance the MRI image and increases the chance of detecting lesions.

Unlike CT scans, MRIs do not cause any exposure to radiation. As noted earlier, certain areas of the brain are best viewed with MRI, including the temporal lobes, the brain stem, the posterior fossa, and subcortical structures. They are especially good for detecting demyelinating lesions, as in multiple sclerosis. If a patient has a normal CT scan yet clinical symptoms point to brain pathology, a follow-up MRI scan may be indicated, especially in patients with seizure disorders and suspected brains aneurysms or arteriovenous malformations. Unfortunately, because MRIs use powerful magnets, they cannot be used in patients with metal aneurysm or surgical clips, residual metallic shrapnel from old injuries, or internal magnetic or mechanical devices like pacemakers. MRIs should be used with extreme caution in the pregnant patient.

Patients who have claustrophobia may find having an MRI more traumatic than a CT scan, because the patient usually has to lie in a narrow tunnel, the scan takes a longer time, and the machine is extremely loud. (There are "open" MRI machines which tend not to cause the same degree of claustrophobia, but most hospitals do not have these.) As with CT scans, sedating medications can be used to help anxious patients tolerate the procedure. Ear plugs and music can also help to calm patients, and patients should be encouraged to keep their eyes closed during the procedure, as opening them can precipitate an anxiety reaction. Unlike CT scans, which cannot be done with others present because of the use of radiation, MRI scans can be done with a family member in the room, which is reassuring to many patients. Of note, injections of gadolinium usually cause no uncomfortable physical sensations or allergic reactions.

Single Photon Emission Computer Tomography (SPECT)

SPECT scanning is a functional neuroimaging technique that produces both quantitative and qualitative measures of cerebral blood flow. It is especially helpful in the diagnosis of dementia, revealing areas of relatively lowered blood flow to certain regions of the brain, corresponding with degeneration of neuronal tissue. It is also useful in the diagnosis of seizure disorders (Mohr et al., 1995).

Positron Emission Tomography (PET)

PET scanning is another functional neuroimaging technique that measures blood flow as well as neurotransmitters and their receptors. Use of the PET scan is limited by the need to be performed near a cyclotron that produces the positron-emitting isotopes. The radioactivity limits how often it can be used in the same patient. It is primarily used in the research setting. PET scans have been especially helpful in understanding normal brain functioning and looking at differences in patients with neuropsychiatric illnesses (Mohr et al., 1995).

Magnetic Resonance Angiography (MRA)

This is a noninvasive technique that is used to visualize the cerebral blood circulation. When used in combination with noninvasive carotid evaluation and transcranial Doppler studies, conventional cerebral angiography can be replaced by MRA (Mohr et al., 1995).

Angiography

This technique is the best method by which to visualize the cerebral circulation. It is performed via an intravenous catheterization and injection of contrast material. It can detect stenosis (blockage of blood flow), formation of thrombus (blood clot), atherothrombotic disease (narrowing of the blood vessels due to plaque), and embolic occlusion (blood clot). All of these conditions can cause stroke and cerebral ischemia (lack of oxygen delivery to the brain tissue). Angiography can identify collateral (alternate) circulation. It carries some risk of complications that occur in 2–12% of patients. These risks are aortic and carotid artery dissection (a tearing and weakening of the inner lining of the blood vessel) and embolic (blood clot-induced) stroke (Mohr et al., 1995).

Unlike the other neuroimaging techniques mentioned, this is an invasive procedure, so the patient may experience genuine physical discomfort as well as realistic anxiety about the procedure. The patient is awake during the procedure, and can be informed in advance of unpleasant physical sensations—like "burning"—that may occur, and be reassured that they are common experiences.

Electrodiagnostic Techniques

Electroencephalogram (EEG)

EEG has been used as a diagnostic tool since the late nineteenth century. It measures electrical activity in the brain by placing electrodes on the scalp. It is noninvasive and causes no discomfort to the patient. The most important use of the EEG is in the diagnosis of seizure disorders. However, EEG can also be helpful in the diagnosis of dementia, encephalitis, drug intoxication, tumor, infarction, delirium, metabolic encephalopathy, or the normal aging of the brain (Emerson, Walczak, & Turner, 1995).

Evoked Potentials

Sensory stimuli provoke an eletrophysiological response in the brain, which can be measured (Emerson et al., 1995). Sensory-evoked potentials are useful in determining whether sensory pathways are intact. For example, a completely deaf person would not have any electrophysiologic response. On the other hand, a person who claimed to have no hearing but was not truly deaf would have an electrophysiologic response. Structural damage, as in multiple sclerosis, or functional impairment, as in delirium, can cause abnormalities in sensory-evoked potentials. Likewise, motor-evoked potentials can demonstrate disruptions in central motor pathways, as in illnesses like multiple sclerosis and motor neuron disease.

Electromyography (EMG) and Nerve Conduction Studies

EMG measures the pattern of electrical activity in muscles. It can provide a guide to the severity of an acute disorder of a peripheral or cranial nerve (Lange & Trujaborg, 1995). In chronic or degenerative disorders, EMG can assess whether the pathological process is of a progressive nature, such as in amyotrophic lateral sclerosis (ALS, also known as Lou Gehrig's Disease).

Nerve conduction studies record the electrical response of a muscle to stimulation of its motor nerve along its course. These studies complement EMG studies. They provide a way to measure the progression and therapeutic response of peripheral nerve disorders. One example of an application of nerve conduction studies is in the evaluation of carpal tunnel syndrome and ulnar and median neuropathy (abnormal functioning of nerves in the arm and hand due to compression of the nerve).

These tests are generally unpleasant, as needles may be placed through the skin in order to precisely deliver electrical current to stimulate muscles or to measure the response, which may cause discomfort and pain.

NONINVASIVE CARTOTID EVALUATION

These studies are done to evaluate the severity, extent and location of atherothrombotic (narrowing of the blood vessels) disease in the carotid arteries (the large arteries that supply blood to the brain). Direct assessment is done using *Doppler assessment* (Mohr et al., 1995). Indirect assessment of pressure and flow in the internal carotid arteries is done by *opthalmodynamometry* and *oculoplethysmography*. There is no pain or discomfort associated with these procedures.

Muscle and Nerve Biopsy

Muscle biopsy is helpful in distinguishing between muscle and nerve pathology. It is helpful in diagnosing muscle diseases like muscular dystrophy, and certain connective tissue diseases like polyarteritis nodosa, certain infections like trichiosis and metabolic defects (Hays & Younger, 1995).

Nerve biopsy can establish whether there is an inflammatory process present. It can distinguish between segmental demyelination (loss of the myelin heath, covering the nerve) and axonal degeneration (nerve cell death), and it can identify specific diseases such as amyloidosis, sarcoidosis, vasculitis, and metabolic neuropathies.

Both of these are surgical procedures, performed under local anesthesia with the patient awake. The patient may experience some physical discomfort when receiving the injection of local anesthetic or if the anesthesia is not adequate to control pain.

Lumbar Puncture (LP) and Cerebrospinal Fluid (CSF) Examination

LP should be considered to measure CSF pressure and to examine the bacterial, cellular, and chemical elements of the CSF, especially in the case of infection (Fishman, 1995). LP can be used also to administer therapeutic medications, including antibiotics, anesthetics, and chemotherapeutic agents. The main complication of LP is a headache caused by a drop in CSF pressure, but it is of a temporary nature.

In order to have a LP done, the patient is usually placed in a fetal position, lying on his/her side, with knees drawn tightly to the chest. This is an awkward position and sometimes the patient feels very exposed. There may also be fear connected to a needle being placed in the spinal spaces. Local anesthesia is given; however, the patient will still experience pushing and may hear the "pop" of the needle penetrating into the space from which the CSF will be drawn. The patient also needs to remain perfectly still, which may be difficult for some individuals.

Neuropsychological Testing

A variety of neuropsychological tests are available that can demonstrate the presence of brain dysfunction and discern the areas and severity of dysfunction. Both cognitive and emotional functioning should be assessed. The neuropsychological evaluation relies on comparisons between the patient's present level of functioning and his premorbid functioning (Stern, 1995). Results of neuropsychological testing can assist in assessing a patient's strengths and weaknesses and help in constructing a realistic, individualized treatment program for the patient (Lezak, 1986).

CONCLUSION

Becoming educated about the basic medical facts of neurological illness is of paramount importance in understanding the physical and psychological impact of these illnesses on patients' lives and well-being. It is often the psychological adaptation by the patient and the family that is the most difficult aspect of living with and recovering from neurological illness. Patients will be referred and will seek support from various mental health care providers to help with this adaptation. Without the basic understanding of the medical facts and psychological sequelae, the mental health provider would lack the necessary tools to assist the patients' recovery and adjustment. This chapter has hopefully provided a basic understanding of effective care of patients with neurological illness.

REFERENCES

Amar, K., & Wilcock, G. (1996). Fortnightly review: Vascular dementia. *British Medical Journal, 312* (7025), 227–231.

Annegers, J. F., Grabow, J. D., Groover, R. V., Laws, E. R. Jr., Elveback, L. R., & Kurland, L. T. (1980). Seizures after head trauma: a population study. *Neurology, 30,* 683–689.

Astrom, M. (1996). Generalized anxiety disorder in stroke patients: A 3 year longitudinal study. *Stroke, 27,* 270–275.

Brooks, N., Campsie, L., Symington, C., Beattie, A., & McKinlay, W. (1986). The five-year outcome of severe blunt head injury: a relative's view. *Journal of Neurology, Neurosurgery, & Psychiatry, 49,* 764-770.

Cash, R., Dennis, T., L'Heureux, R. Raisman, R., Javoy-Agid, F., & Scatton, B. (1987). Parkinson's disease and dementia: Norepinephrine and dopamine in locus ceruleus. *Neurology, 37,* 42–46.

Castillo, C. S., Starkstein, S. E., Federoff, J. P., et al. (1993). Generalized anxiety disorder following stroke. *Journal of Nervous and Mental Disease, 181,* 100–106.

Chan, D., Khandji, A. G., & Hilal, S. K. (1995). CT and MRI. In L. P. Rowland (Ed.), *Merritt's textbook of neurology* (pp. 59-76). Baltimore: Williams and Wilkins.

Clark, M. S., & Smith, D. S. (1997). Abnormal illness behavior in rehabilitation from stroke. *Clinical Rehabilitation, 11,* 162–170.

Commission on classification and terminology of the International League Against Epilepsy. Proposal for revised clinical and electroencephalographic classification of epileptic seizures. Epilepsia 1981; 22-489-501.

Corrigan, J. D. (1995). Substance abuse as a mediating factor in outcome from traumatic brain injury. *Archives of Physical Medicine and Rehabilitation, 76,* 302–309.

Cummings, J. L., & Benson, D. R. (1992). *Dementia: A clinical approach* (2nd ed.). Boston, MA: Butterworth.

Cummings, J. L. (1992). Depression and Parkinson's disease: a review. *American Journal of Psychiatry, 149,* 443–454.

DeJong, G., Branch, L. G., Corcoran, P. J. (1984). Independent living outcomes in spinal cord injury: Multivariate analyses. *Archives of Physical Medicine and Rehabilitation, 65,* 66–73.

Dooneief, G., Mirabello, E., Bell, K., Marder, K., Stern, Y., & Mayeux, R. (1992). An estimate of the incidence of depression in idiopathic Parkinson's disease. *Archives of Neurology, 49,* 305–307.

Elliot, F. A. (1984). The episodic dyscontrol syndrome and aggression. *Neurologic Clinics, 2,* 113–125.

Emerson, R. G., Walczak, T. S., & Turner, C. A. (1995). EEG and evoked potentials. In L. P. Rowland (Ed.), *Merritt's textbook of neurology* (pp. 67–77). Baltimore: Williams and Wilkins.

Epstein, R. S., & Ursano, R. J. (1994). Anxiety disorders. In J. M. Silver, S. C. Yudofsky, R. E. Hales (Eds.), *Neuropsychiatry of traumatic brain injury* (pp. 285–312). Washington, DC: American Psychiatric Press.

Evans, D. A., Funkenstein, H., Albert, M. S., Scheer, P. A., Ostfeld, A. M., Taylor, J. O., et al. (1989). Prevalence of Alzheimer's disease in a community population of older persons: Higher than previously reported. *Journal of the American Medical Association, 262,* 2551–2556.

Fallon, B. A., & Nields, J. A. (1994). Lyme Disease: A neuropsychiatric illness. *American Journal of Psychiatry, 151,* 1571–1582.

Fishman, R. A. (1995). Lumbar puncture and CSF examination. In L. P. Rowland (Ed.), *Merritt's textbook of neurology* (pp. 93–97). Baltimore: Williams and Wilkins.

Frank, J. D., & Frank, J. B. (1991). *Persuasion and healing.* Baltimore: Johns Hopkins University Press.

Geldmacher, D., & Whitehouse, P. (1996). Evaluation of dementia. *New England Journal of Medicine, 335*(5), 330–336.

Genton, P., Bartomolei, F., & Guerrini, R. (1995). Panic attacks mistaken for relapse of epilepsy. *Epilepsia, 36,* 48–51.

Giladi, N., McMahon, D. Przborski, S., Flaster, E., Guillory, S., Kostic, V., et al. (1992). Motor blocks in Parkinson's disease. *Neurology, 42,* 333–339.

Hartelius, L. (1994). Speech and swallowing in Parkinson's disease. *Folia Phoniatr Logop, 46,* 9–17.

Hays, A. P., & Younger, D. S. (1995). Muscle and nerve biopsy. In L. P. Rowland (Ed.), *Merritt's textbook of neurology* (pp. 97-100). Baltimore: Williams & Wilkins.

Hauser, W. A., Rocca, W. A. (1996). Descriptive epidemiology of epilepsy: Contributions of population focused studies from Rochester, Minnesota. *Mayo Clinic Proceedings, 11,* 576–586.

Howell, T., Fullerton, D. T., Harvey, R. F., & Klein, M. (1981). Depression in spinal cord injured patients. *Paraplegia, 19,* 284–288.

Joseph, R. (1996). *Neuropsychiatry, neuropsychology, and clinical neuroscience* (2nd ed.). Baltimore: Williams & Wilkins.

Katerndahl, D. A., & Realini, J. P. (1993). Lifetime prevalence of panic states. *American Journal of Psychiatry, 150,* 246–249.

King, R. B. (1996). Quality of life after stroke. *Stroke, 27,* 1467–1472.

Lange, D. L. & Trojaborg, W. (1995), Electromyography and nerve conduction studies in neuromuscular disease. In L. P. Rowland (Ed.), *Merritt's textbook of neurology* (pp. 77–82). Baltimore: Williams and Wilkins.

Leach, L. R., Frank, R. G., Bouman, D. E., & Farmer, J. (1994). Family functioning, social support and depression after traumatic brain injury. *Brain Injury, 8,* 599–606.

Lezak, M. D. (1986). An individualized approach to neuropsychological assessment. In P. E. Logue & J. M. Schear (Eds.), *Clinical neuropsychology* (pp. 29–49). Springfield, IL: C.C. Thomas.

Marsh, L. (2000). Neuropsychiatric aspects of Parkinson's disease. *Psychosomatics, 41,* 15–23.

Max, W., MacKenzie, E., & Rice, D. (1991). Head injuries: costs and consequences. *Journal of Head Trauma Rehabilitation, 6,* 76–91.

Mayeux, R., & Stern, Y. (1983). Intellectual dysfunction and dementia in Parkinson's disease. In R. Mayeux and W. G. Rosen, (Ed.), *The dementias* (pp. 211–227). New York: Raven.

McKenna, P. J., Kane, J. M., & Parrish, D. (1985). Psychotic syndromes in epilepsy. *American Journal Psychiatry, 142*, 895–904.

Minden, S. L. (1992). Psychotherapy for people with multiple sclerosis. *Journal of Neuropsychiatry, 4*, 198–213.

Minden, S. L., & Schiffer, R. B. (1990). Affective disorders in multiple sclerosis. *Archives of Neurology, 47*, 98–104.

Mohr, E., Mendis, T., & Grimes, J. D. (1995). Late cognitive changes in Parkinson's disease with an emphasis on dementia. *Advances in Neurology, 65*, 97–113.

Mohr, J. R., & Prohovnik, I. (1995). Neurovascular imaging. In L. P. Rowland (Ed.), *Merritt's textbook of neurology* (pp. 82–93). Baltimore: Williams and Wilkins.

Olanow, C. W., Kordower, J. H., & Freeman, T. B. (1996). Fetal nigral transplantation as a therapy for Parkinson's disease. *Trends in Neurosciences., 19*, 102–109.

Pedley, T. A., Scheuer, M. L., & Walczak, T. S. (1995). Epilepsy. In L. P. Rowland (Ed.), *Merritt's textbook of neurology* (pp. 845–884). Baltimore: Williams and Wilkins.

Peguero, E., Abou-Khalil, B., Fakhoury, T., & Mathews, G. (1995). Self-injury and incontinence in psychogenic seizures. *Epilepsia, 36*, 586–591.

Pohjasvaara, T., Leppavuori, A., Siira, I., Vataja, R., Kaste, M., & Erkinjuntti, T. (1998). Frequency and clinical determinants of poststroke depression. *Stroke, 29*: 2311–2317.

Robertson, M. M. (1986). Ictal and interictal depression in patients with epilepsy. In M. R. Trimble & T. G. Bolwig (Eds.), *Aspects of epilepsy and psychiatry* (pp. 213–234). Chichester, England: Wiley.

Robertson, M. M., & Trimble, M. R. (1983). Depressive illness in patients with epilepsy: A review. *Epilepsia, 24* (Suppl 2), S109–S116.

Robinson, R. G., Starr, L. B., Kubos, K. L. et al. (1983). A two year longitudinal study of post-stroke mood disorders: Findings during the initial evaluation. *Stroke, 14*, 736–744.

Robinson, R. G. (1998). *The clinical neuropsychology of stroke.* New York: Cambridge University Press.

Schiffer, R. B., Herndon, R. M., & Rudick, R. A. (1985). Treatment of pathological laughing and weeping with amitriptyline. *New England Journal of Medicine, 312*, 1480–1482.

Schiffer, R. B., Weitkamp, L. R., Wineman, N. M., & Guttormsen, S. (1986). Association between bipolar affective disorder and multiple sclerosis. *American Journal of Psychiatry, 143*, 94–95.

Schubert, D. S., Burns, R., Paras, W., et al. (1992). Increase of medical hospital length of stay by depression in stroke and amputation patients: a pilot study. *Pschotherapy Psychosomatics, 57*, 61–66.

Shadick, N. A., Phillips, C. B., Logigian, E. L., Steere, A. C., Kaplan, R. F., Berardi, V. P., et al. (1994). The long term clinical outcomes of Lyme disease. *Annals of Internal Medicine, 121*, 560–567.

Silver, J. M., Yudofsky, S. C., & Hales, R. E. (1991). Depression in traumatic brain injury. *Neuropsychiatry, Neuropsychology and Behavioral Neurology, 4*, 12–23.

Sinyor, D,. Jacques, R., Kaloupek, D. G., Becker, R., Goldenberg, M., & Coopersmith, H. (1986). Post-stroke depression and lesion location: An attempted replication. *Brain, 109*, 539–546.

Starkstein, S. E., Preziosi, T. J., Bolduc, P. L., et al. (1990). Depression in Parkinson's disease. *Journal of Nervous and Mental Disorders, 178*, 27–31.

Starkstein, S. E., & Mayberg, H. S. (1993). Depression in Parkinson's disease. In S. E. Starkstein & R. G. Robinson (Ed.), *Depression in neurological disease* (pp. 97–116). Baltimore: Johns Hopkins University Press.

Stern, Y. (1995). Neuropsychological evaluation. In L. P. Rowland (Ed.), *Merritt's textbook of neurology* (pp. 100–103). Baltimore: Williams and Wilkins.

Surridge, D. (1969). An investigation into some psychiatric aspects of multiple sclerosis. *British Journal of Psychiatry, 115,* 749–764.

Thomsen, I. V. (1984). Late outcome of very severe blunt head trauma: A 10–15 year second follow-up. *Journal of Neurology, Neurosurgery, and Psychiatry, 47,* 260–268.

Tucker, G. J., & McDavid, J. (1997). Neuropsychiatric aspects of seizure disorders. In S. C. Yudofsky & R. E. Hales (Eds.), *Textbook of neuropsychiatry* (pp. 561–582). Washington, DC: American Psychiatric Press.

Umlauf, R. L. (1992). Psychological interventions for chronic pain following spinal cord injury. *Clinical Journal of Pain, 8,* 111–118.

Weilberg, J. B., Bear, D. A., & Sachs, G. (1987). Three patients with concomitant panic attacks and seizure disorder: Possible clues to the neurology of anxiety. *American Journal of Psychiatry, 144,* 1053–1056.

8

Infectious Diseases

JENIFER A. NIELDS
JOHN A. R. GRIMALDI, JR.

INTRODUCTION

New infectious diseases, and the emergence of drug-resistant strains of old ones, have created formidable challenges to medicine in recent decades. At the same time, we have progressed to a far more subtle and complex understanding of infectious illness, taking us well beyond the simple germ theory of disease. The complex symphony of host immune responses to microbial invasion can become a cacophony of autoimmune, toxic, and neuroendocrine dysregulation with ramifications far beyond the direct effects of the microbe. Such dysregulation can persist even after the infection has seemingly been eradicated. There are diseases such as peptic ulcer disease that have only recently been shown to be infectious in origin and others, such as chronic fatigue syndrome, multiple sclerosis, and even schizophrenia, in whose pathogenesis there are indications that an infectious agent may play a role. Only a few decades ago, antibiotics and vaccination programs seemed to hold the promise of ultimate victory over infectious disease. With the advent of the AIDS epidemic, the battle against microbial invasion has resumed with a vengeance. Concomitantly, we have been sobered by the emergence of resistant strains of tuberculosis, the awareness that stashes of deadly smallpox microbes are held by several nations, and new epidemics such as that caused by Ebola virus, mad cow disease, and Lyme disease. Chronic illness and death due to infectious disease have re-emerged as genuine threats not only to the elderly, the debilitated, and those without access to state-of-the art medical care, but also to the young and healthy.

Given that a chapter of this sort cannot cover the topic of infectious diseases both comprehensively and in depth, we shall concentrate on two diseases: HIV infection and Lyme Disease, and on a clinical symptom complex whose etiology is as yet largely undetermined: chronic fatigue syndrome (CFS). These particular disease entities have been chosen as our focus because of their potential for chronicity, their tendency to affect brain functioning, and the deep and far-reaching psychological effects wrought by certain distinctive features of each one. All three illnesses have been identified, renamed, or become epidemic only within the last two decades. Our understanding of and capacity to treat these diseases is rapidly evolving, thus creating a particular kind of challenge for affected individuals as well as for clinicians. Scientific certainty with regard to diagnosis and treatment is, arguably, more extensive in HIV infection than in Lyme disease, and far less in CFS than in either of the other two.[1] Indeed, the current understanding of CFS resembles an earlier understanding of many diseases: AIDS, Lyme disease, multiple sclerosis, and lupus, to name a few, regarding the pathogenesis of which a multitude of theories, from infectious to psychosomatic to functional to sociocultural, have been promulgated before yielding to scientific evidence and better diagnostic tools.

By describing, comparing, and contrasting HIV, Lyme disease, and CFS we hope to provide a basis for understanding the diverse and complex ways in which a chronic infectious disease or infection-triggered clinical syndrome can affect an individual's life and the multilayered challenges that sufferers face. For each disease entity, we will touch upon the sociocultural context and history of the disease, its epidemiology, the current status of its diagnosis and treatment (including current controversies), specific mental disorders associated with the disease, and other features that impact significantly on the mental health and psychological adjustment of affected individuals.

HIV AND AIDS

Introductory Remarks

Most HIV-positive individuals whom the mental health professional may encounter are quite well-informed about their illness. They may have friends or lovers who had been infected previously and often belong to a community in which HIV prevalence is high. Treatment regimens are complex and require a relatively high degree of sophistication to comply with, let alone choose and understand. The average HIV-positive patient in the United States knows far more about his or her disease than does the average mental health professional. Lack of familiarity with the medical terms associated with HIV and AIDS and their import on the part of mental health professionals can be a significant source of alienation and noncompliance with psychological treatments. This section, there-

---

1. The inclusion of CFS in this chapter should not be construed as suggesting that the etiology of CFS is infectious in all or even most cases The syndrome CFS subsumes many different disease entities, some of them infectious, some "functional," some psychiatric, or of mixed etiology, and the majority as yet unidentified.

fore, will contain more specific medical terminology than do other sections in this book. A glossary of medical terms is provided below in Table 8.1. Given the medical complexity of HIV disease, it is more important than ever that the mental health professional working with HIV-positive individuals be prepared to respectfully learn from the patient.

History and Epidemiology

The epidemic of human immunodeficiency virus Type 1 (HIV-1) began in central West Africa over four decades ago (Gao et al., 1999) and has since spread to virtually every country in the world. It is currently estimated that over 40 million people worldwide are infected with HIV-1 (UNAIDS, 2001) and that the number of deaths globally has reached more than 21.8 million, with 448,060 of those occurring in the United States (CDC, 2000). As of December, 2000, there were an estimated 450,151 people living with HIV and AIDS in the U.S. (CDC, 2000).

How HIV spread from Africa to North America in the 1970s is unknown. But, by the late 1970s, cases of what we now know as AIDS began to appear among gay men in major metropolitan areas in the United States (Grmek, 1990). In 1981 the first cases, mostly young gay men from New York City and San Francisco, were reported to the Centers for Disease Control. All were severely immunocompromised and died of complications of Pneumocystis Carinii Pneumonia (PCP) or Kaposi's Sarcoma (KS) (Gottlieb et al., 1981). Hence, this mysterious new disease was originally called gay-related immunodeficiency or GRID. The etiologic agent, HTLV-3, was identified in 1983 by Robert Gallo (Gallo et al., 1984) in the United States and Luc Montagnier (Barre-Sinoussi et al., 1983) in France. By 1985, a diagnostic blood test to detect antibodies to the virus became available for widespread use. In addition to gay men, injecting drug users (CDC, 1982) and hemophiliacs (Davis et al., 1983) were soon identified as being at risk.

By the start of the second decade, the epidemic, which in the beginning was driven primarily by gay sex, came to rely on substance abuse as a central factor in transmission (CDC, 1995b). Either directly, through needle sharing among intravenuous drug users (IVDUS), or indirectly, by impairing judgment, both IV and non-IV use of psychoactive substances now play a major role in the continued spread of HIV (CDC, 1995a). Additionally, women infected through heterosexual sex with IV drug-using partners are among the fastest growing groups of infected individuals (Wortley & Fleming, 1997). In tandem with this shift, the evolving epidemic has affected an increasingly disproportionate number of people from the black and Hispanic communities (CDC, 1994). Furthering this disproportion, in the mid-1990s, when for the first time new treatment advances resulted in reduced morbidity and mortality, these minorities benefited least in most parts of the country (CDC, 1996)

These epidemiological trends suggest several issues relevant to a discussion

TABLE 8.1. Glossary of Medical Terms of Significance to the Lives
of HIV-Positive Individuals

General Terms

AIDS: Acquired immunodeficiency syndrome. A name given to a condition first noted in the United States in the early 1980s among young gay men in New York and San Francisco consisting of new-onset markedly diminished immune system functioning resulting in infections such as pneumocystis *carinii* pneumonia and cancers such as Kaposi's sarcoma that typically occur only in immunocompromised individuals. AIDS is now known to be caused by HIV infection and refers to the final stage in HIV disease, when immune functioning has become severely compromised and opportunistic infections have begun to occur. It is characterized by numerous opportunistic infections and malignancies and/or a CD4 cell count below 200/mm3 which, in the presence of HIV infection, constitutes a diagnosis of AIDS.

AIDS-defining condition or illness: Opportunistic infections and cancers that occur only in individuals with severely compromised immune systems or markers of severe immune deficiency syndromes that mark the onset of AIDS in HIV-positive individuals. Examples include: PCP, CMV, KS, and CD4 cell counts less than 200.

ARC: Aids-related complex. Condition of an HIV-infected individual who has symptoms (such as swollen lymph nodes and night sweats) but who has not yet developed an opportunistic infection or markedly compromised immune functioning.

CD4 cell count: Concentration of CD4 T helper lymphocytes (a subclass of white blood cells) in the blood at a given time, also of prognostic significance. CD4 cell counts are indicative of how well or how poorly the immune system is holding up within the course of HIV disease. In general, the lower the CD4 cell count the greater the risk of acquiring an AIDS-defining condition.

CD4 T helper lymphocytes: A type of white blood cell that helps the body to fight infection. These cells get invaded by HIV and subsequently both manufacture new HIV particles and are destroyed in the process. Also referred to as, simply, "CD4 cells."

HIV: Human immunodeficiency virus. In common parlance, refers to human immunodeficiency virus type 1 (HIV-1), the etiologic agent of the acquired immunodeficiency syndrome (AIDS). This virus disables the immune system, thereby allowing other infections to harm the body.

opportunistic infections (OIs): Infections that occur only in immunocompromised individuals (due to AIDS, cancer, or immunosuppressive drugs) and that are one of the hallmarks of AIDS. Examples include: Pneumocystis *carinii* pneumonia, cytomegalovirus infection, toxoplasmosis, and others.

undetectable: Refers to viral load. To achieve an "undetectable" viral load is generally the goal of antiretroviral treatment for HIV and means that the level of virus particles in a person's blood falls below the level of detection of the assay used to measure levels of virus in the blood.

viral load: Measurement of HIV virions (viral particles) in the blood plasma of an HIV-infected person at a given time. This number both has prognostic significance for overall survival and serves as a guide to initiation or modification of drug therapy. For example, a rising viral load over 10,000–30,000 may signal failure of the immune system to control viral replication and may serve as an indication to start treatment.

HIV-Related Illnesses

cytomegalovirus (CMV) infection: A viral infection that affects the eyes, the liver, and other vital organs. CMV infection is an AIDS-defining condition.

disseminated mycobacterium avium complex/intracellurare (MAC, a.k.a. MAI)): A serious opportunistic infection which causes symptoms including night sweats, fever, cough, fatigue, weight loss, and malabsorption of food and diarrhea.

Kaposi's Sarcoma (KS): A cancer that, prior to the HIV epidemic, occurred only in the elderly and debilitated and that constitutes an AIDS-defining condition. It is virally mediated and is seen primarily in sexually transmitted HIV disease.

pneumocystis *carinii* pneumonia (PCP): A lung infection seen in immunocompromised individuals. It is an AIDS-defining condition found in nearly 80% of all AIDS patients at some time during the course of the disease and is a major cause of death.

progressive multifocal leuckoencephalopathy (PML): An infection of the central nervous system with a slow virus (JC papovavirus) that occurs in immunocompromised individuals, including 2–5% of AIDS patients. It causes headache, weakness, cognitive dysfunction, visual loss, gait disturbance, and limb incoordination as well as brain lesions on CT or MRI scan. It is an AIDS-defining condition that typically occurs in advanced HIV disease.

toxoplasmosis: A parasitic infection that affects the central nervous system in patients with CD4 cell counts less than 200. Toxoplasmosis is an AIDS-defining condition.

vacuolar myelopathy (VM): Spinal cord disease due to HIV infection.

Drugs Used in the Treatment of HIV

antiretroviral medications: Nucleoside reverse transcriptase inhibitors (NRTIs), nonnucleoside reverse transcriptase inhibitors (NNRTIs), and protease inhibitors (PIs). Newly-developed classes of antimicrobial agents that are effective against HIV, typically used in combinations of three or more drugs.

AZT: The first antiretroviral medication available to combat AIDS.

highly active antiretroviral therapy (HAART): Drug treatment that consists of a combination of three or more potent antiretroviral medications.

nucleoside reverse transcriptase inhibitors (NRTI): These medications were the first effective class of antiretroviral drugs to be developed. They act by incorporating themselves into the DNA of the virus, thereby stopping the replication process. Examples include: zidovudine (AZT and others), didanosine (DDI), stavudine (D4T), and others.

nonnucleoside reverse transcriptase inhibitors (NNRTI): These drugs stop HIV production by binding onto and preventing the functioning of a cellular enzyme, reverse transcriptase, essential to the conversion of RNA to DNA. Examples include: nevirapine, efavirenz, and delavirdine mesylate.

protease inhibitors (PI): These drugs act at the last stage of the virus reproduction cycle. They prevent HIV from being successfully assembled and released from the CD4 cell. Examples include: indinavir, ritonavir, nelfinavir, and others.

of psychological aspects of HIV and AIDS. Despite growing numbers of infected women, the majority of people living with HIV and AIDS are men who must cope with a disease still widely perceived to be associated with homosexual sex and to have originated among a highly stigmatized group, gay men. An appreciation of the psychological and cultural realities confronting blacks, Hispanics, and women affected by HIV and AIDS is more important than ever and essential to stemming the epidemic. As was the case for gay men before them, the growing concentration of HIV among these minorities has further stigmatized already marginalized groups. Substance abuse is often accompanied by psychological distress or psychiatric comorbidity and, unless both the substance abuse and the psychological issues are properly addressed, they may thwart adaptation to illness. Lastly, the same psychological variables that led to primary infection through risk-taking behaviors continue to exert their impact by complicating patients' ongoing struggle to live with HIV and the complex decision-making regarding disclosure, sexual activity, and treatment that HIV imposes.

Pathogenesis, Clinical Course, and Staging of Disease

Understanding of HIV-1 pathogenesis advanced significantly in 1995 with David Ho's elucidation of the dynamics of viral replication and clearance (Ho et al., 1995). Prior theories postulated that the virus entered a latent phase following initial infection and lay dormant until reactivation led to development of clinical manifestations of AIDS. Aided by the development of techniques to measure viral load and potent antiviral pharmacologic agents, Ho's group discovered that from the point of initial infection and throughout the entire course of illness the virus is replicating at a rate of over one billion virions (virus particles) per day (Ho, 1996; Piatak et al., 1993). This discovery and its ramifications, including related advances in treatment, have dramatically changed the perception of HIV/AIDS from an untreatable, uniformly fatal disease to a chronic, manageable illness.

HIV illness has a clinical course that can be divided into three phases. The first phase begins with transmission of the virus, which occurs through the exchange of body fluids. The most common routes of transmission are: (1) sexual (with exchange of blood, vaginal secretions, or semen); (2) needle-sharing (when it results in direct inoculation of blood) between injecting drug-users; (3) perinatal transmission from infected mother to child (in the context of direct exchange of blood) during labor and delivery; and (4) occupational exposure, for example from an accidental needle stick. Once transmission has occurred, the virus enters immune-modulating cells such as CD4 T helper lymphocytes and/or the central nervous system. This initial phase of acute or primary infection usually lasts from a few days to 10 weeks (Kahn & Walker, 1998). Only a small minority of patients experience symptoms during this phase. When symptomatic, this phase is termed the "acute seroconversion syndrome" and is characterized by a rash, swollen glands, sore throat, and/or malaise (Kahn & Walker, 1998).

Central nervous system manifestations occur in a small percentage of persons, with effects ranging from focal weakness to headache and photophobia (sensitivity to light) to delirium. Viral replication rates are initially very high, and a viral load at detectable levels is most often present in the blood. Screening tests, namely the HIV-1 ELISA test followed by confirmatory testing with the Western blot test—the tests that are typically used to make the diagnosis of HIV infection—may be negative at this time. These tests measure the patient's antibodies against the virus, and it may take up to 12 weeks before such antibodies are detectable in the blood (Koup et al., 1994).

Recent studies suggest that during acute infection the level of measurable HIV-1 RNA rises to very high levels and then reaches a set point that has prognostic value. The higher the set point and the lower the corresponding CD4 cell count (see Table 8.1), the more rapidly a person progresses to AIDS, thus shortening overall survival (Mellor et al., 1996). Treatment with combinations of potent antiretroviral medication aims to reduce the set point to the lowest possible levels.

The second phase of illness has a highly variable course and begins with the production of antibodies to HIV. This phase is defined based on absolute CD4 cell counts and clinical features, and encompasses HIV seropositive patients with CD4 > 200 who have not developed an AIDS-defining condition. This phase can be further subdivided into a clinically latent period during which the CD4 cell count remains above 500, and a symptomatic period which usually occurs when the CD4 cell count drops to within the 200–500 range.

Depending on the rate of viral replication as well as host factors, untreated patients may remain in this pre-AIDS phase between 2 and 20 years, with an average of 10 years (Saag, 1997). Viral replication persists, however, even in the presence of undetectable levels of plasma viral RNA, throughout this period. Recent research has attempted to identify the tissue compartments involved in HIV-1 replication. While lymphoid tissue is thought to be the largest reservoir of HIV virus, macrophages, infected but quiescent CD4 cells, and the central nervous system are less well-known tissue reservoirs where HIV may "hide out" (Pantaleo, 1993). Earlier hope and enthusiasm about complete eradication of the virus likely underestimated the longevity of potentially active virus in these lesser compartments, which may not be as accessible to known antiretroviral medications.

The fact that the HIV viral pool is now known to be continuously replicating and very large suggests that viral genetic mutations that can confer resistance to known antiretroviral medications will arise in the course of treatment. We now know that past treatment strategies using single agents did not significantly delay progression to AIDS or increase survival because viral resistance to these agents likely developed rapidly. When combinations of more potent antiretroviral medications are used, the virus must develop multiple simultaneous mutations, leading to multidrug-resistant strains in order to evade treatment. The probability of this occurring in the context of a maximally-suppressive drug regimen is

TABLE 8.2. Opportunistic Infections of the Central Nervous System

Diagnosis	May present with neuropsychiatric signs & symptoms	CD4 cell count	Diagnostic studies	Treatment
		Nonviral OIs		
Toxoplasmosis (protozoa)	Mental status change; focal neurological signs and symptoms; headache	< 100	CT/MRI: multiple enhancing lesions	Bactrim prophylaxis; pyrimethamine plus sulfadiazine or clindamycin for acute infections
Cryptococcal meningitis	Mental status change; headache; mania; malaise	< 50	Positive CSF India ink stain; fungal culture; positive CSF Cryptococcal antigen	Fluconazole; amphotericin B
TB meningitis	Mental status change	Any	CSF AFB-positive smears and cultures	Must take into account problems with MDR TB
		Viral OIS		
CMV encephalitis	Mental status change; seizures; focal or diffuse frontal lobe dysfunction	< 50	MRI: periventricular ependymitis; CMV antigen in CSF	Ganciclovir or foscarnet
Herpes simplex HSV-1	May have slow onset	Any	Brain biopsy; MRI & LP sometimes helpful	Acyclovir

Progressive multifocal leukoencephalopathy (Jakob-Creutzfeldt virus)	Slow onset mental status change; motor, sensory, visual disturbance; lethargy	< 100	CT/MRI: multiple hypodense white-matter lesions better defined than with HAD	HAART
Varicella-zoster	Mental status change; headache	Any	MRI: similar to PML or HAD; VZ difficult to culture from CSF	Acyclovir or famciclovir
Neoplasms				
CNS lymphoma	Memory loss; confusion; focal neurological signs and symptoms	< 100	CT/MRI: enhancing lesions; brain biopsy	Whole brain radiation and intrathecal chemotherapy
KS	Rare in CNS			

Adapted from Simpson & Tagliati, 1994; Goodkin, 1998.

sufficiently low that development of resistant strains of virus may be delayed for several years (Mantaner et al., 1998; Gulick, 1998).

Except in rare cases, untreated HIV infection eventually results in progressive immune system impairment that in turn leads to the development of opportunistic infections and malignancies. The nature and severity of opportunistic illnesses corresponds to the level of immunosuppression as indicated by CD4 cell count. Oral thrush is often the first sign that a person's CD4 cell count has fallen below 500. Other infections that characteristically occur in persons with CD4 cell counts between 200 and 300 include herpes zoster or "shingles," bacterial pneumonia, herpes simplex, and tuberculosis. KS can also occur during this pre-AIDS but clinically immunocompromised phase. Neuropsychological impairments, such as mild deficits in memory, psychomotor speed, attention, and concentration, which do not necessarily interfere with social or occupational functioning, may also manifest during this phase. In general, clinically relevant impairment increases with degree of immunosuppression (Schmitt et al., 1988; Grant et al., 1987).

The final phase of illness, AIDS, is marked by the development of an AIDS-defining condition or illness (see Table 8.1). In 1985, CDC surveillance criteria for AIDS included the following as AIDS-defining illnesses: PCP, KS, cytomegalovirus (CMV), HIV encephalopathy, cryptosporidiosis, and lymphoma (CDC, 1986, 1987). In 1993, CDC surveillance criteria were expanded to include the following: pulmonary tuberculosis, invasive cervical carcinoma, recurrent bacterial pneumonia, and CD4 cell count less than 200 (CDC, 1993). The most commonly seen opportunistic infections and neurologic complications can be grouped according to level of immunosuppression, as indicated by CD4 cell count. PCP pneumonia, the most common initial AIDS-defining illness, occurs in persons with CD4 cell counts between 100 and 200. Once CD4 cell count falls below 100, the likelihood of developing a serious opportunistic fungal or protozoal infection or an opportunistic malignancy is greatly increased. Progressive multifocal leukoencephaolopathy, cerebral toxoplasmosis, peripheral neuropathy, and cervical carcinoma characteristically occur when CD4 cell counts have fallen to between 50 and 100. In end-stage AIDS with CD4 cell counts below 50, disseminated mycobacrenium avium complex, cytomegalovirus, central nervous system lymphoma, and HIV-associated dementia predominate (Phair & Murphy, 1997; Saag, 1997).

Medical Treatment

In December, 1995, the first protease inhibitor, saquinavir, was made commercially available in the United States. This marked the beginning of a new era in the treatment of HIV and AIDS. For the first time, the incidence of HIV-related morbidity and mortality would begin to fall due primarily to the use of combinations of two or more antiretroviral drugs (Palella et al., 1998). Over the ensuing few years, multiple clinical trials have demonstrated the superiority of combinations of three or more antiretroviral agents over combinations of one or two agents (Mantaner et al., 1998; Pialoux et al., 1998; Havlir et al., 1998; Reijers et al., 1998). The combination of three or more highly potent antiretroviral medications is commonly referred to as HAART. In general, HAART has outperformed dual therapy with respect to rise in CD4 cell count, reduction in viral load, progression of disease, and survival (Mantaner et al., 1998). As the number of available antiretroviral medications has increased, so has the complexity of possible medication combinations. Providers and patients are often faced with multiple questions about choice of treatment for which no clear answers exist. When and with which combination of medications should treatment be initiated (Walker & Basgoz, 1998; Cooper & Emery, 1998)? How is treatment failure defined? If failure occurs, which HAART regimen should be substituted? Since viral resistance to one drug may confer resistance to other drugs in the same class, is it better to save protease inhibitors until they are really needed? What is the place of resistance testing in choosing HAART regimens (Flexner, 2000; Hirsch et al., 2000; Boden et al., 1999; Pomerantz, 1999; Hirsch et al., 1998)? Patients often feel bewildered by the uncertainty and the range of choices available and may respond in one of several ways: Some may refuse any treatment at all; others may resist information about medications and their side effects, while asking their physician, a friend, or a family member to make important decisions. Other patients may request, or seek out themselves, vast amounts of information in an effort to reduce their uncertainty. These patients may also find fault with a physician who cannot provide them with needed reassurance and may consult with multiple physicians (Table 8.3).

In the late 1990s, mainstream clinicians in the field generally advocated early, aggressive treatment with HAART in anyone who was symptomatic, immunocompromised, and/or had detectable levels of virus (Ho, 1995; Munsiff, 1999). Several years of experience with treatment and a growing awareness of treatment-associated serious metabolic disturbances and seriously disfiguring side effects have resulted in a shift toward a more conservative approach (Lichtenstein et al., 2001). Many clinicians are now more likely to consider withholding treatment in treatment-naive patients with a more favorable viral load and CD4 cell count (Phillips et al., 2001; Hogg et al., 2001; Pomerantz, 2001). Nevertheless, despite continued controversy about optimal timing of treatment initiation, certain principles still apply. Viral load elevation, CD4 cell reduction, the presence of HIV-related symptoms and an assessment of ability to adhere to medication regimens continue to be the most important parameters used to determine when treatment should optimally begin.

Further adding to the growing complexity of treatment issues, clinical investigators have very recently begun examining the potential benefit of repeated, planned cycles of stopping and restarting HAART. This strategy, termed "structured treatment interruptions" or STI, is presently experimental and not part of standard practice (Lori & Lisziewicz, 2001).

There are presently 18 antiretroviral drugs approved for use against HIV in

TABLE 8.3. HIV Medications

Nucleoside Reverse Transcriptase Inhibitors			
Generic name	Brand name/abbreviation	Central & peripheral nervous system side effects	CNS penetration
Zidovudine	Retrovir/AZT	Anorexia, mania, peripheral neuropathy apathy & fatigue	+4 (43, 28)
Lamivudine	Epivir / 3TC (available in combination with AZT as single tablet, Combivir)	Peripheral neuropathy	+2 (43)
Stavudine	Zerit / d4T	Peripheral neuropathy	+3 (43)
Zalcitabine	Hivid / ddC	Peripheral neuropathy	+1
Didanosine	Videx / ddI	Peripheral neuropathy	+1
Abacavir	Ziagen / ABC (also available in combination with AZT and 3TC as a single tablet, Trizivir)		+4 (44)
Defovir	Preveon / ADV (technically a nucleotide RT inhibitor)	Usefulness limited by renal toxicity	
Tenofovir	Viread (technically a nucleotide RT inhiibitor)	Headache	

Nonnucleoside Reverse Transcriptase Inhibitors			
Generic name	Brand name/abbreviation	CNS side effects / CNS penetration	Drug interactions
Delavirdine	Rescriptor / DLV	/ +1	
Nevirapine	Viramune / NVP	/ +3	May decrease levels of methadone and anti-convulsants by induction of cytP450 hepatic enzymes
Efavirenz	Sustiva / EFV	/ +1 Insomnia, vivid intense dreams, severe anxiety, and mood swings which may subside after 2-4 weeks	avoid triazolam, alprazolam, and midazolam; may decrease levels of methadone

TABLE 8.3. Continued

Protease Inhibitors			
Generic name	Brand name/abbreviation	CNS side effects / CNS pentration	Drug interactions
Indinavir	Crixivan / IDV	/ +3	
Saquinavir	Fortovase (soft gel) / FTV Invirase (hard gel) / SQV	/ +1	
Ritonavir	Norvir / RTV	/+1	Potent inhibitor of cytP450; avoid alprazolam, midazolam, triazolam, diazepam,
Combination of Lopinavir and low-dose Ritonavir	Kaletra	/ +1	flurazepam, zolpidem, clozapine, pimozide, bupropion; may decrease methadone levels
Nelfinavir	Viracept / NFV	/ +1	Use midazolam and triazolam with caution
Amprenavir	Aqenerase / AMV	/ +1	Use midazolam and triazolam with caution

Note: St. John's Wort (hypericum perforatum) may reduce levels of protease inhibitors and lead to loss of their efficiency and development of viral resistance.

the United States. In general, each drug interferes with viral replication by blocking the action of a viral enzyme involved in a crucial step in the virus's life cycle (see Tables 8.1 and 8.2 for details). Since the introduction of HAART, the incidence of opportunistic infections (OIs) and KS has fallen significantly. This reduced incidence is reflected in declining HIV-related deaths and hospitalization rates (Carpenter et al., 2000).

Neuropsychiatric Complications of HIV

HIV-related neuropsychiatric disorders occur commonly in persons infected with HIV. These disorders may result from the direct effect of HIV on the central nervous system or secondarily from HIV-related central nervous system OIs or malignancies (Price & Brew, 1997; Perry, 1990). Below, we will discuss the clinical presentation, differential diagnosis, and treatment of the most commonly encountered primary HIV-related disorders: HIV-1-associated dementia (HAD), minor cognitive motor disorder (MCMD), mood disorders, psychotic disorders, and vacuolar myelopathy (VM).

HIV-Associated Dementia (Formerly AIDS Dementia Complex or HIV Encephalopathy) and Minor Cognitive Motor Disorder

HIV-associated dementia (HAD) is one of the most common neuropsychiatric complications seen in persons infected by HIV. Although HAD may present as the first AIDS-defining condition, the incidence increases with disease progression and decline in CD4 cell count to below 200. An estimated 7.5–27% of patients with AIDS will develop clinical evidence of central nervous system involvement with HIV (Dore et al., 1999; Simpson & Tagliati, 1994).

Patients with HAD present cognitive, motor, behavioral, and affective signs and symptoms, though not all four are necessary to make the diagnosis. The most common presenting complaints are mental slowing, memory loss, and difficulty with concentration. A patient may also complain of losing his train of thought in midsentence or no longer being able to execute complicated or multiple tasks simultaneously. If motor impairment is present, the patient may complain of stumbling while walking, motor incoordination, difficulty with fine motor movements, and clumsiness. Simple tasks such as buttoning a shirt or threading a needle may become difficult to perform (Simpson & Tagliati, 1994; Goodkin, 1998).

A general medical work-up should always include neuroimaging studies (CT and MRI), examination of the cerebral spinal fluid, a metabolic work-up, and consideration of psychoactive substance abuse or side effects of HIV-related medications. Formal neuropsychological testing may be helpful in the differential diagnosis between HAD and depression, psychosis, or mania, since HAD may present with predominantly depressive, manic, or psychotic signs and symptoms. It is essential to note that HAD is a diagnosis of exclusion. Many HIV-related opportunistic infections are treatable and must be ruled out before a diagnosis of HAD can responsibly be made (Simpson & Tagliati, 1994; Goodkin, 1998).

In some cases, patients manifest significant cognitive impairment insufficient to be diagnosed as dementia, typically accompanied by soft neurologic signs; this is termed Minor Cognitive Motor Disorder (MCMD). Like HAD, MCMD is a diagnosis of exclusion.

Mood Disorders and Psychosis Due to Biological Effects of HIV and/or Its Treatments

Depression, hypomania or mania, and/or psychosis may occur either as a direct effect of HIV on the central nervous system or secondarily due to HIV-associated opportunistic infections or malignancies or medications used in the treatment of HIV. Making the clinical distinction between a mood or psychotic disorder due to HIV or HIV-related medical conditions and a "functional" mood or psychotic disorder may not always be possible. Positive neurological findings, such as abnormal reflexes, slowness in rapid successive movements, mild neurocognitive impairment, peripheral neuropathy, or myelopathy (spinal cord damage) suggest HIV CNS involvement.

Vacuolar Myelopathy (VM)

VM is the most common cause of spinal cord disease in AIDS patients. It is thought to be due not to direct effects of HIV infection itself but to indirect metabolic and immune-mediated effects. Clinically, patients with VM present with difficulties in walking and other forms of motor control including, in some cases, urinary problems and/or impotence.

Psychiatric Disorders Associated with HIV but Not Directly Related to Biological Effects

Psychiatric comorbidity among HIV/AIDS patients is quite common and has been studied extensively (Levine, 2001; Treisman, Angelina, & Hutton, 2001). Some studies have found an elevated risk of depression, psychoactive substance use disorders, and suicide among HIV-positive individuals (Bing et al., 2001; Hunt & Treisman, 1999; Edlen et al., 1994; Selwyn & O'Connor, 1992; Marzuk et al., 1988). These findings may, however, reflect an increased risk for psychiatric disorders among persons *at risk* for HIV. For example, one study among predominantly white gay men, regardless of HIV serostatus, found a two-to-seven-times higher rate of non-IV psychoactive substance use disorders, mood disorders, and alcohol dependence and abuse disorders compared to heterosexual HIV-negative controls (Atkinson et al., 1988). Other studies have consistently found an increased risk of psychiatric disorders among intravenous drug abusers (IVDAs), with or without concomitant HIV. One study of suicidality among HIV-positive patients on a general medical inpatient service yielded some remarkable results. The further advanced patients, that is, those with AIDS were significantly *less* suicidal than symptomatic HIV-positive patients without an AIDS diagnosis. AIDS patients were comparable in suicidality to HIV-negative and HIV-unknown patients (McKegney & O'Dowd, 1992). Nevertheless, suicide remains a significant problem among HIV-positive individuals with rates of completed suicides ranging from 16–36 times that of age-matched controls (Rundell et al., 1992; Marzuk, 1988; Beckett, 1998). (See Table 8.4 for specific psychiatric disorders co-occurring with HIV.)

Psychological Issues

The introduction of HAART in 1995 and associated improved prognosis has been a mixed blessing for both patients already infected with HIV and those at risk for infection. While the benefits of better treatments are undeniable, the complexity of psychosocial issues with regard to HIV prevention, treatment, and adjustment to illness has increased with patients' new longevity. Additionally,

TABLE 8.4. Specific Psychiatric Disorders Co-occurring with HIV

Disorder	Clinical presentation	Differential diagnosis	Medications producing signs & symptoms similar to disorder	Treatment
DEPRESSION	Most common psychiatric disorder encountered in clinical settings serving HIV-positive population. Presentation and diagnosis complicated by overlapping signs and symptoms in depression and HIV disease. Therefore, rely on nonsomatic signs and symptoms: dysphoric/depressed mood; guilt or sense of worthlessness; lack of interest; anhedonia; helplessness; hopelessness; suicidal ideation. NOTE: Suicidal ideation may be used as an adaptive strategy enabling patients to feel more in control of an otherwise overwhelming situation. (82, 83)	Psychoactive substance use disorders may be associated with depressed mood. Always inquire about past and recent losses and associated grief. Hypogonadism is a relatively common and easily correctable cause of depression. Anemia, adrenal insufficiency, and low B-12 levels may be associated with depressed mood. CNS toxoplasmosis, PML, and CNS lymphoma can present with apathy, psychomotor slowing and non-focal neurological findings that can be indistinguishable from depression. HAD may present with depressed mood. (84)	Interferon Bactrim Corticosteroids Efavirenz AZT	Cognitive-behavioral therapy, interpersonal therapy, and several antidepressant medications have demonstrated efficacy in clinical trials. Most available antidepressant medications available are safe for use in this population. Subclinical brain disease may increase sensitivity to adverse effects. Therefore, "start low and go slow." Watch for interactions with RTV. Psychostimulants useful in patients with low energy and cognitive impairment 2N to HIV. May want to take advantage of Prozac's long half-life in poorly compliant patients. Sexual dysfunction associated with all SSRI's may limit compliance. (85–92)

MANIA	As many as 8% of AIDS patients may develop mania at some point. Mania increases in incidence with progression of disease. Many times mania occurring in patients with advanced disease will be accompanied by motor and cognitive impairment. Mania may or may not be accompanied by psychosis. Clinical presentation and diagnosis of hypomania and mania are similar to seronegative patients. (63)	Psychoactive substance use disorders may be associated with mania. HAD may present with mania. Any of the commonly occurring OIs affecting the CNS may present with mania.	Corticosteroids Anabolic steroids AZT, DDI Ganciclovir Biaxin Antidepressant medications	If antipsychotic medication is used acutely, "start low and go slow," to avoid EPS, NMS, since this population is more sensitive. Atypical antipsychotic medications offer advantage of fewer side effects. Lithium and valproate are used though watch for neurotoxicity with lithium. (93, 94)
ANXIETY	Anxiety is frequently encountered in this population. Adjustment disorder with anxious mood is frequently seen, though patients at risk for HIV may also be at risk for PTSD as well as panic disorder.	Maintain high index of suspicion for intoxication and/or withdrawal from alcohol, benzodiazepines, cocaine and crack cocaine, opiates, amphetamines, GHB, ketamine, and Ecstasy.	Interferon Interleukin-2 AZT, EFV, D4T, Corticosteroids, Anabolic steroids, Antihypertensive medications, and Bronchodilators	Short-term cognitive-behavioral psychotherapy with or without anxiolytic medications. Longer acting benzodiazepines have lower abuse potential and withdrawal is less of a problem. (89, 95)

Adapted from Beckett, 1998; McDaniel, 1998.

patients' psychological experience differs widely depending on their risk category, ethnic/racial group, and geographic region. A patient's subjective experience is largely determined by his or her phase of illness and the treatment he or she is receiving. Therefore, this section is organized according to stages of disease and associated treatment considerations.

Seroconversion and HIV Antibody Testing

The benefits of HIV antibody testing for people at risk are more compelling than ever before due to the recent introduction of effective combination antiretroviral therapies. Prior to 1995, there was only controvertible evidence that treatment delayed progression of disease. For some individuals, the anguish associated with learning of their HIV-positive status outweighed the benefits. Today, not only are effective treatments available, but very early treatment appears to prevent or at least delay irretrievable loss of essential components of the immune system and may aid immune restitution (Walker & Basgoz, 1998). Despite these improved conditions, several obstacles to testing remain. In increasing numbers of states, physicians and laboratories are legally required to report by name all individuals who test HIV-positive or who come for treatment of HIV disease or HIV-related conditions. In addition, some states' statutes provide for partner notification through local health departments. While there are compelling public health and epidemiologic reasons for enacting these measures, such measures may also deter individuals from receiving both HIV testing and subsequent medical care. HIV and AIDS no longer arouse the degree of fear and loathing they once did, but the associated stigma is still significant. Fear of ostracism by community and/or family, concerns about discrimination in employment and housing and, particularly among younger individuals, the real and poignant fear of never being able to find an understanding partner may also impede testing. Unfortunately, the groups at greatest risk for HIV—poor black women and young black and Hispanic men—are also those least likely to have access to adequate medical care or even information about available medical resources and prevention programs.

Once someone overcomes the obstacles to testing, the testing situation itself provides a rich opportunity to lay the groundwork for future adjustment to a positive test result and to learn to access adequate medical care. The importance of competent pre- and post-test counseling cannot be overemphasized. Earlier studies have demonstrated the benefit of post-test counseling, evidenced in the reduction of suicidal ideation among patients testing HIV-positive to levels comparable to people testing HIV-negative (Perry et al., 1990; Perry, Jacobsberg & Fishman, 1990). Counseling also exposes those who test HIV-negative to educational messages that may help reduce future at-risk behavior.

A person's emotional reaction to hearing he is infected with HIV is highly individual and is determined by a broad range of variables. Most people go through the expectable stages of mourning: shock and denial followed by anger, guilt, depression, anxiety, sadness, and finally acceptance. Others remain fixed in a maladaptive pattern of behavior and feeling. When one's emotional reaction interferes with social, personal, or occupational functioning and/or is associated with prolonged depression, anxiety, or suicidal ideation, a psychiatric consultation may be indicated.

Often, a person's emotional reaction is not expressed verbally but rather is enacted in the form of maladaptive or self-destructive behavior. For example, denial may be expressed by missed medical appointments, poor adherence to medication, and failure to follow up with appointments and paperwork necessary to obtain government HIV-related benefits. Likewise, anger may be expressed through self-destructive behavior, exposing others to risk of infection, or overt hostility toward care providers and concerned family and friends. Increased psychoactive substance abuse is also not uncommon. Guilt may be expressed through self-neglect, depressed mood with loss of self-regard, and feelings of being burdensome to medical providers, family, and friends.

The timing with which a caretaker addresses these potentially maladaptive behaviors is key. For instance, premature confrontation with unsolicited questions about circumstances surrounding transmission may be experienced as critical and judgmental and serve to exacerbate underlying guilt, rage, or depression. However, in time, a patient may benefit from questions about why he may have knowingly put himself at risk. Understanding the reasons behind at-risk behavior may not only help reduce future risky behavior but also facilitate acceptance of HIV by alleviating guilt and shame. Awareness of the fears of both loss of control and dependency that often underlie maladaptive reactions to HIV-positive status can help patients to assume some responsibility for their medical care and to make active life adjustments in the context of their illness. The newly-diagnosed patient must also be given adequate time and space to make decisions about disclosure to friends, family, and/or partners and about his or her medical care. These decisions are usually not urgent, except of course in the setting of acute medical problems or when the patient is knowingly putting others at risk. In nonurgent situations, a patient's anxiety may be greatly alleviated by knowing that disclosure can wait until he has weighed all the pros and cons and is comfortable with the decision reached. Similarly, in choosing a medical provider there is much to consider. Some studies have demonstrated the advantage to patients of seeing a physician with HIV expertise (Kitahata et al., 1986). Often other seropositive patients constitute the primary resource regarding competent medical care in the community. Local AIDS and HIV social service organizations and support groups may also provide information about medical resources. The importance of a good therapeutic relationship with one's doctor, with open, honest communication and mutual trust, cannot be stressed enough. A good therapeutic relationship can facilitate the process of a patient's working through an initial maladaptive reaction to HIV diagnosis.

Initiating Antiretroviral Medications and/or Prophylactic Medication:
Psychological Impact and Patients' Reactions

The decision to begin treatment with antiretroviral medication is charged with significance. A rising viral load, which often is the basis for starting treatment, may recall the initial trauma of testing positive for HIV. Patients often feel the same shock, shame, guilt, and fears about mortality that accompanied their initial diagnosis. On the other hand, those patients starting treatment soon after being diagnosed are faced with the dual psychological tasks of adjusting to both HIV positivity and the prospect of beginning treatment. Overwhelmed by questions about shortened life span and concern about eventual illness and disability, these patients may not be in a position to responsibly evaluate the various available treatment options and may feel deeply ambivalent about taking an active role in any aspect of their care.

For most patients, starting medications is the first outward sign that one is infected with HIV. Up until this point, nothing in the appearance of the person's life had changed except perhaps making doctor visits once every two to four months. After starting antiretroviral medication, the patient's life will be altered forever. Whatever level of denial had sustained him or her will be deeply shaken. It will no longer be possible so easily to conceal from himself or herself, friends, family, or prospective sexual partners the reality of his or her HIV infection. Some medications require refrigeration; others impose dietary restrictions; most must be taken two or three times daily, some with very exact amounts of time between doses and in relation to meals. It therefore becomes impossible for a person to have more than a few hours free of the burden of having to think about one's illness, as many practical and outwardly noticeable adjustments must be made. Many patients anticipate this burden as intrusive, controlling, and unjust. Younger persons in particular may experience the recommendation to start medications as a "life imprisonment," so marked are their experiences of loss of freedom and sense of unfairness. Difficulties in accepting treatment are particularly prominent among patients whose childhood histories have involved sexual and/or physical abuse or neglect. Past experience has taught such patients not to trust their caretakers. Consequently, doctors are often met with hatred and hostility from such patients, and compliance with medical treatments tends to be poor. Patients must be given the opportunity to express their personal reactions to the prospect of beginning treatment, to face the prospect of diminished autonomy, and to integrate the experience lest they be unable to fully engage in treatment. Instead of adhering to complex regimens, patients may rebel by skipping or missing doses, forgetting, or refusing to take medications at all.

Patients who are obsessional by nature may become preoccupied with concerns such as side effects (particularly lipodystrophy, seen with the protease inhibitors) and issues relating to choice of particular combinations of medications. Many such patients are as well or better informed about specific antiretroviral medications and their side effects as are their care providers. These patients may become paralyzed in their decision-making by the abundance of information about efficacy and side effects and/or exhaust the patience of their medical providers with endless ruminations about treatment options. They may use legitimate concerns about cross-resistance among various medications, disfiguring or disabling side effects, and the risk of developing resistant strains of virus to undermine confidence in treatment.

Patients with a major psychiatric disorder and/or psychoactive substance use disorder may show their first obvious signs of difficulty when starting antiretroviral medications. Anxiety and depression can both interfere with decision-making and deplete energy and concentration necessary for compliance with medication regimens. Psychoactive substance use can cloud judgment and increase impulsivity. Patients with severe persistent mental illness such as schizophrenia or poorly controlled bipolar disorder face particular problems with respect to treatment. Some patients fear taking medications, to which they attribute magical or idiosyncratic properties. Patients with schizophrenic disorders may not have the cognitive flexibility and organization and attentional abilities to master complex dosing schedules along with corresponding dietary limitations. These patients may require supervised medication-taking or other types of assistance. Likewise, patients with HIV-related cognitive impairment cannot be expected to adhere to complex medication schedules without assistance.

Finally, there is a small group of patients who have never taken any antiretroviral medications despite having been infected for many years. These patients resisted monotherapy with AZT and other NRTIs when they constituted standard treatment. At the time, these individuals may have insisted that the drugs used for treatment most often did more harm than good. Their refusal may have been viewed as an angry, defiant response stemming from unresolved conflicts about being infected. Today we know that these patients were in some respects correct. Monotherapy is not only ineffective, but also may lead to the development of resistant strains of virus. These patients went against conventional wisdom once, and they were fortunate not only to have survived but also to have been spared medication toxicity and cross-resistance. Unfortunately, many of these patients presently apply the same reasoning to support refusal to take combination medication and do not start treatment until destruction of their immune system is too advanced for antiretroviral medications to be effective.

Treatment Complications and Progression of Disease: Special Considerations

Side Effects and Toxicity. Whereas antiretroviral medications cause immediate unpleasant side effects, clinical benefit is often delayed. Patients, particularly those with limited future orientation, may experience treatment as more harmful than beneficial. It is very important that care providers take the time to explore and empathize with the meaning of particular, distressing side effects and be flexible about changing regimens. For example, a young, gay man may insist upon abandoning a successful therapy because the redistribution of fat from his face and his legs to his abdomen and back (lipodystrophy) due to a protease inhibitor is making him feel physically unattractive and creating stress in a new relationship. Sudden and frequent diarrhea may limit his ability to date or be involved in spontaneous activities with friends. The patient's experience of having his complaints taken seriously can cement a sense of mutual respect between him and his provider that will serve them well at future treatment junctures.

Antiretroviral Treatment Failure and Viral Resistance. Failure of antiretroviral medications due to development of viral resistance always requires a change of medications. In contrast to the days before HAART, when changing therapy was often preceded by a distressing clinical event, change now more often is recommended on the basis of changes in lab values that are imperceptible to patients. Patients who do not have confidence in technologically based Western medicine may question the wisdom of changing treatment when they are feeling well. Usually, however, patients will accept a treatment strategy if they feel their values and input regarding choice of strategies are respected.

Treatment failure should always raise questions about a patient's adherence to his medication regimen. Resistance to medication can develop rapidly, with some studies demonstrating that only several days of missed doses of a protease inhibitor is sufficient. Maintaining a high index of suspicion for substance use, particularly in patients with a known prior history, and assessing for presence of depression, anxiety, and cognitive impairment should be routine with every patient failing antiretroviral medications.

There is a group of patients who have never responded fully to combination antiretroviral medications because of viral resistance. Often, these patients developed resistance prior to 1995 when sequential monotherapy was standard treatment. These patients understandably experience a sense of "missing the train," anger and resentment. Such feelings are intensified by the recent optimistic media coverage of AIDS and HIV treatments, and the resultant conclusion drawn by the general public that HIV disease and AIDS are now treatable. Yet, several social and medical realities suggest a more cautious attitude. There is public health concern about a "second wave" of the epidemic generated by transmission of multidrug-resistant strains of virus.

Opportunistic Infection (OI) and Malignancies. The development of an initial AIDS-defining OI or malignancy can be psychologically devastating for many HIV-infected patients. Before the availability of HAART, patients and providers often felt helpless as the immune system gradually lost its ability to protect against opportunistic diseases. Prophylactic medications were effective up to a point, but they would eventually fail. The anxiety associated with the anticipation of inevitable progression could be unbearable, and many patients experienced, paradoxically, a sense of both relief and profound loss with the onset of AIDS-related illness. The distinction between being HIV-positive and having AIDS was more significant then than it is now, since there was no hope then for patients with AIDS of returning to a more immunocompetent state. That suicidal ideation was more common in patients with ARC (patients with symptoms but not yet AIDS), than with AIDS is testament to the power of the anxiety and fear of the unknown associated with this pre-AIDS condition (McKegney & O'Dowd, 1992). More recently, the clinical context of opportunistic diseases has changed dramatically. Some investigators now believe that both complete eradication of virus and full immune reconstitution are within reach. Additionally, the incidence of infection with PCP and CMV has fallen significantly. Care providers now consider opportunistic diseases preventable and view their occurrence as a failure of HAART rather than a point of no return for the immune system. It is not uncommon now for treatment with HAART to raise CD4 cell levels from below 50 to over 200 and to suppress viral loads to below limits of detection. Many patients have come to expect a return to normal immune functioning, even though it is not known how completely the immune system can regain lost effectiveness.

The "Lazarus Syndrome"

There is a group of patients who developed AIDS before the introduction of HAART. Many had already grieved the loss of their health and physical well-being as well as their ability to work and enjoy leisure time pursuits and had come to terms with their disabled status and eventual premature death. Treatment with combination medications can reverse these losses in some cases. Improvement for some patients has been so dramatic that they have felt as if resurrected from the dead, hence the name "Lazarus Syndrome" (France, 1998). Although most have welcomed the improvement in health and quality of life, many view the change with ambivalence. Hand-in-hand with the hope of living a longer, healthier life come new anxieties about the future. Many resent the pressure placed on them to give up their role as disabled, which had been so painfully acquired. Once having accepted early death as unavoidable, to hope again is frightening and carries the risk of having to face treatment failure and death all over again. Those who had developed AIDS at a time in their lives when they faced very difficult developmental tasks such as establishing financial self-sufficiency and career goals, forming long-term attachments, and separating from families of origin may feel particularly threatened or challenged by having to assume active responsibility for shaping their future. AIDS, in one sense, may have provided a substitute role and identity and relieved them of the responsibility of coping with crucial developmental tasks.

Some patients experience practical dilemmas such as the threat of losing government benefits, entitlements, and social services as their health improves. Many require psychological and/or pharmacologic treatment for anxiety associated with the conflicts posed by returning to work. One patient chose to forego treatment with antiretroviral medications rather than risk the possible loss of financial and social benefits accorded to him by virtue of his illness. For those whose lives had been marked by social, economic, and emotional impoverishment, AIDS provided access not only to important material resources but also to emotional ones. AIDS provided the opportunity for connectedness with caring medical professionals; such relationships have been, for many patients, closer and more supportive than any in their lives before. These are the patients who have had the most to lose from the new combination therapies. Tragically, they are also the ones most likely to be newly infected with HIV.

Facing Death

Although, thanks to the new combination treatments, the number of deaths from AIDS annually in the United States has dropped, people with AIDS continue to face death with the same set of concerns that people with AIDS always have. Although the average age at death is older now, AIDS still affects the relatively young. Many may need to face not only death but also the loss of the opportunity to fulfill their life goals. Some may never accept the reality of their illness and die without ever resolving important developmental and interpersonal issues. Grieving may be more complicated for such patients and for their family and friends. To work through their sense of being cheated out of success with new treatments, these patients need help in clarifying the meaning of their illness and treatment failure and in bearing their sense of loss. Many patients have experienced rejection by family and friends because of lifestyle choices. In such cases, the patient-doctor relationship may become the most positive and meaningful relationship in the patient's life. Conversely, care providers may invest more of themselves with these patients and thus require the opportunity to grieve their deaths (Kagawa-Singer & Blackhall, 2001).

Race/Ethnicity, Gender, Mode of Transmission

A discussion of the psychosocial aspects of HIV disease would be incomplete without acknowledging the impact that race, ethnicity, sex, and transmission categories have on a patient's psychological response. The disproportionate rise in infection rates within the Black and Latino communities poses serious questions about cultural barriers to primary prevention (Shain et al., 1999). Furthermore, the higher incidence in these communities underscores the importance of understanding the cultural influences on ways of coping with this illness. Family and church, for example, by serving as major sources of emotional and financial support to many Blacks and Latinos, may favorably or negatively influence a patient's emotional reaction to infection. The condemnation of homosexuality on the part of some churches as sinful and as a "lifestyle choice" that perhaps can be "cured" by prayer, may painfully alienate many followers, intensifying their sense of guilt and shame. Similarly, in Latino families, close family ties come with a cost. Acknowledgment of one's homosexuality may be perceived as a betrayal or rejection of the family. Because family closeness may mean open sharing of personal information among family members, disclosure of one's sexual orientation to one family member may amount to disclosure to everyone (Carballo-Dieguez, 1989). Many Blacks and Latinos are unwilling to risk open expression of their sexuality, disclosure of their HIV status, and/or full participation in their medical treatment for fear of compromising family bonds.

For Black and Latino homosexual men, the consequences of cultural attitudes toward sexuality and gender roles are manifold. The cultural ideal of machismo places a high value on a man's sexual potency and dominance and is less concerned with the sex of his partners (Carballo-Dieguez, 1989). Since infection with HIV is most commonly associated with being penetrated anally, being infected implies having failed to live up to this masculine ideal. A man may feel more comfortable discussing having sex with other men if it is assumed that he is the dominant partner. Discussion about being penetrated may need to wait until a secure therapeutic alliance has been established. The conflict and guilt generated by the opposition of sexual desires and societal norms are often associated with depression, loss of self-esteem, and internalized homophobia. These negative psychological forces all too often interfere with men's willingness to protect themselves and their partners from infection and to seek appropriate HIV testing and treatment.

For Hispanic women, the flip side of machismo promotes submissiveness and undermines a woman's willingness to protect and care for herself. If a woman insists that her partner use a condom or questions him about his sexual behavior or drug history, she risks undermining his dominance and thereby insulting him. Conversely, a woman may feel compelled to demonstrate her love for and faith in her partner by engaging in unprotected sex. If already infected, she may be afraid to disclose her seropositive status lest she risk rejection or even physical violence. Women are also expected to be responsible for childcare, which may impede adherence to medical visits and complex medication regimens. It is not unusual to see an infected woman caring for both her HIV-positive partner and her children while neglecting her own medical needs.

Lastly, patients with a past and/or present history of intravenous drug use too often face prejudice held by the "majority" population, including, most importantly, the medical community. Some medical providers have an aversion to drug users and view active drug use as an absolute contraindication to treatment with HAART. Patients may feel that any contact with medical providers is suffused with mutual pessimism and mistrust. However, the reality is that drug addiction is a chronic relapsing illness, and, for some, sustained abstinence is an unrealistic goal. For patients with a past or current history of drug addiction, comorbid psychiatric conditions should be treated and harm reduction models of treatment offered. Needle exchange programs, though politically controversial, can effectively reduce rates of viral transmission.

Concluding Remarks

The hope of living a productive, satisfying life is now a real one for many infected with HIV. The latter half of the last decade has witnessed remarkable progress in our understanding of this disease. Recent advances in treatment have significantly lengthened the lives of large numbers of people. Despite these promising developments, important challenges remain. There is as yet no vaccine or cure on the near horizon; therefore, our best chance at the eradication of HIV disease lies in primary prevention. That 40,000 people in the U.S. are newly infected each year suggests that awareness of the disease and of its modes of transmission is insufficient. It will be important for us to develop a deeper understanding of the ways in which psychological, social, and cultural factors interact in a patient's life to create his particular illness experience. Such an understanding will not only render our treatments more acceptable and humane, but also should render our efforts at primary prevention more effective.

LYME DISEASE

Sociocultural Issues and Historical Context

Lyme disease is one of the fastest-growing epidemics in the United States at this time, second only to HIV. It is the most common vector-borne disease in the United States (CDC, 2002). First identified in the late 1970s in its namesake town, Lyme, Connecticut, both the geographic distribution and the range of reported symptomatology associated with Lyme disease have been rapidly expanding. Originally thought to consist of a characteristic "erythema migrans" rash followed months to years later by arthritis (Steere, Broderick, & Malawista, 1978), Lyme disease is now known to affect virtually every organ and system in the body. It has been dubbed "the New Great Imitator" (Pachner, 1989), after the original "great imitator," syphilis, because it can mimic such a great variety of medical conditions and syndromes and is therefore easily missed or mistaken for another disease entity. Because Lyme disease was first described in the United States as a rheumatological illness (Steere et al., 1977, 1978), its neurological and neuropsychiatric presentations—those features that will be the main focus of this section—were slow to be identified.

Because of the diagnostic challenges that it poses, Lyme disease has spawned a major controversy within the medical community (Fallon, Kochevar, Gaiton, & Nields, 1998; Steere et al., 1993). Some doctors view it as an illness that is relatively easily diagnosed and treated. Rarely, if ever, is Lyme disease chronic, and characterized by arthritis and a narrow range of specific neurological and cardiac features (Shadick et al., 1994). Other doctors have seen and reported that Lyme disease in its later stages is most prominently a neuropsychiatric illness whose manifestations are protean (Coyle, 1996; Fallon & Nields, 1994).

According to these doctors, late-stage Lyme disease can require long courses of aggressive antibiotic therapy (Burrascano, 1997) and/or can prove, in rare cases, refractory to treatment (Liegner et al., 1997). The basis of this controversy will be discussed further in subsequent sections on pathogenesis, diagnosis, and treatment. Regardless of its basis, however, the controversy puts patients in a very difficult position. Not only are they met with uncertainty as to how to proceed and whom to believe; they are also are caught in the cross-fire between competing medical authorities. Patients can become the targets of displaced hostility, can be dismissed as being anxious, hypochondriacal, and/or somatizing, and often meet with obstacles in obtaining insurance coverage for needed treatment. The uncertainties as to diagnosis and treatment, coupled with the bizarre, unsettling, and fluctuating array of symptoms that patients with late-stage Lyme disease commonly experience, can leave the sufferer with a profound feeling of alienation: from a once-trustworthy body, from the medical establishment, and even from family and friends. Many have said that the experience of being misunderstood and disbelieved was as devastating, in its way, as the ravages of the disease itself (Fallon et al., 1992).

Epidemiology

Lyme disease has been reported throughout the United States and in numerous countries around the world, including Europe, Asia, and Australia. The geographic spread and incidence in the United States have continued to increase. In the year 2000, 17,730 cases were reported in the United States, the highest figure reported in any year to date (CDC, 2002). The reported incidence of the disease nearly doubled in the decade 1991–2000. Those areas most heavily affected include the Northeast (Connecticut, Massachusetts, New Jersey, New York, Pennsylvania, and Rhode Island), the upper Midwest (Minnesota and Wisconsin), and the Pacific coastal region (California, Oregon, and Washington). It affects all age groups, but most commonly children and young adults, that is, those most likely to spend time outdoors. It is transmitted through the bite of a deer tick (species Ixodes *scapularis*) infected with the Lyme spirochete, *Borrelia burgdorferi* (Steere et al., 1978; Burgdorfer et al., 1982). Lyme disease is most prevalent in suburban and semirural communities where the deer population has been encroaching on relatively densely settled communities. Some areas, such as Block Island, Martha's Vineyard, Lyme, and parts of Minnesota, New Jersey, and New York are very highly endemic, with more than one third of deer ticks being infected with *B. burgdorferi*. It is now known that there are different strains of Lyme spirochetes, that such strains may be localized geographically, and that they can cause differing symptom profiles. For instance, in Europe, infection with *B. burgdorferi* has long been known to produce prominent neurologic symptoms and has been described under a variety of names: Bannworth's Syndrome, Garin-Bujadoux Syndrome, and neuroborreliosis (Bannworth, 1941; Garin &

Bujadoux, 1922; Hellerstrom, 1930). In Europe, at least three different strains of Borrelia have been shown to cause Lyme Borreliosis and its pathognomonic erythema migrans rash, but research has shown that both antibiotic sensitivities (Henneberg, Weinicke, & Neuberg, 1999) and later sequelae (Aberer et al., 1999) tend to differ among these strains. The variability in the biology of the spirochete and the symptoms it causes has undoubtedly contributed to the uncertainty and controversy regarding diagnosis and treatment. Standardization of diagnosis based on one strain of spirochete with its characteristic patterns of antigenic expression and symptom production leads to underdiagnosis of disease caused by other strains; and yet any attempt to be fully comprehensive runs the risk of overdiagnosis. As will be discussed below, coinfection with other tickborne pathogens can be a confounding factor adding to symptom variability and affecting treatment response (Krause et al., 1996, Eskow, Raon, & Mordechai, 2001).

Medical Aspects

Diagnosis

Despite recent advances in laboratory testing, there remains at this time no gold standard laboratory test for Lyme disease. All current testing methods are of limited value in that, for each method, false negative and/or false positive test results occur not uncommonly (Magnarelli, 1989; Bakken, Case, Callister, Borden, & Schell, 1992). Therefore it is crucial to bear in mind that Lyme disease remains a clinical diagnosis (Burlington, 1997). Each case must be evaluated individually, and while laboratory testing can be helpful in confirming a clinical diagnosis or suggesting that alternative diagnoses should be considered, laboratory tests should not be used to rule out Lyme disease where there is strong clinical evidence to support it.

Laboratory Testing. Diagnostic testing includes serologic testing (blood tests), synovial (joint) fluid analysis, cerebrospinal fluid analysis, brain imaging, and neuropsychological testing. The most commonly used serological tests are the ELISA and the Western Blot. The ELISA is often used as a screening test, and the Western Blot is then used to confirm the diagnosis and to rule out false positives on the ELISA. This procedure, advocated by the CDC, is intended to be cost effective but fails to address the problem of false negatives on the ELISA. Many physicians advocate use of the Western Blot in the initial evaluation where there is good clinical evidence for Lyme disease. In evaluating Western Blot results, it is most important to request that the laboratory report all positive bands, not just the CDC-specific bands. The CDC criteria were designed and should be used for surveillance, not clinical, purposes. Some patients who are seronegative by all testing methods seroconvert (from negative to positive) during or following antibiotic treatment (Fein, 1996). Both the ELISA and the Western Blot are indirect testing methods, in that they measure antibody response to the spirochete rather than directly detecting the spirochete itself or parts thereof. Occasionally, *B. burgdorferi* can be cultured out of synovial fluid, but in general it is resistant to culturing and exists only in small concentrations in the blood of infected individuals. One commonly used direct testing method is the Polymerase Chain Reaction (PCR), which detects the presence of DNA specific to *B. burgdorferi* (Rosa & Schwan, 1989; Nocton et al., 1994). A positive PCR suggests the presence of infection, but false negatives are very common, and in less than optimal laboratory conditions contamination can lead to false positives as well. Cerebrospinal fluid (CSF) analysis is an important part of the evaluation of central nervous system Lyme disease, but CSF results, like serologies, are variable (Coyle et al., 1995; Logigan et al., 1997).

Clinical Diagnosis and Staging of Disease. The vast array of possible manifestations of Lyme disease poses a challenge to the diagnostician. For research purposes, the CDC and some academic physicians have held to a relatively narrow clinical definition, thus minimizing the risk of making the diagnosis mistakenly. Other physicians, especially those with extensive clinical experience in Lyme-endemic communities, hold to a broader clinical definition and maintain a higher index of suspicion, with the rationale that a missed or delayed diagnosis of Lyme disease can result in significant and avoidable morbidity. Further detailed clinical observation and a definitive laboratory test are needed in order to fully resolve these differences. The following is a state-of-the art description of clinical diagnosis at the present time.

Early Localized Disease. In about 60% of cases, a characteristic "bullseye" rash occurs within days around the site of the tick bite. Known as *erythema migrans*, the typical form of this rash is a round, red lesion with central clearing, and it is pathognomonic for Lyme disease. Laboratory confirmation is not necessary at this point: treatment should be initiated immediately. It should be noted, however, that variations of this typical form occur not uncommonly.

Early Disseminated Disease. Within days or even hours of infection, spirochetes enter the bloodstream. Typically, flulike symptoms develop within a few days. Given that at least one-third of patients with Lyme disease never notice a rash, the first signs of disease may be fatigue, headache, muscle aches, and lowgrade fever (Steere, 1983). If erythema migrans is present, so-called "satellite lesions" can occur via hematogenous spread. Serological testing generally does not show reactivity until four to six weeks following the tick bite, so treatment is often initiated based on the rash alone.

Central nervous system seeding may occur as early as 24–48 h after infection. Early manifestations include stiff neck, headache, and photophobia. Diagnostic certainty may not be possible at this stage in the absence of the pathognomonic rash, as most other symptoms are nonspecific. Patients whose symptoms are dominated by muscle pain and fatigue may be misdiagnosed as having fibromyalgia. A careful history and thorough symptom inventory are essential. Factors such as a known tick bite in an endemic area or sudden onset following a visit to an endemic area would raise the index of suspicion for Lyme disease.

The presence of multiple symptoms of early disseminated Lyme disease would further weigh in favor of the diagnosis. Symptoms of early disseminated disease can include: headache; fatigue; migrating arthralgia and myalgia (joint and muscle aches); lowgrade fever; nausea; dizziness; fasciculations (muscle twitches); conjunctivitis; photosensitivity; odd visual sensations such as increased floaters, flashing lights, or visual distortions; other sensory hyperacuities; cranial nerve palsies; cardiac conduction disturbances leading to palpitations or skipped beats; pericarditis leading to chest pain; and unusually persistent or recurrent sinus infections (Fallon et al., 1992). Central nervous system involvement at this time typically takes the form of meningitis with recurrent severe headaches, stiff neck, and photophobia or encephalitis with disturbances of mood, concentration, memory, and sleep (Fallon & Nields, 1994). Prominent anxiety and/or panic attacks are also common. Symptoms of encephalitis are easily attributed to a functional psychiatric disorder, most often anxiety and/or depression. Patients often seek psychiatric consultation at this time; clinical tip-offs to CNS Lyme disease include concurrent physical symptoms as described above, tick exposure in an endemic area, failure to respond to previously effective psychotropic medication, and an atypical psychiatric presentation (Nields & Fallon, 1998). A spinal tap may be necessary for relative diagnostic certainty. CSF analysis may show signs of inflammation, intrathecal antibody production, and less commonly PCR positivity. Prognosis is good if treatment is initiated at this time, although relapses can occur even after "adequate" treatment. Symptoms of early disseminated disease may remit on their own, without treatment, or subtle symptoms may persist; symptoms of late-stage disease can appear after a period of relative quiescence during which it may have been presumed that the infection had been eradicated.

Late-Stage Disease. Months to years after infection, symptoms of late-stage disease may develop. Nonneurological symptoms include frank arthritis with effusion and synovial thickening, most typically in the large joints such as the knee. Arthritis occurs in about 60% of untreated cases (Steere et al., 1977a). Cardiac involvement can include the earlier-mentioned symptoms as well as cardiomyopathy. Ophthalmologic involvement can lead to photophobia, odd visual sensations such as increased floaters, visual illusions, flashes of light or shadows, and, rarely, unilateral blindness (usually self-limited or reversible with treatment). Other symptoms can include deafness (also usually reversible) or hyperacusis, tinnitus, labarinthine (inner ear) disorders, endocrinopathies (most commonly thyroid or disturbances in the menstrual cycle), gastrointestinal disturbances, and neuropathies. Peripheral neuropathies (involvement of the spinal nerve roots) manifest as focal weakness, numbness, paresthesias (e.g., tingling sensations), pain syndromes, and fasciculations (muscle twitches). Radiculopathies and autonomic neuropathies can occur as well, leading to lancinating pain, localized piloerection ("goose flesh"), sensations of heat and cold, flushing, low blood pressure, fainting spells, fast heart rate, disturbances in sexual functioning, and/or abnormal gastrointestinal motility. Symptoms may fluctuate from hour to hour, day to day, or week to week (Nields & Fallon, 1998).

Late-Stage Disease: Central Nervous System. Late-stage central nervous system involvement consists of an encephalomyelitis (inflammation of the brain and spinal cord) or encephalopathy (brain involvement). At this stage, CSF analysis is less reliable. In up to 43% of cases, CSF antibody studies may be negative (Coyle, 1995). Whereas there may be mild elevations of protein or cells in the CSF, CSF studies may be entirely normal in up to 20% of cases (Fallon et al., 1998). Encephalopathy is the most common presentation of late-stage Lyme disease. Symptoms include cognitive deficits, disturbances in mood, increased irritability, extreme fatigue, and sleep disturbance. Cognitive deficits range from mild to profound, and like other aspects of late-stage Lyme disease, may fluctuate from day to day or week to week. Occasionally, dementia is severe enough that patients are misdiagnosed as having Alzheimer's disease. This differential diagnosis, although encountered only rarely, is crucial to attend to given that even at this stage Lyme disease-induced dementia is often reversible with antibiotic treatment. Usually there are other concomitant neurological abnormalities: a polyradiculopathy (involvement of many nerve roots) and/or peripheral or autonomic neuropathies. Occasionally psychiatric disturbance is the only obvious symptom (Hess et al., 1999; Nields & Fallon, 1998). Concomitant arthritis may or may not occur. Other common manifestations of late-stage neurologic Lyme disease include sensory hyperacuities (to light, sound, taste, smell, light touch and/or vibration), problems with balance, new onset dyslexia, word-finding problems, parapraxias, and spatial disorientation (Fallon et al., 1992). Given the symptom profile of profound fatigue with disturbances in cognition and mood, patients with Lyme encephalopathy may be misdiagnosed as having Chronic Fatigue Syndrome or primary major depression.

Less commonly, late-stage central nervous system involvement consists of encephalomyelitis, an inflammation of the brain and spinal cord. Clinical presentations are diverse and often quite dramatic: spastic paraparesis; hemiparesis; transverse myelitis; cerebellar syndromes; and movement disorders including chorea, tremors, and motor tics. Seizures occur in rare cases. Patients with Lyme encephalopmyelitis may be misdiagnosed as having multiple sclerosis (MS) because, as in MS, symptoms typically wax and wane, and MRI scans may show white matter intensities similar to those seen in MS. Patients with peripheral neurologic involvement may be misdiagnosed as having amyelotropic lateral sclerosis (ALS) or Guillain-Barre syndrome. Each of these disorders is thought to be autoimmune in etiology, and in Lyme disease, too, autoimmune mechanisms are thought to be involved in the disease process, particularly in late-stage disease. The ongoing presence of *B. burgdorferi* may or may not be necessary to the persistence of autoimmune phenomena in Lyme disease, a question that is pivotal in the debate over the duration of antibiotic treatment.

Late-Stage CNS Disease: Aids to Diagnosis. A number of auxiliary forms of testing are helpful in the diagnosis of late-stage CNS Lyme disease. A spinal tap is indicated whenever there is suspicion of CNS involvement, but a negative spinal tap does not rule out CNS infection. Brain MRI scans may reveal white matter hyperintensities or may be normal. Such lesions are reversible with sufficient and prompt antibiotic treatment. SPECT scans can be helpful in the differential between a primary psychiatric disorder and Lyme encephalopathy. Neuropsychological testing is very helpful both for diagnostic purposes and as a means to identify and quantify cognitive deficits. The areas of cognitive functioning most typically affected in Lyme encephalopathy include short-term memory, memory retrieval ("working" memory), verbal fluency, attention/concentration, visuomotor coordination, and visual memory (Fallon et al., 1997). Also common are new-onset dyslexic changes (reversals of letters when writing or words when speaking) and parapraxias (putting the cereal in the refrigerator and the milk in the cupboard; misjudging the position of the countertop edge and dropping a glass or milk carton on the floor). Along with serial SPECT scans, baseline and follow-up neuropsychological testing can be a helpful gauge of treatment response.

Microbiology

Certain idiosyncracies of the microbiology of *B. burgdorferi* form the foundation of much of the mystery and controversy surrounding diagnosis and treatment of Lyme disease at this time. Like other species of Borrelia, the Lyme spirochete exhibits such extensive antigenic variability that the question has been raised as to whether it is realistic to delineate separate species of Borrelia at all (Felsenfeld, 1971). Where doctors differ in their clinical descriptions and designated laboratory characteristics of Lyme disease, they may in fact be observing the effects of different strains of the organism. Recent data have revealed anomalous forms of *B. burgdorferi*; "cystic" forms and "L" forms that are recognized differently by the immune system and may fail to respond to antibiotics that are effective for conventional forms (Preac-Mursic et al., 1996; Brornson & Brornson, 1998). The organism is also thought to evade immune detection by coating itself with host antigens: by entering a host cell and then, while exiting, dragging a portion of the cell's outer membrane and thereby coating itself with an "immunoprotective shield" (Dorward, 1999). Organisms may evade antibiotic treatment by remaining inside host cells (most antibiotics function only extracellularly) and/or poorly-perfused areas such as joint spaces, the anterior chamber of the eye and the brain parenchyma, where they may remain dormant for long periods of time. The capacity for dormancy and the long replication time of *B. burgdorferi* (24–48 h, compared with 30 min, for example, in the case of Streptococcus) lead to the need for prolonged and/or repeated courses of antibiotics: spirochetes, like other bacteria, are susceptible to antibiotics only during replication (Preac-Mursic et al., 1989; Haupl et al., 1993; Hassler, Reidel, Zorn, & Preac-Mursic, 1991; Liegner et al., 1993). Coinfection with other tick-borne pathogens such as Ehrlichia and Babesia may further compound the problems in diagnosis and treatment (Krause et al., 1996). Most recently, *Bartonella henselae*, more commonly known as the agent of cat-scratch disease, has been identified as a tick-borne pathogen (Schlouls, Van De Pol, Rijkand, & Schot, 1999) and yet another cause of coinfection with Lyme disease (Eskow et al., 2001). As each of these organisms, Ehrlichia, Babesia and Bartonella, may be insensitive or only partially sensitive to the antibiotics prescribed for Lyme disease, it is important to screen for them, particularly in cases of Lyme disease that fail to respond fully to prescribed courses of treatment.

Treatment

In early-stage disease, antibiotic treatment promptly initiated leads to full remission of symptoms in the vast majority of cases. Treatment for early-stage disease consists of oral antibiotics. Specific drug choices include: doxycycline or other tetracyclines, penicillin derivatives such as amoxacillin or ampicillin, cephalosporins such as Ceftin, and the macrolide antibiotics clarithromycin and azithromycin (Biaxin and Zithromax). Duration of treatment should be 4 weeks at minimum. Some physicians may recommend longer durations (6 weeks or more) when symptoms or fever persist. Others may recommend only 7–10 days of antibiotics, but the risk of relapse or partial treatment after such courses is significant. Relapses do occur occasionally, even with optimal treatment, for the reasons outlined in the above section on microbiology. Cases involving coinfection with Ehrlichia are optimally treated with doxycycline; Babesia coinfection requires the use of atovaquone (Mepron) taken concomitantly with azithromycin or clarithromycin; Bartonella coinfection is generally treated with a course of ciprofloxacin (Cipro), but may also respond to other antibiotics that are used in the treatment of Lyme disease .

In late-stage disease and in early disseminated disease with neurological involvement the recommended treatment is intravenous antibiotics. The best-studied treatments are the third generation cephalosporins ceftriaxone and cefotaxime (Rocephin and Claforan), and penicillin derivatives. The recommended duration of treatment in uncomplicated cases is 4–6 weeks. Beyond this, there is significant (and often hot-headed) controversy in the medical community regarding duration of treatment (Legislative Hearing, 1999). Some doctors hold that the need for treatment beyond these guidelines is extremely rare, and that when symptoms persist they are best explained by postinfectious, autoimmune causes, psychological factors, or another disease entity entirely. On the other end of the spectrum are doctors who advocate months and even years of aggressive antibiotic treatment, including IV, sometimes augmented by concomitant oral antibiotics in cases of late-stage disease where symptoms persist or recur. Indeed there is evidence that, at least in some cases, active infection can persist even after extensive antibiotic treatment (Liegner et al., 1997) and that prolonged courses of intravenous antibiotics confer clinical benefit in such cases.

An important caveat, especially in late-stage Lyme disease, is that the differential diagnosis often includes an autoimmune disease (e.g., rheumatoid arthritis, lupus, MS, or ALS) for which systemic steroids are indicated as treatment. While steroids may produce initial symptomatic improvement among patients with Lyme disease, those patients who have been treated with steroids generally have a worse prognosis than those who have not. As in tuberculosis, steroids can allow spread of the disease by suppressing the immune system.

Also notable is that, regardless of the stage of disease when treatment is initiated, effective treatment typically begins with a worsening of symptoms which lasts from a few days to a week or so. This phenomenon parallels the Jarisch-Herxheimer Reaction seen in syphilis: a 24–48 h worsening of symptoms due to lysis of spirochetes, release of toxins, and/or an inflammatory response.

Psychiatric Disorders Associated with Lyme Disease: Biologically Mediated

Lyme disease can cause a wide spectrum of psychiatric disorders. Many of these are thought to be biologically mediated because their frequency in Lyme disease is greater than in other disorders also characterized by chronic pain and by waxing and waning symptomatology, and because psychiatric symptoms typically resolve with antibiotic treatment (Fallon et al., 1992; Fallon & Nields, 1994; Nields & Fallon, 1998). A recent, large-scale study found, furthermore, a higher prevalence of Lyme disease seropositivity in psychiatric patients who were not at the time acutely medically ill than in healthy subjects. Numerous case reports attest to the variety of biologically mediated, antibiotic-responsive psychiatric syndromes seen in Lyme disease (Fallon et al., 1993; Fallon & Nields, 1994; Fallon et al., 1995; Pachner, Durayn, & Steere, 1989; Stein, Solvason, Biggart, & Speigal, 1996; Hess et al., 1999). Most commonly, patients develop anxiety symptoms, major depression, and increased irritability (Fallon & Nields, 1994). Whereas in adults Lyme encephalopathy tends to produce cognitive deficits and depression, in children behavioral problems and attentional difficulties are the most common presentations (Belman et al., 1993; Fallon et al., 1998).

It is only in the past decade or so that the range of psychiatric presentations of Lyme disease has been appreciated. The earliest case reports in the United States included a case of anorexia nervosa in a young boy with a history of Lyme arthritis and evidence of ongoing infection in the CSF (Pachner et al., 1989). He was treated with IV antibiotics and his anorexia and compulsive exercising remitted. Other early case reports have included paranoia, thought disorder, auditory hallucinations, visual hallucinations, olfactory hallucinations, obsessions and compulsions, major depression, violent outbursts, panic attacks, mania, personality changes, catatonia, and dementia (Reik, Smith, Khan, & Nelson, 1985; Waniek, Prohovik, & Kaufman, 1994; Coyle, Schutzer, Behan, Krupp, & Dheng, 1992; Fallon et al., 1993; Omasits, Seiger, & Branin, 1990; Kohler, 1990; Roelke, Barnett, Wilder, Smith, Sigmond, & Hacke, 1992; Pfister et al., 1993; Diringer, Halperin, & Dattwyler, 1987; Burrascano, 1993; Pachner et al., 1989). The range of psychiatric disorders caused or mimicked by Lyme disease has continued to expand (Table 8.5), including Posttraumatic Stress Disorder (PTSD) with and without psychotic features, paranoid schizophrenia, schizoaffective disorder, schizophreniform disorder, obsessive compulsive disorder (OCD), Tourette's syndrome, panic attacks, agoraphobia, attention deficit disorder (ADD), oppositional/defiant disorder, mood disorders, and pervasive developmental delay (PDD) (Nields & Fallon, 1998; Hess et al., 1999). Occasionally the psychiatric disorder is the only symptom present, and not uncommonly in patients who present with psychiatric symptoms it is only after a careful symptom inventory has been taken and appropriate laboratory testing obtained that the link to Lyme disease can be made and appropriate treatment initiated (Nields & Fallon, 1998). Below are some illustrative case vignettes.

In addition, there are psychiatric syndromes that can occur as a result of various treatments used in late-stage Lyme disease. Clarthromycin (Biaxin), albeit very rarely, can cause mania and/or psychosis. It can also raise the blood

TABLE 8.5. Psychiatric Disorders Associated with or Mimicked
by Lyme Disease

Depression
Mood swings/atypical bipolar disorder
Mania
Psychosis
Paranoia
Depersonalization/derealization
Personality change
OCD/Tourette's syndrome
Fugue states
PTSD
Schizoaffective disorder
Dementia
Anorexia nervosa
Conversion disorder
ADD
PDD or specific developmental delays

levels of other medications, for instance certain antidepressants and anticonvulsants that patients may be taking concomitantly. Prior to antibiotic treatment, patients may have idiosyncratic reactions to a variety of psychotropic medications. SSRIs can induce panic attacks prior to antibiotic treatment but become well tolerated in the same patient during or after antibiotic treatment.

Psychiatric Disorders Associated with Lyme Disease Not Directly Due to Biological Effects

Anxiety and Depression

Like those with any chronic illness, patients with late-stage Lyme disease are at increased risk for depression. It is not surprising that the severe psychological stress of having a chronic illness and the limitations it imposes should contribute to symptoms of anxiety and depression. It should be reemphasized, however, that the extent of anxiety and depression in late-stage Lyme disease cannot be accounted for on this basis alone, and often what appears to be a psychologically induced depression remains resistant to either psychotropic drugs or therapy but responds to antibiotics.

Functional Disorders

Especially in children, a functional overlay may develop such that the biologically mediated aspects of the presentation are difficult to sort out from the effects of interpersonal dynamics and primary psychological difficulties. Neurological disorders existing on an organic basis are often accompanied by psychogenic elaboration, thus further compounding the difficulties in diagnosis and treatment. Pseudoseizures occur not uncommonly in patients with EEG-demonstrated seizure disorders (Krumholz & Niedemeyer, 1983), and a combination of medical therapies and psychoeducation may be necessary for relief from symptoms. Pseudopsychoses can occur as well, particularly in children for whom the demarcations between internal sensations and external stimuli, fantasy, and reality are as yet relatively fluid. Patients with bona fide movement disorders may voluntarily if unconsciously exaggerate their movements under certain circumstances. For instance, some children appear more symptomatic in the presence of worried and anxious family members than around medical personnel or caretakers who are relatively calm and relaxed.

PTSD, "Kindling" and Past Trauma

Especially in patients with prominent sensory hyperacuities, a PTSD-like symptom-picture may emerge, with increased startle, vivid nightmares, hyperarousal, avoidance, and numbing. There is good evidence for a biological basis for this symptom cluster (Nields, Fallon, & Jastreboff, 1999). What deserves mention here, however, is that the traumatic aspects of the experience of Lyme disease, whether due to sensory hyperacuities, pain syndromes, or the experience of not being believed, tend to reactivate past trauma. The degree of symptomatology often cannot be accounted for on either a biological or a psychological basis alone, and it may be pointless to try to make a definitive distinction between the two.

Effects of Early Life Experience and Character Structure

Patients with rigid character structures may manifest underlying vulnerabilities when challenged with any chronic disease. The fluctuating symptoms, increased irritability, and erratic behavior that late-stage Lyme disease often produces are reminiscent for some patients of an alcoholic parent and may stir up difficult memories and reawaken latent insecurities. Patients with a history of early physical or sexual abuse may become destabilized and/or experience flashbacks in the context of intrusive medical procedures and recurrent severe pain syndromes.

Personality Disorders

As in any illness, aspects of personality have significant impact both on the illness experience for any given patient and on the physicians's attitude toward the patient and can positively or negatively affect both the quality of the patient-physician relationship and the quality of care. Some personality disorders are notoriously difficult for any practitioner to handle, such as Borderline Personality Disorder (BPD). Such difficulties are compounded in Lyme disease because mood destabilization and volatile temper can be jointly caused by both Lyme disease and BPD. Thus diagnostic and therefore treatment issues become complex and difficult. Lyme disease can become the scapegoat for all the patient's (unrelated and/or lifelong) problems, and, conversely, some patients fail to obtain needed treatment because their behavior is so off-putting and confusing.

Those patients with hysterical defenses may overdramatize their symptoms and appear much sicker than they are; patients with obsessional defenses may find the unpredictability of the illness very difficult to bear.

As will be further elaborated below, a comprehensive approach to treatment, often including multiple modalities, is particularly important in patients with late-stage CNS Lyme disease.

Psychological Issues

Much of the psychological experience of Lyme disease patients relates to aspects of it that have been alluded to in the sections above: the lack of consensus in the medical community regarding diagnosis and duration of treatment, the effects of fluctuating symptoms, and the difficulties in sorting out primary from secondary effects of the disease. For many patients, symptoms develop gradually over months or years, and multiple medical consultations may fail to yield a definitive diagnosis. It is not uncommon for patients to have received numerous seemingly unrelated medical and psychiatric diagnoses before finally arriving at the diagnosis of Lyme disease as the cause of most if not all of their symptoms. Many have been diagnosed, for example, with CFS, fibromyalgia, connective tissue diseases (lupus, rheumatoid arthritis, and mixed connective tissue disease), migraine, sinusitis, Sjogren's syndrome, carpal tunnel syndrome, major depression, somatization disorder, and even MS. Especially patients with a tendency toward self-doubt may experience their bizarre symptoms as their own creation, their own fault. Others may find in the illness an explanation for unrelated problems and in the support group community an outlet for a lifetime of feeling angry at and maltreated by those entrusted with their care and well-being. Even with the current state of medical knowledge, many go for years without being diagnosed, an experience that can be devastating in itself and that renders the disease more refractory to eventual treatment. Multiple medical consultations can place a serious financial burden on the patient and his or her family. Once the diagnosis is made, the search does not end for most patients. Doctors differ in their recommendations. Patients who relapse after a standard four-week course of antibiotics may find themselves searching for a new doctor who will extend their treatment. Even in the course of effective treatment, ups and downs from week to week and daily fluctuations in symptoms are the norm for patients with late-stage disease.

Central to the difficulties for most patients in dealing with late-stage Lyme disease is the experience of not being believed. Women in particular tend to be viewed as depressed, anxious, or hysterical. The expression of normal emotional reactions to an illness can cloud some doctors' views of patients: If a woman cries, her physical symptoms may be dismissed as psychogenic in the absence of strong laboratory evidence to the contrary. Because symptoms can fluctuate so dramatically, it is easy for teachers, spouses, parents, and friends to assume that there is a volitional component to patients' claimed difficulties. A child who seems well and able to participate in school activities one day but irritable, headachey, and unable to concentrate the next is likely to be admonished, whereas he may be responding to genuine changes in brain functioning from day to day. Patients with late-stage Lyme disease may look well but in fact be suffering from significant impairments.

Patients with late-stage CNS involvement—those most likely to have psychiatric presentations and come to the attention of mental health professionals—are at the center of the controversy over duration of antibiotic treatment. Such patients often have persistent symptoms leading to significant disability and are likely to receive conflicting medical advice. Many are referred to mental health professionals for anxiety, depression, or presumed hypochondriasis. The potentially bizarre nature of symptoms in late-stage Lyme disease and the tendency of symptoms to fluctuate dramatically from day to day produce a complex and confusing clinical picture. Many patients have reported they thought they were just going crazy, a feeling compounded by the lack of consensus among their doctors.

Treatment Modalities

Antibiotic treatment for Lyme disease has been discussed above. Adjunctive treatments for late-stage Lyme disease include physical therapy, cognitive remediation, psychotherapies, and various adjunctive medications, including anti-inflammatory agents, pain medications, psychotropic medications, drugs that have been found to be of benefit in the treatment of neuropathic pain including anticonvulsants such as depakote, carbamazepine, and gabapentin, and tricyclic antidepressants such as amitriptyline. Many patients have significant sleep disturbance that may be mitigated by low-dose antidepressants (amitriptyline, imipramine, nortriptyline, doxepin, or trazedone) and/or anxiolytics. Sleep disturbances and psychiatric symptoms should be treated, as the persistence of such difficulties can impede recovery.

Physical therapy can be essential to full recovery. Pain, muscle stiffness, and disuse can produce a downward spiral of disability that will not automatically reverse itself with adequate antibiotic treatment. Active, carefully graded physical therapy with a trained professional or through an informed, self-designed program can produce significant physical and psychological benefits. Some people are helped by yoga, biofeedback, meditation, massage, acupuncture, and other "alternative" approaches, according to their needs and interests. Cognitive remediation can be helpful following medical treatments in those who have residual cognitive deficits.

Individual psychotherapy, couples therapy, and/or group therapy can be of significant benefit to patients suffering from late-stage Lyme disease. Those patients who have been maltreated by caretakers in the past or who have been victims of abuse may find in the experience of Lyme disease a way to approach those earlier experiences and find healing. The present illness can provide a vehicle for therapeutic exploration into areas that had previously been foreclosed, with which the patient had drawn a fragile and often costly peace accord. While some marriages flounder under the stress of the illness and in the context of the role disruptions it imposes, others find a deeper foundation. It can be very reassuring, especially to those who come from broken homes, to discover that their own marriage is able to weather such difficulties. Couples treatment can be instrumental in insuring that the split in the medical community over diagnosis and treatment of Lyme disease not create a split within the couple. Patients have found significant benefit through patient-run support groups as well as through more traditional group therapy approaches. Support groups confirm that one is not alone, that one's illness experience is valid, and function as important clearinghouses for medical information and referrals. In many communities, support groups and task forces have pioneered educational programs for the schools emphasizing prevention and providing information, have sought legislation in favor of patients' rights, and have raised money for research.

The illness experience for any one individual is complex and unique, shaped by the particular strain of the infecting spirochete, the immune responses of the particular person being infected (HLA typing, etc.), that person's physical and psychiatric vulnerabilities and predispositions, and psychological factors based on his or her life history and present life circumstances. For some patients, one or the other of the above considerations may be particularly important. In late-stage disease and in chronic disease, however, psychological factors inevitably come into play. Previously adequate defensive structures are challenged and social roles must be reworked. For such patients, a multimodal approach to both diagnosis and treatment can be essential to their achieving optimal recovery and making peace with whatever level of functioning they are eventually able to achieve.

CHRONIC FATIGUE SYNDROME

Sociocultural Issues and Historical Context

Chronic Fatigue Syndrome (CFS) is characterized by persistent, or relapsing, disabling fatigue of at least six months' duration that does not resolve with rest, as well as associated neuropsychiatric symptoms and pain. Before the diagnosis of CFS can be made, other clinical conditions that can produce similar symptoms must be systematically ruled out. Similar symptoms have historically been described under other names: neurasthenia or nervous exhaustion, epidemic neuromyasthenia, benign myalgic encephalomyelitis, fibromyalgia, chronic Epstein-Barr infection, and others (Beard, 1869, 1880; Henderson & Shelokov, 1959, Acheson, 1959; Anonymous, 1956; Buchwald et al., 1987; Dorfman, 1987; Straus, 1988; Bell, 1991; Schondorf & Friedman, 1999; Wolfe et al., 1990). The etiology of what we now call CFS is likely heterogeneous, the result of lumping together similar symptoms that arise from a variety of causes into a single diagnostic category (Demitrack & Abbey, 1996). Hence issues of uncertainty regarding diagnosis and treatment are even more prominent than in Lyme disease. Historically, various theories about the etiology of chronic fatigue have been propounded. It has been seen in a sociocultural context as the result of poor adaptation to expected social roles (Abbey & Garfinkel, 1991), as psychogenic—as a variant of depression (Abbey & Garfinkel, 1991) or a response to stress (Sternberg, 1993)—as a constitutional "deficiency of nervous strength" (Beard, 1869) and as the result of an infectious process and/or its aftermath (Wesley & Powell, 1989; Straus et al., 1985; Shelokov, Habel, Verder, & Welsh, 1957; Holmes et al., 1987; Trieb et al., 2000). Abnormalities of cell metabolism (DeMeirleir et al., 2000), immune dysregulation (Visser, Dekloet, & Nagelkern, 2000) and markers of inflammation have been noted in more recent studies. The acronym CFIDS (chronic fatigue immune dysfunction syndrome) has been promulgated in recent years to highlight a popular hypothesis that immune dysregulation from whatever cause is a defining feature of the syndrome (Sternberg, 1993). Outbreaks have been identified that have suggested an infectious process in the initiation of CFS (Poskanzer et al., 1957; Shelokov et al., 1957; Medical Staff of the Royal Free Hospital, 1957; Hill, 1955), but hard data supporting such a link are lacking. Doctors who see and treat CFS have been marginalized in various ways (Johnson, 1996), and it was only in the late 1980s that a working case definition was adopted by the CDC (Holmes, 1988), paving the way for research efforts and legitimization of both patients' complaints and their doctors' observations. This case definition has been revised and expanded over the subsequent years (Demitrack & Abbey, 1996b). Until the various causes of CFS have been identified and distinguished from one another, there will be controversies and polarizations within the medical community, with some doctors emphasizing possible links to infection or immune dysregulation and others the similarities to "functional" disorders such as neurasthenia and psychiatric disorders such as depression.

Epidemiology

The prevalence of CFS is difficult to assess, given changing diagnostic criteria and potential overlap with other syndromes. Early studies estimated it in the range of 3 to 10 per 1000 in a general medical clinic population (Bates et al., 1993) and 4 to 10 per 100,000 in the general population (Gunn et al., 1993). More recent studies have suggested a much higher prevalence. A recent study of the Seattle area estimated a prevalence of 75 to 265 per 100,000 in the general population and another study conducted in San Francisco found a prevalence of "CFS-like disease" of approximately 200 per 100,000 (CDC, 2000). In practice, CFS is recognized increasingly as a "legitimate," albeit mystifying ,diagnosis that is associated with significant morbidity and disability.

Medical Aspects

CFS is currently defined as: (1) clinically evaluated, unexplained, persistent or relapsing fatigue (six or more months' duration) that is of new or definite onset (has not been lifelong), is not the result of ongoing exertion, is not substantially alleviated by rest, and results in substantial reduction in previous levels of occupational, educational, social, or personal activities; and (2) concurrent presence for six or more months of four or more symptoms, including impaired memory or concentration, sore throat, tender cervical or axillary lymph nodes, muscle pain, multijoint pain, new headaches, unrefreshing sleep, and postexertion malaise (CDC, 1994, Revision of Chronic Fatigue Syndrome Definition quoted in Demitrack & Abbey, 1996b). In addition to poor memory and concentration, patients may complain of other subtle neuropsychiatric difficulties such as photophobia, irritability, and depression. Its etiology is unknown, and there is ample evidence that it is a heterogeneous disorder. Psychological, neurological, endocrinological, biopsychosocial, sociocultural, and infectious causes have been postulated. There is evidence to show that at least some cases fit into each of these disparate categories. CFS is included in this chapter in light of an infectious etiology in some cases, but other postulated causes of CFS will also be addressed. It is important to note that CFS is a diagnosis of exclusion, after hypothyroidism, acute mononucleosis, certain neoplasms, and Lyme disease, for example, have been ruled out. Some people have been diagnosed with CFS as part of a "Post-Lyme Syndrome." There is data to show that a portion of such patients in fact still harbor the organism (Coyle, 1994), although the connection between Lyme disease and CFS remains controversial (Treib et al., 2000; Schutzer & Natelson, 1999). For the moment, CFS remains an extremely debilitating disorder for which no definitive treatment exists.

Diagnosis

Given that CFS is a clinical syndrome and not a disease entity with a discrete cause, diagnosis consists in taking an accurate history as well as doing a physical and mental status exam and ruling out by history, physical examination, and laboratory testing other medical diagnoses that can present with similar symptoms. Prominent in the differential are endocrine disorders such as hypothyroidism and adrenal insufficiency, anemia from a variety of causes, autoimmune disorders, psychiatric disorders, Lyme disease and other chronic infections, cardiovascular disease, metabolic disorders, and occult malignancies. Exclusionary clinical diagnoses are: any present medical condition that could explain the chronic fatigue; any such past medical condition about the full remission of which there is reasonable doubt; psychiatric disorders including psychotic major depression; bipolar affective disorder; schizophrenia; delusional disorders; dementias; anorexia nervosa; bulimia nervosa; and alcohol or other substance abuse within two years prior to the onset of the chronic fatigue or at any time thereafter (CDC, 1994, CFS definition revision).

The most commonly reported symptoms associated with CFS (reported in > 75% of subjects) are: fatigue, postexertional severe intensification of fatigue, headaches, myalgia, cognitive problems, sore throat, painful lymph nodes, mild fever/chills, muscle weakness, sleep disturbance, and arthralgias.

It is important to note that nonpsychotic major depression is not an exclusionary clinical diagnosis, as there is significant overlap, both phenomenologically and epidemiologically, between depression and CFS. Many studies have been devoted to distinguishing and/or delineating the relationship between the two (Taerk, Toner, Salit, Garfinkel, & Ozersky, 1987; Wessely & Powell, 1989; Gold et al., 1990; Hickie et al., 1990; Katon, Buchwald, Simon, Russo, & Mease, 1991; Wood, Bentall, Gopfert, & Edwards, 1991). Nevertheless, it is important to note that patients with major depression who present with mainly somatic complaints may be clinically almost indistinguishable from those with CFS, including impairments in concentration, headaches, muscle aches, and nonrefreshing sleep, and that this differential is very important to make. Patients with underlying depression as the sole cause of their chronic fatigue have a much better chance of reverting to their normal state with the help of antidepressant medication and/or psychotherapy.

Etiology

Infectious. Although infectious agents have been implicated in the etiology of CFS, definitive data supporting such a link are lacking. Early reports linked the newly identified syndrome to Epstein-Barr infection, suggesting that chronic EBV infection was the cause of a number of "clusters" of CFS in discrete geographical areas (Johnson, 1996). Among these cases, a significant proportion showed elevated EBV titers. Further research, however, showed that elevated EBV titers are not uncommon in the general population, and that antibody levels do not correlate with severity of symptoms. The evidence suggestive of an infectious etiology for CFS consists of the presence of sudden onset of flulike symptoms, often including lymphadenopathy and sore throat or gastrointestinal symptoms in a majority of patients who go on to develop CFS, and the fact that in some instances cases have been clustered among individuals who shared a common workplace or geographic location. There have been studies suggesting a link to enteroviruses (Archard, Bowles, Behan, Bell, & Doyle, 1988; Cunningham, Bowles, Lane, Dubowitz, & Archard, 1990; Gow et al., 1991; Yousef et al., 1988) and to herpes virus-6 (Buchwald et al., 1992; Patnaik, Komaroff, Conley, Ojo-Amaise, & Peter, 1995; Strayer et al., 1994) and to *Borrelia burgdorferi* (Treib et al., 2000). It remains unclear, however, whether the elevated antibody titers to such organisms in some patients relate to active disease, specific autoimmune phenomena, or nonspecific immune activation. There is growing support for the hypothesis that an infectious agent such as EBV, CMV, parvovirus (Leventhal et al., 1991), or even *B. burgdorferi* (Coyle & Krupp, 1990; Dinerman & Steere, 1992) may trigger a cascade of immunomodulatory effects resulting in chronic immune dysregulation and the symptoms of CFS (Komaroff & Fagioli, 1996).

In addition to such "mainstream" speculations and observations, "alternative" theories as to an infectious etiology of CFS abound. Among the most popular are "stealth" virus and systemic yeast infection. As with any hypothesized cause of CFS, such theories may prove true in some cases. A number of books written for the lay person enumerate the CFS-like symptoms that can accompany systemic yeast infection and present symptom checklists and treatment options, including dietary regimens, for those who identify themselves as possible sufferers. A handful of doctors are treating "stealth" virus infections with aggressive courses of antiviral agents.

Immune Dysregulation. Most mainstream theories regarding the etiology of CFS include some immune dysregulation syndrome. Some suggest autoimmune phenomena, and others varying degrees of subtle immunodeficiency (Gupta & Vayuvegula, 1991; Klimas, Saluato, Morgan, & Fletcher, 1990; Lloyd, Wakefield, Broughton, & Dwyer, 1989; Murdoch, 1988). Indeed, the Australian definition of CFS includes among its criteria abnormal cell-mediated immunity as indicated by reduction in absolute count of T8 and/or T4 lymphocyte subsets, and/or cutaneous anergy (The Australian Definition of Chronic Fatigue Syndrome, 1988, as outlined in Demitrak & Abbey, 1996; Lloyd et al., 1989). Conversely, a number of studies have implicated abnormal overactivation of the immune system rather than—or in addition to—immunodeficiency in CFS (Bates et al., 1995; Landlay, Jessop, Lennette, & Levy, 1991; Straus et al., 1985; Sternberg, 1993; Visser et al., 2000). Other studies have found immune activation consistent with the notion that in CFS the body is reacting to a "perceived" pathogen, whether or not such a pathogen actually persists in the body and regardless of what the pathogen may be or has been (Komaroff & Fagioli, 1996). While there is good consensus in the American literature that some form of immune dysregulation is a common feature of CFS, a full understanding of the nature and implications of such dysfunction is yet to come. Recent work on the immunological, neurochemical, neuroendocrine, and behavioral effects of cytokines (so-called "hormones of the immune system") (Kronfol & Remick, 2000; Moss, Mercandetti, & Vojdani, 1999) may in time shed light on the pathophysiology and treatment of CFS. For example, interleukin-1 (IL-1), a cytokine, is produced both in the brain in response to psychological stress and by white blood cells in response to infection; IL-1 in turn produces "somnogenic activity" in the brain (Krueger & Majde, 1994) and, along with other cytokines, results in "sickness behavior," such as increased sleep, decreased appetite, and decreased sexual drive (Kronfol & Remick, 2000). The current burgeoning of research into the many complex linkages between the brain and the immune system should provide clues to the various etiologies of CFS, but specific implications for treatment are as yet unknown.

In the popular literature, various "allergic" etiologies have been postulated. Indeed, mainstream studies, too, have shown that a substantial proportion of CFS patients (up to 64%) have a history of allergies (Straus et al., 1988b) and one recent study suggested a link between CFS and allergy to nickel (Marcussen, Lindh, & Evergard, 1999), but the relationship of CFS to allergies is a subject that has received more attention among naturopaths and in the lay literature than among medical practitioners and researchers. Extensive batteries of tests for various allergies are available, along with recommendations for elimination diets aimed at symptom reduction in patients with undiagnosed food allergies. The term "allergy" is often used loosely, not in the specific medical sense of a documented IgE or IgG-mediated event but rather as an idiopathic adverse reaction. Even more than those with Lyme disease, people with CFS may feel confused by the plethora of remedies touted in the popular press and by well-meaning friends who have experienced a "miraculous" recovery and will swear by their particular methods.

Neurohumeral Dysregulation. One cause of CFS that has been relatively well documented in some patients and for which there appears to be effective treatments is neurally mediated hypotension (NMH) (Rowe & Calkins, 1998). NMH is a dysregulation of the autonomic nervous system. Symptoms of NMH include nausea, hypotension, lightheadedness, diaphoresis (sweating), abdominal discomfort, and blurred vision. Chronically, NMH can lead to significant fatigue. NMH is diagnosable on the basis of a positive "tilt-table test." A positive tilt table test result is characterized by a paradoxical precipitous decrease in blood pressure often accompanied by syncope following prolonged upright posture (the patient is strapped to the "tilt table" which is then tilted to 90 degrees from the horizontal) and is present in 60–90% of CFS patients according to some studies (Bou-Holaigah, Rowe, Han, & Calkins, 1995; Clauw, Radulovic, Katz, Baraniuk, & Barbay, 1995; Rowe, Bou-Holaigah, Han, & Calkins, 1995). Prolonged upright posture, exercise, warm ambient temperature, anxiety, and hot showers can all be triggers for a rise in pulse rate and reactive overcompensation by the parasympathetic nervous system leading to low blood pressure and symptoms of NMH. Recent studies at Johns Hopkins have suggested that, for a subset of patients with CFS who have NMH, medications aimed to counteract NMH may lead to relief from CFS (Bou-Houlaigah et al., 1995; Rowe & Calkins, 1998). It is thought that NMH can occur spontaneously or can manifest following an infectious illness such as Lyme disease in genetically predisposed individuals.

Neuroendocrine. A number of studies have found neuroendocrine dysregulation in patients with CFS (Poteliakhoff, 1981; Demitrack et al., 1991; Bakheit et al., 1992, 1993; Bearn et al., 1995), which in turn may lead to alterations in immune regulation (Visser et al., 2000). One of the most intriguing hypotheses emergent from such studies is of a dysregulation of the hypothalamic-pituitary-adrenal (HPA) axis with consequent hypocortisolemia (Poteliakhoff, 1981; Demitrack et al., 1991; Demitrack, Blair, Chambers, & Wessley, 1993; Cleare, 2001). Demitrack has observed that such dysregulation may contribute to both the abnormalities in mood and cognition and the immune activation characteristic of CFS (Demitrack, 1996). His observations are intriguing in that they link together a number of disparate findings (fatigue, arthralgias, myalgias, depressed mood, cognitive dysfunction, sleep disturbance, immune activation, exacerbation of allergic responses) characteristic of CFS that are also hallmarks of glucocortcoid insufficiency (Baxter & Tyrell, 1981; Demitrack & Greden, 1991; Demitrack, 1996).

Psychiatric. Multiple articles in the medical literature have suggested a link between CFS and depression (Abbey, 1996; Abbey & Garfinkel, 1991; Abbey, 1996;

Kruesi, Dale, & Straus, 1989; Lam, 1991; Manu et al., 1989; Ray, 1991; Taerk et al., 1987). Some suggest that CFS is in fact a variant of depression and that patients are best served by a combination of antidepressant medication and cognitive-behavioral approaches. Irrespective of a causal link in either direction between CFS and depression, studies have suggested that there may be concomitant depression in up to two-thirds of patients with CFS (Taerk et al., 1987; Gold et al., 1990; Kreusi et al., 1989; Hickie et al., 1990a).

Clinical trials of antidepressant medications in patients with CFS have yielded inconsistent results. There is some evidence of two distinct subgroups of CFS patients, one with significant cognitive deficits, relatively sudden onset of illness and little psychiatric comorbidity, and the other with minor if any cognitive deficits, gradual onset of symptoms and a greater incidence of comrobid Axis I psychiatric disorders (DeLuca et al., 1997a, 1997b).

Recent articles continue to raise the question of role adjustment difficulties as a cause of CFS in some cases and recommend cognitive-behavioral treatments with the aim of reducing feelings of helplessness and encouraging the patient to abandon the sick role (Butler, Chandler, Rob, & Wessely, 1991; Sharpe, 1996; Wessely, 1996). The success of such therapies in some cases and not in others is testimony to the heterogeneity of CFS. Even among patients whose CFS is not "cured" by such treatments, significant improvements in mood, level of functioning, and psychological adjustment can result. For other patients, however, such treatments produce little benefit, and the belief of some doctors and of friends and family in a psychogenic or sociocultural etiology of CFS can be devastating. Compounding the misery of being severely debilitated is the feeling in such patients that they are being held somehow to blame for their condition, that it represents a neurotic maladjustment or weakness of character and that, given sufficient willpower, they ought to be able to "snap out of it." Unfortunately, a referral to a psychiatrist is often seen by both doctor and patient as a negative moral judgment. It is therefore extremely important to distinguish clearly between the notion that increasing coping skills can improve clinical status (Ax, Gregg, & Janes, 2001) and the notion of a psychogenic or "functional" etiology for the disorder.

Cognitive deficits in CFS typically include difficulty with concentration and poor short-term memory (Grafman et al., 1993, Grafman, 1995). The presence of such deficits has been interpreted in some cases as secondary to depression, but such deficits can exist in CFS patients independently. Neuropsychological testing can be very helpful in delineating the deficits, making the differential diagnosis between CFS and depression, and providing an objective measure that can be helpful to patient, physician, and family members alike in validating a patient's subjective complaints.

Physical Deconditioning. Some have suggested that CFS can become a chronic and severe condition because of a combination of negative beliefs about the prognosis of the illness and the physical deconditioning that is known to result from extreme inactivity (Riley, O'Brien, McClusky, Bell, & Nicholls, 1990; Straus, 1996).

Medically Oriented Treatment

Treatments for CFS fall, broadly speaking, into two categories, one based on specific suppositions regarding etiology and aimed at addressing the underlying cause, and others based on symptom reduction, irrespective of etiology. Of course, given these parameters, there is significant overlap.

Treatments Related to Specific Etiologies. Some of these treatments have been alluded to in the above sections on etiology.

Infectious. Treatments based on a presumed infectious etiology include antiviral agents, antibiotics, and antifungals such as nystatin for systemic yeast infection. No clear data supporting such agents in general for CFS exist; nevertheless, patients with undiagnosed Lyme disease or those with "post-Lyme syndrome" who continue to harbor *B. burgdorferi* may benefit from antibiotic treatments, and others diagnosed with CFS may indeed harbor indolent viral or other infections for which appropriate antimicrobial treatment could prove effective. For example, some patients with CMV IgG positivity may benefit from treatment with i.v. gancyclovir. By contrast, however, controlled studies of acyclovir and of systemic nystatin for CFS have yielded negative results (Straus et al., 1988a; Dismukes, Wade, Lee, Dockery, & Hain, 1990).

Immune System Overactivation. Occasionally, patients with demonstrated generalized immune activation have been treated empirically with i.v. gamma globulin based on the theory that the body's negative feedback response to excess IgG would help reverse generalized immune activation. This treatment is currently being pioneered in known autoimmune disorders such as Pediatric Autoimmune Neurologic Disorders associated with Streptococcal Infection and Systemic Lupus Erythematosis (SLE). Studies of its value in CFS have yielded some positive short-term results (Lloyd, Hickie, Wakefield, Boughton, & Dwyer, 1990; Peterson et al., 1990), but side effects are common and longer term outcome is as yet unknown (Straus, 1990). One controlled study suggested that steroids may be effective for fibromyalgia in some cases, but another suggested that deterioration rather than improvement occurred more commonly (Clark, Tindall, & Bennett, 1985). Again, the possibility that such conflicting results may reflect the heterogeneity of the disorder rather than ruling out the effectiveness of steroids for a subset of patients with a variant of CFS must be considered.

Systemic Yeast and Food Allergies. Naturopathic practitioners may prescribe a variety of elimination diets and nutritional supplements aimed at changing the intestinal flora, relieving symptoms of food allergies, and improving strength and stamina. While systemic nystatin has been recommended by some doctors and affirmed by some patients as effective treatment for CFS due to systemic yeast infection, a controlled study of treatment of nystatin for CFS failed to show positive results (Dismukes et al., 1990).

Neurally Mediated Hypotension. For patients with CFS-associated neurally mediated hypotension, increased intake of fluids and salt is a cornerstone of treatment, and may in itself yield significant benefit. Florinef, B-blockers, and disopyramide have also been used with some efficacy in these patients (Bou-Holaigah et al., 1995; Rowe & Calkins, 1998).

Psychiatric. Antidepressants and cognitive-behavioral therapies (CBT) are used where underlying depression is suspected. Controlled studies of antidepressants for CFS have produced variable results. Several case reports of fluoxetine for the treatment of CFS have shown "complete remission of symptoms" (Geller, 1989; Finestone & Ober, 1990), but controlled studies have not borne out such dramatically positive results (Vercoulen et al., 1996). Tricyclic antidepressants, most often amitriptyline, have been shown in some studies to yield improvement in pain, sleep and overall functioning. One controlled study showed significant reductions in illness severity and improved functional status in patients treated with the monoamine oxidase inhibitor phenelzine (Natelson et al., 1996). It is important to note that benefit from antidepressant medication does not implicate depression as an etiological factor, as antidepressants have known beneficial effects for sleep and pain disorders unrelated to depression. CBT will be discussed further under "therapies."

Nonspecific Treatments. Early studies targeting fatigue, depressive symptoms, and cognitive difficulties using antidepressants (sertraline and bupropion) suggested mild benefit across all these symptom categories. Subsequent studies have not consistently borne out a role for antidepressants in the treatment of CFS per se, although, as noted above, some antidepressants are very effective for the treatment of neuropathic pain and for some sleep disorders. Stimulants have also been tried with mixed results.

Muscle relaxants, including cyclobenzaprine (Flexoril) and the three agents carisprodol (Soma), acetaminophen, and caffeine in fixed proportions (Somadril) have each been associated with subjective improvement in pain, sleep quality, fatigue, and general well-being in controlled studies (Bennett et al., 1988; Quimby, Gratwok, Whitney, & Block, 1988; Vaeroy, Abrahamson, Forre, & Kass, 1989). One placebo-controlled study of CFS following viral infection showed significant improvement in patients treated with high doses of essential fatty acids (Behan, Behan, & Horrobin, 1990).

Amantadine, shown in controlled studies to be of help in alleviating fatigue associated with multiple sclerosis (Murray, 1985; Canadian MS Research

Group, 1987; Cohen & Fisher, 1989), has resulted in a diminution of fatigue in some patients with CFS as well.

A number of "alternative" remedies and nutritional supplements have been advocated by a subgroup of physicians, naturopaths, and patient groups. Such treatments include: CoQ10 (synthesized by the body except in deconditioned states; used experimentally in patients with heart failure) to restore energy and proper metabolic functioning, ginkgo bilboa for cognitive difficulties, and s-adenosyl methionine (SAMe, pronounced "Sammy") for pain, fatigue, sleep problems, and depression (Brown, Bottiglier, & Colman, 1999).

Of these treatments, SAMe appears the most promising. It has been used successfully for depression in Europe for a number of years, and is the most commonly prescribed anti-inflammatory agent in Germany. There are extensive studies, mainly in the European medical literature, demonstrating its efficacy as an antidepressant, as an analgesic, and as an anti-inflammatory agent. It has the advantage of having no known side effects to date. Ginkgo bilboa is thought to function by increasing blood flow to the brain. Mainstream medical research suggests that benefit from CoQ10 is likely limited to deficiency states such as Kearn-Sayre syndrome (KSS), mitochondrial myopathy, encephalopathy, lactic acidosis, strokelike episodes (MELAS) and other mitochondrial encephalomyopathies (Abe et al., 1991.; Goda et al., 1987; Ogashara, Engel, Frens, & Mack, 1986). It deserves mention, however, that mitochondrial myopathies can be difficult to diagnose or recognize and that associated symptoms are very similar to those of CFS. Patients who demonstrate "miraculous" responses to CoQ10 may have undiagnosed metabolic myopathies (Engleberg, 1996).

Biological Effects on the Central Nervous System

While CFS is defined primarily in terms of fatigue, many patients experience changes in mood and cognition. The etiology of such changes is unknown, but at least in some cases there is evidence suggestive of an encephalopathic process. It is not uncommon to see SPECT scan patterns (diffuse decreased uptake/patchy hypoperfusion) in CFS patients that are similar to those typical of Lyme disease, vasculitis, and chronic cocaine abuse. One study showed two distinct groups of patients, one with relatively severe cognitive deficits and the other without cognitive deficits; the former group with little psychiatric comorbidity and the latter group with a significant incidence of Axis I psychiatric disorders. This study suggests that, at least in some patients, CFS-associated cognitive difficulties are not simply a by-product of depression (DeLuca et al., 1997b).

Psychiatric Disorders Associated with CFS

The psychiatric disorders most commonly associated with CFS are anxiety and depression. Additionally, the question of various somatoform disorders often comes up, as with any disease with scant objective findings, no definitive test, "nonspecific symptoms," and uncertain etiology.

Psychological Issues

One of the most difficult features of CFS for patients is the fact of having significant disability in the context of "nonspecific" symptoms and an absence of clearly demonstrable physical signs and laboratory abnormalities. The fact that the disability imposed by CFS cannot be externally validated has far-reaching effects on the patient's relationships with friends and family, the physician-patient relationship, and the patient's sense of self. For many, there is a constant, nagging question regarding to what extent the illness is "real" versus "all in one's head." For healthy people, too, energy levels may fluctuate based on life circumstances and mood; for those with CFS, these normal fluctuations take on exaggerated significance. If one can feel a little more energetic in the context of low-stress situations or following a fulfilling or successful life event, does that mean that the nagging fatigue at other times is "all in one's head?" Conversely, if one feels depleted after failing at something or when a loved one departs, is this a sign that the underlying illness is getting worse, and that one should withdraw from work endeavors and social activities?

The significant disability without clearly defined medical cause can lead to stigma in the workplace, although this has been lessening in recent years as CFS has increasingly been recognized as a "legitimate" disorder and as more people have friends, family members, and/or colleagues with CFS. Still, in the absence of a dramatic presentation and clear prognosis around which friends and family can rally, many CFS patients experience a lack of psychosocial support and understanding. This is an illness that is, by its nature, private and isolating. No one else is privy to the levels of fatigue and/or pain to which the sufferer is subject. There are no gross outward physical manifestations and no laboratory values by which an outside observer can assess the severity of one's condition. There is no moment of definitive diagnosis. CFS is an illness that creeps up on one: unlike cancer or HIV infection, there is no single moment at which patients come to know that they have a disorder that will change their life. This awareness dawns only slowly, when the passage of months and then years makes the chronicity of the disorder apparent. Until then, the expectation of physician, patient, and family is that the condition will remit in due course, like most viral syndromes, colds, and flu. The patient is left to explain himself or herself to an often disbelieving medical establishment. Loved ones who have reason not to want their cherished and needed friend or family member to be sick may minimize his or her condition, wishing or assuming that it can be overcome given the right psychological orientation. Additionally, chronic fatigue leads to social isolation simply by virtue of decreased participation in social and occupational activities.

It is difficult to cope courageously, let alone heroically, with an indolent disease characterized substantially by fatigue, malaise, and depression. This is where psychotherapies can be of tremendous value, because there are, of course, ways of coping that involve courage and that lead to greater life satisfaction and higher functioning whether or not these differences are externally apparent. Patients must adapt their standards to their capabilities and neither despair when they cannot live up to wellness standards nor assume that they can no longer live a meaningful and productive life.

The presence of abnormalities on SPECT scans and/or neuropsychological testing can be helpful to patients, treaters, family, employers, and insurers in providing at least some form of external validation for the patient's difficulties. These tests may also be helpful in guiding therapies. For example, a patient with evidence of hypoperfusion on SPECT scan might benefit from treatment with ginkgo bilboa, and someone with specific cognitive deficits on neuropsychological testing might benefit from cognitive remediation.

Treatment Modalities

In addition to the medically-oriented treatments outlined above, a number of therapies have been tried in CFS, each of which has proven valuable in some cases. Such treatments include: CBT, "psychological reverse deconditioning," physical therapy, cognitive remediation, yoga and meditation, insight-oriented individual therapies, couples therapy, group therapy, and support groups.

CBT functions on the premise that patients with CFS are ill largely as a result of maladaptive cognitions about the etiology of their symptoms and about their functional potential. Advocates of CBT fall into two camps: one using a psychosocial etiological model for CFS who recommend CBT as potentially curative, and the other without commitment to a specific etiological model who view CBT as of potential help in maximizing functioning in the context of the illness. The belief that one is suffering from an occult viral infection for which there is no cure can lead some patients to adopt an unnecessarily passive and defensive approach to daily life. Believing that no initiative on their part can improve their condition and believing also that even mild activity can prove harmful, some patients enter a vicious cycle of pain and chronic fatigue leading to withdrawal and inactivity, leading to physical deconditioning and demoralization, leading to more profound levels of fatigue and pain. CBT can be instrumental in breaking such maladaptive cycles.

"Psychological reverse deconditioning" shares a number of precepts with CBT, including a proactive orientation toward one's illness, aimed at reversing those patterns that serve to perpetuate and exacerbate symptomatology. This treatment is an adaptation of a treatment for low back pain developed by Dr. John Sarno (Sarno, 1991). Pain syndromes often lead to inactivity, which in turn leads to deconditioning, weakness, and increased levels of pain. Even after the initial injury has healed, patients may continue to experience significant pain simply as a result of deconditioning. "Reverse" deconditioning consists in a graded program of rehabilitation. "Psychological reverse deconditioning" aims to reverse the patterns of "learned helplessness" that illness can entail and, using a carefully graded and individually adapted program, to increase levels of functioning and confidence. To aim for, and achieve, "small successes" increases one's sense of competence and restores a sense of oneself as an active—and effective—agent. Both CBT and psychological reverse deconditioning operate under the tenet that, even if the illness was triggered by an external, biological agent, there are aspects of the patient's cognitions and behaviors that conspire to perpetuate in the patient an unnecessarily debilitated and demoralized state.

SUMMARY/CONCLUDING REMARKS

This chapter has focused on three diseases, ranging from lethal to indolent, from clearly infectious to nebulous in origin, one the most highly publicized and politicized disease in contemporary American culture, another barely classified as a disease. All have the potential to become chronic. All impose far-reaching changes on an individual's life. These diseases exemplify the growing complexity of our understanding of host-pathogen interactions. While once the "germ theory" of disease suggested that antimicrobial agents could "cure" infectious diseases in an uncomplicated and reliable way, it is now known that infections can alter immune responsiveness, creating immune deficiency syndromes as in HIV or autoimmune postinfectious conditions such as Sydenham's Chorea and PANDAS. Increasing numbers of diseases such as peptic ulcer disease, multiple sclerosis, schizophrenia, and certain cancers are known or suspected of being triggered, at least in some cases, by an infection. Host factors such as HLA typing may drastically alter the clinical course of an infection. Patients with HLA DR4 have been shown to have a greater risk of severe arthritis when infected with *B. burgdorferi,* and the presence of the DR8/17 haplotype seems to correlate positively with the incidence of PANDAS. Many of the difficulties encountered by patients suffering from the three diseases discussed above relate to this kind of complexity, which is only now beginning to be elucidated.

As with any chronic illness, sufferers from these diseases on the one hand may take the opportunity to galvanize latent psychological resources in coping with a new challenge, and on the other hand may find themselves foundering in radically changed physical, psychological, and/or occupational circumstances, their old resources and old defensive structures proving inadequate, and may sink into suicidal depression. There is, therefore, enormous potential for mental health professionals to help these individuals find new, original, courageous, creative, and adaptive ways of coping in the context of diseases that can otherwise all too often lead to despair.

REFERENCES

Abbey, S. E. (1996). Psychiatric diagnostic overlap in chronic fatigue syndrome. In *Chronic fatigue syndrome: An integrative approach to evaluation and treatment* (pp. 3–35). New York: Guilford Press.

Abbey, S. E., & Garfinkel, P. E. (1991). Chronic fatigue syndrome and depression: Cause, effect or covariate. *Reviews of Infectious Diseases, 13*(Suppl. 1), S73–S83.

Abbey, S. E., & Garfinkel, P. E. (1991). Neurasthenia and Chronic Fatigue Syndrome: The role of culture in the making of a diagnosis. *American Journal of Psychiatry, 148*(12), 1638–1646.

Abe, K., Fujimura, Y., Yorifuji, S., Mezaki, T., Hirono, N., Nishitani, N., & Kameyama, M. (1991). Marked reduction in CSF lactate and pyruvate levels after CoQ therapy in a patient with mitochondrial myopathy, encephalopathy, lactic acidosis and stroke-like episodes (MELAS). *Acta Neurologica Scandinavica, 83,* 356–359.

Aberer, E., Grabmeier, E., Kinaciyan, T., & Stunzer, D. (1999). Typing of Borrelia *burgdorferi s.l.* strains isolated from the skin of patients with different manifestations of Lyme borreliosis in Austria. *VIII International Conference on Lyme Borreliosis and other Emerging Tick-Borne Diseases, Munich, Germany,* June, 1999 (Abstract #O58, p. 18).

Acheson, E. D. (1959). The clinical syndrome variously called benign myalgic encephalomyelitis, Iceland disease and epidemic neuromyesthenia. *American Journal of Medicine,* 569–595.

Anonymous (editorial). (1956). A new clinical entity? *Lancet, May 26,* 789–790.

Archard, L. C., Bowles, N. E., Behan, P. O., Bell, E. J., & Doyle, D. (1988). Postviral fatigue syndrome: Persistence of enterovirus RNA in muscle and elevated creatine kinase. *Journal of the Royal Society of Medicine, 81,* 326–329.

Atkinson, J. H., Grant, I., & Kennedy C. J., et al. (1988). Prevalence of psychiatric disorders among men infected with HIV. *Archives of General Psychiatry, 45,* 859–64.

Ax, S., Gregg, V. H., & Jones, D. (2001). Coping and illness cognition: chronic fatigue syndrome. *Clinical Psychological Review, 21*(2), 161–182.

Bakheit, A. M., Behan, P. O., Dinan, T. G., Gray, C. E., & O'Keene, V. (1992). Possible upregulation of hypothalamic 5-hydroxytryptamine receptors in patients with postviral fatigue syndrome. *British Medical Journal, 304*(6833), 1010–1012.

Bakheit, A. M., Behan, P. O., Watson, W. S., & Morton, J. J. (1993). Abnormal arginine vasopressin secretion and water metabolism in patients with postviral fatigue syndrome. *Acta Neurologica Scandinavica, 87*(3), 234–238.

Bakken, L. L., Case, K. L., Callister, S. M., Bourdeau, N. J., & Schell, R. F. (1992). Performance of 45 laboratories participating in a proficiency testing program for Lyme disease serology. *Journal of the American Medical Association, 268,* 891–895.

Baldowicz, T. T., Brouwers, P., Goodkin, K., Kumar, A. M., & Kumar, M. (2000). Nutritional contributions to the CNS pathophysiology of HIV-1 infection and implications for treatment. *CNS Spectrums, 5*(4), 61–72.

Bannworth, A.(1941). Chronische lymphocytare meningitis, enzundliche polyneurotis and "rheumatisms." *Arch Psychiatr Nervenk, 113,* 284–376.

Barbour, A. G., & Garon, C. F. (1987). Linear plasmids of the bacterium Borrelia burgdorferi have covalently closed ends. *Science, 237,* 409–411.

Barre-Sinoussi, F., Chermann, J.-C., Rey, F., et al. (1983). Isolation of T-lymphotropic retrovirus for a patient at risk for acquired immune deficiency syndrome (AIDS). *Science, 220,* 868.

Bates, D. W., Buchwald, D., Lee, J., Kith, P., Doolittle, T., Rutherford, C., et al. (1995). Clinical laboratory test findings in patients with the chronic fatigue syndrome. *Archives of Internal Medicine, 155,* 97–103.

Bates, D. W., Schmitt, W., Buchwald, D., et al. (1993). Prevalence of fatigue and chronic fatigue syndrome: A prospective primary care practice. *Archives of Internal Medicine, 153,* 2759–2765.

Baxter, J. D., & Tyrell, J. B. (1981). The adrenal cortex. In P. Felig, J. D. Baxter, A. E. Broadus, L. A. Frohman (Eds.), *Endocrinology and metabolism* (pp. 385–510). New York: McGraw-Hill.

Beard, G. M. (1869). Neurasthenia or nervous exhaustion. *The Boston Medical and Surgical Journal, III*(13), 217–221.

Beard, G. M. (1880). *A practical treatise on nervous exhaustion (Neurasthenia). Its symptoms, nature, sequences, treatment* (2nd edition). New York: William Wood.

Bearn, J. A., Allain, T., Coskeran, P., Munro, N., Butler, J., McGragor, A., et al. (1995). Neuroendocrine responses to D-fenfluramine and insulin-induced hypoglycemia in chronic fatigue syndrome. *Biological Psychiatry, 37*(4), 245–252.

Beckett, A. (1988). Mood Disorders. In *HIV-related neuropsychiatric complications and treatment, HIV/AIDS training curriculum* (pp. 1–28). American Psychiatric Association, AIDS Program Office.

Behan, P. O., Behan, W. M. H., & Horrobin, D. (1990). Effect of high doses of essential fatty acids on the postviral fatigue syndrome. *Acta Neurologica Scandinavica, 82,* 209–216.

Belman, A. L., Iyer, M., Coyle, P. K., et al. (1993). Neurologic manifestations in children with North American Lyme Disease. *Neurology, 43,* 2609–2614.

Bennett, R. M., Gatter, R. A., Campbell, S. M., Andrews, R. P., Clark, S. R., & Scarola, J. A. (1988). A comparison of cyclobenzaprine and placebo in the management of fibrositis. *Arthritis and Rheumatism, 31*(12), 1535–1542.

Bing, E. G., Burnam, M. A., Longshore, D. et al. (2001). Psychiatric disorders and drug use among Human Immunodeficiency Virus-infected adults in the United States. *Archives of General Psychiatry, 58,* 721–728.

Boden, D., Hurley, A., Zhang, L. et al. (1999). HIV-1 drug resistance in newly infected individuals. *Journal of the American Medical Association, 282,* 1135–1141.

Bou-Holaigah, I., Rowe, P. C., Kan, J., & Calkins, H. (1995). The relationship between Neurally Mediated Hypotension and the Chronic Fatigue Syndrome. *Journal of the American Medical Association, 274*(12), 961–967.

Brornson, O., & Brornson, S. H. (1998). In vitro conversion of Borrelia *burgdorferi* to cystic forms in spinal fluid and transformation to motile spirochetes by incubation in BSK-H medium. *Infection, 26*(3), 144–150.

Brown, R., Bottiglieri, & Colman, C. (1999). *Stop depression now.* New York: G. P. Putnam's Sons.

Buchwald, D., Cheney, P. R., Peterson, D. L., Henry, B., Wormsley, S. B., Greiger, A., et al. (1992). A chronic illness characterized by fatigue, neurologic and immunologic disorders, and active human herpesvirus type-6 infection. *Annals of Internal Medicine, 116,* 103–113.

Buchwald, D., Sullivan, J. L., & Komaroff, A. L. (1987). Frequency of "chronic active

Epstein-Barr virus infection" in general medical practice. *Journal of the American Medical Association, 257*(17), 2303–2307.

Burgdorfer, W., Barbour, A., Haye, S., et al. (1982). Lyme disease: A tick-borne spirochetosis? *Science, 216,* 1317–1319.

Burlington, D. B. (1997). *FDA public health advisory: Assays for antibodies to Borrelia burgdorferi: Limitations, use and interpretation for supporting a clinical diagnosis of Lyme disease.* Rockville, MD: Department of Health and Human Services, Food and Drug Administration.

Burrascano, J. J. (1993). Lyme disease presenting as organic psychosis (abstract). Sixth Annual Lyme Disease Scientific Conference. Hartford, CT: Lyme Disease Foundation.

Burrascano, J. J. (1997). Lyme disease. In *Conn's current therapy* (pp. 140-143). Philadelphia: W. B. Saunders Company.

Butler, S., Chalder, T., Ron, M., & Wessely, S. (1991). Cognitive behavioral treatment in the chronic fatigue syndrome. *Journal of Neurology, Neurosurgery, and Psychiatry, 54,* 153–158.

Canadian MS Research Group. (1987). A randomised controlled trial of amantadine in fatigue associated with multiple sclerosis. *Canadian Journal of Neurological Science, 14,* 273–278.

Carballo-Dieguez, A. (1989). Hispanic culture, gay male culture, and AIDS: Counseling implications. *Journal of Counseling and Development, 68,* 29.

Carpenter, C. C., Cooer, D. A., Fischel, M. A., Gatell, J. M., Gazzard, B. G., Hammer, S. M., et al. (2000). Antiremoviral therapy in adults: Updated recommendations of the International AIDS Society—USA Panel. *Journal of the American Medical Association, 283*(3), 381–390.

Center for Disease Control and Prevention. (2002). Revision of the CDC surveillance case definition for acquired immunodeficiency syndrome. *MMWR, 36* (suppl 15), 15.

Centers for Disease Control and Prevention. (1982). Centers for Disease Control Task Force on Kaposi's sarcoma and opportunistic infections. *New England Journal of Medicine, 306,* 248.

Centers for Disease Control and Prevention. (1986). Classification system for human T-lymphotropic virus type III/lymphadenopathy-associated virus infections. *MMWR, 35,* 334.

Centers for Disease Control and Prevention. (1992). 1993 Revised classification system for HIV infection and expanded surveillance of definition for AIDS among adolescents and adults. *MMWR, 41* (RR-17), 1.

Centers for Disease Control and Prevention. (1994). AIDS among racial/ethnic minorities—United States. *MMWR, 43,* 644–647, 653–655.

Centers for Disease Control and Prevention. (1995a). AIDS associated with injecting-drug use—United States, 1995. *MMWR, 45,* 392–398.

Center for Disease Control and Prevention. (1995b). First 500,000 AIDS cases—United States, 1995. *MMWR, 44,* 849–855.

Centers for Disease Control and Prevention. (1996). Update: Trends in AIDS incidence, deaths, and prevalence—United States, 1996. *MMWR, 46,* 165–173.

Centers for Disease Control and Prevention. (2002). Lyme disease—United States, 2000. *MMWR Weekly, 51*(02), 29–31.

Centers for Disease Control and Prevention. (2000). U.S. HIV and AIDS cases reported through December, 2000. *HIV/AIDS surveillance report, 12*(2), (Year End Edition).

Centers for Disease Control and Prevention, National Center for Infectious Diseases. (2000). CFS Information, CFS Homepage. http://www.cdc.gov/ncidod/diseases/cfs/info.htm September 7, 2000.

Clark, S., Tindall, E., & Bennett, R. M. (1985). A double blind crossover trial of prednisone versus placebo in the treatment of fibrositis. *Journal of Rheumatology, 12*(5), 980–983.

Clauw, D. J., Radulovic, D., Katz, P., Baraniuk, J., & Barbay, J. T. (1995). Tilt table testing as a measure of dys autonomia in fibromyalgia. *Journal of Musculoskeletal Pain, 3*(Suppl. 1), 10.

Cleare, A. J., Miell, J., Heap, E., Sookdeo, S., Young, L., Malhi, G. S., & O'Keane, V. (2001). Hypothalamo-pituitary-adreanal axis dysfunction in chronic fatigue syndrome and the effects of low-dose hydrocortisone therapy. *Journal of Clinical Endocrinology and Metabolism, 86*(8), 3545–3554.

Cleare, A. J., Blair, D., Chambers, S., & Wessely, S. (2001). Urinary free cortisol in chronic fatigue syndrome. *American Journal of Psychiatry, 158*(4), 641–643.

Cohen, R. A., & Fisher, M. (1989). Amantadine treatment of fatigue associated with multiple sclerosis. *Archives of Neurology, 46,* 676–680.

Cooper, D. A., & Emery, S. (1998). Therapeutic strategies for HIV infection—time to think hard. *New England Journal of Medicine, 339,* 1319.

Coyle, P. K. (1996). Lyme disease and Chronic Fatigue Syndrome. Symposium Abstract #102D. *Syllabus and Scientific Proceedings of 149th Meeting of the American Psychiatric Association in New York.* Washington, DC: American Psychiatric Association.

Coyle, P. K., & Krupp, L. (1990). Borrelia burgdorferi infection in the chronic fatigue syndrome. *Annals of Neurology, 28,* 243–244.

Coyle, P. K., Schutzer, S. E., Belman, A. L., Krupp, L. B., & Dheng, Z. (1992). Cerebrospinal fluid immunologic parameters in neurologic Lyme disease. In S. E. Schutzer (ed.), *Lyme disease: Molecular and immunologic approaches* (pp. 31–43). Cold Spring Harbor, NY: Cold Spring Harbor Laboratory Press.

Coyle, P. K., Schutzer, S. E., & Deng, Z. (1995). Detection of Borrelia burgdorferi-specific antigen in antibody-negative cerebrospinal fluid in neurologic Lyme disease. *Neurology, 45,* 2010–2015.

Cunningham, L., Bowles, N. E., Lane, R. J. M., Dubowitz, V., & Archard, L. C. (1990). Persistence of enteroviral RNA in chronic fatigue syndrome is associated with the abnormal production of equal amounts of positive and negative strands of enteroviral RNA. *Journal of General Virology, 71,* 1399–1402.

Davis, K. C., Horsburgh, C. R., Jr., Hasiba, V., et al. (1998). Acquired immunodeficiency syndrome in a patient with hemophilia. *Annals of Internal Medicine, 98,* 284.

DeLuca, J., Johnson, S. K., Ellis, S. P., & Natelson, B. H. (1997a). Cognitive functioning is impaired in patients with chronic fatigue syndrome devoid of psychiatric disease. *Journal of Neurology, Neurosurgery, and Psychiatry, 62*(2), 151–155.

DeLuca, J., Johnson, S. K., Ellis, S. P., & Natelson, B. H. (1997b). Sudden vs. gradual onset of chronic fatigue syndrome differentiates individuals on cognitive and psychiatric measures. *Journal of Psychiatric Research, 31*(1), 83–90.

DeMeirleir, K., Bisbal, C., Campine, I., DeBecker, P., Salehzada, T., Demettre, E., et al. (2000). A 37 kDa 2-5A binding protein as a potential biochemical marker for chronic fatigue syndrome. *American Journal of Medicine, 108*(2), 99–105.

Demitrack, M. A., & Greden, J. F. (1992). Chronic fatigue syndrome: The need for an integrative approach. *Biological Psychiatry, 32*, 1065–1077.

Demitrack, M. A. (1993). Chronic fatigue syndrome: A disease of the hypothalamic-pituitary-adrenal axis? *Annals of Medicine, 26*(1), 1–5.

Demitrack, M. A., Dale, J. K., Straus, S. E. et al. (1991). Evidence for impaired activation of the hypothalamic-pituitary-adrenal axis in patients with chronic fatigue syndrome. *Journal of Clinical Endocrinology and Metabolism, 73*, 1224–1234.

Demitrack, M. A., & Abbey, S. E. (1996). *Chronic fatigue syndrome: An integrative approach to evaluation and treatment.* New York: Guilford Press.

Demitrack, M. A., & Abbey, S. E. (1996). Historical overview and evolution of contemporary definitions of chronic fatigue states. In *Chronic fatigue syndrome: An integrative approach to evaluation and treatment* (pp. 3–35). New York: Guilford Press.

Demitrack, M. A. (1996). The psychobiology of chronic fatigue: The central nervous system as a final common pathway. In *Chronic fatigue syndrome: An integrative approach to evaluation and treatment* (pp. 72–109). New York: Guilford Press.

Dinerman, H., & Steere, A. C. (1992). Lyme disease associated with fibrromyalgia. *Annals of Internal Medicine, 117*, 281–285.

Dismukes, W. E., Wade, J. S., Lee, J. Y., Dockery, B. K., & Hain, J. D. (1990), A randomized, double-blind trial of nystatin therapy for the candidiasis hypersensitivity syndrome. *New England Journal of Medicine, 323*, 1717–1723.

Diringer, M. N., Halperin, J. J., & Dattwyler, R. J. (1987). Lyme meningoencephalitis: a report of a severe, penicillin-resistant case. *Arthritis and Rheumatism, 30*, 705–707.

Donta, S. T. (1999). Fibromyalgia, Lyme disease and Gulf War Syndrome. *12th International Conference on Lyme Disease and Other Spirochetal and Tick-Borne Diseases,* New York, NY, 1999.

Dore, G. J., Correll, P. K., Li, Y. et al. (1995). Changes in AIDS dementia complex in the era of highly active antiretroviral therapy. *AIDS, 13*, 1249–53.

Dorward, D. W. (1999). Lymphotropism by B. *burgdorferi* in vitro and in vivo. *VIII International Conference on Lyme Borreliosis and other Emerging Tick-Borne Diseases, Munich,* Germany, June, 1999 (Poster #P205, p.5 7).

Edlen, B. R., Irwin, K. L., Faruque, S., et al. (1994). Intersecting epidemics—crack cocaine use and HIV infection among inner-city young adults. *New England Journal of Medicine, 331*, 1422–1427.

Engleberg, N. C. (1996). Medically-oriented therapy for chronic fatigue syndrome and related conditions. In *Chronic fatigue syndrome: An integrative approach to evaluation and treatment* (pp. 3–35). New York: Guilford Press.

Eskow, E., Rao, R. V., & Mordechai E. (2001). Concurrent infection of the central nervous system by Borrelia burgdorferi and Bartonalla henselae: Evidence for a novel tick-borne disease complex. *Archives of Neurology, 58*(9), 1357–1363.

Fallon, B. A., Das, S., Plutchok, J. J. et al. (1997). Functional brain imaging and neuropsychological testing in Lyme disease. *Clinical Infectious Disease, 25*(S), 57–63.

Fallon, B. A., Kochevar, J. M., Gaito, A. G., & Nields, J. A. (1998). The underdiagnosis of neuropsychiatric Lyme disease in children and adults. *Psychiatric Clinics of North America, 21*(3), 693–703.

Fallon, B. A., & Nields, J. A. (1994). Lyme disease: A neuropsychiatric illness. *American Journal of Psychiatry,, 151*, 1571–1583.

Fallon, B. A., Nields, J. A., Burrascano, J. J., et al. (1992). The neuropsychiatric manifestations of Lyme borreliosis. *Psychiatric Quarterly, 63*, 95–115.

Fallon, B. A., Neilds, J. A., Parsons, B. P., Liebowitz, M. R., & Klein, D. F. (1993). *Journal of Clinical Psychiatry, 54*(7), 263–268.

Fallon, B. A., Schwartzberg, M., Bransfield, R., Zimmerman, B., Scotti, A., Weber, C. A., et al. (1995). Late stage neurologic Lyme disease: Differential diagnosis and treatment. *Psychosomatics, 36,* 295–300.

Fein, L. A. (1996). Multivariate analysis of 160 patients with Lyme disease [abstract]. *In Program and Abstracts of the 9th Annual International Conference on Lyme Borreliosis and Other Tick-Borne Disorders.* Boston: Lyme Disease Foundation.

Felsenfeld, O., (1971). *Borrelia.* St. Louis, MO: Warren Green Press.

Finestone, D. H., & Ober, S. K. (1990). Fluoxetine and fibromyalgia. *Journal of the American Medical Association, 264*(22), 2869–2870.

Flexner, C. (2000). Genotype and phenotype–arresting resistance? *Journal of the American Medical Association, 283,* 2442–2444.

France, D. (1998, October 10). Holding AIDS at Bay, only to face "Lazarus Syndrome." *The New York Times,* p. F7.

Gallo, R. C., Salahuddin, S. Z., Popovic, M., et al. (1984). Frequent detection and isolation of cytopathic retroviruses (HTLV-III) from patients with AIDS and at risk for AIDS. *Science, 224,* 500.

GAO. (1998). *HIV/AIDS: USAID and UN Responses to the Epidemic in the Developing World.* GAO Report to Congressional Request; July 27, 1998. (Report No. NSIAD-98-202). Washington, DC: GAO.

Gao, F., Bailes, E., Robertson, D. L., et al. (1999). Origin of HIV-1 in the chimpanzee Pan troglodytes. *Nature, 397,* 436–41.

Garin, C. H., & Bujadoux, A. (1922). Paralyse par les tiques. *J Med Lyon, 3,* 765–767.

Geller, S. A. (1989). Treatment of fibrositis with fluoxetine hydrochloride (Prozac). *American Journal of Medicine, 87,* 594–595.

Goda, S. K., Hamada, T., Ishimoto, S., Kobayashi, T., Goto, I., & Kuroiwa, Y. (1987). Clinical improvement after administration of coenzyme Q10 in a patient with mitochondrial encephalomyelopathy. *Journal of Neurology, 234,* 62–63.

Gold, D., Bowden, R., Sixbey, J., Riggs, R., Katon, W. J., Ashley, R., et al. (1990). Chronic fatigue: A prospective clinical and virologic study. *Journal of the American Medical Association, 264*(1), 48–53.

Goldenberg, D. L., Simms, R. W., Geiger, A., & Komaroff, A. L. (1990). High frequency of fibromyalgia in patients with chronic fatigue seen in a primary care practice. *Arthritis and Rheumatism, 33,* 381–387.

Goodkin, K. (1998). Complications of the central and peripheral nervous system. In *HIV-related neuropsychiatric complications and treatments, HIV/AIDS training curriculum* (pp. 1–93). American Psychiatric Association AIDS Program Office.

Gottlieb, M. S., Schroff, R., Schanker, H. M., et al. (1981). Pneumocystis carinii pneumonia and mucosal candidiasis in previously healthy homosexual men: evidence of a new acquired cellular immunodeficiency. *New England Journal of Medicine, 305,* 1425.

Gow, J. W., Behan, W. M. H., Clements, G. B., Woodall, C., Riding, M., & Behan, P. O. (1991). Enteroviral RNA sequences detected by polymerase chain reaction in muscle of patients with postviral fatigue syndrome. *British Medical Journal, 302,* 692–696.

Grafman, J. (1995). Neuropsychological features of chronic fatigue syndrome. In S. Straus (Ed.), *Chronic fatigue syndrome.* New York: Marcel Dekker.

Grafman, J., Schwartz, V., Dale J. K., et al. (1993). Analysis of neuropsychological functioning in patients with chronic fatigue syndrome. *Journal of Neurology, Neurosurgery, and Psychiatry, 56*(6), 684–689.

Grant, I., Atkinson, J. H., Hesselink, J. R., et al. (1987). Evidence for early central nervous system involvement in the acquired immunodeficiency syndrome (AIDS) and other human immunodeficiency virus (HIV) infections: Studies with neuropsychological testing and magnetic resonance imaging. *Ann Intern Med, 107,* 828–36.

Grmek, M. D. (1990). *History of AIDS, emergence and origin of a modern pandemic* (pp. 1–12). Princeton, NJ, Princeton University Press.

Gulick, R. (1998). HIV treatment strategies, planning for the long term. *Journal of the American Medical Association, 279,* 957.

Gunn, W. J., Connell, D. B., & Randall, B. (1993). Epidemiology of chronic fatigue syndrome: The Centers for Disease Control study in chronic fatigue syndrome. *Ciba Foundation Symposium, 173,* 83–93.

Gupta, S., & Vayuvegula, B. (1991). A comprehensive immunological study in chronic fatigue syndrome. *Scandinavian Journal of Immunology, 33,* 319–327.

Hajek, T., Paskova, B., Janovska, D., Bahbouh, R., Hajek, P., Libiger, J., et al. (2002). Higher prevalence of antibodies to Borrelia *burgdorferi* in psychiatric patients than in healthy subjects. *American Journal of Psychiatry, 159,* 297–301.

Hanner, L. (1991). *When you're sick and don't know why.* Minneapolis, MN: DCI Publishing.

Hassler, D., Riedel, K., Zorn, J., & Preac-Mursic, V. (1991). Pulsed high-dose cefotaxime therapy in refractory Lyme borreliosis (letter). *Lancet, 338,* 193.

Haupl, T., Hahn, G., Rittig, M., et al. (1993). Persistence of Borrelia burgdorferi in ligamentous tissue from a patient with chronic Lyme borreiosis. *Arthritis and Rheumatism, 36,* 1621–1626.

Havlir, D. V., Mauchner, I. C., Hirsh, M. S., et al. (1998). Maintenance antiretroviral therapies in HIV-infected subjects with undetectable plasma HIURNA after triple-drug therapy. *New England Journal of Medicine, 339,* 1261–1268.

Hellerstrom, M. (1930). Erythema chronicum migrans Afzelii. *Acta Derm Venereol (Stockh), 11,* 315–321.

Henderson, D. A., & Shelokov, A. (1959). Epidemic neuromyesthenia—A clinical syndrome? *New England Journal of Medicine, 260*(15), 757–764; *260*(16), 814–818.

Hill, R. C. J. (1955). Memorandum on the outbreak amongst the nurses at Addington Hospital. *South American Medical Journal, 9,* 344–345.

Henneberg, J. P., Wienecke, R., & Neubert, U. (1999). Borrelia *burgdorferi* sensu stricto (s. s.), B. *afzelii* and B. *garinii*—comparison of their antibiotic sensitivities in vitro. *VIII International Conference on Lyme Borreliosis and other Emerging Tick-Borne Diseases, Munich, Germany,* June, 1999 (Poster #P324, p. 86).

Hess, A., Buchmann, J., Zetti, U. K., Henschel, S., Schlaefke, D., Grau, G. , et al.. (1999). Borrelia *burgdorferi* central nervous system infection presenting as an organic schizophrenialike disorder. *Biological Psychiatry, 45*(6), 795.

Hickie, I., Lloyd, A., Wakefield, D., et al. (1990). The psychiatric status of patients with the chronic fatigue syndrome. *British Journal of Psychiatry, 156,* 534–540.

Hickie, I., Silove, D., Hickie, C., Wakefield, D., & Lloyd, A. (1990). Is there immune dysfunction in depressive disorders? *Psychological Medicine, 20,* 755–761.

Hirsch, M. S., Conway, B., D'Aguila, R. T., et al. (1998). Antiretroviral drug resistance testing in adults with HIV infection, implications for clinical management. *Journal of the American Medical Association, 279,* 1984.

Hirsch, M., Brun-Vezinet, F., D'Aquila, R. et al. (2000). Antiretroviral drug resistance testing in adult HIV-1 infection: Recommendations of an international AIDS society–USA panel. *Journal of the American Medical Association, 283,* 2417–2426.

Ho, D. D. (1995). Time to hit HIV, early and hard. *New England Journal of Medicine, 333,* 450–451.

Ho, D. D., Neumann, A. V., Perelson, A. S., Chen, W., Leonard, J. M., & Markowitz, M. (1995). Rapid turnover of plasma virions and CD4 lymphocytes in HIV-1 infection. *Nature, 373,* 123.

Ho, D. D. (1996). Viral counts count in HIV infection. *Science, 272,* 1124–1125.

Hogg, R., Yip, B., Chan et al. (2001). Rates of disease progression by baseline CD4 cell count and viral load after initiating triple-drug therapy. *Journal of the American Medical Association, 286,* 2568–2577.

Holmes, G. P., Kaplan, J. E., Gantz, N. M. et al. (1988). Chronic fatigue syndrome: A working case definition. *Annals of Internal Medicine, 108,* 387–389.

Holmes, G. P., Kaplan, J. E., Stewart, J. A., Hunt, B., Pinsky, P. F., & Schonberger, L. B. (1987). A cluster of patients with a chronic mononucleosis-like syndrome: Is Epstein-Barr virus the cause? *Journal of the American Medical Association, 257*(17), 2297–2302.

Hunt, P. H., & Treisman, G. J. (1999). Diagnosis and treatment issues of mood disorders in HIV-infected patients. *Primary Psychiatry, 6,* 47–50.

Jelliffe, S. (1905). Dispensary work in nervous diseases. *The Journal of Nervous and Mental Diseases, 32,* 449–453.

Johnson, H. (1996). *Osler's web: Inside the labyrinth of the chronic fatigue epidemic.* New York: Penguin Books.

Kagawa-Singer, M., & Blackhall, L. J. (2001). Negotiating cross-cultural issues at the end of life. *Journal of the American Medical Association, 286,* 2993–3001.

Kahn, J. O., & Walker, B. D. (1998). Acute human immunodeficiency virus type 1 infection. *New England Journal of Medicine, 339,* 33.

Katon, W., Buchwald, D. S., Simon, G. E., Russo, J. E., & Mease, P. J. (1991). Psychiatric illness in patients with chronic fatigue and rheumatoid arthritis. *Journal of General Internal Medicine, 6,* 277–285.

Kitahata, M. M., Koepsell, T. D., Deyo, R., et al. (1986). Physicians' experience with the acquired immunodeficiency syndrome as a factor in patients' survival. *New England Journal of Medicine 334,* 701–706.

Klimas, N. G., Salvato, F. R., Morgan, R., & Fletcher, M. (1990). Immunologic abnormalities in chronic fatigue syndrome. *Journal of Clinical Microbiology, 28,* 1403–1410.

Kohler, V. J. (1990). Lyme disease in neurology and psychiatry. *Fortschritte der Medizin, 108,* 191–194.

Komaroff, A. L., & Fagioli, L. (1996). Medical assessment of fatigue and chronic fatigue syndrome. In *Chronic fatigue syndrome: An integrative approach to evaluation and treatment* (pp. 3–35). New York: Guilford Press.

Koup, R. A., Safir, J. T., Cao, Y., et al. (1994). Temporal association of cellular immune response with the initial control of viremia in primary human immunodeficiency virus type 1 syndrome. *Journal of Virology, 68,* 4650.

Krause, P. J., Telford, S. R., Spielman, A., et al. (1996). Concurrent Lyme disease and babesiosis. Evidence for increased severity and duration of illness. *Journal of the American Medical Association, 275,* 1657–1660.

Kreuger, J. M., & Majde, J. A. (1994). Microbial products and cytokines in sleep and fever regulation. *CRC Critical Reviews in Immunology, 14,* 355–379.

Kreusi, M. J. P., Dale, J., & Straus, S. E. (1989). Psychiatric diagnoses in patients who have chronic fatigue syndrome. *Journal of Clininical Psychiatry, 50,* 53–56.

Kronfol, Z., & Remick, D. G. (2000). Cytokines and the brain: Implications for clinical psychiatry. *American Journal of Psychiatry,, 157*(5), 683–694.

Krumholz, A., & Niedemeyer, E. (1983). Psychogenic seizures: a clinical study with follow-up data. *Neurology, 33,* 498–502.

Lam, R. W. (1991). Seasonal affective disorder presenting as chronic fatigue syndrome. *Canadian Journal of Psychiatry, 36,* 680–682.

Landlay, A. L., Jessop, C., Lennette, E. T., & Levy, J. A. (1991). Chronic fatigue syndrome: Clinical condition associated with immune activation. *Lancet, 338,* 707–712.

Lawrence, C., Lipton, R. B., Lowy, F. D., & Coyle, P. K. (1995). Seronegative chronic relapsing neuroborreliosis. *European Neurology, 35,* 113–117.

Legislative Hearing on Insurance Coverage for the Treatment of Lyme Disease. (1999). Hartford, Conn, February, 1999.

Leventhal, L. J., Naides, S. J., & Freudlich, B. (1991). Fibromyalgia and parvovirus infection. *Arthritis and Rheumatism, 34*(10), 1319–1324.

Lichtenstein, K., Ward, D., Moorman, A., et al. (2001). Assessment of HIV-associated lipodystrophy in an ambulatory population. *AIDS, 15,* 1389–1398.

Liegner, K. B., Duray, P., Agricola, M., et al. (1997). Lyme disease and the clinical spectrum of antibiotic-responsive meningoencephalomyelitides. *Journal of Spirochetal and Tick Borne Diseases,* vol. 4, pp. 61–73.

Liegner, K. B., Shapiro, J. R., Ramsay, D., et al. (1993). Recurrent erythema migrans despite extended antibiotic treatment with minocycline in a patient with persisting Borrelia burgdorferi infection. *Journal of the Americn Academy of Dermatology, 28,* 312-314.

Logigan, E. L., Johnson, K. A., Kijewski, M. F. et al. (1997). Reversible cerebral hypoperfusion in Lyme encephalopathy. *Neurology., 49,* 1661–1670.

Levine, J. M. (2001). Psychiatric aspects of HIV care. *AIDS Clinical Care, 13,* 101–109.

Lloyd, A., Hickie, I., Wakefield, D., Broughton, C., & Dwyer, J. (1990). A double-blind, placebo-controlled trial of intravenous immunoglobulin therapy in patients with chronic fatigue syndrome. *American Journal of Medicine, 89,* 561–568.

Lloyd, A. R., Wakefield, D., Boughton, C. R., & Dwyer, J. M. (1989). Immunological abnormalities in the chronic fatigue syndrome. *The Medical Journal of Australia, 151,* 121–124.

Lori, F., & Lisziewicz, J. (2001). Structured treatment interruptions for the management of HIV infection. *Journal of the American Medical Association, 286,* 2981–2987.

Lyketsos, C. G., Hanson, A. L., Fishman, M., Rosenblatt, A., McHugh, P. R., & Treisman, G. J. (1983). Manic syndrome early and late in the course of HIV. *American Journal of Psychiatry, 150,* 326–327.

Magnarelli, L. A. (1989). Laboratory diagnosis of Lyme disease. *Rheumatic Diseases Clinica of North America, 15,* 735–745.

Mantaner, J. S. G., Reiss, P., Cooper, D., et al. (1998). A randomized, double-blind trial comparing combinations of revirapine, didanosine, and zidovudine for HIV-infected patients. *Journal of the American Medical Association, 279,* 930.

Manu, P., Matthews, D. A., Lane, T. J., Tennen, H., Hesselbrock, V., Mendola, R., &

Affleck, G. (1989). Depression among patients with a chief complaint of chronic fatigue. *Journal of Affective Disorders, 17,* 165–172.

Marcussen, J. A., Lindh, G., & Evergard, B. (1999). Chronic fatigue syndrome and nickel allergy. *Contact Dermatitis, 40*(5), 269–272.

Martinez, E., Mocroft, A., Garcia-Viajo, M., et al. (2001). Risk of lipodystrophy in HIV-1- infected patients treated with protease inhibitors: A prospective cohort study. *Lancet, 357,* 592–98.

Marzuk, P. M., Tierney, H., Tradiff, K., et al. (1988). Increased risk of suicide in persons with AIDS. *Journal of the American Medical Association, 259,* 1333–1337.

McDaniel, J. S. (1998). Anxiety Disorders. In *HIV-related neuropsychiatric complications and treatment: HIV/ AIDS training curriculum* (pp. 1–21). American Psychiatric Association, AIDS Program Office.

McKegney, F. P., & O'Dowd, M. A. (1992). Suicidality and HIV status. *American Journal of Psychiatry, 149,* 396–398.

Medical Staff of the Royal Free Hospital. (1957). An outbreak of encephalomyelitis in the Royal Free Hospital Group, London, in 1955. *British Medical Journal, 19,* 895–904.

Mellor, J. W., Rinaldo, C. R. Jr., Gupta, P., White, R. M., Todd, J. A., & Kingsley, L. A. 1996). Prognosis in HIV-1 infection predicted by the quantity of virus in plasma. *Science, 272,* 1167–1170.

Moss, R. B., Mercandetti, A., & Vojdani, A. (1999). TNF-alpha and chronic fatigue syndrome. *Journal of Clinical Immunology, 19*(5), 314–316.

Munsiff, A. V. (1999). *Antiretroviral treatment and dosing guide for adults* (3rd ed.) Feb. 1999.

Murdoch, J. C. (1988). Cell-mediated immunity in patients with myalgic encephalomyelitis syndrome. *New Zealand Medical Journal, 101,* 511–512.

Murray, T. J. (1985). Amantadine therapy for fatigue in multiple sclerosis. *Canadian Journal of Neurological Science, 12,* 251–254.

Natelcon, B. H., Cheu, J., Pareja, J., Ellis, S. P., Policastro, T., & Findley, T. W.(1996). Randomized, double blind, placebo-phase in trial of low dose phenelzine in the chronic fatigue syndrome. *Psychopharmacology, 124,* 226–230.

Nields, J. A., & Fallon, B. A. (1998). Differential diagnosis and treatment of Lyme disease with special reference to psychiatric practice. *Directions in Psychiatry, 18,* 209–228.

Nields, J. A., Fallon, B. A., & Jastreboff, P. J. (1999). Carbamazepine in the treatment of Lyme disease-induced hyperacusis. *Journal of Neuropsychiatry and Clinical Neurosciences, 11,* 97–99.

Nields, J. A., & Kveton, J. F. (1991). Tullio phenomenon and seronegative Lyme borreliosis (letter). *Lancet, 338,* 128–129.

Nocton, J. J., Dressler, F., Rutledge, B. J., Rys, P. N., Persing, D. H., & Steere, A. C. (1994). Detection of Borrelia burgdorferi DNA by polymerase chain reaction in synovial fluid from patients with Lyme arthritis. *New England Journal of Medicine 330,* 229–234.

Ogashara, S., Engel, A. G., Frens, D., & Mack, D. (1989). Muscle coenzyme Q10 deficiency in familial mitochondrial encephalomyelopathy. *Proceedings of the National Academy of Sciences USA, 86,* 2379–2382.

Omasits, M., Seiser, A., & Brainin, M. (1990). Recurrent and relapsing borreliosis of the nervous system. *Weiner Klinische Wochenschrift, 102,* 4–12.

Pachner, A. R. (1989). Neurologic manifestations of Lyme disease, the new "Great Imitator." *Reviews of Infectious Diseases, 11*(Suppl 6), S1482–S1486.

Pachner, A. R., Duray, P., & Steere, A. C. (1989). Central nervous system manifestations of Lyme disease. *Archives of Neurology, 46,* 790–795.

Palella, F. J., Delaney, K. M., Moorman, A. C., et al. (1998). Declining morbidity and mortality among patients with advanced human immunodeficiency virus infection. *New England Journal of Medicine 338,* 853.

Pantaleo, G. (1993). HIV infection is active and progressive in lymphoid tissue during the clinically latent stage of disease. *Nature, 362,* 355.

Patnaik, M., Komaroff, A. L., Conley, E., Ojo-Amaise, E. A., & Peter, J. B. (1995). Prevalence of IgM antibodies to human herpes-6 early antigen (p41/38) in chronic fatigue syndrome. *Journal of Infectious Diseases, 172,* 1364–1367.

Perry, S. W., Jacobsberg, L. B., Fishman, B., et al. (1990). Psychological responses to serological testing for HIV. *AIDS, 4,* 145–152.

Perry, S. W. (1990). Organic mental disorders caused by HIV: Update on early diagnosis and treatment. *American Journal of Psychiatry, 147,* 696–710.

Perry, S. W., Jacobsberg, L. B., & Fishman, B. (1990). Suicidal ideation and HIV testing. *Journal of the American Medical Association, 263,* 679–682.

Peterson, P. K., Shepard, J., Macres, M., Schenk, C., Crosson, J., Rechtman, D., et al. (1990). A controlled trial of intravenous immunoglobulin G in chronic fatigue syndrome. *American Journal of Medicine, 89,* 554–560.

Pfister, H. W., Preac-Mursic, V., Wilske, B., Rieder, G., Forderreuther, S., Schnidt, S., et al. (1993). Catatonic syndrome in acute severe encephalitis due to Borrelia burgdorferi infection. *Neurology, 43,* 433–435.

Phair, J. P., & Murphy, R. L. (1997). *Contemporary diagnosis and management of HIV/ AIDS infections* (pp.17–27). Newtown, PA: Handbooks in Health Care Co.

Phillips, A., Staszewski, S., Weber, R. et al. (2001). HIV viral load response to antiretroviral therapy according to the baseline CD-4 cell count and viral load. *Journal of the American Medical Association, 286,* 2560–2567.

Pialoux, G., Raffi, F., Brun-Vezinet, F., et al. (1998). A randomized trial of 3 maintenance regimens given after 3 months of induction therapy with zidovudene, iamivudene, and indinaur in previously untreated HIV-1-infected patients. *New England Journal of Medicine, 339, 1269*–1276.

Piatak, M., Saag, M. S., Yang, L. C., et al. (1993). High levels of HIV-1 in plasma during all stages of infection determined by competitive PCR. *Science, 259,* 1749.

Pomerantz, R. (1999). Primary HIV-1 resistance: A new phase in the epidemic? *Journal of the American Medical Association, 282,* 1177–1179.

Pomerantz R. (2001). Initiating antiretroviral therapy during HIV infection: Confusion and clarity. *Journal of the American Medical Association, 286,* 2597–2599.

Poskanzer, D. C., Henderson, D. A., Kunkle, E. C., et al. (1957). Epidemic neuromyesthenia: An outbreak in Punta Gorda, Florida. *New England Journal of Medicine, 257*(8), 356–364.

Poteliakhoff, A. (1981). Adrenocortical activity and some clinical findings in acute and chronic fatigue. *Journal of Psychosomatic Research, 25*(2), 91–95.

Preac-Mursic, V., Weber, K., Pfister, H. W., et al. (1989). Survival of Borrelia burgdorferi in antibiotically-treated patients with Lyme borreliosis. *Infection, 17,* 355–359.

Preac-Mursic, V., Wanner, G., Reinhardt, S., et al. (1996). Formation and cultivation of Borrelia *burgdorferi* spheroplast-L-form variants. *Infection, 24*(3), 218–225.

Price, R. W., & Brew, B. J. (1997). Central and peripheral nervous system complications. In V. T. De Vita, Jr., S. Hellman, & S. A. Rosenberg (Eds.), *AIDS, etiology, diagnosis, treatment and prevention.* (4th ed., 331–353). Philadelphia: Lippincott-Raven Publishers.

Quimby, L. G., Gratwok, G. M., Whitney, C. D., & Block, S. R. (1989). A randomized trial of cyclobenzaprine for the treatment of fibromyalgia. *Journal of Rhematology, 16*(Suppl 19), 140–143.

Ray, C. (1991). Chronic fatigue syndrome and depression: Conceptual and methodological ambiguities. *Psycholical Medicine, 21,* 1–9.

Riley, M. S., O'Brien, C. J., McClusky, D. R., Bell, N. P., & Nicholls, D. P. (1990). Aerobic work capacity in patients with chronic fatigue syndrome. *BMJ (Clinical Research), 301,* 953–956.

Reijers, M. H., Weverling, G. J., Jurriaans, S., et al. (1998). Maintenance therapy after quadruple induction therapy in HIV-1 infected individuals: Amsterdam Duration of Antiretroviral Medication (ADAM) study. *Lancet, 352,* 185–190.

Reik, L., Smith, L., Khan, A., & Nelson, W. (1985). Demyelinating encephalopathy in Lyme disease. *Neurology, 35,* 267–269.

Roelcke, U., Barnett, W., Wilder-Smith, E., Sigmund, D., & Hacke, W. (1992).Untreated neuroborreliosis: Bannworth's syndrome evolving into acute schizophrenia-like psychosis. *Journal of Neurology, 239,* 129–131.

Rosa, P. A., & Schwan, T. G. (1989). A specific and sensitive assay for the Lyme disease spirochete, borrelia burgdorferi, using the polymerase chain reaction. *Journal of Infectious Diseases, 160,* 1018–1029.

Rowe, P. C., Bou-Houlaigah, I., Kan, J. S., & Calkins, H. (1995). Is neurally mediated hypotension an unrecognised cause of chronic fatigue? *Lancet, 345,* 623–634.

Rowe, P. C., & Calkins, H. (1998). Neurally-mediated hypotension and chronic fatigue syndrome. *American Journal of Medicine, 105*(3A), 15S–21S.

Rundell, J. R., Kyle, K. M., Brown, G. R., & Thomason, W. L. (1992). Risk factors for suicide attempts in a human immunodeficiency virus screening program. *Psychosomatics, 33,* 24–27.

Saag, M. S. (1997). Clinical spectrum of human immunodeficiency virus diseases. In V. T. De Vita, Jr., S. Hellman, & S. A. Rosenberg (Eds.), *AIDS, etiology, diagnosis, treatment and prevention.* (4th ed., 202–213). Philadelphia: Lippincott-Raven Publishers.

Sarno, J. (1991). *Healing back pain: The mind-body connection.* New York: Time Warner Books.

Schmitt, F. A., Bigley, J. W., McKinnis, R., et al. (1988). Neuropsychological outcome of zidovudine (AZT) treatment of patients with AIDS And AIDS-related complex. *New England Journal of Medicine, 319,* 1573–1578.

Schondorf, R., & Freeman, R. (1999). The importance of orthostatic intolerance in the chronic fatigue syndrome. *American Journal of Medical Sciences, 317*(2), 117–123.

Schouls, L. M., Van De Pol, I., Rijpkema, S. G., & Schot, C. S. (1999). Detection and identification of Ehrlichia, Borrelia burgdorferi seusu lato and Bartonella species in Dutch Ixodes ricinus ticks. *Journal of Clinical Microbiology, 37*(7), 2215–2222.

Schutzer, S. E., & Natelson, B. H. (1999). Absence of Borrelia burgdorferi-specific immune complexes in chronic fatigue syndrome. *Neurology, 53*(6), 1340–1341.

Selwyn, P. A., & O'Connor, P. G. (1992). Diagnosis and treatment of substance users with HIV infection. *Primary Care, 19,* 119–156.

Shain, R. N., Piper, J. M., Newton, E. R., et al. (1999). A randomized, controlled trial of a behavioral intervention to prevent sexually transmitted disease among minority women. *New England Journal of Medicine, 340,* 93–100.

Shadick, N. A., Phillips, C. B., Logigan, E. L. et al. (1994). The long-term clinical outcomes of Lyme disease. *Annals of Internal Medicine, 1221,* 560–567.

Sharpe, M. C. (1996). Cognitive-behavioral therapy for patients with chronic fatigue syndrome: How? In *Chronic fatigue syndrome: An integrative approach to evaluation and treatment* (pp. 3–35). New York: Guilford Press.

Shelokov, A., Habel, K., Verder, E., & Welsh, W. (1957). Epidemic neuromyesthenia: An outbreak of poliomyelitis-like illness in student nurses. *New England Journal of Medicine 257*(8), 345–355.

Simpson, D. M., & Tagliati, M. (1994). Neurologic manifestations of HIV Infection. *Annals of Internal Medicine, 121,* 769–785.

Steere, A. C., Taylor, E., & McHugh, G. L., et al. (1993). The overdiagnosis of Lyme disease. *Journal of the American Medical Association, 269,* 1812–1816.

Steere, A. C., Malawista, S. E., Snydman, D. R., et al. (1977b). Lyme arthritis: An epidemic of oligoarticular arthritis in children and adults in three Connecticut communities. *Arthritis and Rheumatism, 20,* 7–17.

Steere, A. C., Broderick, T. F., Malawista, S. E. (1978). Erythema chronicum migrans and Lyme arthritis: Epidemic evidence for a tick vector. *American Journal of Epidemiology, 108,* 312–321.

Steere, A. C., Bartenhagen, N. H., Craft, J. E., Hutchinson, G. J., Newman, J. H., Rahn, et al. (1983). The early clinical manifestations of Lyme disease. *Annals of Internal Medicine, 99,* 76–82.

Steere, A. C., Malawista, S. E., Hardin, J. A., Ruddy, S., Askenase, P. W., & Andiman, W. A. (1977). Erythema chronicum migrans and Lyme arthritis: the enlarging clinical spectrum. *Annals of Internal Medicine, 86,* 685–698.

Stein, S. L., Solvason, H. B., Biggart, E., & Spiegal, D. (1996). A 25-year-old woman with hallucinations, hypersexuality, nightmares and a rash. *American Journal of Psychiatry, 153*(4), 545–551.

Sternberg, E. M. (1993). Hypoimmune fatigue syndromes: Diseases of the stress response? *Journal of Rheumatology, 20*(3), 418–421.

Strayer, D. R., Carter, W. A., Brodsky, I., Cheney, P., Peterson, D. L., Salvato, P., et al. (1994). A controlled clinical trial with a specifically configured RNA drug, poly (I):poly(C 12U) in chronic fatigue syndrome. *Clinical Infectious Diseases, 18,* S88–95.

Straus, S. E. (1988). Intravenous immunoglobulin treatment for the chronic fatigue syndrome. *American Journal of Medicine, 319*(26), 1692–1698.

Straus, S. E. (1990). Intravenous immunoglobulin treatment for the chronic fatigue syndrome. *American Journal of Medicine, 89*(5), 551–553.

Straus, S. E. (1996). Chronic Fatigue Syndrome. *British Medical Journal, 313*(7061), 831–832.

Straus, S. E., Dale, J. K., Tobi, M., et al. (1988). Acyclovir treatment of the chronic fatigue syndrome: Lack of efficacy in a placebo-controlled trial. *New England Journal of Medicine, 319*(26), 1692–1698.

Straus, S. E., Dale, J. K., Wright, R., & Metcalfe, D. D. (1988). Allergy and the chronic fatigue syndrome. *Journal of Allergy and Clinical Immunology, 81,* 791–795.

Straus, S. E., Tosato, G., Armstrong, G., Lawley, T., Preble, O. T., Henle, W., et al. (1985). Persisting illness and fatigue in adults with evidence of Epstein-Barr virus infection. *Annals of Internal Medicine, 102,* 7–16.

Taerk, G. S., Toner, B. B., Salit, I. E., Garfinkel, P. E., & Ozersky, S. (1987). Depression in patients with neuromyasthenia (benign myalgic encephalomyelitis). *International Journal of Psychiatry Medicine, 17,* 49–56.

Treib, J., Grauer, M. T., Haass, A., Langenbach, J., Holzer, G., & Woessner, R. (2000). Chronic fatigue syndrome in patients with Lyme borreliosis. *European Neurology, 43*(2), 107–109.

Treisman, G. J., Angelino, A. F., & Hutton, H. E. (2001). Psychiatric issues in the management of patients with HIV infection. *Journal of the American Medical Association, 286,* 2857–2864.

Tyber, M. A. (1990). Lithium carbonate augmentation therapy in fibromyalgia. *Canadian Medical Association Journal, 143*(9), 902–904.

UNAIDS Joint Nations Programme on HIV/AIDS. (2001). AIDS Epidemic update. December, 2001.

Vaeroy, H., Abrahamsen, A., Forre, O., & Kass, E. (1989). Treatment of fibromyalgia (fibrositis syndrome): A parallel double blind trial with carisoprodol, paracetamol and caffeine (somadril comp) versus placebo. *Clinical Rheumatology., 8,* 245–250.

Vercoulen, J. H., Swanink, C. M., Zitman, F. G., Vreden, S. G., Hoofs, M. P., Fennis, J. F., et al. Randomised, double-blind, placebo-controlled study of fluoxetine in chronic fatigue syndrome. *Lancet, 347,* 858–861.

Visser, J. T., DeKloet, E. R., & Nagelkern, L. (2000). Altered glucocorticoid regulation of the immune response in the chronic fatigue syndrome. *Annals of the New York Academy of Science, 917,* 868–875.

Walker, B. D., & Basgoz, N. (1998). Treat HIV-1 infection like other infections—treat it. *Journal of the American Medical Association, 280,* 91.

Waniek, C., Prohovnik, I., & Kaufman, M. A. (1994). Rapid progressive frontal type dementia associated with Lyme disease and subcortical degeneration. In *Abstracts of the VII Annual International Scientific Conference on Lyme Borreliosis.* Hartford, CT: Lyme Disease Foundation.

Wessely, S. C. (1996). Cognitive-behavioral therapy for patients with chronic fatigue syndrome: Why? In *Chronic fatigue syndrome: An integrative approach to evaluation and treatment* (pp. 3–35). New York: Guilford Press.

Wessely, S., & Powell, R. (1989). Fatigue syndromes: A comparison of chronic "postviral" fatigue with neuromuscular and affective disorders. *Journal of Neurology, Neurosurgery, and Psychiatry, 52,* 940–948.

Wolfe, F., Smythe, H. A., Yunus, M. B., Bennett, R. M., Bombardier, C., Goldenberg, D. L., et al. (1990). The American College of Rheumatology 1990 criteria for the classification of fibromyalgia. *Arthritis and Rheumatism, 33*(2), 160–172.

Wood, G. C., Bentall, R. P., Gopfert, M., & Edwards, R. H. T. (1991). A comparative psychiatric assessment of patients with chronic fatigue syndrome and muscle disease. *Psychological Medicine, 21,* 619–628.

Wortley, P. M., & Fleming, P. (1997). AIDS in women in the United States, recent trends. *Journal of the American Medical Association, 278,* 911.

Yousef, G. E., Bell, E. J., Mann, G. F., Murugesan, V., Smith, D. G., McCarney, R. A., et al. (1988). Chronic enterovirus infection in patients with postviral fatigue syndrome. *Lancet, 1,* 146–150.

9

Women's Health

MINDY E. WEISS
ELIZABETH H. W. RICANATI
ELSA-GRACE V. GIARDINA

INTRODUCTION

Why Women's Health?

Gender-based medicine has become a reality throughout the last decade. Expanding our knowledge in this area will affect further research, clinical practices, medical education, and public policy. In delineating women's health as a separate entity, we acknowledge that women are not little men. Rather, disease affects each gender differently. Certain diseases affect women exclusively or disproportionately. Surprisingly, the concept of women's health as a distinct medical discipline/phenomenon is relatively new, with its roots in the late twentieth century. Until recently, the majority of clinical trials enrolled predominantly male subjects. It was assumed that the results were similarly applicable to women, a fact that has since been disproved (Shelton, 1997).

How to Choose a Doctor—Gender Matters

The 1990s have witnessed an explosive interest in women's health as both the public and scientific communities have started to address this issue. An example is the Women's Health Initiative, a multimillion-dollar research effort on behalf of the National Institutes of Health, which will be completed in the next several years. This landmark series of research protocols addresses medical problems in women, an area that has been historically neglected. Women are learning that gender matters, and this is reflected in their healthcare choices, including their selection of a physician. Increasingly, women are choosing female physicians. A recent study demonstrates increased adherence to preventive health care protocols by female physicians.

Female internists and family practitioners recommended or offered cancer screening with Pap smears and mammography more frequently than their male counterparts. The researchers noted that historically the most common reason a woman patient did not undergo these preventive tests was that they were not recommended or offered by their physicians.

THE REPRODUCTIVE YEARS

Sexual Interview

There are many important reasons to obtain a sexual history. Patients' sexual health affects overall well-being as many sexual problems often reflect underlying disease processes or psychological morbidity (i.e., anger, anxiety, and depression). Obtaining a sexual history also facilitates dialogue about topics such as sexually transmitted diseases and pregnancy. It is essential that the practitioner maintain a nonjudgmental approach as she inquires about sexual orientation, contacts, practices, and problems.

Physical and sexual violence is common, often affecting women more than men. Intimate partners or relatives with a normally protective role may also perpetrate violence against women. It is imperative to inquire about all forms of abuse, including emotional, physical, and sexual abuse. Health care providers must be aware that somatic disorders, such as eczema, eating disorders, sexual dysfunction, substance abuse, and depression may reflect a history of abuse.

Reproductive history includes age of menarche, last menses, and regularity and duration of menses. Relevant obstetrical history includes inquiring about number of pregnancies, number of deliveries, miscarriages, abortions, and complications of pregnancy.

Vaginitis, Cervical Infections, and Pelvic Inflammatory Disease

Vaginitis

Normal vaginal secretions are usually odorless and clear or white and homogenous. Vaginitis presents with abnormal vaginal discharge, as well as vaginal odor, vulvar irritation and itching, or pain with urination or sexual intercourse. Common causes of vaginitis include candidiasis, bacterial vaginosis, trichomonas, or atrophic vaginitis. Important history includes the color, consistency, volume of discharge, and presence of itching or odor, as well as history of previous infections, past treatments, and last sexual contact. After a careful examination, a wet mount preparation should be made to facilitate diagnosis.

Candidiasis. Candida, usually C. *albicans*, is part of the normal vaginal flora; alterations in this milieu often result in infection. Common predisposing factors include diabetes, pregnancy, use of oral contraceptives with high estrogen content, immunosuppression, and various medications (i.e., antibiotics). Thus, most women experience candidiasis at some point in their lives. Typical symptoms include a thick, curdlike, sometimes malodorous, white discharge accompanied by vulvar itching and inflammation. Diagnosis is confirmed by both physical exam and laboratory findings, including a normal vaginal pH, which is less than four and a half, and pseudohyphae on a potassium hydroxide-stained wet mount. Treatment with either over-the-counter or prescription antifungal creams, suppositories, or prescription oral preparation result in symptomatic relief within one to two days. Occasional patients experience chronic yeast infections and may benefit from prophylactic oral antifungals.

Bacterial Vaginosis. Also called nonspecific vaginitis, bacterial vaginosis is a polymicrobial infection that has been associated with *Bacteriodes, Corynebacterium, Eubacterium, Gardnerella vaginalis, Mycoplasma hominis,* and *Peptococcus.* It is the most common cause of vaginitis in childbearing women. Symptoms include a thin, homogenous, grayish discharge without vulvar irritation. The accompanying odor smells fishlike or musty and is especially prominent after sexual intercourse; it is usually not sexually transmitted. Diagnosis is confirmed by vaginal fluid pH between five and six and the presence of clue cells on microscopic examination of a saline-stained wet mount. Normally, asymptomatic patients do not require treatment; however, recent data supports treating pregnant women to reduce the incidence of preterm labor. The treatment of choice is metronidazole.

Trichomonas. This infection, unlike the other causes of vaginitis, is often sexually transmitted; however, it can also be transmitted through contaminated clothing or water. Symptoms, if present, include a frothy, greenish discharge with vaginal burning and occasional spotting. Pregnant women with trichomonas risk premature rupture of membranes, preterm birth, and posthysterectomy cellulitis. Patients may also complain of urinary symptoms, including increased urinary frequency, dysuria and urgency, secondary to periurethral inflammation. Rarely, patients complain of a malodorous discharge. Physical examination is notable for mild vulva-vaginal erythema and inflammation. The cervix often has a "strawberry" appearance. Laboratory analysis demonstrates an elevated pH between six and seven motile flagellated organisms on saline-stained wet mount and an increased number of polymorphonuclear cells. Both patients and their partners must be treated with antibiotics. The treatment of choice is metronidazole.

Atrophic Vaginitis. This condition generally occurs in postmenopausal women and is secondary to estrogen deficiency. Symptoms, if present, include dryness and blood-tinged discharge. On physical examination, vulvar skin is often thin and shiny with a lack of hair; erythema may be present. Vaginal walls often lack the normal rugal folds. Treatment with estrogen creams offers acute, local relief; long-term treatment may utilize oral estrogens.

Cervical Infections

Chlamydia Trachomatis. This is the most common sexually transmitted disease in America. Unfortunately, in most women it is asymptomatic. When present, symptoms include vaginal discharge secondary to mucopurulent cervicitis; the cervix in this case is friable, edematous, and covered with discharge. A large proportion of patients present with pelvic inflammatory disease (see next section). Given the high incidence of asymptomatic patients and the risk of serious sequelae, widespread screening is beneficial. Cultures are the gold standard for diagnosis and doxycycline is the medicine of choice for treatment.

Neisseria Gonorrhea. Gonorrhea has been described throughout civilization and humans have been found to be the only natural hosts for this species. Symptoms vary widely and women may remain asymptomatic for a while; nonspecific symptoms such as a vaginal discharge, painful intercourse, irregular bleeding, and lower abdominal discomfort are infrequently accompanied by a mucopurulent cervical discharge. Some women do not present until they have already developed pelvic inflammatory disease (see next section). Gram-stain and culture diagnose this organism. Treatment with antibiotics is warranted, usually with ceftriaxone. Often patients receive medications for both gonorrhea and chlamydia simultaneously given the high rate of coinfectivity.

Pelvic Inflammatory Disease (PID). PID is caused by the ascension of bacteria that have colonized the endocervix. Common sexually transmitted organisms include *Chlamydia* and *Gonorrhea*; anaerobic organisms include *Peptococcus* and *Bacteroides*; and facultative aerobes include *E. Coli, Group B Streptococcus, Gardnerella vaginalis*, and *Haemophilus*. The spectrum of upper genital sexually transmitted diseases includes inflammation of the lining of the uterus or pelvis, inflammation of the fallopian tubes, and tubo-ovarian abscesses. Unfortunately, at least one-fourth of those affected experience serious sequelae including infertility, ectopic pregnancy, or chronic pelvic pain.

Personal behaviors and sexual practices are two risk factors for PID. Barrier methods of contraception help to decrease risk, whereas multiple sex partners, frequent intercourse, and the recent acquisition of a new partner increase risk. Unfortunately, no historical, physical, or laboratory finding can conclusively diagnose PID; clinical suspicion and empiric therapeutic interventions are required to avoid serious complications.

Minimal criteria for diagnosis include lower abdominal tenderness, adnexal tenderness, and cervical motion tenderness; additional criteria used to increase specificity include elevated temperature, abnormal discharge, elevated erythrocyte sedimentation rate or C-reactive protein and laboratory confirmation of chlamydia or gonorrhea. The gold-standard diagnostic test is laparoscopy. Treatment mandates empiric, broad-spectrum antibiotic usage, usually outpatient but sometimes requiring hospitalization. In addition, patients must prevent further exposure to sexually transmitted diseases (Heath & Heath, 1995; Judson, 1990; Newkirk, 1996; Reife, 1996; Sobel, 1996).

Contraception

Short of abstinence, no birth control option offers 100% efficacy. However, the second half of this century has seen the development of a multitude of safe birth control options for women. Making a decision remains complex and is dictated by each method's effectiveness, potential risks and benefits, the cost and lifestyle considerations—values, future fertility, beliefs, and so on. A number of options will be addressed including hormonal contraception, barriers, spermicides, intrauterine devices, sterilization, and natural methods.

Hormones

With the discovery that progesterone blocks ovulation, hormonal contraception first developed in the 1950s. Subsequently, many variations have been introduced, including pills, injections, and implants. Most commonly, women take combined synthetic estrogen and progesterone oral contraception pills, which inhibit ovulation, induce changes in the cervical mucus that affect sperm transport, and alter the endometrial surface to disrupt implantation. Benefits include increased regularity of the menstrual cycle with overall decreased flow, decreased cramps/pain associated with menses, and reduced risk of functional ovarian cysts, ovarian and endometrial cancers, and pelvic inflammatory disease. The potential risks include thromboembolic disease (blood clots), cardiovascular disease, liver adenomas, benign breast disease, and cervical cancer.

Absolute contraindications include a history of thromboembolism, heart attack, stroke, clotting disorder, high cholesterol, severe liver disease, undiagnosed irregular vaginal bleeding, known/suspected pregnancy, known/suspected genital tract or breast cancer, smoker over age thirty-five, and hypertension. Relative contraindications include history of migraines, diabetes, depression, seizures, sickle cell anemia, and Crohn's disease.

The two broad methods of treatment include (1) a fixed dose of hormones for 21 days followed by a seven-day hormone-free period and (2) a triphasic dose that attempts to mimic a woman's natural menstrual cycle. Both are equally effective. A third, less reliable oral form of hormonal contraception is the "mini-pill," or progesterone-only pill. This does not inhibit ovulation in every woman; rather, it alters the cervical mucus. Given its decreased efficacy, it is used in either women with decreased fertility or when the combined pill is contraindicated.

Injectable medroxyprogesterone acetate provides another option; it prevents ovulation. As this circumvents the liver, some of the pill's side effects are avoided and lower amounts of hormone can be used. Additionally, since it is injected every three months, compliance is improved. Alternatively, implants containing synthetic progesterone provide alternative hormonal contraception. They are effective for five years, and work by preventing ovulation and thickening the cervical mucus. Benefits include the absence of estrogen-related side effects, improved compliance, low cost amortized over the five years, high efficacy, and an immediate return of fertility after removal. Risks include initial irregular bleeding, progesterone-related side effects such as acne, infection at the insertion site, and initial increased costs. Contraindications include active thrombophlebitis/thromboembolic disease, undiagnosed vaginal bleeding, acute liver disease, breast cancer, and suspected/confirmed pregnancy.

Finally, the "morning-after" pill, Ovral, has recently been approved. This consists of supranormal doses of combined oral estrogen and progesterone taken within 72 hours of unprotected intercourse.

Barrier Methods

Barrier methods include the diaphragm and the female condom for women and the condom for men. Diaphragms cover the cervix and should be used in conjunction with a spermicidal cream or jelly. The female condom consists of an internal ring that covers the cervix, polyurethane sheeting that covers the vaginal walls, and an outer ring. The male condom is also an effective protective device when used correctly. Both condoms not only protect against pregnancy, but also against sexually transmitted diseases (STDs) and in addition, they decrease the risk of cervical cancer. Adversely, they require daily forethought.

Spermicides

Spermicides kill sperm. They are usually placed in the vagina proximate to the cervix just prior to intercourse; condoms now also come coated with them. A variety of preparations exist, including foams, jellies, and creams. Most contain nonoxynol-nine as the active ingredient, which is also effective against STDs.

Intrauterine Devices

Intrauterine devices (IUDs) prevent pregnancy, although what their mechanism of action is has not been clearly determined. Benefits include effectiveness, reversibility, and obviation of a daily preparation. Risks include increased risk of infection, menstrual cramping, heavy bleeding, and increased risk of ectopic pregnancy.

Sterilization

Sterilization methods, vasectomy for men and tubal ligation for women, are often permanent. Although hysterectomy also results in sterilization, this procedure is not generally performed for this indication.

Natural Methods

Finally, natural methods including withdrawal and periodic abstinence are methods of contraception; these however do not protect against STDs and are significantly less effective than previously described alternatives (Baird & Glaser, 1953).

Pregnancy

The optimal time for pregnancy, physiologically, is the age between eighteen and thirty-five. Very young women risk bearing low-birth weight infants and older women are at increased risk of bearing children with congenital anomalies. Realistically, though, the optimal time for pregnancy is when the woman and her partner are ready.

Prior to conception, if possible, a woman should prepare herself physically and psychologically. Avoiding alcohol and tobacco are important for the developing fetus, as is the administration of a daily multivitamin with folic acid to prevent neural tube defects. In addition, other prescriptions or over-the-counter medicines should be reviewed as these may pose teratogenic risk to the developing fetus.

Conception occurs when the fertilized egg implants in the uterus. The surrounding tissues then begin producing a hormone, human chorionic gonadotropin (HCG), which enters the bloodstream and is secreted in the urine. HCG is the basis of the urine pregnancy test and may be positive as early as one week after a missed period. Symptoms of pregnancy emerge as this hormone level increases. The most common first sign of pregnancy is a missed period. Other signs include full and swollen breasts, fatigue, frequent urination, and a sensation of pelvic pressure. Additionally, about 50% of women experience some degree of morning sickness, with accompanying nausea and occasional vomiting. Significantly, this can occur at any time of the day, not just the morning!

Routine prenatal examinations should begin once a woman realizes that she is pregnant. These help ensure the health of both mother and fetus, preventing complications and facilitating early treatment if they arise. The first prenatal visit is often the most involved, with the physician performing a complete history and physical examination, including pelvic examination. A Pap test is completed and laboratory tests drawn, including a complete blood count to rule out anemia, a rubella test, blood typing, and tests to rule out syphilis and, depending on the situation, an HIV test.

The subsequent monthly visits are shorter, usually involving a weight and blood pressure checks, examination of the urine for protein and glucose, fetal heart sound evaluation and time to answer questions. By week 32, office visits become more frequent, initially biweekly and then for the last month, weekly. When clinically mandated, additional testing may include alpha-fetoprotein, ultrasonography, and amniocentesis when warranted.

Weight gain during pregnancy is a concern for most women. Current guidelines recommend that women of an average weight gain twenty-five to thirty pounds; thin women need to gain more and heavy women less. About 25% of weight gain are attributable to the fetus; the remainder is distributed among the placenta, amniotic fluid, uterus, breasts, and increased blood and body fluids.

Nutrition is very important during pregnancy. In addition to increased caloric requirements, the woman needs to ensure adequate increases in certain vitamins and minerals. Specifically, additional protein is required to build fetal tissues, calcium for bone and tooth development, and iron for hemoglobin production. The latter is important not only for the fetus, but also for the mother. Most women need iron supplementation, often difficult when morning sickness is present. Dividing the pills and taking half in the morning and half at night can help. Conversely, taking the entire dose at bedtime may be beneficial. Early in the first trimester, folic acid is important to prevent neural tube defects. Current guidelines recommend that all women of childbearing age take a multivitamin with folic acid.

Exercise is important during pregnancy; it not only prepares for labor, but also promotes overall well-being. Later in pregnancy, nonweight-bearing exercise is best avoided to decrease knee, ankle, and abdominal muscle strain. Additionally, after the fourth month, exercising on the back should be avoided as the pressure might affect blood flow to the fetus. As the pregnancy progresses, a woman's center of gravity shifts and sports that might result in falling should be avoided.

Many hormonal changes occur during pregnancy and women may experience sudden changes in mood. In addition to morning sickness, common physical changes that occur include heartburn and constipation. Heartburn occurs more frequently in later pregnancy as progesterone increases, causing greater muscle relaxation of the lower esophageal sphincter. In addition, progesterone has also been implicated in constipation by slowing down the smooth muscle action of the bowel.

Infertility

Infertility is defined as the inability to conceive after one full year of unprotected sexual intercourse. It affects approximately 10–15% of U.S. couples, and its frequency is increasing. The reasons for the increase are multifactorial: first, women are delaying childbirth with resultant difficulties in conception (i.e., ovulatory dysfunction, etc.); second, the prevalence of sexually transmitted disease is increasing, with subsequent increased potential for fallopian tube damage and uterine adhesions; and third, more people are turning earlier towards infertility treatments. Studies have shown that the root of infertility can be traced to the woman in 30% of the cases, the man in 30%, and a combination or unexplained cause in 40%. A successful work-up therefore includes assessment of both partners.

The Woman

Criteria for defining infertility are dependent on the woman's age. The woman's anatomy and physiology should be evaluated to look for causes of her infertility. Prior to age 35, it is the inability to conceive for one full year that constitutes infertility; thereafter, only six months confers that diagnosis.

History and Physical. Eliciting from a patient whether she has a basic understanding of conception is important (i.e., ovulation will most likely occur two weeks prior to the next menstrual cycle and therefore, sexual intercourse on alternate days around this time is optimal for conception). Determination of ovulation may be accomplished through history alone. For example, a woman may note changes in her cervical mucus during her menstrual cycle or she may note characteristic ovulatory discomfort. In addition, ovulation predictor kits can be useful. Assessing previous alterations in pelvic anatomy are important, too, including a history of pelvic inflammatory disease, previous insertion of an intrauterine device, or previous pelvic surgeries.

Hormonal imbalances affect fertility; this may be evident if a patient has hirsutism, acne, obesity, or abdominal striae on examination. Also, on physical examination, pelvic masses or nodularities in the cul-de-sac may be detected.

Laboratory and Radiology. Following the history and physical examination, evaluation of ovulation should be completed. If irregular menses are present, then a pregnancy test is warranted. If not, serum progesterone should be measured seven days after ovulation; this marks ovulation for that specific cycle. If ovulation is present, further labs may not be indicated and treatment may proceed. However, if there is no ovulation, further testing is warranted, including thyroid studies to rule out hypothyroidism, prolactin levels to rule out pituitary adenomas, empty-sella syndrome, medication interactions or renal disease, and FSH to rule out premature ovarian failure or a hypergonadotropic state. If the partner's semen analysis is within normal limits, then hysterosalpingography (HSG) can be ordered to evaluate the patient's anatomy. This is the most facile test to evaluate for shape and patency of the uterus and fallopian tubes.

The Man

History and Physical. Relevant information includes review of his general health, including a history of childhood mumps, crytporchidism, pelvic radiation, and chemotherapy. A testicular examination should be performed to look for varicoceles.

Laboratory. A semen analysis should be performed, ideally prior to any invasive testing of the woman. If this is abnormal, then referral to an urologist for further work-up should be made.

Therapy. If both partners have been evaluated and the cause of infertility is deemed either anovulation or irregular ovulation, then pharmacological interventions such as clomiphene citrate can be introduced during the menstrual cycle. This results in ovarian stimulation. Clomiphene citrate can also be used if the woman is ovulatory, but other regimens are superior. At this point, it is appropriate to refer to a reproductive endocrinologist for further evaluation and potential therapies (Hanson & Dumesic, 1998).

Menstrual Irregularities

Premenstrual Syndrome

Premenstrual syndrome (PMS) is cyclic, and occurs during the luteal phase of menses, with a variety of changes in mood, behavior, and somatic function. The pathophysiology is multifactorial, involving both biological and psychosocial factors. Resolution of this syndrome occurs with menopause. The nature and severity of these symptoms vary from patient to patient. Up to 40% of women are estimated to experience symptoms sufficient to impair daily activity and affect relationships, with 5% of women severely affected. An accurate diagnosis is essential for successful management; other conditions can present with or be exacerbated by PMS symptoms.

Initial evaluation must include prospective charting of symptoms for at least two cycles; less than 50% of symptomatic women actually meet this diagnostic criterion. Physical symptoms include headache, bloating, and breast tenderness; psychological symptoms include irritability, depression, and decreased concentration. These must occur more frequently during the luteal phase in order to meet diagnosis for PMS.

A variety of treatments exist to ameliorate the symptoms. Addressing the most serious symptoms is usually the most effective short-term goal, while developing a comprehensive care approach is the long-term goal. Treatment may target either the luteal phase or the entire cycle. Nonspecific treatments include education about lifestyle, diet, and behavior modifications. Women who adopt these self-care measures have significant short- and long-term relief of symptoms. Luteal-specific medicines include vitamins (i.e., B_6) alone or in combination with evening of primrose oil, diuretics, nonsteroidal anti-inflammatory medicines such as ibuprofen, or anxiolytics such as diazepam. Continuous cycle medications include serotonergic antidepressants such as fluoxetine or anovulatory hormones. Some patients may also benefit from cognitive therapy.

Dysmennorhea

The two most common causes of amenorrhea and dysmenorrhea in women of reproductive age are pregnancy and chronic anovulation (dysfunctional uterine bleeding). Thus, if there is any bleeding abnormality, pregnancy must be ruled out. Chronic anovulation is a diagnosis of exclusion. There are five major classes of abnormal vaginal bleeding: (1) organic gynecologic diseases (i.e., cancer of endometrium, cervix, myometrium, or ovary; inflammation of vagina, cervix, endometrium, or fallopian tubes; pregnancy—intrauterine or ectopic), (2) systemic diseases (i.e., hypothyroidism, liver disease, chronic renal failure, and blood dyscrasias), (3) iatrogenic causes (i.e., contraceptives, other drugs, and intrauterine devices), (4) trauma, or (5) chronic anovulation.

As with most other diagnoses, a careful history and physical examination often elucidates the correct diagnosis. The first step requires determining ovulation status, based on prodromal symptoms and timing of bleeding. Confirmation may be obtained by charting basal body temperature, measuring serum progesterone during the luteal phase, or doing an endometrial biopsy during this time. Other laboratory tests include a pregnancy test, Pap smear, and complete blood count. Treatment depends on the diagnosis. For anovulatory bleeding (metrorrhagia), hormonal therapy is appropriate. For heavy bleeding (menorrhagia), standard oral contraceptive doses or high-dose nonsteroidal anti-inflammatory medicines may be effective.

Primary amenorrhea is defined as (1) no spontaneous uterine bleeding by age 14 in the absence of other secondary sexual characteristics or (2) no spontaneous uterine bleeding by age 16 with normal development. The definition of secondary amenorrhea requires the absence of uterine bleeding for 6 months in a woman with regular menses or 12 months in a woman with oligomenorrhea. The menses require a feedback mechanism between the hypothalamic-pituitary axis, the hormonally responsive uterus and the intact outflow tract; problems at any point in the pathway may cause amenorrhea. Common causes include organic gynecologic causes (congenital anomalies, pregnancy, premature ovarian failure, and intrauterine adhesions), other systemic diseases (thyroid disease, hyperprolactinemia, and hypothalamic or pituitary lesions), iatrogenesis (contraceptive steroids, gonadotropin suppressants, and psychoactive drugs), and chronic anovulation (related to excessive weight gain/loss or exercise, stress, or androgen excess).

The work-up is multistep: After the history and physical, laboratory tests should include a pregnancy test and thyroid and prolactin levels; if normal, then a progesterone-withdrawal test should be done to determine outflow tract patency and estrogen status. If withdrawal bleeding is present, then the patient is anovulatory. If no bleeding occurs, the patient has hypoestrogenic amenorrhea and follicle stimulating hormone and leutenizing hormone levels should be measured; if high, they signify premature ovarian failure and if low, they signify a hypothalamic or pituitary disorder. Common causes of hypothalamic amenorrhea include a history of weight loss, stress, or vigorous exercise. Treatment for those patients with adequate estrogen is cyclic progesterone; for those without adequate levels it should include hormonal therapy and calcium supplementation (Chadraiah, 1998; Daugherty, 1998; Kiningham, Apgar, & Shenk, 1996; Klein, 1996).

Breast Disease

Fibrocystic Changes

These are the most common of all benign breast conditions and are present in up to half of all premenopausal women. Approximately half of those affected are symptomatic. Fibrocystic changes are thought to be associated with an exaggerated response to estrogen and progesterone, hence their increased prevalence during the reproductive years. On biopsy, there are three definitive histological phases of breast tissue. Initially, the upper-outer quadrant is affected, with proliferation of stromal tissue sometimes causing induration and tenderness. The second stage involves the development of small cysts, which may be painful. In the late stage, the cysts enlarge and the pain abates. The most common presentation involves cyclic, bilateral breast pain and engorgement. Often, this pain is diffuse with multiple nodules on examination. Findings are most prominent prior to menstruation. The approach to treatment varies. Some benefit from needle aspiration of the cysts; others are aided by eliminating caffeine from their diet or switching to a low-salt diet; and yet others find relief with vitamin E or evening primrose oil supplements.

Fibroadenoma

After fibrocystic changes, fibroadenomas are the most common form of benign breast disease. Unlike fibrocystic changes, fibroadenomas remain constant throughout the menstrual cycle. They are generally slow-growing, firm, painless, and freely mobile masses comprised of a mixture of proliferating epithelial and supporting fibrous tissue. Generally, they are small in size, approximately two to three centimeters. As with other breast masses, after examination and imaging, they are usually biopsied and/or excised to definitively rule out malignancy (Beckmann et al., 1995).

Eating Disorders

These biopsychosocial syndromes encompass anorexia nervosa, bulimia, binge-eating disorders, and their variants. The morbidity and mortality of these illnesses are very high and are frequently potentiated by delay between the onset of symptoms and initiation of treatment. Noteworthy epidemiological factors include: (1) females are affected more commonly than males, usually during adolescence or young adulthood; and (2) industrialized societies across socio-economic (though usually upper and upper-middle class) and ethnic lines (though usually white) are affected more than nonindustrialized societies. Approximately half recover. An additional 30% of those affected have partial recovery. It is often a fluctuating illness, with periods of remission.

Strict diagnostic criteria exist for each category. For anorexia, the following four criteria must be met: (1) body weight < 85% of expected weight, (2) intense fear of weight gain, (3) inaccurate perception of own body, size, or shape, and (4) amenorrhea. For bulimia, there are also four criteria: (1) recurrent binge eating (at least two times a week for three months), (2) recurrent purging, (3) excessive exercise or fasting (at least two times a week for three months), and (4) absence of anorexia. For binge-eating disorders, the following four criteria exist: (1) recurrent binge eating, (2) marked distress with at least three of the following—eating very rapidly, eating until uncomfortably full, eating when not hungry, eating alone, feeling disgusting or guilty after a binge, (3) no recurrent purging, excessive exercise or fasting, and (4) absence of anorexia. Finally, atypical eating disorders exist when some, but not all, of the above criteria are present.

Anorexia usually develops in young women who perceive themselves as overweight. This perception becomes a preoccupation, with subsequent development of altered eating patterns. These alterations include either extreme restriction of food intake or restriction alternating with binge eating (binge-purge cycle) that ends with self-induced emesis, laxatives, or excessive exercise. Bulimia usually occurs in late adolescence after multiple failed diet attempts. Here, too, variations exist, with some inducing postprandial emesis, and others binging. Bingers often have accompanying feelings of guilt, shame, and low self-esteem. These latter symptoms make it easier to treat bulimics as their disease upsets them.

The complications of anorexia are primarily related to starvation, whereas those of bulimia are more related to the sequelae of the binge-purge cycle. Altered nutritional status can cause many physical problems, and careful history and physical examination, with additional laboratory tests as needed, are required. The examiner must inquire not only about dietary habits and weight fluctuations, but also about exercise habits and purging. The use of laxatives, enemas, and/or other medications must be addressed. On examination, height, weight, and body mass index should be evaluated. There are many signs and symptoms. They include orofacial effects (i.e., dental caries, enlargement of the parotid glands), cardiovascular effects (i.e., hypotension, prolonged QT, arrhythmias), gastrointestinal effects (i.e., decreased intestinal motility, constipation), endocrine and metabolic disarray (i.e., amenorrhea, hypokalemia, hyponatremia, hypoglycemia, hypothermia, and osteoporosis), renal effects (i.e., calculi) and integumentary effects (i.e., dry skin and hair, hair loss, lanugo, yellow-tinged skin). Overall, the clinical picture of anorexia suggests hypothyroidism or hypopituitarism, whereas that of bulimia depends on whether it is primarily a binge-illness or a purge-illness.

Psychological assessment is paramount to the evaluation of eating disorders as their pathophysiology includes not only genetic, neurochemical, and sociocultural parameters but also psychological ones as well. A culture of thinness pervades our society and women are constantly bombarded with this message, especially those in occupations/recreations that stress thinness (i.e., athletes, models, ballerinas, and actresses). Additionally, eating disorders are usually accompanied by other comorbid psychiatric illness, such as depression, which must be evaluated as well.

Treating existing problems and preventing further complications is the primary medical treatment goal. This is usually done on an outpatient basis; occasionally, inpatient management is required. A large component of treatment is educational. These illnesses exemplify how a multidisciplinary model involving physicians, nutritionists, and psychologists working together can treat a disease entity with a physician coordinating the medical/nutritional therapy and a psychiatrist/psychologist coordinating the psychosocial care of the patient. Psychotherapy has been shown to be quite helpful, be it individual or group psychotherapy, cognitive therapy, or family therapy. Finally, the selective serotonin-reuptake inhibitors have some use in the treatment of bulimia as this is often accompanied by an obsessive-compulsive disorder (Becker, Grinspoon, Klibanski, & Herzog, 1999; Herzog & Copeland, 1985).

Anxiety Disorders

Many people are affected by anxiety disorders, most commonly generalized anxiety disorders, panic attacks and social phobia. Often, symptoms are similar making differentiation between the various disorders difficult. Symptoms may be cardiac (i.e., chest pain, hyperventilation, tachycardia, and palpitations), neurologic (i.e., tremulousness, dizziness, lightheadedness, faintness, and headache), or gastrointestinal (i.e., nausea, vomiting, diarrhea, and abdominal pain). The disorders may overlap, as with panic disorder and accompanying anxiety. They are often chronic, with a remission-relapse cycle, and require a long-term treatment strategy. Symptoms commonly flare during times of stress or depression. Of note, patients may present with somatic complaints. Conversely, an underlying medical or different psychiatric condition may present with symptoms consistent with an anxiety disorder. Optimal treatment requires a combination of pharmacology and psychotherapy. Pharmacological intervention includes benzodiazepines, beta-blockers, tricyclic antidepressants, and selective serotonin reuptake inhibitors. Psychotherapeutic methods include brief interventions (i.e., supportive and cognitive approaches) and behavioral therapies (i.e., biofeedback and systematic desensitization).

Generalized Anxiety Disorders

This is the most common anxiety disorder. It is defined as unrealistic or excessive anxiety or worries about two or more life circumstances for greater than six months. Specific symptoms are categorized based on their relationship to motor tension, autonomic hyperactivity, and excessive vigilance. Often, this is a diagnosis of exclusion.

Panic Disorder

Diagnosis of panic disorder requires four spontaneous panic attacks within a four-week period, or one or more attacks followed by at least one month of persistent anxiety. Each attack is characterized by the sudden onset of multiple physical and psychological symptoms; all of these are related to adrenergic excess. Patients report fear of immediate death or loss of control. Episodes are self-limited and are normally short-lived, often resolving within 10–30 min. Panic disorder is often underdiagnosed since its clinical picture mimics many other medical conditions. Between episodic attacks, patients often suffer from anticipatory anxiety and agoraphobia.

Social Phobia

Patients with social phobia have a persistent, irrational fear of situations that may provoke embarrassment or humiliation, such as public speaking. Diagnosis requires an immediate phobic response to the specific situation with a recognized interference in subsequent work or social activity. These patients characteristically fear criticism, overreact to embarrassment, and uphold rigid ideas of appropriate behaviors (Walley, Beebe, & Clark, 1994; Weinstein, 1995).

THE MATURE YEARS

Menopause

Signs and Symptoms

Menopause may be surgical, with abrupt cessation of menses, or natural, with gradual decline in estrogen production when a woman is in her 30s and complete when no menses have occurred for a year. The average age of menopause in the United States is 52. There appears to be a genetic predisposition as to when women undergo menopause, as they tend to experience this at approximately the same age as their female relatives.

Initially, women notice a change in their usual cycle with irregular menses and either increased or reduced blood flow. Concurrently, vasomotor symptoms appear and include hot flashes, night sweats, and palpitations. Other symptoms that may be troubling are vaginal dryness and itching. These develop several years after menopause and may lead to an increased susceptibility to vaginitis and dyspareunia. There is an increased risk of urinary tract infections and stress incontinence. Emotional difficulties often appear at this time with wide mood swings, irritability, depression, and forgetfulness. These symptoms may be related to hormonal changes and/or related to lifestyle changes that happen to coincide with menopause.

Treatment Options

In 1992 the American College of Physicians (ACP) published clinical guidelines for counseling postmenopausal women about preventive hormone therapy. Differentiation must be made when beginning therapy for therapeutic reasons—symptoms of menopause versus prevention. The decision to begin hormone replacement therapy (HRT) should be a consensus between the patient and her physician and a discussion should be held discussing the merits and potential harms of therapy. Current recommendations include: (1) regardless of race, all postmenopausal women should consider HRT; (2) in women who have undergone hysterectomy, an estrogen without progestin should be given; (3) HRT should be continued in women with coronary heart disease who have been taking hormonal replacement for at least one year, although its role for primary prevention of coronary disease remains a subject of ongoing research and controversy; (4) HRT risks may outweigh benefits in women at risk for breast cancer.

Therapy Regimens. For those women without an intact uterus, estrogen monotherapy is sufficient. However, estrogen plus a progestin should be used in all other women. The progestin reduces the increased risk of endometrial cancer associated with unopposed estrogen in women with intact uteri. This can either be administered for 10–14 days per month or estrogen plus continuous progestin can be prescribed throughout the month.

When to Initiate Treatment and Treatment Duration. The ACP guidelines were developed with the 50-year-old woman as the prototypical patient. Commonly in clinical practice HRT is offered during the perimenopausal period. However, as most of the diseases that we are attempting to prevent are found later in life, there may even be benefit in initiating therapy in older women. When treating for menopausal symptoms, therapy should be limited secondary to the small, but probably real, increased risk for breast and endometrial cancers. The risk of these cancers rises with increased therapy duration. However, in those on HRT for risk reduction of cardiac disease, stoke, osteoporosis, and possibly Alzheimer's disease, long-term therapy should be advocated, as longer therapy is associated with maximal risk reduction.

Surveillance. For women taking estrogen plus progestin, pelvic examinations should be performed prior to initiation of treatment; however, there is no need for routine endometrial evaluation. If vaginal bleeding occurs (a) in women on cyclic estrogen plus progestin, other than at days 10–15 of the month (if the progestin is given on days 1–10) or (b) in women on continuous estrogen plus progestin therapy, and the bleeding is heavier, lasts longer, the cycle occurs more frequently than prior to HRT, or persists for longer, then endometrial evaluation by endometrial sampling, or alternatively monitoring by transvaginal ultrasound, should be performed.

Alternatives to HRT. There is a vast array of herbal and supplemental substances available in health food and drug stores that are unregulated by the FDA. These products are not regulated by the FDA, not standardized, and do not undergo the same rigorous testing as do regulated pharmaceuticals. Nonetheless, many of these products are in wide use. While some may confer potential benefit, others may cause terrible harm.

The FDA has not approved any herbal substance for use in the peri- or postmenopausal period. Black Cohosh (*Cimicufuga racemosa*) has been promoted in the lay press as effective for menopausal symptoms. There is some scientific evidence demonstrating estrogen-like activity with some efficacy in treating vasomotor symptoms, such as hot flashes, night sweats, palpitations. Long-term safety, however, has not been established. Another herb widely touted in the lay press is Dong Quai (*Angelica sinensis*); there is no evidence of its effectiveness in treating hot flashes when compared with placebo. Phytoestrogens, however, which are found in soy products and legumes, contain estrogenic substances and may have some of the beneficial effects of estrogen without the risks of synthetic hormones. There is currently intense scientific interest in this and studies are underway to determine the effectiveness and safety of these substances.

In addition to herbs, there are several natural hormones that are directly marketed to the public for control of perimenopausal symptoms. Melatonin, a product of the pineal gland, is produced in response to light-dark cycles. Its level declines with age and may be responsible for altered sleep cycles in the elderly. As perimenopause can be associated with sleep difficulty, women have used melatonin to improve sleep. There is no study to date that has evaluated the optimal dose of melatonin, and current evidence does not support its use. A note of caution should be mentioned when using unregulated natural hormones and amino acids. In 1989, tainted lots of an amino acid, L-tryptophan, led to disability and death.

Androgens have also been promoted for use during the peri- and postmenopausal period. Both DHEA and DHEA-S decline with age, regardless of menopausal status. Animal studies suggest that DHEA have age-attenuating effects. These effects include insulin-sensitivity, antiosteoporotic, antiobesity, cognition-enhancing, and immunity-augmenting. Recent data, however, shows that oral supplementation may lead to significant reduction in HDL cholesterol, the good form of cholesterol (Management of Perimenopause, 1999).

Cardiac Disease

The leading cause of death in the United States among women is heart disease, which accounted for 52% of all female mortality in 1992. Following menopause the risk of cardiovascular disease increases dramatically, presumably due to the waning protection of estrogen. Nonetheless, heart disease is underdiagnosed and undertreated in women. In addition, women have a worse prognosis than men following a heart attack. They are twice as likely to die than are males and have a higher mortality rate following coronary bypass surgery and angioplasty. Since women are generally older than men when they develop heart disease, they are more likely to have more significant comorbid illness.

The risk factors that contribute to cardiac disease in women are similar to those found in men. They include elevated blood pressure, cigarette smoking, elevated lipid levels, diabetes, family history of cardiac disease (in male relatives heart disease prior to age 50 and in female relatives prior to age 60), and increasing age. Several other factors that contribute to cardiac disease are obesity and sedentary lifestyle.

Hypertension

After age 50, women develop hypertension more than twice as frequently as men. Treatment of hypertension in women may reduce the incidence of coronary artery disease; however, the reduction in men is significantly greater.

Cigarette Smoking

Smoking cessation reduces the risk of heart attack by approximately 50%. It also reduces the risk of lung cancer, which accounts for approximately 61,000 deaths annually among women. Lung cancer is now the leading cancer cause of death in women, as it is in men, having recently surpassed deaths secondary to breast cancer.

Elevated Lipids

Men and women under the age of 20 have approximately similar lipid profiles. From the ages of 20 to 55, most men have higher total cholesterol levels than women; however, after the age of 55, cholesterol levels in women increase rapidly, presumably related to the decline in their estrogen levels. Of note, greater than 50% of women have elevated cholesterol and greater than 30% are candidates for drug therapy.

High-density lipoproteins (HDL, "good" cholesterol) and triglycerides (TG) levels have been shown to be more powerful predictors of coronary events in women than men. Recent guidelines set forth by the American Heart Association in conjunction with the American College of Cardiology recommend aggressive targets for HDL (≥ 45 mg/dl) and TG (≤ 150 mg/dl). Until more data is available, first line therapy should continue to be with HMG-CoA reductase inhibitors (the –statins) as hormone replacement therapy has not been shown to significantly benefit women with coronary heart disease.

Osteoporosis

Characterized as low bone mass and microarchitectural bone tissue deterioration, osteoporosis affects approximately 10 million women in the United States. Fifty percent of all white women will experience an osteoporotic fracture at some point in their lifetime. In 1995 osteoporotic fractures were responsible for 432,000 hospital admissions and cost $13.8 billion.

The World Health Organization defines osteoporosis as bone mineral density (BMD) two and one half or more standard deviations below that of a "young normal adult." There are nonmodifiable and modifiable risk factors for osteoporotic fractures. Among the nonmodifiable risks are history of adult fracture, family history of fracture in a first-degree relative, Caucasian race, increasing age, female sex, and dementia. Modifiable risks include low body weight (< 127 lbs.), current cigarette smoking, estrogen deficiency, sedentary life style, alcoholism, low calcium intake, and impaired eyesight. Additionally, there are a variety of medical conditions and medications associated with increased risk of osteoporosis. Some of the more common medical conditions include: chronic obstructive lung disease, hyperparathyroidism, insulin dependent diabetes mellitus, multiple sclerosis, pernicious anemia, rheumatoid arthritis, sarcoidosis, and severe liver disease. Medications that may increase risk of osteoporosis are aluminum, anticonvulsants, excessive thyroid hormone, glucocorticosteroids, heparin, lithium, and premenopausal use of tamoxifen.

Screening Recommendations

Bone mineral density testing is warranted in: (1) all postmenopausal women under age 65 with one or more risk factors for osteoporosis; (2) all women over age 65 regardless of additional risk factors; (3) postmenopausal women presenting with fractures; (4) women who are weighing benefits of therapy for osteoporosis and want to use BMD to aid in decision making, and (5) women who have been on HRT for prolonged periods.

Treatment

There are several different options currently available to women with osteoporosis. FDA-approved pharmocologic treatments include hormone replacement therapy, alendronate, raloxifene and calcitonin. HRT use decreases vertebral fractures 50–80% and reduces nonvertebral fractures approximately 25% when used for five years or more. With greater than 10 years of use there is an even greater reduction in fracture rate (see above discussion for the benefits and potential risks of HRT).

An option to HRT, alendronate sodium, a bisphosphonate that has been shown in well-conducted, randomized, controlled clinical trials, reduces the risk of osteoporosis. Alendronate must be administered on an empty stomach, first thing in the morning, 30 min prior to eating or drinking, with a large glass of water, to minimize esophageal symptoms such as heartburn and swallowing difficulties. Esophageal ulceration has been reported in less than 1% of recipients.

Raloxifene is the first drug in its class of SERMS, or selective estrogen receptor modulators, to be approved for prevention of osteoporosis. This "designer estrogen" not only reduces the risk of vertebral fractures in patients with osteoporosis but seems to decrease the risk of breast cancer as well. Similar to estrogen there is an increased risk of deep vein thromboses. In addition, hot flashes may occur with use (Cummings et al., 1999; Eastell, 1998; National Osteoporosis Foundation, 1998).

Incontinence

Urinary incontinence is defined as involuntary loss of urine sufficient to affect daily life. It affects approximately 10–35% of adults and is twice as prevalent in women as in men. Despite this high prevalence, most people do not seek medical attention since they feel uncomfortable discussing it with their caregivers. Many different factors have been implicated, including anatomical, physiological, and others. Once the specific risk factor has been identified, treatment can be targeted appropriately.

The work-up of incontinence includes a thorough assessment of the patient and identification of risk factors and reversible conditions. A complete history focusing on medical, neurological, and genitourinary function should be obtained; characteristics of the incontinence should be elicited, including duration, frequency, precipitants, other urinary tract symptoms, prior treatments, and treatment expectations. The physical examination should highlight the abdominal, rectal, and pelvic examinations, as well as direct observation of urine loss. Laboratory assessments should include a measurement of postvoid urine residual volume and a urinalysis. This basic evaluation often suffices.

The four most common types of urinary incontinence include urge, stress, mixed, and overflow incontinence. Others to consider include functional and unconscious or reflexive incontinence. Urge incontinence is defined as an abrupt involuntary loss of urine associated with a strong sensation of urinary urgency. Stress incontinence is characterized by involuntary urination with coughing, lifting objects, or sneezing. It is associated with weakness or invagination of the bladder. Mixed incontinence is a combination of both urge and stress incontinence. Finally, overflow incontinence occurs with bladder overdistention. Reversible conditions that either cause or contribute to urinary incontinence include: (1) drugs (i.e., diuretics, caffeine, anticholinergics, narcotics, alpha and beta adrenergics, and calcium channel blockers); (2) increased urine production (i.e., metabolic, increased fluid intake, volume overload); (3) lower urinary tract problems (i.e., urinary tract infection, vaginitis or atrophic urethritis, pregnancy/vaginal delivery/episiotomy, and stool impaction); and (4) impaired ability or willingness to reach a toilet (i.e., delirium, psychological, and restricted mobility).

Some patients require further evaluation, including women with uncertain diagnoses, treatment failures, those considering surgical intervention, those with hematuria without infection, or those with comorbid conditions. Specialized tests, including urodynamics, endoscopic, and imaging tests may all be utilized.

Treatment options include behavioral, pharmacological, and surgical modalities. Behavioral interventions include developing specific toileting programs and pelvic muscle rehabilitation. Supportive devices, such as catheters, may be needed. Pharmacological interventions include anticholinergics, tricyclic antidepressants, alpha-adrenergics, and estrogen replacement agents. Surgical options include various suspension procedures, implanting slings, and artificial sphincters (AHCPR, 1998; Bruskewitz, Ruoff, & Chancellor, 1999).

AGELESS ISSUES

Violence Against Women

In the United States approximately 4.5 million women between the ages of 18 and 65 are victims of domestic violence each year. Greater than 90% of domestic violence involves women abused by men, and approximately one in four women using the emergency department has a history of partner violence within the past year. During pregnancy, one in six women is abused every year in the United States and over 3 million children between ages 3 and 17 witness parental abuse. Violence cuts across all age, race, education, and socioeconomic lines. In 1994, the government enacted a federal law, the 1994 Violence Against Women Act, that provides measures for preventing violence against woman and includes a national toll-free hotline for information and referrals, the National Domestic Violence Hotline (1-800-799-SAFE). This law, while important for initiating action in those who break the law, serves an even greater role in signaling to those in need that they need not suffer in silence. The framework now exists to lend support and aid. Key, however, is primary prevention.

Although domestic violence is so widely prevalent, most medical professionals fail to recognize it in clinical practice due to a lack of clinical guidelines and discomfort in discussing the topic. Diagnosing domestic violence may be difficult due to its varied presentation. Findings range from specific physical signs, such as dental trauma and head and neck injuries, to more general complaints, i.e., chronic abdominal, pelvic, or chest pain, somatic disorders, irritable bowel syndrome, sexually transmitted diseases, or HIV exposure. Psychological symptoms, such as depression, anxiety and panic disorders, eating disorders, substance abuse or post-traumatic stress disorder may be the first manifestations of domestic violence. Other clinical indicators of abuse include delaying treatment for or poor explanation of injuries, repeat emergency room or clinic visits, and an overly attentive or verbally abusive partner. Simple, but important, screening questions include: "Do you ever feel unsafe at home?" and, "Has anyone at home hit you or tried to injure you in any way?"

Once abuse is admitted, caregivers must carefully document as precisely as possible evidence of abuse as the information may be needed for future medical practitioners and potential legal proceedings. It is imperative not to include the patient's address or phone number in the medical record as the abuser may be inadvertently given access to the patient's chart and seek retaliation. Providers should inform patients of resources and advocates that are available. Patients should be provided with the number of National Domestic Violence Hotline (see above) (Eisenstat & Bancroft, 1999; Leiman, Rothschild, Meyer & Kolt, 1998).

Cancer

Breast

The fear of breast cancer is universal among women despite the fact that it ranks second to heart disease as the leading cause of death in western society. In 1997, approximately 182,000 new cases of breast cancer were diagnosed and 44,000 people died of the disease. The most important risk factor for developing breast cancer is a positive family history. Other risk factors include increasing age, early menarche, late menopause, nulliparity, early exposure to ionizing radiation, long-term postmenopausal HRT, and alcohol ingestion.

Screening. Screening mammography and clinical examination by a trained practitioner have resulted in early diagnosis and a 25–30% reduction in mortality in women over the age of 50. Currently, controversy surrounds the efficacy of screening women below the age of 50. This has led to discrepancies in guideline recommendations as to when to initiate screening in patients with standard risk of developing breast cancer. The decision to screen women before the age of 50 should be individualized on a patient to patient basis after discussion of the risks and benefits of the screening test. Women from high-risk families, especially those who have the BrCa1 or 2 mutation should be screened beginning at age 25, or five years prior to the earliest age at which breast cancer was detected in a relative.

Diagnosis and Staging. For palpable masses, the standard diagnostic modality is fine needle aspiration or core needle biopsy. For suspicious, nonpalpable masses other modes such as ultrasound-guided core needle biopsy, stereotactic biopsy, and magnetic resonance-directed biopsy are useful. Staging is based on the internationally recognized TNM (tumor, node, metastasis) classification and groups patients according to the extent of their disease, for example, tumor extent, lymph node involvement, and the presence of metastatic spread to other areas of the body.

Therapy. Most breast cancer presents with subclinical metastatic disease in all but a small percentage of women. Therefore, treatment with adjuvant modalities, such as radiation and/or chemotherapy, is warranted in addition to surgical lumpectomy or modified mastectomy. It has now been established that breast-conserving lumpectomy with radiotherapy is adequate treatment for those with early breast cancer. This is contrary to past practice mandating treatment with radical mastectomy.

For women with noninvasive tumors greater than 2 cms in size or invasive tumors, lymph node dissection remains the standard of care. Newer modalities are being tested as alternatives to lymph node dissection because this is an invasive procedure and only useful as a prognostic modality and does not aid in treatment. However, until these alternatives are validated, lymph node dissection remains the standard of care.

Postmastectomy radiotherapy has been shown to decrease the incidence of local and regional recurrences by 50–75%. Until recently, however, this has not been shown to improve survival. In recent randomized trials in premenopausal women with high-risk breast cancer, survival was improved with radiotherapy when added to chemotherapy. In 1999, optimal treatment for women with primary breast cancer includes systemic chemotherapy and hormonal treatment. Using this approach has resulted in reduction in recurrence and improved survival. In addition to using chemotherapy postoperatively, it is now being used to shrink tumors preoperatively, thus allowing for a lumpectomy to be performed instead of the more disfiguring mastectomy.

Adjuvant systemic therapy, either chemotherapy or systemic hormonal therapy (tamoxifen in postmenopausal women, ovarian ablation in premenopausal women), given in the absence of demonstrated metastases has been shown to improve overall survival beyond 15 years. The indications for adjuvant therapy include invasive ductal or lobular carcinoma greater or equal to 1 cm in largest diameter with negative lymph nodes, invasive carcinoma greater or equal to 3 cm in largest diameter with negative lymph nodes, and invasive breast cancer with positive axillary lymph nodes regardless of size or histologic type. Combination chemotherapy has been shown to be more effective than individual agents and reduces the annual death risk by approximately 20%. This benefit persists for patients up to age 69, although the benefits are more substantial in younger patients.

Tamoxifen therapy significantly improves survival in all age groups, especially when given for five years and in those who have tumors with positive estrogen receptors. Treatment for greater than five years has not increased survival. Combination of chemotherapy and hormonal therapy further improves survival, especially for women with a high risk of disease recurrence. Discussion of therapy for metastatic breast cancer is beyond the scope of this chapter.

Ovarian

Screening. Epithelial cancer of the ovary predominantly affects postmenopausal women in their fifties and is the fifth most common malignant condition among women in the U.S. It is a lethal cancer, largely because it produces few initial symptoms and therefore most women present with advanced disease. Risk factors include family history, especially if two or more first-degree relatives have been affected, and uninterrupted ovulation, such as with nulliparity or a first birth after age 35. Conversely, a woman's risk can be decreased with childbirth, especially prior to age 25, or with oral contraceptives.

Two familial syndromes have been described, the hereditary breast-ovarian cancer syndrome and the Lynch syndrome II. Both of these, which occur in less than 5% of all ovarian cancers, have autosomal dominant inheritance patterns and tend to occur in younger women. The BrCa1 gene has been implicated in the former syndrome. For women at high risk, frequent screening includes measurement of Ca-125 and pelvic ultrasonography; these have not yet been recommended for general screening. Additionally, high-risk women may consider prophylactic oophorectomy after childbearing is complete.

Clinical presentation is often late in the course of this illness and varies based on the extent of disease. Common symptoms include abdominal fullness and early satiety secondary to ascites and omental tumor implants. On examination, these patients may have ascites, abdominal fullness, umbilical hernias, or lymphadenopathy (Sister Mary Joseph's node). Asymptomatic women are often diagnosed on routine pelvic exam. Occasionally, women may present with paraneoplastic symptoms. Studies utilized to evaluate a pelvic mass include Ca-125 measurements and pelvic ultrasonography. On ultrasound, suspicious masses are often complex and multicystic.

Diagnosis. Diagnosis requires exploratory surgery. Upon pathologic confirmation of epithelial ovarian cancer, staging and surgical treatment commence with a total abdominal hysterectomy, bilateral salpingo-oophorectomy, and omentectomy. Additionally, all of the serosal surfaces are examined, biopsies are taken of grossly involved areas, and peritoneal washings/ascites are sampled. Adverse prognostic factors include advanced stage of disease, high tumor grade, presence of residual disease after surgery, older age, and certain histologic subtypes.

Treatment. After staging laparotomy, chemotherapy may be considered. The standard regimen includes combination therapy with a platinum analog. For limited disease, Stages 1A and 1B, adjuvant chemotherapy does not improve survival. However, adjuvant chemotherapy does decrease recurrence in Stage 1C or 2. The majority of women present with Stage 3 and 4 disease. Despite advances in adjuvant chemotherapy protocols, overall five-year survival is still poor. Carboplatinum and taxol are often used in combination. In the past, second-look laparotomy was used to detect persistent disease. However, this is no longer routinely performed as it does not convey survival benefit. A newer therapeutic approach involves dose intensification. However, given the increased rates of toxicity with this therapy, many physicians are opting instead for high-dose carboplatinum followed by bone marrow transplantation with autologous peripheral blood progenitor cells. Theoretically, this allows for higher chemotherapy doses while ameliorating subsequent side effects.

Ovarian cancer that relapses is generally not amenable to cure. Following Ca-125 is a useful way to monitor relapses. Options for relapsed cancers include a second debulking surgery and second-line chemotherapy, intravenously or intraperitoneally (Cannistra, 1993).

Cervical

Screening. Invasive cervical cancer has become relatively uncommon since the development of widespread screening with the Pap smear in the United States. However, worldwide, especially in third-world countries, it remains a major cause of morbidity and mortality. This screening method detects precursor lesions in the cervical epithelium, often years before invasive cancer actually develops. Cervical cancer, has in effect, become preventable.

Precursor, intraepithelial lesions occur in younger women, often under age 40. The transformation into malignant invasive carcinoma has a long latency period and does not appear until the fifth or sixth decade of life. The intraepithelial lesions, also known as cervical intraepithelial neoplasia (CIN), are defined as a wide range of dysplastic changes confined to the epithelial layer. Multiple risk factors for CIN have been identified: sexual intercourse at an early age, multiple male sexual partners, male sexual partners who have had multiple sexual partners, and smoking. Immunosuppression may confer added risk.

Human papillomavirus has been found in both CIN and invasive cancer. Many subtypes of this virus are prevalent in the general population. Types 16, 18, 31, 33, and 35 are often associated with moderate dysplasia (CIN 2), severe dysplasia, or carcinoma in situ (CIN 3). They are also prevalent in the majority of patients with cervical cancer.

The data supporting the success of the Pap smear is retrospective data from both the U.S. and Europe. These data overwhelmingly demonstrate the effectiveness of mass screening, despite not utilizing the gold standard of scientific evidence, the randomized control trial. For example, the mortality in the U.S. decreased by 70% between 1947 and 1984. The results of the test are dependent on both the quality of the specimen and the accuracy of the cytological interpretation. In addition, the proper technique in obtaining the specimen must be utilized; specifically, the transformation zone must be adequately sampled. This is the boundary between the squamous epithelium of the exocervix and the columnar epithelium of the endocervix. However, since malignant transformation requires a long time, the shortcomings of obtaining and processing the sample are minimized, as there are multiple opportunities to perform the test. There is debate on the frequency of testing. Current guidelines recommend screening all women at 18 or after initiation of sexual activity; thereafter, after three consecutive negative smears, a low-risk woman can be tested less frequently.

Pap smears only indicate patients with premalignant or malignant changes, and a biopsy must be performed to definitively diagnose CIN or invasive cervical cancer. Currently, the Bethesda classification is used. This system uses two broad categories to define cytologic changes. First, low-grade squamous intraepithelial lesions (LGSIL) are associated with a heterogeneous group of histologic changes. Biopsies of these lesions often reveal CIN 1, which can spontaneously resolve or may reveal HPV without a CIN lesion. Occasionally, LGSIL is associated with the more severe forms of CIN, 2 and 3, which may transform into malignancy. Secondly, high-grade squamous intraepithelial lesions (HGSIL) usually correspond to CIN 2 and 3, and sometimes represent invasive carcinoma. In addition, a third category exists: atypical squamous cells of uncertain significance, ASCUS.

Once a Pap smear documents LGSIL, HGSIL, or ASCUS, further evaluation is required with colposcopy, a low-power magnifier, which identifies mucosal abnormalities characteristic of CIN or carcinoma. This procedure can both help identify suspicious areas that can be biopsied and determine the extent of atypia.

The treatment of CIN depends on histologic diagnosis and extent of disease. Biopsy-proven CIN 1 usually resolves spontaneously, requiring no further therapy. In contrast, CIN 2 and 3 require treatment to prevent malignant transformation. This can be accomplished with conservative, outpatient modalities, such as cryotherapy, laser vaporization, or loop electric excision procedure (LEEP). If these criteria cannot be met then a more aggressive, surgical approach, cervical conization or cone biopsy, with resection of a portion of cervical tissue, including the part of the endocervical canal, is appropriate.

Diagnosis. Unfortunately, invasive cervical cancer is often asymptomatic, with occasional reporting of vaginal discharge and postcoital bleeding. If patients present with extensive disease involving the pelvic lymph nodes, they may have lower extremity deep venous thromboses or ureteral obstruction. Again, biopsy is required for diagnosis and staging. Stage 1 disease is limited to the cervix. Stage 2 disease extends beyond the cervix to the upper two thirds of the vagina or the parametrial tissue but not to the pelvic sidewalls. In stage 3, the disease has spread to the pelvic sidewall, the pelvic nodes, or the lowest third of the vagina. Finally, in stage 4 disease, invasion of the mucosa of the bladder or the rectum or to distant sites occurs.

Treatment. Stage 1A, microinvasive disease, does not require extensive treatment. Often, a simple hysterectomy is sufficient; pelvic lymph-node dissection is not indicated because of the low likelihood of metastasis. Survival five years post-treatment surpasses 95%.

Most patients, however, who present with cervical cancer have stage 1B or 2A disease and must therefore undergo clinical staging with a pelvic exam, cystoscopy, proctoscopy, chest X-ray, and urinary tract imaging. Treatment consists of surgery, with radical hysterectomy and pelvic-node dissection, and/or radiotherapy, to decrease local recurrence. Five-year survival is 80–90%. In contrast, those with pelvic-node metastases have only a 45% five-year survival rate. Because radiotherapy may cause vaginal stenosis, women wishing to remain sexually active often opt for the hysterectomy.

Stage 2B, 3, and 4 must have radiotherapy, as surgery results in a high-risk of recurrence. Five-year survival is 65%, 40%, and 20%, respectively. Stage 4, in addition, often requires chemotherapy in an attempt to control systemic disease. Unfortunately, cervical cancer often relapses, either locally with pelvic and para-aortic adenopathy or distantly such as with lung and bone involvement. Most recurrences are both local and distant. Cisplatin is the agent of choice; palliative care is the goal. Chemotherapy has another use, too: studies show that it may have a role in the future in previously untreated patients with locally advanced disease as it may facilitate local resection, may eradicate micrometastases, and may function as a radiosensitizer (Cannistra & Niloff, 1996).

Uterine

Epidemiology. Uterine cancer is the fourth most common cancer in women in the U.S. Of the 10 most prevalent cancers in women, it is the most curable. The most common uterine type is endometrial cancer, which arises from the endometrial glands. Usually, it presents postmenopausally, on average in the seventh decade and its incidence increases with age. Risk factors include obesity, nulliparity, late menopause, diabetes, unopposed estrogen therapy, tamoxifen therapy, and the use of sequential oral contraceptives. Of note, most of these risks are related to elevated levels of estrogen, which stimulates the endometrium, resulting in endometrial hyperplasia. In addition, environment (i.e., diet, tobacco) and genetic factors (i.e., Lynch Syndrome II) are thought to play a role.

Diagnosis. Unlike ovarian cancer, endometrial cancer is usually diagnosed in its early stages because it generally presents with postmenopausal bleeding. As a woman ages, the likelihood that postmenopausal bleeding is a symptom of endometrial carcinoma increases. Therefore, postmenopausal bleeding must be evaluated with pelvic examination, Pap smear with endocervical evaluation, and endometrial biopsy. In addition, transvaginal ultrasound effectively measures endometrial thickness. Normal values depend on race and use of tamoxifen.

Treatment. Initial treatment is surgery with prognosis determined by the surgical and pathological findings. There are four stages: Stage 1A is limited to the endometrium; Stages 1B and C affect the myometrium. Stage 2A has endocervical glandular involvement and 2B has cervical stromal invasion. Stage 3A invades the serosa or adnexa, and may have malignant peritoneal cytology; 3B has vaginal metastases and 3C has pelvic or para-aorta lymph node involvement. Stage 4A involves the bowel or bladder mucosa, while 4B is characterized by distant metastases. There are three clinically significant histologic subtypes: endometrioid adenocarcinoma, clear-cell carcinoma, and papillary serous carcinoma. The latter two types present in older women. The last type, papillary serous, is extremely malignant. In addition to staging, a grade is given based on tumor architecture and reflecting the amount of nongland-forming tumor present. Grade correlates with extent of disease and is a predictor of survival. Vascular space invasion in the hysterectomy specimen portends adverse outcome and also correlates with depth of invasion and tumor differentiation. Finally, tumor size contributes to prognosis and rate of recurrence.

Clinically, endometrial cancer behaves differently in various cohorts. Younger women generally fare better, having better-differentiated tumors. However, there is some data to suggest that these same women present later and thus may not do as well. African-American women tend to have more poorly differentiated carcinomas despite decreased incidence. They also have other poor prognostic indicators, including deeper myometrial invasion, nodal metastases, and malignant peritoneal cytology.

Biologic markers for endometrial carcinoma include both estrogen and progesterone receptors with high levels correlating with better differentiation, less myometrial invasion, and decreased amount of nodal metastases. In addition, chromosomal measurements of tumor activity and mutations of the p53 tumor-suppressor gene are associated with a poor prognosis. The HER-2/*neu* gene, an important prognosticator in breast and ovarian cancer, is present in over 25% of patients with metastatic endometrial cancer.

The majority of women are treated surgically with total abdominal or vaginal hysterectomy and bilateral salpingo-oophorectomy, peritoneal cytologic sampling, and abdominal exploration. Depending on the pathology, further classification is made into low, intermediate, or high risk of recurrence. This helps determine appropriateness of adjuvant chemotherapy. High-risk cancers in stages 1–3 are offered radiotherapy; stage 4 may also benefit from chemotherapy or progestin therapy (Rose, 1996).

HIV Disease

Diagnosing and treating the human immunodeficiency virus (HIV) is similar in men and women, with the exception of pregnant women. Notably, throughout the 1990s, the proportion of women affected with HIV has continued to increase, predominantly through heterosexual intercourse. As this trend has continued to emerge, gender-specific issues have developed in the areas of disease transmission, reproductive concerns, and gender-specific infections and neoplasms.

Injection drug use was the predominate mode of transmission in the past. However, recently heterosexual intercourse has become the primary route of infection. Transmission from men to women is greater than from women to men. Although abstinence is the most effective mode of prevention, latex condoms when used correctly and consistently have helped to decrease the rate of transmission.

The majority of women infected with HIV are of childbearing age. Pregnancy outcomes do not appear to differ between women with and without HIV. The high-risk categorization of pregnant women with HIV relates more to coexisting high-risk factors such as injection drug use, poorer access to health care, and malnutrition than to the infection itself. Three modes of vertical transmission exist: across the placenta, through intrapartum spread, or while breastfeeding. Currently, zidovudine (AZT) is recommended to decrease the risk of transmission, as studies have shown that it reduces transmission rates by up to two-thirds.

Gynecologic health management decisions are quite considerable. Common gynecologic infections, such as candidiasis, HPV-associated diseases, and pelvic inflammatory disease (PID), require different treatment strategies in women with HIV. Candidiasis is the most common opportunistic mucosal infection in women; vaginal candidiasis of new onset or with increased frequency may be a woman's first sign of infection with HIV. In addition, the incidence and severity of PID depends more on a patient's high-risk behaviors than on merely being infected with HIV. In 1993, the CDC included invasive cervical carcinoma as an AIDS-defining diagnosis. More than their HIV-negative counterparts, these patients have cervical squamous abnormalities as well as greater frequency of concomitant HPV infection. The severity of the neoplasm correlates with the degree of immunosuppression; in addition, these patients have a greater degree of recurrence. Therefore, a more aggressive screening program exists for this population (Saglio, Kurtzman, & Radner, 1996).

Thyroid Disease

Hypothyroidism

Overt Hypothyroidism. Hypothyroidism is a result of an underproducing thyroid-gland, resulting in an elevation of thyroid stimulating hormone. The most widely prescribed treatment is levothyroxine, with the goal of restoring serum thyrotropin levels to normal. It often takes several weeks to titrate to the appropriate dose. Weight reduction and increases in pulse rate and blood pressure occur early on in treatment, but hoarseness, anemia and changes in skin and hair may take longer to resolve. Appropriate thyroid hormone replacement dose varies depending on the etiology of hypothyroidism. Thyroid levels need to be closely monitored as overtreatment may occur. If this happens, then clinical hyperthyroidism can occur. Over replacement increases the risk of decreased bone mineral density and the possible risk of osteoporotic fractures; under-replacement increases the risks of hypercholesterolemia and ischemic heart disease.

Subclinical Hypothyroidism. This condition results from either inadequate replacement therapy or spontaneously, most commonly as a result of chronic autoimmune thyroiditis. It is more prevalent in postmenopausal women than in the adult population as a whole. Diagnosis is made via detection on routine follow up of patients receiving replacement therapy or by screening patients with nonspecific symptoms, such as fatigue and weight gain. Although there is debate as to the benefits of treating subclinical disease, studies show that treatment leads to symptomatic relief and prevents progression to overt hypothyroidism.

Transient Hypothyroidism. Multiple etiologies exist for transient hypothyroidism, a mild asymptomatic hypothyroidism that lasts for several weeks. It may be secondary to the recovery phase of subacute or painless thyroiditis, spontaneously remitting chronic autoimmune hypothyroidism, the use of iodine-containing antiseptics applied vaginally during labor or topically to the skin of newborns, untreated or inadequately treated Addison's disease, or following subtotal thyroidectomy.

Ischemic Heart Disease. A small percentage of patients with long-standing hypothyroidism report angina. In patients who receive replacement therapy, this symptom may not remit; myocardial infarction and sudden death are well-recognized complications of hypothyroidism, even in patients on lose-dose replacement therapy.

Pregnancy. Hypothyroidism may occur during pregnancy, with increase in both fetal and maternal morbidity. Women with chronic autoimmune thryroiditis usually require less replacement therapy secondary to improvement during pregnancy. However, in most pregnant women, the serum thyrotropin levels increase, likely a result of an increase in the concentration of thyroxine-binding globulin during pregnancy. Also, transient hypothyroidism affects a small percentage of all women in the first six months postpartum; those with pre-existing chronic autoimmune thyroiditis are at greatest risk (Toft, 1994).

Hyperthyroidism

As opposed to hypothyroidism, hyperthyroidism is a result of an overactive thyroid gland. This condition is common, affecting women more than men. Treatment includes antithyroid medications, radioiodine, or surgery. If symptoms are absent, then serum thyrotropin and total or free thyroxine should be measured.

Graves' Disease. Graves' disease is the most common cause of hyperthyroidism, and it is an obvious diagnosis if the presenting signs include a diffuse goiter and ophthalmopathy.

Antithyroid agents include methimazole, carbimazole, and propylthiouracil. Their principle mechanism of action is inhibition of the organification of iodide and coupling of iodothyronines. Additionally, the former two have immunosuppressive actions and the latter drug inhibits peripheral conversion of T4 to T3. Treatment goals in Graves' disease are (1) to induce a remission during treatment or (2) to achieve an euthyroid state prior to radioiodine therapy or surgery. If compliance is not an issue, antithyroid drugs are an effective means of controlling hyperthyroidism. Beta-adrenergic antagonists, i.e., propranolol, can be used in the short term to treat some of the symptoms of hyperthyroidism, including tremor, anxiety, and palpitations.

Radioiodine therapy aims to destroy enough thyroid tissue to cure hyperthyroidism. It can be first-line therapy for Graves' hyperthyroidism and it is also used for recurrent hyperthyroidism and after antithyroid agents have been used. The ultimate goal of this modality is eu- or hypothyroidism. If hypothyroidism develops, then thyroid hormone replacement with levothyroxine is necessary. Subsequent withdrawal of medication and reassessment of levels should occur, as continued therapy may not be indicated.

Subtotal thyroidectomy can be performed after maintaining an euthyroid state on medications, thus reducing the risk of postoperative thyrotoxic crisis. Relapse after surgery may occur or hypothyroidism may develop.

Toxic Adenoma or Toxic Nodular Goiter. These conditions are suspected in patients with hyperthyroidism but no goiter or ophthalmopathy and are more common in the middle-aged and the elderly populations. Physical examination followed by a radionuclide scan confirms the diagnosis; uptake into a single nodule or patchy uptake into more than one hyperfunctioning nodule may be present.

Since these are permanent causes of hyperthyroidism, without spontaneous remission, long-term medical therapy is inappropriate. The most appropriate treatment is radioiodine with adjunctive medical therapy such as beta-blockers when needed.

Thyroiditis. Subacute thyroiditis should be suspected when thyroid pain and tenderness accompany hyperthyroidism. Silent thyroiditis should be suspected

when hyperthyroidism lasts several weeks, without goiter or extrathyroidal manifestations of Graves' disease. These latter symptoms typify postpartum thyroiditis, which occurs in the first six months postpartum. The mechanism of action
in all these various forms of thyroiditis involves unregulated, inflammation-in-
duced release of stored T4 and T3. On uptake studies, radioiodine is low and
treatment with antithyroid medicines or radioiodine is ineffective. Fortunately,
the disease is usually mild and transient, often requiring no treatment. The pain
and inflammation of subacute thyroiditis can be treated with salicylates and
glucocorticosteroids. In all forms of thyroiditis, transient hypothyroidism usually occurs, occasionally requiring short-term thyroid replacement therapy.

Pregnancy. Hyperthyroidism may occur in pregnancy. The preferred treatment
is with an antithyroid medication at the lowest possible dose. Propylthiouracil is
preferred over methimazol for both pregnant and lactating women since less
crosses the placenta and only small amounts are found in breast milk.

Thyrotoxic Crisis (Thyroid Storm). Thyrotoxic crisis is a medical emergency defined as severe clinical hyperthyroidism, with marked tachycardia, fever, agitation, and weakness. Supportive measures, including fluids and
glucocorticosteroids, should be given in addition to treatment with antithyroid
medicines, potassium and beta-blockers (Franklyn, 1994).

Alternative Health Issues

Current surveys now suggest that as many as 40% of Americans use alternative
health options, and therefore alternative health has become an important adjunct to Western medicine. A variety of therapies exist, both behavioral and clinical. The National Institutes of Health Office of Alternative Medicine has defined
seven categories of alternative health: mind-body interventions,
bioelectromagnetic therapies, alternative systems of medical practice (i.e., acupuncture, homeopathy), manual healing methods (i.e., chiropractice, infant
massage), pharmacological (i.e., herbs) and biologic treatments, herbal medicine,
and diet and nutrition.

Most of the people who seek alternative health models have already tried
conventional, Western approaches. When these fail, patients may look for something new. Sometimes, patients are merely looking for complementary therapies.

Mind-Body Intervention

Common interventions include biofeedback, relaxation, meditation, hypnosis,
and imagery all based on the mind-body connection. Research has shown some
efficacy with treating common medical conditions such as hypertension, asthma,
and chronic pain. More body-oriented therapies, such as t'ai chi and yoga, have

been shown to enhance cardiovascular and immune function while simultaneously improving balance and flexibility. These are important factors in potentially decreasing the fall rate in elderly patients. These techniques may be individualized or may be used by support groups.

Electromagnetic Therapies

The utilization of bioelectromagnetic therapies involves multiple modalities. Electrical current has helped heal fractures. Transcutaneous electrical nerve stimulation has been used to treat pain. Some researchers also feel that effects of bioelectromagnetism may be involved with other alternative therapies, such as acupuncture and homeopathy.

Alternative Systems of Medical Practice

Indian Ayurveda and classical Chinese medicine are examples of alternative systems of medical practice. Research has attempted to prove their efficacy. In addition, a relatively newer system that developed as a reaction to conventional practices, homeopathy, was created in the 1700s. It is based on a "doctrine of similars" and utilizes tiny doses of various substances that in larger doses would create the symptoms that it is trying to treat.

Manual Healing Methods

Therapy with osteopathy, chiropractic manipulation, physical therapy, and massage therapy are some of the manual healing methods currently available. In addition, therapeutic touch has been shown to enhance physiologic function.

Pharmacological and Biologic Treatments

Most of these treatments are not accepted in conventional practices; rather, they are reserved for patients with life-threatening conditions desperate for any therapeutic intervention. Examples include chelation and shark cartilage therapy.

Herbal Medicine

Herbs are the original healing system and are still the mainstay in many indigenous populations throughout the world. Traditional herbalists use small amounts of many different herbs to treat a specific individual disease.

Diet and Nutrition

This approach is either used for prevention or treatment and dates back to Hippocrates. Pesticides and modern techniques of food preparation have been implicated in multiple illnesses, thus encouraging alternative dietary approaches. Diet modification or the use of supplements is used. Most of existing research supports individual therapies, such as the current recommendation that women of childbearing age take folic acid to help prevent neural tube defects (Gordon, 1996).

Lifestyle Issue

Obesity and Exercise

Over 3 out of 5 of American women are overweight and only 20% regularly exercise. Research has shown that exercise improves overall health and quality of life. Unfortunately, most Americans maintain sedentary lifestyles. The burden, then, is on health care professionals to encourage patients to participate in physical activity, be it structured or not. Patients should accumulate 30 min or more a day on most days of the week to achieve maximum benefit. Exercise impacts on longevity, heart disease, diabetes, obesity, osteoporosis, and mental health.

Sedentary lifestyle is a significant risk factor for heart disease. In addition, patients with inactive lifestyles have increased mortality and reduced quality of life. Healthy People Initiative 2000 aims to have 30% of those over six years of age engaged in light to moderate activity daily and 20% of adults involved at least three times a week in activity sufficiently rigorous enough to sustain their cardiorespiratory fitness.

Office visits provide a unique opportunity to educate patients about exercise. Only a selected group of high-risk individuals merit pre-exercise testing. Selection of the appropriate activity is important, taking into account the patient's fitness level, interests and resources. Patients also need instruction on duration, intensity, and frequency of exercise (Jones & Eaton, 1995).

Alcoholism

Women drink less than men, have lower rates of alcohol problems, and account for approximately one-third of all alcoholics. Because of this, female alcoholics are less likely to be diagnosed than males. The highest rates of alcohol-related problems (i.e., driving under the influence or interpersonal conflicts) occur in the youngest age group, ages 21 to 34. Married women tend to have the lowest overall problem rate. Generally, women begin drinking at a later age than their male counterparts but enter treatment at the same age. Additionally, they are more likely to have a history of depression with or without suicide attempts, anxiety disorders, abuse of other substances (especially abuse of sedatives, tranquilizers, and amphetamines), and low self-esteem. Women alcoholics have a higher mortality rate than their male counterparts and nonalcoholic women (Blume, 1986).

TABLE 9.1. Current Screening Recommendations

	> 18 years old	> 40 years old
Physical	Height and weight every one to three years Blood pressure every two years Skin exam not recommended unless suspicious lesions noted	Breast exam every year
Laboratory	Cholesterol every five years Syphilis, gonorrhea, and, if multiple sexual, partners Tuberculin skin test (ppd) If exposed or high-risk Chest X-ray not recommended PAP smear every one to three years	Urinalysis for > 60 years Bone mineral density if high-risk or estrogen therapy being considered for osteoporosis prophylaxis Mammography every two years between 40 and 49, and yearly > 50 years old Stool for occult blood > 50 years old every one year Sigmoidoscopy > 50 years every three to five years
Counseling	Well-balanced diet, behavioral modification and exercise to maintain prevent obesity, including a low-fat diet high in fiber and low in salt Calcium intake to equal 1200 mg per day, through food or supplements All menstruating women should have adequate iron intake Counsel re: STD prevention, unintended pregnancy, and contraceptive options Actively counsel patients re: smoking cessation, alcohol consumption, and illicit drug use Counsel re: seatbelts, maintenance of smoke detectors, guns, and violent behavior Encourage dental hygiene every year Remain alert for signs and symptoms of stress, depression, abuse	Encourage safety in home and community to decrease risk of falls
Immunizations	Tetanus-diphtheria vaccine every ten years	Influenza vaccine each fall Pneumovax > 65 years old and revaccinate in five years

CURRENT SCREENING RECOMMENDATIONS

Over the years, the annual physical examination has evolved from a head to toe evaluation to a rational, tailored periodic health visit based on a particular patient's risk of disease. When screening for disease, the aim is prevention of morbidity and mortality, thus necessitating tests that are highly sensitive and specific for disease. Therefore, prior to recommending preventive services, careful evaluation of the evidence supporting various screening tools must be undertaken.

Three expert panels, the U.S. Preventive Services Task Force, the American College of Physicians and the Canadian Task Force, in addition to other specialized societies (i.e., the American Cancer Society), have evaluated preventive health services based on the strength of scientific evidence currently available. What follows is a brief overview of current evidence-based screening recommendations in low-risk females (Table 9.1).

Physical examination should include measurement of blood pressure at every physical visit and at least every two years in all patients regardless of age. For women older than 40, annual breast examination is recommended. Beginning in early adulthood, serum cholesterol should be measured every five years. While there is a consensus of opinion on the need for annual mammography in all women over the age of 50, controversy still surrounds the recommendation for screening mammography between the ages of 40 and 49. All panels recommend cervical cytology screening for sexually active women every one to three years, beginning at the age of first intercourse. Colon cancer screening over the age of 50 either with three fecal occult blood tests or with flexible sigmoidoscopy should be performed every three to five years. In the future, screening colonoscopy may become the preferred method of screening. However this is currently controversial. After age 65, if there has been regular screening with normal results, further testing is unnecessary. Annual influenza vaccination should be offered to all females over the age of 65. Pneumococcal vaccination should be administered at age 65 and at five-year intervals thereafter. Counseling on smoking cessation, alcohol and drug use, seatbelt use, adequate nutrition (including calcium) and exercise, injury prevention, daily dental hygiene, and functional assessment (elicitation of marital and sexual problems) should be performed (Mosca et al., 1999b; Sox, 1994).

REFERENCES

AHCPR Urinary Incontinence in Adults Guideline Update Panel. (1996). Clinical practice guidelines: Managing acute and chronic incontinence. *American Family Physician, 54*, 1661–1672.

Baird, D. T., & Glaser, A. F. (1993). Hormonal contraception. *New England Journal of Medicine, 328*, 1543–1549.

Becker, A. D., Grinspoon, S. K., Klibanski, A., & Herzog, D. B. (1999). Eating disorders. *New England Journal of Medicine, 340,* 1092–1098.

Beckmann, C. R. B., Ling, F. W., Barzansky, B. M., Bates, G. W., Herbert, W. N. P., Laube, D. W., et al. (1995). *Obstetrics and gynecology* (2nd ed., pp. 235–237). Baltimore: Williams and Wilkins.

Blume, S. B. (1986). Women and alcohol: A review. *Journal of the American Medical Association, 256,* 1467–1470.

Bruskewitz, R. C., Ruoff ,G. E., & Chancellor, M. B. (1999). Ending the silence about urinary incontinence: New treatment options for bladder control disorders. Proceedings of a symposium. *Consultant, 39,* 56–59.

Cannistra, S.A. (1993). Medical progress: Cancer of the ovary. *New England Journal of Medicine, 329,* 1550–1559.

Cannistra, S. A., & Niloff, J. M. (1996). Cancer of the uterine cervix. *New England Journal of Medicine, 334,* 1030–1038.

Chandraiah, S. (1998). Premenstrual syndrome—An update. *Resident Staff Physician, 44,* 67–69.

Cummings, S. R. et al. (1999). The effect of raloxifene on risk of breast cancer in postmenopausal women: Results from the MORE randomized trial. *Journal of the American Medical Association, 281*(23), 2184–2197.

Daugherty, J. E. (1998). Treatment strategies for premenstrual syndrome. *American Family Physician, 58,* 183–192.

Eastell, R. (1998). Treatment of postmenopausal ssteoporosis. *New England Journal of Medicine, 338,* 736–746.

Eisenstat, S. A., & Bancroft, L. (1999). Domestic violence. *New England Journal of Medicine, 341,* 886–892.

Franklyn, J. A. (1994). Drug therapy: The management of hyperthyroidism. *New England Journal of Medicine, 330,* 1731–1738.

Gordon, J. S. (1996). Alternative medicine and the family physician. *American Family Physician, 54,* 2205–2212.

Hanson, M. A., & Dumesic, D. A. (1998). Initial evaluation and treatment of infertility in a primary-care setting. *Mayo Clinic Proceedings, 73,* 681–685.

Harris, J. R., Lippman, M. E., Veronesi, U., & Nillett, W. (1992). Medical progress: Breast cancer. *New England Journal of Medicine, 327,* 319–328.

Heath, C. B., & Heath, J. M. (1995). *Chlamydia trachomatis* infection update. *American Family Physician, 52,* 1455–1461.

Herzog, D. B., & Copeland, P. M. (1985). Eating disorders. *New England Journal of Medicine, 313,* 295–303.

Hotobagyi, G. B. (1998). Treatment of breast cancer. *New England Journal of Medicine, 339,* 924–1018.

Jones, T. F., & Eaton, C. B. (1995). Exercise prescription. *American Family Physician, 52,* 543–550.

Judson, F. N. (1990). Sexually transmitted diseases: Gonorrhea. *Medical Clinics of North America, 74,* 1353–1365.

Kiningham, R. B., Apgar, B. S., & Shenk, T. L. (1996). Evaluation of amennorhea. *American Family Physician, 53,* 1185–1194.

Klein, T. A. (1996). Office gynecology for the primary care physician, part two: Pelvic pain, vulvar disease, disorders of menstruation, premenstrual syndrome, and breast disease. *Medical Clinics of North America, 80,* 325–332.

Leiman, J. M., Rothschild, N., Meyer, J. E., & Kolt, A. (1998). *Addressing domestic violence and its consequences: Report of the commonwealth fund commission on women's health,* New York: Columbia University.

Lurie, N., et al. (1993). Preventive care for women—Does the sex of the physician matter? *New England Journal of Medicine, 329,* 478–482.

Management of perimenopause: Focus on alternative therapies. (1999). *Cleveland Clinic Journal of Medicine, 66,* 213–218.

Mosca, L., Grundy, S. M., Judelson, D., King, K., Limacher, M., Oparil, S., et al. (1999a). *Circulation, 33,* 1751–1775.

Mosca, L, Grundy, S. M., Judelson, D., King, K., Macher, M., Oparil, S., et al. (1999b). Guide to preventive cardiology for women. *Circulation, 99,* 2480–2484.

National Osteoporosis Foundation. (1998). *Physician's guide to prevention and treatment of osteoporosis.*

Newkirk, G. R. (1996). Pelvic inflammatory disease: A contemporary approach. *American Family Physician, 53,* 1127–1135.

Reife, C. M. (1996). Office gynecology for the primary care physician, part 1: Vaginitis, the papanicolaou smear, contraception, and postmenopausal estrogen replacement. *Medical Clinics of North America, 80,* 299–303.

Rose, P. G. (1996). Medical progress: Endometrial cancer. *New England Journal of Medicine, 335,* 640–649.

Saglio, S. D., Kurtzman, J. T., & Radner, A. B. (1996). HIV infection in women: An escalating health concern. *American Family Physician, 54,* 1541–1548.

Schwartz, M. H. (1994). *Textbook of physical diagnosis: History and examination* (2nd ed., pp. 19–20). Philadelphia: W. B. Saunders.

Shelton, D. L. (1997). Not just little men. *American Medical News, 2,* 14–17.

Sobel, J. D. (1997). Vaginitis. *New England Journal of Medicine, 337,* 1896–1903.

Sox, H. C. (1994). Preventive health services in adults. *New England Journal of Medicine, 330,* 1589–1595.

Toft, A. D. (1994). Drug therapy: Thyroxine therapy. *New England Journal of Medicine, 331,* 174–180.

Walley, E. J., Beebe, D. K., & Clark, J. L. (1995). Management of common anxiety disorders. *American Family Physician, 50,* 1745–1753.

Weinstein, R. S. (1995). Panic disorder. *American Family Physician, 52,* 2055–63.

Treatment

10

The Impact of Stress
and the Objectives
of Psychosocial Interventions

LUIZ R. A. GAZZOLA
PHILIP R. MUSKIN

This chapter will review the impact of stress on people as well as the impact of medical illness as a stressor. The goals of all psychosocial interventions are determined by the stress on the individual and the coping skills available to that person. The objectives of the interventions are to increase the patient's experience of control, to reduce stress, to enhance the person's resilience, to enable the person to use the most effective coping skills, and to maximize the support available from family and friends. These objectives must take into account the individual's prior abilities, his or her personality style, and the existing support system. We will describe these various components and the research that has been done in each of these areas. The role of the physician responsible for the care of the patient and the role of mental health professionals in providing psychological support to medically ill patients will be described briefly.

SCOPE AND LIMITATIONS OF SUPPORT

An insufficient amount of attention is paid to the consequences caregivers face in providing support. The deleterious consequences of support provision may be substantial. Those close to the recipient may become emotionally drained from the long-term provision of support that the recipient may be unable or unwilling to reciprocate (Belle, 1982). Women are at particular risk because they are more likely to be called upon as caregivers. It is important to assess these risks and assist in developing mechanisms for reducing them when evaluating patients and their families.

ASSESSING SUPPORT POTENTIAL

No one gets far or feels well for long without drawing on someone significant or something held valuable that sustains the effort to cope. When assessing support potential, the professional must pay attention to a large number of social and psychological issues in order to identify both resources and pressure points where trouble might arise. We will examine some of these areas.

Resources and Pressure Points

Health and Well-Being

It is important to assess the patient's general health, paying attention to organs and systems not involved in the current injury or illness. As a rule, the healthier the patient is, the better and faster recovery will be. Equally important is to determine the level of well-being prior to the present crisis. Overlooking the fact that a patient was already functioning at a lesser level of self-satisfaction could create unrealistic expectations. Intervention in a crisis situation will be successful if the prior level of functioning is restored, leaving to more long-term management the effort to raise the baseline well-being.

Support Providers

These same aspects must be assessed in potential support providers. Persons who have low levels of well-being are often ineffective supporters. They may feel resentful in switching roles and being called on to provide support when they feel entitled to being supported themselves. The health of providers plays a significant role in the potential to give support. A young and healthy spouse may be more likely to be effective than a frail, elderly grandmother. There is the potential for guilt feelings in the patient when there is a perception that support will drain someone who is already burdened with his or her own issues.

Family Responsibility

Patients may react differently to illness according to their status in their families. Bread winners or parents with young children may feel devastated and guilty when they anticipate the consequences of their illness to the welfare and safety of their family members. Persons who identify themselves as authority figures may be able to draw upon their inner resources and adopt a serene, reassuring attitude. Regarding the support provider's side, it is important for the health professional to understand the patient's family structure, identify the main players, and identify the ultimate sources of authority who can be called upon to assure the stability of the family. Cultural aspects of family structure are crucial in the accurate evaluation.

Marital and Sexual Roles

Few resources are as powerful to pull someone through a difficult illness than a supportive spouse or significant other. The opposite is also true; troubled relationships may be aggravated by illness in one of the partners. A number of conditions interfere profoundly with sexual capacity and with one's self-image as a sexual being, such as cardiovascular illness, surgical procedures involving ostomies, and strokes that result in paralysis. Even in the absence of these objective difficulties, the simple fact that one is ill may generate insecurities and performance anxiety. Both the patient and his/her partner may need counseling and reassurance to overcome these concerns.

Employment and Money

Employers and coworkers can be either a resource or a threat to the patient. Job security will aid in keeping a sense of self-worth and importance throughout the illness. The absence of knowing that one's job awaits increases the distress associated with illness, especially when the outcome of the illness itself can impact on the patient's professional capacities. It is important to assess the availability of vocational rehabilitation services. Financial burdens from lost revenue and medical expenses will play an equally important role in the patient's recovery. Thus the identification of potential sources of financial support in certain cases deserves as much consideration as psychological support. Twenty-four percent of patients exhaust their life savings in treatment for serious illness (Covinsky, Landefeld, Tero, & Connors, 1996).

Community Expectations and Approval

These are potential sources of both support and stress. The patient's social status in his or her environment can be very important in fostering a sense of being surrounded and of having an uninterrupted identity and self worth. However, the fear that these expectations will not be met because of limitations imposed by the illness can add to the patient's discomfort. Certain conditions are heavily stigmatized by society and can be sources of shame, such as AIDS, mental illness, and substance-induced disorders. Issues of confidentiality and disclosure will be paramount in addressing these concerns therapeutically.

Religious and Cultural Demands

Religion can be an extremely powerful force in maintaining someone through difficult times. Religious beliefs can conflict with medical care (e.g., Jehovah Witnesses, or believing that treatment is unnecessary). Cultural mistrust of health care providers in favor of various kinds of naturalistic healing techniques is another example of the issues that may have to be considered. Family members may support convictions that are deleterious to the patient's care. Respect for beliefs combined with a patient's guidance on the medical realities of health care will be instrumental in exploring how religion can be of support to the patient.

Self-Image and the Patient's Sense of Adequacy

A positive self-image is highly predictive of the patient's adaptability, but it can be profoundly shaken by illness. It is important for most people to perceive themselves as competent, adequate adults. Regression to more dependent and infantile positions is a possible consequence of illness. Grief for actual or anticipated loss of capacities may damage a patient's self-image. The health care provider must convey the sense that the core of one's worth is not directly related to illness, and when possible also provide reassurance that with recovery the person will return to his or her former self.

Existential Issues

Life and death have different meanings for different people and relate to their ethical, religious and cultural background and standards. Such issues are often not discussed in day-to-day medical practice but can be incorporated without an undue burden of time. Understanding how the patient situates himself or herself in regard to these issues is one essential step to maximize support. These issues cannot be adequately addressed without the physician engaging in a more thorough discussion and understanding of areas not typically a part of routine history taking, such as the meaning of life. In the absence of such discussions an angry response from a patient receiving a diagnosis of cancer may be mistaken as evidence of a "difficult patient." This response might actually reflect the person's belief that prior suffering in life should exempt him from other of life's misfortunes.

Group Differences and Psychosocial Support

In assessing and fostering support, the health care provider must take these important differences into consideration.

Social Class Differences

It was once believed that people with lower socioeconomic status were exposed to more stressful life experiences than those with more advantaged social status, and that this accounted for higher rates of psychiatric disorders in socially disadvantaged classes. Empirical demonstration of this assumption failed. Stressful life experiences, although not more prevalent in the lower socioeconomic class, do have a greater capacity to provoke mental health problems in members of the lower socioeconomic class than in members of the middle class (Kessler, 1979). One of the most plausible explanations is that one's experience as a member of a particular class leads to the development of individual differences in coping capacity as well as to differences in access to interpersonal coping resources. There is also some evidence that personality characteristics associated with vulnerability to stress, such as low self-esteem, fatalism, and intellectual inflexibility, are more common among people in lower socioeconomic class (Wheaton, 1980). It was also documented that people in lower socioeconomic class have fewer confidants than those in the middle class (Brown & Harris, 1978), which contributes to their vulnerability to undesirable life events.

Gender Differences

Community surveys show that adult women are twice as likely as men to report extreme levels of distress (Kessler & McRae, 1981). It has been speculated that women are disadvantaged relative to men because their roles expose them to more chronic stress. Female role stresses are particularly pronounced in traditional role situations. Although aggregate analysis of life-event inventories show that women are, on the average, more vulnerable than men, there are some events for which this is not true. Research on widows, for example, shows that women adjust better than men. Women also adjust as well or better than men to divorce. Financial difficulties do not affect women as much as men. Their greater vulnerability is primarily associated with events that occur to people close to them—death of a loved one other than a spouse being the most commonly reported event. One component of this difference is linked to the fact that women provide more support than men and that this creates stresses and demands that can lead to psychological impairment (Belle, 1982). Another speculation is that women might be more empathic than men, or might extend their concern to a wider range of people (Kessler, Price, & Wortman, 1985).

Ethnic Differences

Studies have shown greater exposure and vulnerability to undesirable life events among non-whites (Kessler, 1979). Minority status and the life experiences associated with it are not themselves instrumental in creating mental health problems once socioeconomic factors are controlled (Kessler, 1983). A way to understand this observation is that minority status, although related to experiences of prejudice and discrimination, is also related to structural resources that can help protect against the adverse effect of these stresses (Kessler & Neighbors, 1983). There seems to be a stress-buffering effect of group solidarity among members of deprived groups. The group provides cognition that identifies responsibility for their deprivation with structural conditions, thus removing any self-blame. The group also provides emotional support that can buffer the effects of stress in a variety of ways.

PERCEPTION OF PERSONAL CONTROL

Types of Control

Control over Ones Personal Environment, Power, and Position

To control is to exercise authoritative or dominating influence over something. Human beings learn from the very beginning of their existence how to control their body and their environment. The ability to control is closely linked to one's survival. In all aspects of life this central function can be identified. A person starts by controlling bodily functions such as bowel and bladder movements, ingestion of food and water, motor coordination, and so forth, up to the control of one's personal environment including clothing, shelter, territorial limits, proximity of other human beings, etc. Personal power in family and social structures therefore become one of the most important aspects of one's identity. Changes in the structure of how a person's experience of being in or out of control are profoundly unsettling.

Impact of Illness on the Experience of Control

Physical illness, and therapies, may disrupt physical and mental functions that were previously under the patient's control. Occasionally these changes are permanent and/or progressive. Patients frequently lose physical strength secondary to their illness or to bed rest. They occasionally lose control of bowel and/or bladder function, or experience changes in motor coordination or the ability to speak articulately. Secondary to illness, medication, and sleep deprivation, they lose the ability to adequately regulate both their emotions and the expression of emotion. These losses are particularly distressing for patients. Patients whose medications (directly or as a side effect) are centrally active, or patients who are recovering from general anesthesia, CNS disorders, or endocrine disorders, can find themselves unable to adequately express what they think and feel to friends, family, and physicians. These distressing circumstances can cause a decompensation in patients whose self-esteem is dependent upon an image that can tolerate no loss of control in any sphere of life.

The Sick Role—Who is in Charge?

The doctor-patient relationship is a dyadic interaction in which both the physician and the patient have roles and responsibilities. The doctor's responsibilities are to diagnose, cure disease whenever possible, maximize functioning, minimize pain, provide solace, and palliation. The name given to the patient's responsibility is the *sick role*, defined as follows (Parsons, 1951):

1. The sick person is exempt from normal social-role responsibilities and activities. Thus, the breadwinner is not expected to work nor is the mother/housewife expected to care for family/home if sick.
2. The sick person is not to be blamed for his illness and not to be expected to recover by himself. His illness therefore requires medical attention.
3. The sick person is obliged to want to get well and to cooperate with appropriate care givers.
4. The sick person is obliged to seek technically competent help.

The most striking element of the sick role is the fact that the patient must relinquish control over a myriad of functions and delegate to the doctor the task of being in charge of the treatment. For some patients, their cultural expectations help to accept the fact that the physician must be in charge of many decisions. Modern medical care cannot be delivered by physicians alone. In the complex environment of a tertiary medical center, a large number of professionals are in charge of many aspects of the patient's care. The head nurse is responsible for the functioning of the whole ward, and the patient's individual nurse has enormous control over the patient's entire schedule, to the point of determining even when the patient is able to sleep. Visiting hours, dietary requirements, and interactions with the hospital administration or with the patient's employer are all functions that will be controlled by nurses, dietitians, and social workers. Even the degree of territorial liberty of patients will be determined by various factors that may dictate that one be restricted to bed, or to a room, or to a ward. Physicians themselves have complex hierarchic structures that impact on how much each one of them is actually in charge. Attendings, chief residents, residents, interns, and medical students interact with the patient with different levels of responsibility. The particularities of call schedules and work shifts are such that patients may be seen each day by a different nurse, or a different doctor. The impact of managed care has shifted power from health care providers to the agents of insurance companies that can interfere with health care decisions. Patients may wonder, "Who is in charge?" generating a significant degree of insecurity and anxiety. This is exacerbated when the question is unclear for the care providers themselves. Such pulverization of power may lead to conflicting medical decisions, internal dissension, and inappropriately reacting to patients who have a tendency to split the team into "bad" and "good" people.

Sick Role in Acute Illness

It is relatively easy for most patients to accept the sick role when they are acutely ill. It is more socially and psychologically acceptable to retire from the usual exercise of power and control when the situation appears to be transient. The perspective of a quick return to "normal" life will facilitate the willingness to break from the patient's usual pattern of behavior. However, acuteness also often means little time to adapt to changes and less awareness of the limitations that an illness may impose. A person may try to keep going as if nothing had happened and may not recognize an illness through lack of knowledge or psychological inability to face illness (Strauss, Spitzer, & Muskin, 1990). Similarly, acuteness often goes along with the severity of illness and life-threatening situations. The patient may be unprepared to cope with illness and will react negatively to being placed in the sick role. Single parents or sole wage-earners may be particularly vulnerable experiencing their responsibilities as preventing them from having the "luxury" of being ill.

Sick Role in Chronic Illness

Although chronic patients will be often more aware of the limitations that they face and have had more time to adapt, different problems may interfere with their compliance with the sick role. One of the most common obstacles is a sense of helplessness leading to low motivation to keep up the fight in patients that have gone through many defeats and disappointments. Patients who were previously compliant with the therapeutic regimen may turn against the health provider out of fatigue and despair. Chronic illness can lead to changes in personality, exacerbating pre-existing negative character traits, when patients become bitter and resentful. It is essential that the health care provider develop a long term relationship with chronic patients. This aids in recognizing changes and assisting patients in appropriately reacting to the burdens of chronic illness.

The Hospitalized Patient

Unlike the staff of a hospital, patients and their families do not have time to adapt to the system and therefore may experience both the impact of the illness and the hospitalization with distress.

The physical structure of the hospital is an important factor that contributes to the stress for patients and staff. Negotiating this physical plant can be a bewildering experience. As the size of the health care setting increases, patients report themselves as experiencing greater degrees of anxiety (Lucente & Flec, 1972). The initial experience of negotiating the transportation to the hospital, the emergency room, or the admitting office contributes to the stress of the hospitalization as well.

Various parts of the hospital may have different odors. In addition to the numerous disinfectants there are others which are associated with pain, suffering and death, loss of bowel control, and sexuality. Health care workers may become habituated to the olfactory stimuli but patients and their families are greeted by this sensory stimulation, even if it is not a conscious experience. The impact of the olfactory experience may contribute to the stress of hospitalization and to the regressive pull illness and hospitalization exert upon patients.

Admission to the hospital means the relinquishing of the comfort of and the control over one's personal environment. Not only does the patient leave home, he or she is asked to give up personal belongings. Most importantly, patients are asked to relinquish their clothing. In giving up their clothes, their belongings and their home, individuals attain a new status, that of "patient." The individual must adapt to this new patient role. All patients are viewed as the same in the health care setting.

How an individual copes with the inescapable stress of hospitalization will determine the difficulty of the illness experience for that person. How the hospital structure, the personnel, and the resources of the patient (financial, social, and cognitive) limit the ability of the patient to cope with the stress of hospitalization may determine whether a particular patient successfully copes with illness and a hospital stay. The interaction of these various components requires systems analysis and reflects the biopsychosocial approach to medical care (Miller, 1973). It seems reasonable to conclude that serious illness and hospitalization create a situation of psychological stress for all patients and their families (Kornfeld, 1979). Psychological stress is anything that destabilizes a person's life. Serious illness, a sudden financial change, the illness or death of an important person, and many other expected and unexpected occurrences all cause stress. Patients will vary in their vulnerability to this stress and will vary in their ability to adapt to the situation. How a patient adapts to the stress will depend upon prior experiences with illness and doctors, the characteristic manner of coping with stress, and the particular type and severity of stress that the patient is experiencing. The individual's particular character style and the resources of the family play a powerful role. An illness severe enough to require hospitalization will be experienced and modulated by the childhood life of the individual. The remnants of the past, no matter how distant, will be reflected in this current life crisis. Strain and Grossman (1975) have noted that the vast majority of patients are able to cope and to assume the role of patient without difficulty.

What Do Patients Experience When They Feel They Have Lost Control

Regression

The most common effect of loss of control is regression. This means that the individual is placed in a situation of dependency which replicates the experience of childhood. Behavior, coping skills, experience of and expression of emotion all take on qualities from previous stages of the person's development. This may range from the temporary loss of recent gains in the patient's psychological make-up to a style more appropriate for a young child. Unfortunately, regression evokes a negative image, but this is not necessarily the case. Regression might be better thought of as a dedifferentiation of the individual such that he or she is in a more plastic state but one that is simultaneously more primitive. As such, regression offers the person more flexibility to adapt to the environment and the potential for positive change. It also suggests that, for some period of time, the person may function in a manner different from his or her usual way which exerts a stress upon friends, family, and caregivers. Regression implies that the person is using defenses that are less reality-oriented, based more upon unresolved conflicts from childhood, less stable and less adaptive to the demands of the environment (Field, 1979).

The regressed adult is operating with a defensive structure more appropriate for someone who typically functions at a lower level of psychological health. The adequacy with which the individual negotiated the stresses and conflicts of development, and the strengths and/or deficiencies of his or her parental relationships, will play a crucial role in how this adult will cope with illness and hospitalization. This is the starting point for the patient. The lower the starting point, the more primitive the defensive structure to which the patient regresses. Simultaneous with this process are patients' reactions to their regression and the attempts to return to the usual level of function and control. The attempts at regaining control are frequently what generates concern among the health care providers rather than the regression itself.

Acting-Out and Noncompliance

Maladaptive attempts to regain control can often result in acts that are impulsive and only partially understood by patients. These are similar to the classical concept of *acting-out* in which patients in therapy will act outside the frame of the treatment, as a result of unconscious forces stirred up by the therapeutic process. Patients can appear overdemanding, aggressive, challenging, querulous, dramatic, and so forth. Patients may act violently, threaten suicide, or try to leave the hospital while their medical condition is critical. They may defiantly refuse to cooperate with diagnostic and therapeutic procedures or with hospital rules such as smoking restrictions or visiting hours. This generates a response from the therapeutic team, which may range from inadequate to appropriately therapeutic.

Therapeutic Responses

The remedy for most inadequate patient behavior depends on establishing open staff communication, which enables staff to get a well-rounded view of the patient. Adler (1973) recommends firm, nonpunitive limit setting as crucial for inpatient treatment of challenging patients. As it is a natural human instinct to confront such patients angrily, Adler and Buie (1972) offer a useful set of restrictions and precautions for the management of patients' inappropriate behavior:

1. Acknowledge the real stresses in the patient's situation.
2. Avoid breaking down needed defenses.
3. Avoid overstimulation of the patient's wish for closeness.

4. Avoid overstimulation of the patient's rage.
5. Avoid confrontation of narcissistic entitlement.

Communication with the patient needs to be simple and truthful. Brief daily staff conferences may help planning the patient's treatment to reach a consensus about what is to be told to the patient. Ideally, one person should make all decisions and negotiate them with the patient. However, constant personnel shifts are difficult to avoid in the real world. Just bearing in mind that the patient feels scared at each change of shift can help, and at the beginning of each shift one staff member should familiarize himself or herself with the patient, introduce himself or herself to the patient, ask how things are, and tell how long he or she will be on duty. Understanding of patient entitlement as one of the last defenses that a scared patient is able to use is useful to increase awareness and self-control of the negative feelings that such behavior provokes among the staff. Rather than confronting this behavior, competent staff should repeat to the patient that his or her demands are understood but because he or she deserves the best possible care, staff are going to continue to pursue the course dictated by experience and good judgement.

Restoration of Partial Control

This balanced approach will usually enable patients to reach better control of their own behavior. Once both patient and staff reach a point of equilibrium, it is easier to restore the patient's much needed feeling that he or she is able to gain partial control over his or her care.

One of the best ways to demonstrate to patients that they are able to keep some control is a frank discussion about the treatment plan. Informed consent refers to the patient's right to choose among treatment options or diagnostic procedures for his or her disorder based on a thorough understanding of the potential benefits and risks. As much as possible, the patient must be encouraged to exercise this control. There are limitations to a patient's capacity to make health care decisions. The treatment options must be explained by the physician in a manner understandable to a lay person. Such communications can be impeded by fluctuating levels of consciousness, impaired cognition due to various causes such as a dementing disorder or delirium, ambivalence, or distorted reality-testing due to a psychiatric disorder or anxiety. The physician must assess if the patient is able to understand the essential information regarding the treatment or procedure, is able to appreciate the situation within the context of the disease, is able to clearly communicate a choice, and is able to base his or her decision on a reasonable analysis of the information given. As long as an adult patient demonstrates these four elements, his or her decisions must be respected. The more this communication between patients and physicians is exercised, the more patients will feel in control and the less they will adopt regressive and maladaptive behaviors.

Patients should also be offered as much control of apparently minor aspects of their care as possible. As part of a reasonable negotiation and in the setting of gentle but firm limit setting, patients can be offered small privileges that will be very important to them. Measures as simple as allowing patients to keep personal belongings and to rearrange and decorate their rooms (within reasonable limits) will foster a feeling of control over their environment. Efforts to rearrange patients' schedules for procedures, vital signs checking, and visiting hours, in order to improve their comfort and to allow longer hours of tranquility help build a therapeutic alliance. The pay-off provided by the patients gratitude and appreciation for being treated as deserving human beings will often outweigh the trouble that such effort may bring to the nursing staff.

METHODS OF COPING WITH ILLNESS: ENHANCING RESILIENCE

Definition of Coping

One of the most important tasks of health care providers dealing with acutely or chronically ill patients is the fostering of better coping skills (Kessler, Price, & Wortman, 1985; Druss, 1995; Weisman, 1997). The coping process can be defined as the cognitive and behavioral effort made to master, tolerate, or reduce demands/stressors that tax or exceed a person's resources (Kessler, Price, & Wortman, 1985). Coping is a problem-solving behavior that is intended to bring about relief, reward, quiescence, and equilibrium (Weissman, 1997). Among individuals exposed to a particular stressful experience, variation in coping strategies is associated with variation in emotional adjustment. For example, Coyne, Aldwin, and Lazarus (1981) found that depressed individuals were more likely to appraise situations as requiring more information in order to act, to seek emotional support, and to engage in wishful thinking. Coping strategies of depressed people are characterized by negative self-preoccupations that may hamper their ability to deal decisively and effectively with their problems.

The more varied an individual's coping repertoire, the more protected he or she is from distress. Pearlin and Schooler (1978) found that the most effective coping strategies are more likely to be employed by men, by the educated, and by the affluent members of society, which suggests that the groups most exposed to hardship are also least equipped to deal with it.

The vast majority of studies of coping with specific life crises have focused on the process of coping with physical health problems or with major surgery (Lazarus & Cohen, 1977). In almost all cases, the studies have focused on the impact of denial on recovery, showing in general that reappraisal of the situation was more effective in ameliorating the consequences of stress than attempts to deny the stress (Cohen & Lazarus, 1979; Mullen & Suls, 1982).

In the majority of cases, those who experience life crises rarely turn to professionals for help. Victims are much more likely to turn to informal support systems, such as family, friends, and neighbors (Veroff, Douvan, & Kulda, 1981), which may be at times unfortunate because there is evidence that those informal systems are not always particularly helpful (Wortman & Lehman, 1984).

Assessing How Someone Copes

Who Copes Well? Who Copes Poorly?

Individuals who cope well are those with special skills or with personal traits that enable them to master many difficulties (Weisman, 1997). Although it is rare to encounter such idealized good copers, and no one copes superlatively at all times, these are some of their characteristics:

1. They are optimistic and maintain high morale despite setbacks.
2. They tend to be practical in focusing on immediate problems before tackling more remote ones.
3. They are resourceful in selecting from a wide range of strategies and tactics.
4. They are flexible and open to suggestions without relinquishing the final say in decisions.
5. They are vigilant in avoiding emotional extremes that could impair judgment.

People who cope poorly are not incorrigibly ineffective people, but they will tend to have the following traits:

1. They tend to be excessive in self-expectation, and are rigid, inflexible, and reluctant to compromise or ask for help.
2. They show little tolerance toward other people's behavior.
3. Although prone to preconceptions, they may be suggestible on specious grounds with little cause.
4. They are inclined to excessive denial, elaborate rationalizations, and are unable to focus on salient problems.
5. They may be more passive and fail to initiate action because they find it difficult to weight alternatives.
6. When the rigidity lapses they may make impulsive judgments.

Personal Styles Responding to Illness

In addition to these general traits, personal styles or even personality disorders will impact on how people react to illness, and consequently on how they cope with it. Druss (1995) identifies six common problems or styles that lead patients to cope poorly with illness.

Illness as Punishment Leading to a Sense of Being Unlovable. In many religious traditions, illness has been seen as divine punishment for the commission of sins. Many patients do not participate or cooperate in the fight against their illness because of a conviction that they deserve it. Depression, unlike grief, is a maladaptive response to the crisis of illness, of which irrational guilt and self-accusation are a common feature. The feeling of being unloved and unlovable are the signal hallmarks of these traits.

Illness Leading to a State of Hopelessness. Disease is experienced as humiliating and demeaning. The loss of control, the taking away of status and position in the hospital, as discussed above, all contribute to the sense of helplessness. Each individual has a secret fantasy of the end point of an illness—to become very ugly and repellent, to be alone, to be racked with pain—generating feelings of helplessness, humiliation, and shame.

Illness as Betrayal. Perfectionist, narcissistic individuals demanding bodily perfection do badly with any illness or even the aging process. These individuals say to themselves: "Why me?" They are angry at everyone, at the diagnostician for discovering the disease, at the surgeon for mutilating them, at the clinician for the continuance of their disability, and with the side effects of treatments. They are angry at family and friends, envying others' good health.

Illness and Alteration in the Self. Some patients may have enormous difficulty in dealing with new boundaries in their selves as consequence of body changes such as surgery, prostheses, or disfiguring illnesses. Presumed positive changes such as rhinoplasty or breast augmentation or reduction can also result in a difficult psychological adjustment.

Illness as a Preoccupation. Chronic illness has the capacity to become a central focus of an individual's life by its realistic intrusions. Chronic illness is hard to ignore and reminds us of our bodily entrapments. Illness can become a preoccupation as well, allowing little conflict-free ego to attend to other matters. Some consequences of illness can be promoted to the central issues in someone's life, such as the location of bathrooms for patients with colitis, steps and revolving doors for wheelchair-bound persons, and so forth.

Illness as a Cause of Loss. Illness is poorly handled when it involves a change from better to worse and a loss ensues. It has been noted, for example, that women who undergo breast reconstruction immediately after a mastectomy, therefore changing from a whole breast to a reconstructed one, are less content with their reconstructed breast than those who wait a whole year before reconstruction, who then change from an absent breast to a reconstructed one (Druss, 1995).

Impact of Personality on Coping Ability

More specifically than these general problems that may affect anyone, personality disorders will have a profound impact on a patient's reaction to illness. Even when patients do not have personality disorders, they can still show character styles that may influence their experience of illness and hospitalization. Character style does not mean character pathology but instead is a characteristic manner by which an individual will experience the world and behave in the world. We all have a personality which has certain typical features. While there are pathological concomitants to the personality types, health care providers should not overemphasize the "diagnosis" versus the patient's characterological reactions (Geringer & Stern, 1986). Character style thus plays an important role in understanding a particular patient/staff dyad as the staff member is engaged positively or negatively by the patient's character. A review of the seven personality types, as described by Kahana and Bibring (1964), and the conceptualization of how their anxieties should be approached, will be presented.

People Who Are Dependent and Overdemanding (Oral). The individual seems to need special attention and has an urgency about his or her needs. Such people can be impulsive, seemingly naive, and demanding of care without limitations from their doctors. There is the potential for anger, depression, and inappropriate use of medications or drugs stemming from a low tolerance for frustration. The individual's conflict centers around fears of abandonment and wishes for unlimited care. Illness reawakens the desire to exist in a secure, infantile state where all needs are provided for by another. Acute illness is perceived as the result of a failure of protection and caring by others. Staff needs to structure their interactions to convey the intent to help the patient recover. The inevitable setting of limits should be presented not as punishment for the patient's inexhaustible demands but as a way to best aid the patient to obtain his or her return to health.

People Who Are Orderly and Controlled (Compulsive). "Knowledge is power!" might best describe these people who seek to control their anxiety by finding out as many "facts" as they can. The orderly, neat, conscientious patient may be quite obstinate in dealings regarding health. Defenses against impulses to soil, be aggressive, or act hedonistically are threatened by the person's illness. This increases the necessity to be orderly and to contain emotions, the outcome of which results in ritualized or intensely formal behavior. In an effort to gain control through knowledge the patient asks questions repeatedly. Never satisfied they have enough information they may become indecisive when they have to make decisions regarding their care. "Informed consent" can become a caricature with such patients. The provision of details of what the physician plans, why a procedure is required, and the science of the medical approach is reassuring to these patients. Giving adequate, but not overwhelming, detail permits the patient to use intellectualization to calm anxiety and the fear of losing control of impulses. When practically possible, patients benefit from active participation in treatment planning and in carrying out appropriate components of their treatment.

People Who Are Dramatizing and Captivating (Histrionic). These patients are often charming, interesting, and pleasurably challenging. They behave in a personal and warm manner. The dramatic, sometimes teasing or seductive manner of such patients, and their attempts to form idealized and intimate relationships with staff, protects them from their fears of punishment for forbidden unconscious wishes. Illness means that they are weak, unattractive, and unloved and it is experienced as a threat to their masculinity or femininity. Attempts to master their fears may result in displays of their strength, power, and sexuality. Such attempts at re-establishing control typically overstimulate, frighten, anger, and distance doctors and nurses from the patient. Establishing a comfortable degree of appreciation for the patient's attractiveness and strength, while remaining aware of the possibility of their seeking intense emotional involvement, is the ideal way for the staff to treat such patients. The often quoted clinical pearl of the physician telling the counterphobic body builder with a recent myocardial infarction that he has to be "strong enough" to lie in bed doing "specialized" finger and toe exercises, as opposed to vigorous calisthenics, is the insightful comment to the anxious patient with a hysterical character style.

People Who Are Long-Suffering and Self-Sacrificing (Masochistic). This personality style is perplexing to medical staff who cannot understand how unfortunate events seem to "occur" to the patient. There is often the suspicion that the patient plays some role in the misfortunes and there is often "evidence" that this is the case (though the causation is on an unconscious basis). These patients are exhibitionistic about their suffering, in contrast to their humble manner. The need to prepay for pleasure, or pay for experienced or fantasized pleasure fuels this patient's experience and behavior. They wish to be loved and cared for but feel unworthy and guilty. Thus they expect to either not get what they want, or to be punished for having gotten their wishes gratified. Such patients can cause great frustration in their doctors who find the patient seemingly worsened by news of their positive progress. While the patient does not malinger or create illness, he or she is disheartened by the good news. Acknowledgment of the patient's difficulties and suffering, demonstrating an understanding of the "burden," works far better for these patients. Structuring recovery as a tough ordeal, or to benefit others for whom the patient feels responsible, may enable the person to resolve conflicts regarding the attention and care from the medical staff.

People Who Are Guarded and Querulous (Paranoid). The suspicious, watchful individual who reacts to the most minimal of slights is obvious to even the least psychologically minded observer. This person overreacts to any criticism and seem to expect an attack at any moment. Everything is externalized, that is, nothing is the person's fault. This can be particularly problematic in the hospital setting where there is much in the way of bad news, unexpected discomfort, lost laboratory results, or incorrect meals. It follows from this that such a patient blames others for the illness. His or her fears of being harmed intensify when ill, which increases the aggressive impulses. The anxiety thus stimulated is defended by an increase in the guardedness, suspiciousness, and need to control others, principally the doctors and nurses who are responsible for the patient's care. These are patients for whom care needs to be taken that they not be surprised by what happens in the hospital. Particular attention needs to be paid towards informing them of what is expected to happen at each step in the diagnostic and therapeutic process. There should be an attempt to acknowledge how the patient feels rather than a hostile confrontation of his or her "perceptions." This can be particularly difficult for an exhausted intern or resident. It is sometimes possible to ally with the patient to enlist cooperation in "putting up" with the realities of the hospital, thus gaining cooperation in a continued stay and recovery.

People Who Have a Feeling of Superiority (Narcissistic). These people see themselves as being powerful and important, whether or not their station in society substantiates this feeling. Overtly they may appear quite humble or modest, but this facade is seen through by others. Relating to a staff member, upon whom the patient must depend, can be a difficult task, especially if the health care provider does not reinforce the patient's special status by having a special status. Illness threatens this patient's need to be perfect and invulnerable. The patient's increased grandiosity and entitlement is a defensive maneuver. He easily finds fault with his caretakers but fears the staff might not be able to help him. The fantasy that he must have the "great professor" can be demoralizing for the intern or resident who feels devalued. The tactful, not defensive, acknowledgment of one's knowledge, training, and abilities is reassuring to the patient who can idealize the doctor and contain overwhelming anxiety.

People Who Are Aloof and Not Involved (Schizoid). These patients seem eccentric or odd in their behavior on the ward, uninvolved with their doctors and nurses, and seemingly "too calm" regarding their illness. They do not seem easily swayed by things and appear quite independent. This external calm conceals a fragile interior which requires a withdrawal from everyday life to manage otherwise overwhelming anxiety. While they may function apparently well in their regular lives, and may have VIP status resultant from their accomplishments, their illness and hospitalization present a stress with which they cannot cope. This may result in a denial that they are ill, in spite of hard evidence to the contrary, as illness disrupts their carefully balanced system. Though the impulse to "break through" to these patients may be strong, a better management technique acknowledges their need to remain safe, with the physician and family doing the large portion of the decision-making.

Improving Coping Skills: Strategies That Are Effective or Ineffective

The courage to cope means a wish to perform competently and to be valued as a significant person, even when threatened by risk. It is important to recognize that in evaluating how patients cope, one should learn his or her own coping styles and learn from patients. In trying to comfort distressed patients, it is not enough to mean well, have a warm heart, or possess scientific information. It is essential to foster open communication and self-awareness. No technique for coping is applicable to everyone.

The essential step in helping patients to cope better is to understand their coping strategies. A careful and thorough interview that will explore the use of these strategies is both diagnostic and therapeutic because of its psychoeducational value. The physician can simultaneously show to the patient what his or her strategies have been and which ones are more or less adaptive.

Weisman has suggested a hierarchy of effectiveness in coping strategies (Weisman 1974). The most mature and effective strategies include a rational or intellectual approach in order to undermine unrealistic fears. These people use ventilation to relieve anxiety and distress and redefinition as an effort to accept, but change the meaning of the problem to something more manageable. They search for feasible alternatives and can comply with directives from appropriate authority sources.

Partially successful strategies that may or may not have positive impact include changing emotions in an attempt to make light of problems and to try to laugh them off. Sometimes counterphobic maneuvers by which patients deliberately do not avoid the subject of their illness with silence and secrets but rather voice them out loud are helpful. Suppression and denial by trying to put the problem out of one's mind may work well if the person can still comply with treatment. Displacement, an attempt to distract oneself from painful situations by doing other things, usually brings only temporary relief.

The clarification of a person's coping effectiveness may require many encounters to be actually understood and incorporated by patients. Confidence in being able to cope can be enhanced only through repeated self-appraisal, self-instruction, and self-correction. In addition to pointing out which strategies are effective, discussing with patients the characteristics of good and bad copers may also foster more appropriate adaptation.

Preventive interventions can address patients' concerns before dreaded interventions or procedures. What is most frightening in approaching a surgical procedure—the diagnosis, anesthesia, possible invalidism, failure, pain, abandonment by physician or family? Frank discussion with the patient allows for correction of unrealistic fears and helps to reduce anxiety.

Few people readily admit their tendency to fail, shirk, or behave in unworthy ways. Nevertheless, a skillful interview gets behind denial, rationalization, posturing, and pretense without evoking a threat to security or self-esteem. The key for such an interview is empathy. This comes from the awareness that vulnerability is present in all humans and shows up at times of crisis, stress, calamity, and threat to well-being and identity.

Patients who are ashamed of their conditions feel relieved when health care providers show that the disfiguration or disability is accepted. Physical contact, such as a handshake with patients with transmissible diseases, or looking at dreadful facial anomalies, inoperable tumors, bladder extrophies, and other malformations, makes patients feel worthwhile.

It is essential to realize and respect the uniqueness of each patient's disabilities. Each person has his or her own way to cope with and master illness. Staff members must respect each pathway, regardless of their own theoretical orientation or belief system, and must refrain from judging the patient or disavowing his or her defense mechanisms. The danger of minimizing someone's suffering with the apparent good will of making them feel better most often fails. Disability that may not seem so important to the health care provider may be very significant for the patient. For example, for people whose face is their fortune, a skin lesion would terrify him or her more than it might others; for others for whom mobility is necessary, bed rest, paralysis, or even a limp becomes their Achilles' heel.

The establishing of staff-patient partnership is another instrumental step in maximizing coping effectiveness and in dissolving fears of abandonment and helplessness. Patients who are dying often have the fear that others will turn their backs on them. It is extremely important for these patients to realize that although their doctors cannot cure them, they will remain at their side to minimize pain and discomfort and allow them to die with dignity. When a health care provider can say, and mean it, "whatever happens, I will be here with you," the comfort that the patient will derive is priceless.

The help of a knowledgeable, caring professional who faces adversity with serenity will provide a role model for better coping. People who admire robustness and self-reliance in themselves will be effective in reinforcing these qualities in others and will present gentle opposites of regression and pessimism. A limited and controlled degree of self-disclosure may enhance the modeling of these qualities to patients.

A useful technique (Druss, 1995) is the fostering of a reduction of the boundaries of the Self such that the sickness is viewed as external to one's essence rather than as a part of the Self. Patients benefit from believing that the battle between the disease and a drug or surgery occurs outside some central core self, which remains inviolable. This is most obvious in a condition like breast cancer, in which a woman comes to the understanding that she has not changed in any fundamental way, she is the same; it is only a sick breast that has been removed. This approach may be less effective when the diseased organ is central to life (such as the heart or brain) or the illness is disseminated in a wide-spread infection, immunodeficiency, or metastasized cancer (Fishman, 1988). Nonetheless, the individual avers something like, "They can have my leg or heart or strength, but they can't have me." This conveys the notion that the core of human worth is not affected by illness, that the patient remains a dignified human being in spite of sickness. The attack can reach the perimeter, which may have to be sacrificed, but the soul or the central core remains intact. Prisoners of war and Holocaust survivors have reported a similar state of mind (Druss, 1995).

STRESS

Stress is a state of psychological or physical strain that imposes demands for internal and external adjustments. Stress can give rise to feelings of anxiety and trigger a series of physiological reactions. The concept of stress popularized by Selye (1956) describes it as a nonspecific response of the body to external demands. Stress is now seen as a complex, multilevel process of an interaction with the external world with a series of integrated responses (Kasl, 1984). An individual's response is largely determined by the way the person perceives a stressful situation.

The Life Event Approach versus Chronic Stress

Evidence shows that some severe life event stresses are significant in producing psychopathology, for example, post-traumatic stress disorder. Thoits (1983) has concluded that the features of any specific life event that are most important for the development of psychopathology are undesirability, magnitude, time clustering, and uncontrollability. Investigators have suggested that exposure to life events can undermine feelings of self-esteem by disrupting the person's repertoire of coping responses. It has been also suggested that life events may exert noxious influence by increasing the number of chronic stressors to which one is exposed (Pearlin, Lieberman, Meneghan, & Mullen, 1981).

Stress and Its Effect on Health

Stress is a process central to the relationship between behavior and health because it helps to explain how psychologically relevant events translate into health-impairing physiological changes and illness. Although definitions of stress are often imprecise, a number of direct physiological effects of stressors (e.g., immunosuppression, increased blood pressure) have been identified. The indirect effects of stress may also provoke behavioral changes that are harmful, such as cigarette smoking, alcohol abuse, or drug abuse (Elliott & Eisdorfer, 1982).

The Physiologic Response to Stress

Mediators of physiologic response to stress. The neuroendocrinophysiology of stress can be very grossly summarized as follows (Morihisa & Rosse, 1990): Limbic system activation by stress causes the hypothalamus to release corticotrophin releasing factor (CRF), which stimulates the release of adrenocorticotropic hormone (ACTH) from the pituitary gland. This stimulates the adrenal gland to release cortisol. The limbic system control of the hypothalamus may be mediated through cholinergic or serotonergic stimulatory pathways, or both, and through adrenergic inhibitory pathways. Stress can be associated with increases in heart and respiratory rates, blood pressure, muscle tension, body oxygen consumption, and an increase in serum levels of lactate, cortisol, catecholamines, and cholesterol (Morihisa & Rosse, 1990). Stress can also be associated with changes in skin conductance, decreased blood flow, and decreased temperature of the extremities, and it has been reported to be associated with decreased immune function. There is also a reduction in alpha wave frequency on the electroencephalogram (Morihisa & Rosse, 1990). Stress brings adaptation to strain, but paradoxically the physiologic systems activated by stress cannot only protect and restore but also damage the person (McEwen, 1998).

Allostasis and Allostatic Load. Allostasis is the ability to achieve stability through change, and it is critical to survival. Through allostasis, the autonomic nervous system, the hypothalamic-pituitary-adrenal (HPA) axis, and the cardiovascular, metabolic, and immune systems protect the body by responding to internal and external stress. The price of this accommodation is the wear and tear that results from chronic overactivity or underactivity of allostatic systems (McEwen, 1998).

Over weeks, months, or years, exposure to increased secretion of stress hormones can result in allostatic load and its pathophysiologic consequences. Four situations are associated with allostatic load:

1. *Frequent stress.* In primates repeated elevations of blood pressure over weeks and months accelerate atherosclerosis, and surges in blood pressure can trigger myocardial infarction (Muller, Tofler, & Stone 1989).
2. *Failure of adaptation to repeated stressors of the same type.* This results in prolonged exposure to stress hormones. Normally, repeated exposure attenuates the stress response, but some people are prone to a prolonged response (Kirschbaum, Prussner, & Stone, 1995).
3. *Inability to shut off allostatic responses after a stress is terminated.* The failure to turn off the HPA axis and sympathetic activity efficiently after stress is a fea-

ture of age-related functional decline in laboratory animals (McCarty, 1985; Sapolsky, 1992; McEwen, 1992), although evidence in humans is still limited (Seeman & Robbins, 1994; Wilkinson, Peskind, & Raskind, 1997). One speculation is that allostatic load over a lifetime may cause the allostatic system to wear out or become exhausted (Seeman & Robbins, 1994). A vulnerable link in the regulation of the HPA axis is the hippocampal region. According to the "glucocorticoid-cascade hypothesis," wear and tear on this region of the brain leads to dysregulation of the HPA axis (Sapolsky, 1992).

4. *Inadequate responses by some allostatic systems.* This triggers compensatory increases in others, and may lead to an enhanced inflammatory response and autoimmune disturbances. HPA hyporesponsiveness in humans has been related to conditions such as fibromyalgia, chronic fatigue syndrome, and atopic dermatitis (Crofford, Pillemer, & Kalogeras, 1994; Poteliakhoff, 1981; Buske-Kirschbaum et al., 1997). In patients with post-traumatic stress disorder, basal HPA activity is low (Yehuda, Teicher, Trestman, Levengood, & Silver, 1996). Intrusive memories of a traumatic event can produce a form of chronic stress which drives physiologic responses (Baum, Cohen, & Hall, 1993).

Effects of Stress on Health

Stress and Lifestyle. Certain forms of behavior are closely related to the way people cope with a challenge. It is common to see people reacting to chronic stress by smoking, drinking alcohol, eating high-fat foods, and decreasing the amount of exercise. All these behaviors can affect allostatic load. A high-fat diet accelerates atherosclerosis and progression to noninsulin-dependent diabetes by increasing cortisol secretion, leading to fat deposition and insulin resistance (Brindley & Rolland, 1989). Smoking elevates blood pressure and accelerates atherogenesis (Verdecchia, Schillaci, & Borgioni, 1995). Exercise protects against cardiovascular disease, and the lack of exercise removes this protection (Bernadet, 1995).

Stress and Cardiovascular Disorders. The best-studied system of allostasis and allostatic load is the cardiovascular system (McEwen, 1998). In nonhuman primates, the incidence of atherosclerosis is increased among the dominant males of unstable social hierarchies and in socially subordinate females (Shively & Clarkson, 1994). In humans, lack of control on the job increases the risk of coronary heart disease (Bosma, Marmot, Hemingway, Nicholson, Brunner, & Stansfeld, 1997), and job strain results in elevated ambulatory blood pressure (Schnall, Schwartz, Landsbergis, Warren, & Pickering, 1992). Chronic stress and hostility are linked to increased reactivity of the fibrinogen system and of platelets, both of which increase the risk of myocardial infarction (Raikkonen, Lassila, Keltikangas-Jarvinen, & Hautanen, 1996).

Stress and the Brain. Repeated stress affects brain function, especially in the hippocampus, which has a high concentration of cortisol receptors (Markowe et al.,

1985). The hippocampus participates in verbal memory, and its impairment decreases the reliability and accuracy of contextual memories, which may exacerbate stress (Sapolsky, 1990). Acute stress increases cortisol secretion, which suppresses mechanisms in the hippocampus and temporal lobe that serve short-term memory (McEwen & Sapolsky, 1995). Repeated stress results in the atrophy of dendrites of pyramidal neurons in the hippocampus. This atrophy is reversible if the stress is short-lived, but stress lasting many months or years can kill hippocampal neurons (Uno, Tarara, Else, Suleman, & Sapolsky, 1989). Magnetic resonance imaging has shown that post-traumatic stress disorder and recurrent depressive illness are associated with atrophy of the hippocampus (McEwen & Margarinos, 1997). Early experiences are believed to set the level of responsiveness of the HPA axis and autonomic nervous system. These systems overreact in animals subjected to early unpredictable stress, which accelerates the aging of the brain (Meaney, Tannenbaum, & Francis, 1994).

Stress and the Immune System. Acute stress has the effect of calling immune cells to their battle stations, and this form of allostasis enhances responses for which there is an established immunologic "memory." If the memory is of a pathogen, the result of stress is presumably beneficial. However, if the response leads to an autoimmune or allergic reaction, then the effect is harmful (Dhabar & McEwen, 1996). When allostatic load is increased by repeated stress, the outcome is completely different; the delayed hypersensitivity response is substantially inhibited rather than enhanced (Dhabar & McEwen, 1997). Thus the immunologic consequences of chronic stress include increased severity of the common cold (Cohen, Tyrrel, & Smith, 1991). In laboratory animals, chronic stress causes recurrent endotoxemia, which decreases the reactivity of the HPA axis to a variety of stimuli and decreases production of the cytokine tumor necrosis factor alpha, potentially increasing the risk for cancer (Hadid, Spinedi, Giovambattista, Chautard, & Gaillard, 1996).

Stress and Other Medical Disorders. It has been suggested that stress may play a role in the early development or appearance of cancers in humans (Sklar & Anisman, 1981). Several studies have examined survival differences as a function of psychological characteristics of patients (Fox, 1978). Results seem to suggest that states such as depression and helplessness are associated with worse survival rates, whereas psychological responses of anger and hostility are related to more favorable outcomes (Barofsky, 1981). Interventions that increase social support and enhance coping prolong the life span of patients with breast cancer, lymphomas, and malignant melanoma (Spiegel, Bloom, Kraemer, & Gottheil, 1989; Richardson, Shelton, Krailo, & Levine, 1990; Fawzy, Fawzy, & Hyun, 1993). Abdominal obesity has been positively correlated with chronic stress and is related to a number of conditions such as diabetes, arthrosis, pulmonary hypertension, sleep apnea, and impotence (Larson, Seidell, & Suardsudd, 1989). Indirect effects of stress include behavioral changes that are harmful, for example, cigarette smoking and alcohol abuse, which have several health implications such as peripheral vascular disease, lung cancer, hepatic dysfunction, and so forth (Elliot & Eisdorfer, 1982).

Psychosocial Risk Factors

Certain conditions, such as excessive workload, job responsibility, and dissatis-factions, may enhance coronary risk (House, 1975). Hypertension is a sensitive index of job stress among factory workers, workers with repetitive jobs and time pressures, and workers whose jobs were unstable because of the concern over layoffs (Kasl & Cobb, 1970; Pickering, Devereux, & James, 1996).

Techniques to Reduce Stress

Medical illness itself is a source of stress, producing anxiety about prognosis, treatment, disability, and interference with social roles and relationships. Physi-cians and other health care providers can help patients reduce allostatic load by helping them learn coping skills. Specific techniques for stress reduction, psychoeducation, and health hygiene are all important. Patients need to be alerted to the risks of a high-fat diet, the role of smoking and drinking alcohol, and the beneficial effects of exercise. Two important causes of allostatic load appear to be isolation (Seeman & McEwen, 1996) and lack of control in the work environ-ment (Bosma et al., 1997). Interventions designed to increase a worker's control over his or her job have improved health and attitudes toward work (Melin, Lundberg, Soderlund, & Granquist, 1998).

   A number of specific techniques have been used to reduce stress. The fol-lowing sections detail some examples.

Traditional Psychotherapy

Short-term psychotherapeutic interventions usually involve a gradation of goals. The initial objective of the sessions is to obtain the patient's perceptions of re-cent life events and to assess psychological defenses and responses to stressful events. The therapy strives to find more successful response management tech-niques. The typical duration of this psychotherapeutic intervention is between six and twelve sessions. Psychoeducation is as important as the identification of psychological defenses and response patterns.

   Traditional psychotherapy models involving longer-term techniques and deep psychodynamic exploration are not indicated to manage acute stress related to life events (e.g., acute illness, hospitalization). These techniques often stir up repressed material and induce a temporary increase in stress and anxiety. How-ever, in patients experiencing chronic stress, long-term dynamically oriented psychotherapy may be effective.

Cognitive-Behavioral Therapy

Behavioral therapy draws on learning theories and the operant conditioning paradigm, using the basic concepts of reward, reinforcement, punishment, stimulus generalization, and extinction.

The term cognitive-behavioral therapy, often used instead of the term behavioral therapy, denotes the current interest in the cognitive mechanisms involved in behavior and the use of specific procedures to alter distorted cognition (Agras, 1995). This should not be confused with cognitive therapy as proposed by Beck, which draws from cognitive and social psychology, information-processing theory, and psychoanalytic theory (Beck, Rush, Shaw, & Emery, 1979).

Behavioral therapy is an effective treatment to reduce stress. Teaching patients to practice specific behaviors is the cornerstone of all behavioral therapies. The therapist begins by defining the behavior to be changed and the one that should replace it, then a monitoring procedure is instituted. This is followed by instructions that constitute a graduated therapeutic program (a behavioral plan) in which the undesirable behavior is extinguished via aversive conditioning, positive reinforcement and extinction, systematic desensitization, and modeling. The patient is encouraged to increase the frequency and the strength of the desired behavior. Self-monitoring and reporting is used to gauge progress and to identify obstacles which need to be overcome. There is initial behavior change, then generalization and maintenance of the new behavior, and finally prevention of relapse. Specific modalities of behavioral therapy have been validated by studies showing their efficacy in a number of conditions (Franks, Wilson, Kendall, & Foreyt, 1990).

Relaxation

Initial interest in the role of relaxation training was sparked in the 1930s by the work of Edmund Jacobson, who demonstrated that patients taught to relax their skeletal musculature reduced their blood pressure. In the 1970s, the procedure was rediscovered. Relaxation techniques have been successfully used to treat anxiety disorders, sleep disorders, hypertension, panic disorder and post-traumatic stress disorder (Agras, 1995).

Relaxation reduces the stress response, probably by reducing sympathetic nervous system arousal (Agras, 1995). The typical training involves 10 sessions in which patients are first taught to tense and relax each muscle group to achieve a state of deep relaxation. Various relaxing images and meditative techniques, such as the use of a simple mantra, are usually added. When a satisfactory state of relaxation has been achieved, the patient is trained to bring on this state more rapidly, often simply by visualizing the word "relax." They are then taught to apply the rapid relaxation procedure in the natural environment and to practice relaxation several times each week at home for some 20 min. The mental focusing involved in relaxation is also effective in reducing stress (Benson, 1997).

Biofeedback

This technique uses instruments to provide visual or auditory measurements of physiological processes, such as small-muscle contractions, heart rate, skin temperature, and blood pressure. Patients are able to voluntarily control these processes by making changes in their behavior. This can be used to teach patients to relax and to reduce stress levels. The therapist usually augments feedback by specific instructions and reinforcement.

Biofeedback has been successfully used to treat tension headache, migraine headache, essential hypertension, pain associated with muscle tension, fecal incontinence, enuresis, Raynaud's disease, and has been considered promising in approaching cardiac arrhythmia and bruxism (Agras, 1995; Schwartz, 1987).

The use of biofeedback to treat stress relies on the fact that physiologic responses to stress involve increased heart rate, blood pressure, and increased occipitofrontal muscle tension, which are all measurable by biofeedback instruments.

Hypnosis

Hypnosis is a state in which a subject is induced to respond to suggestions that involve alterations in perception, memory, or mood. It has variously been described as being an altered state of consciousness, a dissociated state, an access to the unconscious, a form of conditioning, and a compliant response to suggestion or social cues (Rhue, Lynn, & Kirsch, 1988; Brown & Harris, 1987; Crasilneck & Hall, 1985). The person appears to be in a state of relaxed wakefulness but not sleep. There are many misconceptions such as the common belief that the hypnotist is able to gain control over the subject's behavior. All hypnosis is ultimately self-hypnosis, necessitating the patient's active participation. Medical use of hypnosis has been directed to control of pain syndromes, recovery of repressed memories during psychotherapy, treatment of dissociative disorders, control of psychological factors affecting medical conditions (e.g., asthma attacks), treatment of anxiety disorders and PTSD, and so forth (Orne, Dinges, & Bloom, 1995).

Hypnosis is a technique, not a psychotherapy (Spiegel, 1993), and can be used in different psychotherapeutic approaches. It is easy and effective to teach patients self-hypnosis, which can be practiced outside of the office. Hypnosis is also a useful bedside procedure in general hospital settings. The relaxation and feelings of comfort are effective in treating stress syndromes. Self-hypnosis can provide a tool that permits the patient to relax and to control or eliminate the response to stressful stimuli. Hypnosis is more a function of the subject's abilities than of the hypnotist's skills. Therefore, the induction of hypnosis in a cooperative subject requires some but not tremendous expertise. The techniques are simpler and easier to learn than most people believe. Induction of hypnosis is often a question of establishing a good rapport with the patient, and providing information to counteract fears. Statements such as "most people who have good powers of concentration are able to respond," or "it is the patient who chooses to go into hypnosis," are often useful to reassure the patient. Once appropriate rapport is established, standard speeches to foster concentration and relaxation are used. Specific suggestions are made, for example, it can be suggested that a patient will perceive warmth or cold instead of pain, or will feel a floating sensation. The patients are then instructed to return to normal consciousness feeling relaxed and refreshed.

Hypnosis can be used as an adjunct to the treatment of numerous disorders, but it has its contraindications (Orne, Dinges, & Bloom, 1995). Hypnosis is not appropriate for psychotic disorders or severe depressive disorders. Paranoid patients may react very strongly to the possibility of being hypnotized. In more general terms, one should be aware that hypnosis, when used as part of a psychotherapeutic process, will share the same issues of transference and countertransference that are seen in therapy.

Meditation

Meditation is an exercise of contemplation, in which one attempts to think deeply and quietly. Religions and spiritual disciplines that practice meditation include Asceticism, Confucianism, Hinduism (including Yoga), Buddhism, Tibetan Buddhism, and Zen Buddhism, among others (Webb, 1997). The two systems of meditation from Eastern cultures that have been most diffused in the Western world are Zen and Yoga.

Zen is a Buddhist school that developed in China and later in Japan as the result of a fusion between the Indian form of Buddhism (Mahayana) and the Chinese philosophy of Taoism. Zen is the Japanese way of pronouncing the Sanskrit term *dhyana*, which designates a state of mind roughly equivalent to contemplation or meditation. Zen is a way of seeing the world just as it is, i.e., with a mind that has no grasping thoughts or feelings. This attitude is called "no-mind," a state of consciousness wherein thoughts move without leaving any trace. Zen students meditate by sitting and observing, without mental comment, whatever may be happening (Watts, 1997).

Yoga (Sanskrit *yuga*, "yoke"), is one of the six classic systems of Hindu philosophy, distinguished from the others by the marvels of body control ascribed to its advanced devotees. Yoga affirms the doctrine that one may achieve liberation from the limitations of flesh, the delusions of sense, and the pitfalls of thought and thus attain union with the object of knowledge. Yoga practice forms a ladder leading to perfect knowledge through eight stages. The process is said to lead to an inner illumination, the ecstasy of the true knowledge of reality (Watts, 1997).

Systems of meditation like the ones just described can help practitioners to adjust to adversity provoked by illness by fostering acceptance of the ways of the natural world. They also constitute effective means of stress reduction.

Medication

The prescription of medications is too often the sole involvement of physicians with their patients' coping processes. Medications are helpful to treat acute anxiety and reduce stress. Over-reliance on medication can prevent physicians from listening to their patients and from achieving a deeper understanding of the different aspects involved in trauma and stress.

Psychiatrists treating soldiers with acute stress in wartime described the dramatic relief that short-term hypnotics and anxiolytics could provide. These drugs were typically used for two to three days following the event. Most soldiers were sufficiently recovered to allow discontinuation of the treatment. The same general principle is useful in treating many stress-related conditions: Medication therapy is a powerful adjunct but should be as brief as possible (Schatzberg, 1990). Treatment with benzodiazepines or buspirone should be considered when the patient is too anxious to engage in the process of talking about ways to cope with the distress.

PSYCHOSOCIAL TREATMENTS OFTEN FAIL

The Relapse Problem

Many patients do not respond to psychosocial interventions as much as would be desirable. The gains obtained through psychosocial interventions are often difficult to maintain once the treatment ends. Though better health habits can be attained, patients often relapse. A characteristic pattern of relapse is found in many different treatment approaches for addictive behavior (heroin, smoking, alcohol) (Hunt, Barrett, & Ranch, 1971). In the three months following treatment, 40% of patients remain abstinent; in six months about 30%, after 12 months 20% are still abstinent. These relapse curves seem to apply not only to addiction but also to exercise habits, diet modifications, and preventive dental care.

Intrapsychic Factors

Intrapsychic factors can be major obstacles to sustained change in patients. Viewed from a behavioral perspective, treatment failure occurs because immediate rewards and punishments are more effective than delayed ones. The health threats posed by smoking, overweight, lack of exercise, unhealthy diet, and so on, are experienced as remote compared to the immediate pleasures that one gets from these behaviors. The inconvenience and effort involved in more healthful behaviors act as further deterrents to therapeutic success. Viewed from a psychodynamic perspective, the ability to alter one's lifestyle or change health behaviors may be influenced by whether the behavior is maintained by a neurotic symptom which avoids conflicts that would be even more upsetting (primary gain). Illness may provoke modifications in interpersonal relations that are appealing to the patient, such as gaining more tenderness and attention (secondary gain) which can also mitigate against change.

Forces in the Social Environment

A second major set of barriers to lifestyle modification are forces in the social environment, these are cultural influences in society and family factors. Family dynamics are constructed around complex role systems which are refractory to change. At an unconscious level, family members may sabotage psychosocial interventions that change these role dynamics. Advice and psychoeducation, which make sense when seen from the standpoint of the cultural group to which the provider belongs, may be highly inconsistent with the beliefs and values typical of the patient's culture. Patients may give token agreement and show some initial compliance with their doctor, only to promptly become noncompliant at home.

PROMOTING ADHERENCE TO MEDICAL PROTOCOLS AND LIFESTYLE MODIFICATIONS

Health Attitude

The failure of patients to follow medical advice or prescriptions reduces the effectiveness of health care and increases its cost. Estimates of noncompliance vary, but up to 50% of patients may fail to adhere to medicine-taking regimens (Ley, 1977). Compliance with preventive regimens or long-term lifestyle change is even worse. Long-term treatment for an asymptomatic illness (e.g., hypertension) is particularly problematic (Haynes, 1979). Moderate levels of fear about negative consequences of poor hygiene are optimal to change health attitudes (Krantz, Baum, & Singer, 1983). Positive incentives are also effective in promoting dietary change and reduction in heart disease risk (Foreyt, Scott, Mitchell, & Gotto, 1979; Meyer, Nash, McAllister, Maccoby, & Farquhar, 1980). Studies have shown that the simple fact that primary care practitioners encourage patients to think about smoking can double the chances of not smoking six months later (Goldstein et al., 1997; Prochaska & Goldstein, 1991).

SUMMARY AND CONCLUDING COMMENTS

We have emphasized that psychosocial factors such as support resources, vulnerability to stress, control issues, and coping ability (or lack thereof) may influence both illness and curative and/or preventive care. Health care workers possess a variety of strategies and tools that can be used to minimize the negative impact of some of these psychosocial factors, while making better use of the therapeutic properties of personal, professional, and social relationships. The well informed, competent, and flexible health care provider will be able to explore these tools to maximize treatment success while enhancing patient adherence to medical protocols and lifestyle modifications.

REFERENCES

Adler, G., & Buie, D. H. (1972). The misuses of confrontation with borderline patients. *International Journal of Psychoanalytic Psychotherapy, 1,* 109–120.

Adler, G. 1973. Hospital treatment of borderline patients. *The American Journal of Psychiatry, 130,* 105–122.

Agras, W. S. (1995). Behavior therapy. In H. I. Kaplan & B. J. Sadock (Eds.), *Comprehensive textbook of psychiatry* (6th ed., pp. 1788–1806). Baltimore: Williams and Wilkins.

Barofsky, I. (1981). Issues and approaches to the psychosocial assessment of the cancer patient. In C. K. Prokop & L. A. Bradley (Eds.), *Medical psychology: Contributions to behavioral medicine* (pp. 57–64). New York: Academic.

Baum, A., Cohen, L., & Hall, M. (1993). Control and intrusive memories as possible determinants of chronic stress. *Psychosomatic Medicine, 55,* 274–286.

Beck, A. T., Rush, A. J., Shaw, B. F., & Emery, G. (1979). *Cognitive therapy of depression.* New York: Guilford.

Belle, D. (1982). The stress of caring: Women as providers of social support. In L. Goldberger & S. Breznitz (Eds.), *Handbook of stress: Theoretical and clinical aspects* (pp. 496–505). New York: Free Press.

Benson, H. (1997). The relaxation response: Therapeutic effect [letter]. *Science, 278*(5344), 1694–1695; also comment in *Science, 278*(5338), 561.

Bernardet, P. (1995). Benefits of physical activity in the prevention of cardiovascular diseases. *Journal of Cardiovascular Pharmacology, 25*(Suppl 1), S2–S8.

Bosma, H., Marmot, M. G., Hemingway, H., Nicholson, A. C., Brunner, E., & Stansfeld, S. A. (1997). Low job control and risk of coronary heart disease in Whitehall II (prospective cohort) study. *British Medical Journal, 314,* 558–565.

Brindley, D. N., & Rolland, Y. (1989). Possible connections between stress, diabetes, obesity, hypertension and altered lipoprotein metabolism that may result in atherosclerosis. *Clinical Sciences, 77,* 453–461.

Brown, D., & Fromm, E. (1987). *Hypnosis and behavioral medicine.* Hillsdale, NJ: Erlbaum.

Buske-Kirschbaum, A., & Jobst, S. (1997). Attenuated free cortisol response to psychosocial stress in children with atopic dermatitis. *Psychosomatic Medicine, 59,* 419–426.

Cohen, F., & Lazarus, R. S. (1979). Coping with the stresses of illness. In G. S. Stone, F. Cohen, & N. Adler (Eds.), *Health psychology* (pp. 217–254). San Francisco: Jossey-Bass.

Cohen, S., Tyrrel, D. A. J., & Smith, A. P. (1991). Psychological stress and susceptibility to the common cold. *New England Journal of Medicine, 325,* 606–612.

Covinsky, K. E., Landefeld, C. S., Tero, J., & Connors, A. F. (1996). Is economic hardship on the families of the seriously ill associated with patient and surrogate care preferences? *Archives of Internal Medicine, 156,* 1737–1741.

Coyne, J. C., Aldwin, C., & Lazarus, R. S. (1981). Depression and coping in stressful episodes. *Journal of Abnormal Psychology, 90*(5), 439–447.

Crasilneck, H., & Hall, J. (1985). *Clinical hypnosis: Principles and applications* (2nd ed.). Orlando: Grune & Stratton.

Crofford, L. J., Pillemer, S. R., & Kalogeras, K. T. (1994). Hypothalamic-pituitary-adrenal axis perturbations in patients with fibromyalgia. *Arthritis and Rheumatism, 37,* 1583–1592.

Dhabar, Fs., & McEwen, B. S. (1996). Stress-induced enhancement of antigen-specific cell-mediated immunity. *Journal of Immunology, 157,* 2608–2615.

Dhabar, Fs., & McEwen, B. S. (1997). Acute stress enhances while chronic stress suppresses, cell-mediated immunity in vivo: A potential role for leukocyte trafficking. *Brain, Behavior, and Immunity, 11*(4), 286–306.

Druss, R. G. (1995). *The psychology of illness: In sickness and in health.* Washington DC: American Psychiatric Press.

Elliott, G. R., & Eisdorfer, C. (1982). *Stress and human health: Analysis and implications of research.* New York: Springer.

Fawzy, F. I., Fawzy, N. H., & Hyun, C. S. (1993). Malignant melanoma: Effects of an early structured psychiatric intervention, coping, and affective state on recurrence and survival six years later. *Archives of General Psychiatry, 50,* 681–689.

Field, H. L. (1979). Defense mechanisms in psychosomatic medicine. *Psychosomatics, 20,* 690–700.

Fishman, S. (1988). *A bomb in the brain.* New York: Charles Scribner.

Forety, J. P., Scott, L. W., Mitchell, R. E., & Grotto, A. M. (1979). Plasma lipid changes in the normal population following behavioral treatment. *Journal of Consulting and Clinical Psychology, 47,* 440–452.

Fox, B. H. (1978). Premorbid psychological functions as related to cancer incidence. *Journal of Behavioral Medicine, 1,* 45–133.

Franks, C. M., Wilson, G. T., Kendall, P. C., & Foreyt, J. P. (1990). *Review of behavior therapy: theory and practice* (vol. 12). New York: Guilford.

Geringer, E. S., & Stern, T. A. (1986). Coping with medical illness: The impact of personality types. *Psychosomatics, 20,* 690–700.

Goldstein, M. G., Niaura, R., Willey-Lessne, C., DePue, J., Eaton, C., Rakowski, W., et al. (1997). Physicians counseling smokers: A population-based survey of patient's perceptions of health care provider-delivered smoking cessation interventions. *Archives of Internal Medicine, 157*(12), 1313–1319.

Hadid, R., Spinedi, E., Giovambattista, A., Chautard, T., & Gaillard, R. C. (1996). Decreased hypothalamo-pituitary-adrenal axis response to neuroendocrine challenge under repeated endotoxemia. *Neuroimmunomodulation, 3,* 62–68.

House, J. S. (1975). Occupational stress as a precursor to coronary disease. In W. D. Gentry & R. B. Williams (Eds.), *Psychological aspects of myocardial infarction and coronary care* (1st ed., pp. 24–36). St. Louis: Mosby.

Hunt, W. A., Barnett, L. W., & Ranch, L. G. (1971). Relapse rates in addiction programs. *Journal of Clinical Psychology, 27,* 455–456.

Kahana, R. J., & Bibring, G. L. (1964). Personality types in medical management. In N.

Zinberg (Ed.), *Psychiatry and medical practice in a general hospital* (pp. 108–123). New York: International Universities Press.

Kasl, S. V. (1984). Stress and health. *Annual Review of Public Health, 5,* 319–341.

Kasl, S. V., & Cobb, S. (1970). Blood pressure changes in men undergoing job loss: A preliminary report. *Psychosomatic Medicine, 32,* 19–38.

Kessler, R. C. (1979). Stress, social status, and psychological distress. *Journal of Health and Social Behavior, 20,* 259–272.

Kessler, R. C., & McRae, J. A., Jr. (1981). Trends in the relationship between sex and psychological distress: 1957–1976. *American Sociological Review, 46,* 443–452.

Kessler, R. C., & Neighbors, H. W. (1983). *Special issues related to racial and ethnic minorities in the U.S.* Institute of Social Research, University of Michigan. Unpublished paper.

Kessler, R. C., Price, R. H., & Wortman, C. B. (1985). Social factors in psychopathology: Stress, social support, and coping processes. *Annal Review of Psychology, 36,* 351–372.

Kessler, R. C. (1983). Methodological issues in the study of psychosocial stress: Measurement, design, and analysis. In H. B. Kaplan (Ed.), *Psychosocial stress: Recent developments in theory and research* (pp. 267–341). New York: Academic.

Kirschbaum, C., Prussner, J. C., & Stone, A. A. (1995). Persistent high cortisol responses to repeated psychological stress in a subpopulation of healthy men. *Psychosomatic Medicine, 57,* 468–474.

Kornfeld, D. S. (1979). The hospital environment: Its impact on the patient. In C. A. Garfield (Ed.), *Stress and Survival.* St. Louis: Mosby.

Kranz, D. S., Baum, A., & Singer, J. E. (Eds.). (1983). *Handbook of psychology and health. Vol. 3: Cardiovascular disorders and behavior.* Hillsdale, NJ: Erlbaum.

Larson, B., Seidell, J., & Svardsudd, K. (1989). Obesity, adipose tissue distribution and health in men—The study of men born in 1913. *Appetite, 13,* 37–44.

Lazarus, R. S., & Cohen, J. B. (1977). Environmental stress. In I. Altman & J. F. Wohlwill (Eds.), *Human behavior and the environment: Current theory and research.* New York: Plenum.

Ley, P. (1977). Psychological studies of doctor-patient communication. In S. Rachman (Ed.), *Contributions to medical psychology* (vol. 1). Oxford: Pergamon.

Lucente, F. E., &Flec, S. (1972). A study of hospitalization anxiety in 408 medical and surgical patients. *Psychosomatic Medicine, 34,* 304–312

Markowe, H. L. J., Marmot, M. G., & Shipley, M. J. (1985). Fibrinogen: A possible link between social class and coronary heart disease. *British Medical Journal, 291,* 1312–1314.

McCarty, R. (1985). Sympathetic-adrenal medullary and cardiovascular responses to acute cold stress in adult and aged rats. *Journal of the Autonomic Nervous System, 12,* 15–22.

McEwen, B. S. (1998). Protective and damaging effects of stress mediators. *New England Journal of Medicine, 338*(3), 171–179.

McEwen, B. S, & Margarinos, A. M. (1997). Stress effects on morphology and function of the hippocampus. *Annals of the New York Academy of Sciences, 821,* 271–284.

McEwen, B. S., & Sapolsky, R. M. (1995). Stress and cognitive function. *Current Opinion in Neurobiology, 5,* 205–216.

McEwen, B. S. (1992). Re-examination of the glucocorticoid hypothesis of stress and aging. In D. F. Swaab, M. A. Hofman, M. Mirmiran, R. Ravid, & F. W. van Leeuwen

(Eds.), *Progress in Brain Research vol. 93: The human hypothalamus in health and disease* (pp. 365–383). Amsterdam: Elsevier Science.

Meaney, M. J., Tannenbaum, B., & Francis, D. (1997). Early environmental programming; hypothalamic-pituitary-adrenal responses to stress. *Seminars in Neuroscience, 6*, 247–259.

Melin, B., Lundberg, U., Soderlund, J., & Granqvist, M. (1998). Psychological and physiological stress reactions of male and female assembly workers: A comparison between two different forms of work organization. *Journal of Organizational Behavior, 20*(1), 47–61.

Meyer, A. J., Nash, J. D., McAllister, A. L., Maccoby, N. , & Farquhar, J. W. (1980). Skills training in a cardiovascular education campaign. *Journal of Consulting and Clinical Psychology, 48*, 129–142.

Miller, W. B. (1973). Psychiatric consultation: Part I. A general system approach. *Psychiatry in Medicine, 4*, 135–145.

Morihisa, J. M., & Rosse, R. B. (1990). Psychophysiology. In *Behavioral science*. Baltimore: Williams and Wilkins.

Mullen, B., & Sulss, J. (1982). The effectiveness of attention and rejection as coping styles: A meta-analysis of temporal differences. *Journal of Psychosomatic Research, 26*(1), 43–49.

Muller, J. E, Tofler, G. H., & Stone, P. H. (1989). Circadian variation and triggers of onset of acute cardiovascular disease. *Circulation, 79*, 733–743.

Orne, M. T., Dinges, D. F., & Bloom, P. B. (1995). Hypnosis. In H. I. Kaplan & B. J. Sadock (Eds.), *Comprehensive textbook of psychiatry* (6th ed., pp. 1807–1821). Baltimore: Williams and Wilkins, Baltimore.

Parsons, T. (1951). *The social system*. New York: Free Press.

Pearlin, L. I., Lieberman, M. A., Meneghan, E. G., & Mullen, J. T. (1981). The stress process. *Journal of Health and Social Behavior, 22*, 337–356.

Pearlin, L. I., & Schooler, C. (1978). The structure of coping. *Journal of Health and Social Behavior, 19*, 2–21.

Pickering, T. G., Devereux ,R. B., & James, G. D. (1996). Environmental influences on blood pressure and the role of job strain. *Journal of Hypertension, 14*, S179–S185

Poteliakhoff, A. (1981). Adrenocortical activity and some clinical findings in acute and chronic fatigue. *Journal of Psychosomatic Research, 25*, 91–5.

Prochaska, J. O., & Goldstein, M. G. (1991). Process of smoking cessation: Implications for clinicians. *Clinics in Chest Medicine, 12*(4), 727–735.

Raikkonen, K., Lassila, R., Keltikangas-Jarvinen, L., & Hautanen, A. (1996). Association of chronic stress with plasminogen activator inhibitor-1 in healthy middle-aged men. *Arteriosclerosis, Thrombosis, and Vascular Biology, 16*, 363–367.

Rhue, J., Lynn, S., & Kirsch, I. (1988). *Handbook of clinical hypnosis*. Washington, DC: American Psychological Association.

Richardson, J. L., Shelton, D. R., Krailo, M., & Levine, A. M. (1990). The effect of compliance with treatment on survival among patients with hematologic malignancies. *Journal of Clinical Oncology, 8*, 356–64.

Sapolsky, R. M. (1990). Stress in the wild. *Scientific American, 262*, 116–123

Sapolsky, R. M. (1992). *Stress, the aging brain and the mechanisms of neuron death*. Cambridge, MA: MIT Press.

Schatzberg, A. F. (1990). Anxiety and adjustment disorder: A treatment approach. *Journal of Clinical Psychiatry, 51S*, 20.

Schnall, P. L., Schwartz, J. E., Landsbergis, P. A., Warren, K., & Pickering, T. G. (1992). Relation between job strain, alcohol, and ambulatory blood pressure. *Hypertension, 19,* 488–494

Schwartz, M. S. (Ed.). (1987). *Biofeedback: A practitioner's guide.* New York: Guilford.

Seeman, T. E., & McEwen, B. S. (1996). The impact of social environment characteristics on neuroendocrine regulation. *Psychosomatic Medicine, 58,* 459–471

Seeman, T. E., & Robbins, R. J. (1994). Aging and hypothalamic-pituitary-adrenal response to challenge in humans. *Endocrine Review, 15,* 233–260.

Selye, H. (1956). *The Stress of life.* New York: McGraw-Hill.

Shively, C. A., & Clarkson, T. B. (1994). Social status and coronary artery atherosclerosis en female monkeys. *Arteriosclerosis, Thrombosis, and Vascular Biology, 14,* 721–176.

Sklar, L. S., & Anisman, H. (1981). Stress and cancer. *Psychology Bulletin, 89,* 369–406.

Spiegel, D. (1993). *Living beyond limits.* New York: Times Books.

Spiegel, D., Bloom, J. R., Kraemer, H. C., & Gottheil, E. (1989). Effect of psychosocial treatment on survival of patients with metastatic breast cancer. *Lancet, 2,* 888–891.

Strain, J. J., & Grossman, S. (1975). *Psychological care of the medically ill.* New York: Appleton-Century-Croft.

Strauss, D. M., Spitzer, R. L., & Muskin, P. R. (1990). Maladaptive denial of physical illness: A proposal for DSM-IV. *The American Journal of Psychiatry, 31,* 426–433.

Thoits, P. A. (1983). Dimensions of life events that influence psychological distress: An evaluation and synthesis of the literature. In H. B. Kaplan (Ed.), *Psychological stress: Trends in theory and research* (pp. 33–103). New York: Academic.

Uno, H., Tarara, R., Else, J. G., Suleman, M. A., & Sapolsky, R. M. (1989). Hippocampal damage associated with prolonged and fatal stress in primates. *Journal of Neuroscience, 9,* 1705–1711.

Verdecchia, P., Schillaci, G., & Borgioni, C. (1995). Cigarette smoking, ambulatory blood pressure and cardiac hypertrophy in essential hypertension. *Journal of Hypertension, 13,* 1209–1215

Veroff, J., Douvan, E., & Kulda, R. A. (1981). *The inner American: A self portrait from 1957–1976.* New York: Basic Books.

Watts, A. W. (1997). Zen. In *Microsoft encarta 1997 encyclopedia CD-ROM.* Redmond, CA: Microsoft Corporation.

Webb, W. B. (1997). States of consciousness. In *Microsoft encarta 1997 encyclopedia CD-ROM.* Redmond, CA: Microsoft Corporation.

Weisman, A. D. (1974). *The realization of death: A guide for the psychological autopsy.* New York: Jason Aronson.

Weisman, A. D. (1997). Coping with illness. In N. H. Cassem (Ed.), *Handbook of general hospital psychiatry* (pp. 25–34). St. Louis: Mosby.

Wilkinson, C. W., Peskind, E. R., & Raskind, M. A. (1997). Decreased hypothalamic-pituitary-adrenal axis sensitivity to cortisol feedback inhibition in human aging. *Neuroendocrinology, 65,* 79–90.

Yehuda, R., Teicher, M. H., Trestman, R. L., Levengood, R. A., & Siever, L. J. (1996). Cortisol regulation in posttraumatic stress disorder and major depression: A chronobiological analysis. *Biological Psychiatry, 40,* 79–88.

Treatment

KATHLEEN ULMAN

Psychosocial interventions for medical patients start with the first visit to a health care provider. Communications between patients and clinicians are not only a means of exchanging medical information, they also are human interactions. For example, the health care provider's approach to questions about symptoms and details of everyday life, the emotional and behavioral advice offered, and the empathy and support conveyed to the patient, all may have an impact on the patient's psychosocial functioning (Greenfield, Kaplan, & Ware, 1985). The first mention of a referral to a mental health professional is the start of a formal psychosocial intervention.

As many health care providers have discovered, making a successful referral for a psychosocial intervention is complex. Clinical experience informs us that the timing and manner in which the referral is introduced and implemented has a bearing on the success of the intervention. As with all patient-physician communication, referrals made in an empathic open-ended way that give the patient time to digest the particular medical diagnosis and its psychosocial implications have the best chance for success (Greenfield, Kaplan, & Ware, 1985). The medical clinician may need to bring a patient back for several follow-up visits to complete the referral to a mental health professional.

INITIAL CONSIDERATIONS

Once the referral for a psychosocial intervention has been made, the treating mental health clinician needs to gather information about the patient. The clinician will use this information to develop the most appropriate treatment plan for this particular patient. Clinical experience has shown that the mental health clinician must determine and understand the expectations of the referring health care provider. This includes obstacles to compliance with his medical recommendations as well as his perception of the difficulties the patient may experience. Consideration of optimal ways to prepare the patient for the psychosocial intervention is an integral part to a successful treatment plan. Preparation includes explanations of the rationale for the choice of intervention, details of how this particular intervention will be implemented, and time for patient questions.

EVALUATING A PATIENT'S APPROPRIATENESS FOR PSYCHOSOCIAL INTERVENTION

The mental health clinician will meet with the patient for at least one or two intake sessions to evaluate the patient's appropriateness for a psychosocial intervention. In these initial sessions, the mental health clinician will obtain general information that would be gathered in any mental health intake, but may vary the amount of detail obtained in particular areas. For example, a brief family and social history may be gathered with an added focus on the role illness in general has played in the psychosocial context of the individual. It is essential that the clinician be alert to symptoms of depression. Major and minor depressions often go unrecognized in medical settings (Magruder-Habib et al., 1989). Medical patients who are depressed have increased morbidity and mortality (Broadhead, Blazer, George, & Tse, 1990; Coulahan, Schulberg, Block, Janosky, & Arena, 1990; Wells et al., 1989). The mental health clinician may be the only health care provider who directly asks about a patient's symptoms of depression. Additionally, the clinician may ask for a very detailed medical history along with specific information about current social supports. Knowledge of life-style choices, such as nutrition and exercise, and coping styles in past crises will be helpful in choosing the most effective intervention.

It is also useful for the clinician to ask about the patient's attitude towards his illness, his understanding of its causation, and possible treatment. Extensive clinical experience tells us that exploration of the patient's emotional responses to his illness will help the clinician to assess how this patient's reactions compare with what might be expected of most people in the same situation and evaluate the degree to which neurotic conflicts and characterological functioning may have distorted the patient's reaction to his illness. The clinician may use this information to assess the degree of awareness the patient has regarding his or her own psychological history and current medical status and his or her ability to use both medical and psychological treatment (Taylor & Aspinwall, 1990; Brown & Fromm, 1987). It is not necessary to have psychological insight to benefit from many psychosocial interventions, but the presence of insight and curiosity may determine the particular psychosocial intervention chosen (Roth, 1990).

Detailed information on the patient's current use of coping skills will be essential in choosing a psychosocial intervention (Brown & Fromm, 1987). For example: what does the patient typically do in the face of loss or stress? What has the patient done in response to the current illness to improve his or her condition or the quality of her life? What is the patient willing to do now to address her illness? Can the patient take an active stance? Is the patient willing to use psychosocial resources such as support from friends, family, medical clinicians, support groups, or counseling? Is the patient interested in adopting new behaviors? Is the patient able to set goals and try new approaches to the new problems created by his or her illness?

A crucial part of the evaluation for a psychosocial intervention is the determination of the patient's wishes and expectations (Lazare, & Eisenthal, 1979; Lazare, Eisenthal, & Frank, 1979). How does he or she imagine that you will help him or her? How does he or she want to be different when he or she comes to the end of the intervention? Additionally, it is important to determine the expectations of the referring physician.

CHOOSING THE MOST EFFICACIOUS APPROACH

The clinician may choose the most efficacious approach for each individual patient from a number of possible psychosocial interventions. Usually, a particular treatment plan is comprised of a mixture of available interventions (Brown & Fromm, 1987).

Psychoeducation

Psychoeducation is often one of the first psychosocial interventions used with medical patients. It can be very effective in providing a cognitive framework to help reduce the patient's anxiety (Simonton & Sherman, 2000). The intervention may include: (1) information on the impact of psychosocial variables on the patient's particular illness; (2) general information regarding the impact of social supports on health, and (3) discussion of the positive impact symbolic expression of affect can have on immune function (Kiecolt-Glaser et al., 1985; Pennebaker, 1992; Pennebaker, Kiecolt-Glaser, & Glaser, 1988). The patient can also be taught about the potential influence of the stress response on illness and the benefits of stress reduction (Benson, Beary, & Carol, 1974). This knowledge can increase the patient's awareness of current behavior that may aggravate his or her symptoms and may interfere with recovery. It may also serve as a springboard for developing more adaptive coping skills with the goal of increasing the patient's sense of control over his or her situation (Domar & Dreher, 1996; Simonton & Sherman, 2000).

Ideally, psychoeducation will be a multidisciplinary effort with physicians, nutritionists, physical therapists, clergy, and others working together with mental health professionals to provide the patient with information about the illness and options for managing its personal, emotional, interpersonal, social, and occupational impact (Simonton & Sherman, 2000).

Psychotherapy

Supportive Psychotherapy

Supportive psychotherapy is an appropriate psychosocial intervention for medical patients who are feeling overwhelmed and in need of a place to express feelings and receive validation and support. It is particularly helpful for those individuals who lack social support, who have had previous difficulty coping day-to-day, or who appear to have significant psychiatric disorders (House, Landis, & Umberson 1988; Karasu, 1995).

Supportive psychotherapy offers medical patients a place to express and to have validated intense feelings that they may not feel free to share with family or friends. Giving verbal expression to traumatic affect can have a beneficial effect on the course of illness (Pennebaker, 1992) and, when accompanied by supportive and clarifying responses from the therapist, may lead to relief and increased insight (Uchino, Cacioppo, & Kiecolt-Glaser, 1996). For example, supportive psychotherapy may provide a patient with the opportunity to put into words the terror he or she experienced during a heart attack; a feeling he or she might have been reluctant to share with his or her spouse.

Cognitive Psychotherapy

Cognitive psychotherapy is appropriate for those individuals who demonstrate distortions and pessimism about themselves or their illness and who express interest in changing their thought patterns (Beck & Rush, 1995; Brown & Fromm, 1987). Those medical patients who experience troublesome, intrusive, and repetitive thoughts often find cognitive psychotherapy useful. Research has shown that cognitive treatment has resulted in improvements in distress and attitudes towards health in medical patients (Fawzy, Fawzy, Arndt, & Pasnau, 1995).

Clinical experience has demonstrated that cognitive psychotherapy is not appropriate for those who are reluctant to entertain the notion that their thoughts may have an influence on their physical or emotional state. Nor is it appropriate for those who currently feel overwhelmed or who have an immediate need to receive support and validation and express intense affects such as anger. However, after an initial supportive psychosocial intervention, such individuals may benefit from cognitive psychotherapy.

Behavioral Psychotherapy

Behavioral psychotherapy is ideal for those individuals who want to make changes in their behavior and who are willing to collaborate with a therapist to identify specific behaviors that are contributing to their distress (Brown & Fromm, 1987; Agras, 1995). Those patients with specific behaviors that aggravate their illness or create a life-threatening situation may find behavioral interventions particularly helpful. Target behaviors would include the eating patterns of an obese medical patient with high blood pressure or smoking for a patient with decreased pulmonary function.

Behavior therapy is also useful for those who seek to increase their sense of control over a personal or medical situation and is not appropriate for those who externalize blame for their illness or other life situations and are uninterested in being a participant in their health care.

Cognitive and behavioral interventions usually are offered together by one psychotherapist and often represent an integrated approach to psychological distress related to illness (Agras, 1995).

Insight-Oriented Psychotherapy

Insight-oriented psychotherapy is an appropriate psychosocial intervention for those medical patients who describe some psychic pain related to their illness and who express an interest in changing their psychological state (Karasu, 1995; Roth, 1990). It can also be an efficacious intervention for patients who demonstrate functional defenses which allow them to express and bear some affect, and who show some capacity for insight and curiosity about themselves.

Insight-oriented psychotherapy is not appropriate for those individuals who see themselves as psychologically "fine" before their illness or for those who see themselves as passive recipients of medical care. It is also not appropriate for patients whose primary goal is to learn techniques to manage physical symptoms. However, at the completion of a structured intervention such as a time-limited cognitive behavioral group, a small number of individuals will have begun the process of internal exploration and may benefit from a referral for insight-oriented psychotherapy (Ulman, 2000).

Relaxation-Stress Management

Teaching relaxation techniques together with stress management are an appropriate psychosocial intervention for any interested patient (Agras, 1995; Caudill, Galluci, & Bevus, 1996). Benson, Beary, and Carol (1974) describe a stress reaction as an acute or chronic increase in adrenaline or noradrenaline and subsequent physiological changes such as elevated blood pressure, increased muscle tension, and increased heart rate. This stress reaction occurs in response to a real or perceived threat which may be an external event or an internal feeling. Inducing a state of relaxation can help to re-establish physiological equilibrium in anyone who has been experiencing a stress reaction. A state of relaxation can be induced by performing a repetitive exercise, whether physical or mental (Benson et al., 1974; Domar & Dreher, 1996; Kabat-Zinn, 1990). Patients often find focusing on breathing to be the easiest relaxation technique. Other effective relaxation techniques are repetition of a syllable, progressive muscle relaxation, yoga, and mindfulness meditation and body scan, which involves focusing one's attention on successive areas of the body. Walking, meditation, and t'chi are useful techniques for those who cannot tolerate sitting quietly. Regular practice of relaxtion is associated with decreased responsivity (Hoffman et al., 1982). The most important ingredient is for the individual to find the relaxation technique that suits him or her best (Ulman, 2000).

The stress management programs described by Benson and Stuart (1982), Kabat-Zinn (1992), and Ulman (2000) are particularly useful combinations of psychosocial interventions. These programs combine psychoeducation, relaxation, cognitive and behavioral interventions, and, at times, written expression of affect. Cognitive interventions are often focused on repetitive, stress-inducing, negative thoughts. Behavioral interventions focus on identifying and reducing stress-inducing situations and on increasing behaviors which produce relaxation, such as exercise, social recreation, or listening to music. With this combination of psychosocial interventions, medical patients often have their first opportunity to focus their attention on their own internal experience (physical, cognitive, and/or affective) and to make connections between external events, physical sensations, and internal psychological events (Ulman, 2000).

Visualization

Visualization, also called guided imagery, is frequently used in combination with a state of relaxation or hypnosis (Orne, Dinges, & Bloom, 1995). When used with medical patients, generally this technique involves using the mind to create a sense of physical well-being and health (Altshuler, 1995). The clinician uses verbal suggestions to structure the imagery for the patient. For example, the clinician may suggest that the patient imagine a place in her mind where he or she feels specific things that would relieve his or her symptoms such as: peaceful, calm, and healthy. Visualization often helps individuals gain a sense of control over seemingly involuntary physiological functions such as breathing or gastric motility. It can also be very useful in helping patients manage anxiety related to medical procedures such as chemotherapy, dentistry, and surgery (Baker, 1996; Simonton & Sherman, 2000). In these cases the clinician can suggest that the patient imagines himself going through a procedure comfortably with positive results (Baker, 1996).

Factors Influencing Choice of Treatment

The choice of psychosocial treatment must be done on an individual basis (Brown & Fromm, 1988). The severity, stage, and type of illness will be considered in making a treatment recommendation (Simonton & Sherman, 2000). The final choice should always be a mutual decision between patient and clinician.

In presenting a recommendation for psychosocial treatment to the medical patient, it is important that the clinician clearly describe the treatment and the reasons for his or her recommendation. For many medical patients who have ongoing medical conditions which are not terminal or acute and whose emotional reactions to their illness are not significantly distorted by neurotic or characterological factors, an initial referral to a time-limited psychoeducation group that includes cognitive, behavioral, and stress-reducing interventions would be a useful choice (Simonton & Sherman, 2000). However, for a patient who experiences emotional lability and a sense of urgency as a result of his or her illness, an initial referral for individual supportive treatment would be the best choice (based on extensive clinical experience). For those patients who feel unable to participate in a group, individual psychoeducational and supportive treatment is appropriate. A few medical patients may seek insight-oriented psychotherapy at the outset, and others may request it after participating in another psychosocial intervention. At times, the clinician may decide to recommend insight-oriented psychotherapy to a patient who demonstrates insight and curiosity about his psychological functioning even if he or she has not requested insight-oriented psychotherapy.

Combining Interventions

Often a combination of interventions is the most appropriate and effective treatment (Brown & Fromm, 1987; Spira, 1997). Offering the patient a well thought out succession of psychosocial interventions gives the patient experience with a variety of approaches to modifying his response to illness (Simonton & Sherman, 2000). It is hard to anticipate, at the outset, which interventions the patient will prefer and be able to tolerate. For example, some individuals have dysphoric experiences when using imagery, some prefer to talk, and others cannot sit still.

In the case of a serious acute illness, a patient may feel overwhelmed, vulnerable, and ashamed and be unwilling at the outset to be in a group. Clinical experience has demonstrated that for this type of patient supportive treatment often is initially appropriate and is sometimes followed by psychoeducation. Further into the course of illness, after the turmoil of the initial reaction has diminished, the patient may wish to move to a combination of cognitive and behavioral interventions that may include relaxation and stress management. At that point the patient may even feel able to participate in a group. In the case of a chronic illness such as diabetes or heart disease, for a patient who is not in acute emotional crisis treatment often starts with psychoeducation. Treatment may then move to a combination of cognitive and behavioral interventions or stress management to address the anxiety and isolation that often accompanies chronic illnesses. At the same time, the patient may benefit from individual supportive treatment to bolster his usually effective defenses and to help him move forward with his or her everyday life while dealing with the challenge of meeting the demands of his or her illness. The clinician remains alert to signals from the patient that he or she might want to pursue more intensive insight-oriented psychotherapy.

CHOOSING A SPECIFIC TYPE OF INTERVENTION

Once an approach is determined (i.e., cognitive-behavioral, supportive counseling, or psychotherapy), the choice of the type of psychosocial intervention (i.e., individual, group, or family) depends a variety of factors, including individual wishes, patient's psychosocial situation, availability of services, type of illness, stage of illness, and therapist's expertise and comfort with a particular mode of intervention.

Individual Intervention

The psychosocial interventions previously mentioned can be offered on an individual basis. Initially, individual supportive treatment is particularly useful after a serious diagnosis or an event such as a myocardial infarction, stroke, or serious accident (Taylor & Aspinwall, 1990). Individual cognitive and behavioral interventions are appropriate for those interested. However, these interventions often provide additonal benefits when offered in a group format (Speigel, 1993; Ulman, 2000). As stated earlier, for some patients with the motivation to learn about and change their personality individual insight-oriented psychotherapy may be the psychosocial treatment of choice from the start (Karasu, 1995). However, the availability of any open-ended individual treatment is often limited by financial resources. Thus, for both clinical and financial reasons, often the most efficacious psychosocial treatment may be a brief individual intervention followed by a group .

Couple/Family Interventions

Illness affects everyone in a family system. The choice of intervention will depend on the make-up and dynamics of the family.

Couple interventions may be helpful when the patient's illness has a significant influence on the marital relationship and/or the spouse's ability to carry out usual daily tasks. Examples of such situations include illnesses that influence sexual functioning, cause changes in physical appearance, or place limitations on the patient's ability to carry out basic daily tasks inside or outside the home. Clinical experience demonstrates that couple interventions are especially appropriate when the patient indicates to the clinician that conflicts in the marriage are interfering with the patient's ability to cooperate with medical treatment or that the medical treatment is interfering with the couple's relationship.

Couple interventions are indicated when the couple is experiencing difficulty discussing feelings or behavior related to the illness, or when the illness activates previously unresolved conflicts which the couple are not able to discuss on their own. For example, couples who have been unable to discuss feelings regarding sexuality and body image often need help in resuming sexual intimacy after breast or prostate surgery. Some spouses often have difficulty discerning their partners' needs. Several meetings between the couple and a skilled clinician can be helpful in clarifying the situation, enlisting the spouse's cooperation, and in reducing anxiety. Couple interventions are also particularly effective when an illness is terminal and the couple needs help addressing grief, in making plans, and in saying good-bye.

Family interventions may be helpful when a child is seriously ill. At such times, the family's functioning is affected and siblings may suffer. The usefulness of a family intervention is determined by the nature of the illness, the make-up of the family, the ages of the children, the ability of the parents to communicate with the children and to allow the expression of feelings. For example, when children have chronic illnesses that are managed easily by parents who are able to communicate openly their feelings, there may be no need for a family intervention. On the other hand, family interventions may be particularly useful when illness activates previously unresolved conflicts.

Many medical settings offer groups for couples and families. The groups can be effective in providing information, support, and the opportunity to express thoughts and feelings, as well as reducing the sense of isolation and shame that many families experience.

Group Interventions

Groups are an ideal psychosocial intervention for most medical patients at some point in the course of their illness (Allen & Scheidt, 1981; Lonergan, 1985; Speigel, 1993; Spira, 1997; Ulman, 1993). Groups of all types (self-help, support, or psychotherapy) provide opportunities to reduce isolation and shame by bringing patients together with others who also have had similar health experiences (Ulman, 1993). Groups can also provide an opportunity for expression, reduce isolation and shame, provide a sense of hope, and, at times, decrease depressive symptoms that may aggravate the particular medical condition (Speigel, 1992). Groups for medical patients vary in structure, schedule, and membership requirements (Gick, McClelland, & Budd, 1997; Hellman, Budd, Borysenko, et al., 1990; Simonton and Sherman, 2000; Toner et al., 1998; Ulman, 1993). Whatever their complexion, these groups should be an integral part of most treatment plans. They may help the patient develop a sense of competence and self-efficacy related to the illness, help interested patients to mobilize psychosocial supports, and improve the quality of their lives (Spira, 1997; Ulman, 2000).

Some patients are uncomfortable in groups and refuse a group referral. In such cases, the clinician may explain the organization of the particular group, encourage the patient to try a single session drop-in group to get the feel of being with others in a similar situation, and/or reintroduce the group referral in a low-key way periodically in the future. However, it is counterproductive to push medical patients into a group that they do not want. Frequently, patients who reluctantly join groups merely to comply with their clinician's suggestion do not fully participate in the group and may end up feeling traumatized by the experience (Rutan & Stone, 1993).

Time-Limted Groups

Time-limited groups that combine emotional support, instruction in relaxation techniques, cognitive and behavioral interventions, and self-selected goals provide the best short-term opportunity for medical patients to accomplish desired changes (Sobel, 1995). Such groups offer patients a psychosocial experience not possible with individual intervention. In addition to providing an opportunity for expression of affect and reducing isolation and shame, these groups can address negative attitudes and encourage active problem-solving related to managing the illness. Time-limited groups are particularly useful for those medical patients who do not take on the identity of a chronic patient, but who, instead, want to manage their illness as well as possible and move on with their lives (Ulman, 1993).

Family Groups

Groups can provide similarly positive psychosocial experiences for families and significant others. Illness affects everyone in the family system. Coming together with others in a similar situation often creates a sense of community and social support for these individuals who may be feeling isolated, sad, anxious, depressed, and depleted. Family groups vary in terms of membership and schedule. They may meet once, several times, or many times. They may be drop-in groups or require regular attendance.

Open-Ended Groups

Some clinicians report success with open-ended groups which initially combine psychoeducation with cognitive or behavioral interventions such as relaxation or pain management, and then gradually move to the expression and exploration of affect (Ulman, 1993). Such groups have also been effective among patients suffering other chronic conditions for whom the patient-identity has become syntonic (Ulman, 1993). David Spiegel (Spiegel, Bloom, Kramer, & Gottheil, 1989) has reported success with his supportive expressive model for patients with breast cancer.

Traditional open-ended psychodynamic groups use the interactive process among group members and between group members and the group therapist to understand the historic roots of members' current psychological functioning (Rutan & Stone, 1993). Such groups may be useful for two types of medical patients. The first are individuals for whom the identity as a chronic medical patient is syntonic (Ulman, 1993). Often these patients will attend a time-limited group and then move to an open-ended group for medical patients. The second category are those who discover in the course of their illness or as a result of cognitive behavioral treatment that there are intrapsychic and interpersonal factors which interfere with their health or quality of life that they would like to change. Patients with a variety of medical conditions who participate in such open-ended groups have been found to use less medication and have fewer doctor's visits (Ulman, 1993).

ARRANGING THE TREATMENT REGIMEN

Given the various combinations of psychosocial treatments available to medical patients, a treatment regimen often involves utilizing interdisciplinary treatment teams (Simonton & Sherman, 2000). Such an approach allows for assessment from a variety of vantage points, enriches each clinician's point of view, adds breadth to the treatment options, and allows for the possibility of consecutive or simultaneous treatment with a variety of psychosocial interventions. To avoid misunderstandings between members of the treatment team, careful attention should be paid to maintaining clear communication and respecting each clinician's area of expertise. The ability to employ an interdisciplinary treatment team may be limited by financial considerations or by the patient's unwillingness or inability to be involved with a number of clinicians.

Managed Care Considerations

Seldom does the clinician welcome managed care. At times it limits the options for intervention, intrudes on the confidentiality of the clinician-patient relationship, and requires additional administrative work. However, in many parts of the United States, the majority of patients currently are covered by managed care plans, and treatment plans must be designed with insurance carriers requirements in mind.

For many patients the most effective use of their limited medical benefits is a time-limited group intervention incorporating a variety of techniques designed to: provide psychosocial support; teach coping skills; promote an awareness of internal states, an increased sense of control, and self-efficacy; decrease the patient' feelings of isolation; and provide a sense of universality and hope (MacKenzie, 1990; Sobel, 1995). In addition to the financial benefits, many clinicians (Benson, Beary, & Carol, 1974; Kabat-Zinn, 1982; Sobel, 1995) believe that cognitive-behavioral and stress-reducing interventions are more effective when delivered in a group. Open-ended group psychotherapy is clinically effective and financially practical for those medical patients who need a more extended psychotherapeutic intervention due to mood and personality factors which influence the course of their illness. As stated previously, researchers have reported decreases in medical visits and medication usage for medical patients engaged in open-ended group psychotherapy (Ulman, 1993). Open-ended individual insight-oriented psychotherapy may be available through managed care only when the patient demonstrates significant impairment in functioning.

Patient Preparation

Ideally, the mental health clinician who performed the initial assessment will meet with the patient to review the treatment recommendations. Clinical experience has shown that these initial sessions set the stage for future interventions. If there is a possibility that the patient will be referred to another mental health clinician for treatment, it is best that this be mentioned at the first meeting. A brief review of data on the usefulness of various psychosocial interventions for individuals attempting to manage an acute illness or those living with chronic illness is helpful. The clinician can then present to the patient an outline of the treatment recommendations, including a discussion of the rationale for each particular intervention and an estimated time frame. The clinician will also take time to clarify the conditions of confidentiality, make plans for communication with other health care professionals, set the fee structure, determine the role of managed care, and clarify his or her availability throughout the treatment (Roth, 1990). A good portion of the preparation session can be set aside to allow the patient to ask questions and to express reactions to the recommendation. A recommendation for a couple or family intervention is often received best if it is first mentioned to the medical patient and then presented to all individuals who will be involved in the treatment. The meeting can conclude with an agreement between the clinician and patient as to the particular type of interventions to be pursued, expected length of treatment, and responsibilities of each party.

If the treatment recommendation involves a referral to another clinician, the evaluating clinician should review the reasons for choosing this particular individual. A referral to another clinician can be difficult for medical patients who already may have several health care professionals. Ideally, the mental health professional responsible for the assessment will communicate all necessary details to the clinician responsible for treatment. Meanwhile, a relationship will be maintained with the patient until the referral process has been completed and the patient is engaged in the psychosocial intervention.

At the initial meeting, the clinician responsible for treatment will review many of the details already discussed with the evaluating clinician. In spite of the repetitiveness, the patient usually finds the opportunity to discuss his medical situation, expectations, and history helpful in making the difficult transition from the evaluating clinician to the treating clinician. A portion of the session may be set aside to give the patient an opportunity to discuss his reactions to the evaluation and referral process as well as to review the plan of the intervention.

Consideration of Group Composition

Time-Limited Groups

The composition of time-limited groups may be homogeneous or heterogeneous, according to medical and/or psychiatric diagnosis. As with individual interventions, all members need to be informed as to what is expected of them and agree to work on the group's designated goals (MacKenzie, 1990).

Homogeneous groups can be most helpful when patients have specific educational needs or when they experience isolation and shame related to their particular symptoms, as do patients with irritable bowel syndrome, most forms of cancer, or premenstrual syndrome (Simonton & Sherman, 2000; Spira, 1997; Toner et al., 1998; Ulman, 1993).

Groups consisting of members with heterogeneous diagnoses are more effective when patient complaints involve stress-related illnesses or adaptation to chronic illness (Ulman, 1993; Ulman, 2000). A heterogeneous group helps patients to focus on similarities related to the condition of having an illness rather than on particular symptoms.

Open-Ended Groups

Research has shown that medical patients do well in either heterogeneous or homogeneous open-ended psychotherapy groups (Ulman, 1993; Spiegel et al., 1989). The clinician may make a recommendation based upon the individual needs and wishes of each patient and the current availability of specific groups. Many cancer patients prefer a homogeneous group as described by Spiegel et al. (1989) and Simonton and Sherman (2000). Groups with a variety of diagnoses are more effective for many patients with chronic medical conditions, such as diabetes and arthritis (Ulman, 1993). It is difficult for members of a heterogeneous group to focus on particular symptoms or medications as a defense against dealing with feelings. Rather, the heterogeneous group composition encourages members to explore the shared similarities of their varied existential situations. Clinical experience also has shown that some medical patients may prefer a heterogeneous open-ended psychotherapy group in which the majority of members have no significant medical problems.

In putting together homogeneous or heterogeneous groups, the overall mix of individual patients' styles is an important consideration. An open-ended group of any type works best when each member has at least one other group member with whom they can identify and a few group members from whom they can learn new ways of responding to emotional challenges (Rutan & Stone, 1993). Having only one of any particular category such as one angry member, one male, one very young individual, or one passive member, does not provide optimal therapeutic opportunities for all group members.

TREATMENT CONSIDERATIONS

Distinguishing Psychosocial Treatment from Psychotherapy

In undertaking psychosocial interventions for medical patients it is useful for the clinician to clearly distinguish psychotherapy from other types of psychosocial interventions. Among psychosocial interventions, psychotherapy is the only intervention whose primary aim is personality change (Karasu, 1995). As stated previously, most medical patients see themselves as having a condition that has interfered with their everyday life. They seek psychosocial treatment to help them cope with the challenges brought on by the medical condition. Generally, they do not see themselves as needing to change their personality and do not seek psychotherapy. Thus, it is important that once a treatment plan has been agreed upon, the clinician employ techniques which are congruent with the goals of the treatment plan. If a clinician is conducting supportive treatment, he will neither deliberately foster nor interpret the development of negative transference. This may be particularly difficult on those occasions when it becomes clear to the clinician that one patient is experiencing negative interactions with his health care provider which may be interfering with treatment. However, if during treatment a patient decides he would like to explore the sources of his reactions to his illness and to his health care provider, he and the mental health clinician may jointly agree to modify the treatment plan to include insight-oriented psychotherapy. Similarly, if as a result of participation in a support group a patient comes to recognize that he has repetitive negative thoughts which aggravate his medical condition, he may choose to participate in some cognitive psychotherapy.

Similarities

Clear Definition of Goals and Boundaries

For all psychosocial interventions including psychotherapy,the clinician and patient need to come to a clear agreement regarding the boundaries and goals of treatment (Roth, 1990; Rutan & Stone, 1993). This includes the time, place, and frequency of meetings, cost, estimated length of treatment, availability of the clinician between meetings, and focus of treatment. For open-ended interventions, the clinician and patient will come to an agreement as to how they will know when the goals have been accomplished (Rutan & Stone, 1993). For time-limited treatment, the patient and clinician will agree together on the date of the final meeting (MacKenzie, 1990).

Therapeutic Stance

The mental health clinician always seeks to provide a therapeutic experience by creating a sense of predictability and safety for the medical patient. The therapist is careful to observe the agreed-upon boundaries of therapy such as starting and ending the sessions on time and keeping the patient's information confidential. Additionally, the therapist tries to behave consistently by presenting a similar demeanor to the patient in each session and by listening attentively and respectfully each session (Karasu, 1995).

Symptoms Requiring Change in Treatment Plan

All clinicians need to remain alert to the possibility that the patient may demonstrate changes in mood and behavior which require a change in the treatment plan. This may happen even with patients seeking the least complicated psychosocial interventions. Any indication of suicidal or homicidal ideation or symptoms indicative of a depression or an anxiety disorder need to be taken seriously. In such instances, the other health care professionals involved with the patient need to be informed and an appropriate referral should be made. Depression is often under-recognized and undertreated in medical settings.

Differences

One difference between most forms of psychosocial treatment and psychodynamic psychotherapy is that insight regarding the role of psychological functioning is necessary only for patients participating in psychotherapy (Karasu, 1995). As stated previously, clinical experience has demonstrated that most patients seeking psychosocial interventions see their problems as arising as a result of their physical illness. Their goal is to learn to cope with the changes in their everyday life brought about by their illness.

Another difference is that in undertaking most psychosocial interventions, the clinician takes a supportive stance and seeks to diminish anxiety and to support the patients' defenses. In psychodynamic psychotherapy, however, the clinician seeks to increase the level of anxiety and challenge the patient's defenses (Karasu, 1995). When conducting many types of psychosocial treatment, the clinician may address issues of social support sooner and more directly than when psychodynamic psychotherapy is a part of the psychosocial intervention. Additionally, the clinician seeks out unconscious material only when defenses appear to support attitudes, moods, and coping styles that interfere with recovery from or management of the illness. To this end, the clinician seeks to enhance the positive transference and does not encourage the development of negative transference as he or she does in psychodynamic psychotherapy (Karasu, 1995). If a negative transference develops the clinician seeks to address it immediately. Additionally, the clinician takes a more active stance in introducing topics and strategies, and in providing direct interventions. Generally, within this framework, the clinician and patient together define the goals and specific behaviors to be addressed.

Creating a Therapeutic Environment

It is the clinician's responsibility to create a therapeutic environment (Roth, 1990). As in all treatment, the clinician should provide a safe, consistent, and private physical space. If the treatment takes place in a medical setting, the clinician may have to take a more active role in securing the space. This is particularly true when the treatment takes place in a medical inpatient setting. It is often a challenge to secure a private room which is free from intrusive interruptions. As stated previously, the therapist should address with the patient, the conditions of confidentiality in relation to the patient's physician and family as well as other members of the treatment team.

A VARIETY OF INTERVENTIONS PROVIDES OPTIMAL PSYCHOSOCIAL TREATMENT

For optimal psychosocial treatment of medical patients, the therapist must draw upon a variety of interventions ranging from psychoeduction to open-ended psychotherapy (Brown & Fromm, 1987; Simonton & Sherman, 2000). Clinical judgement determines the timing and choice of anxiety-reducing or anxiety-promoting interventions, when to promote open exploration and elaboration of affect, when to support defenses, and when to invite the patient's curiosity regarding particular self-defeating behaviors. The flow of the treatment becomes smoother when the therapist is comfortable in using a variety of techniques. Ideally, a treatment team is assembled that includes specialists such as nutritionists and exercise specialists whenever appropriate.

STRATEGIES TO AID IN DIFFICULT SITUATIONS

Consult with Colleagues

As in all clinical work, individuals providing psychosocial treatment for medical patients may need, at times, to consult with colleagues. A large number of variables impinge on medical patients and complicate the therapist's job. Clinical experience has demonstrated that a consult is particularly appropriate when the clinician feels anxious, unsure, or is puzzled by an increase in the patient's psychological distress.

Difficult Situations

Therapists working with medical patients often confront difficult situations related to a tragic unexpected illness. Often families and caretakers look to the mental health provider to help them bear unbearable feelings. Such situations force the therapists to confront their own difficult feelings related to helplessness and mortality. Clinical experience has demonstrated that a strong professional and social network is important for all clinicians to call upon when working with seriously medically ill patients.

Difficult Patients

Medically ill patients who are not ready to give up life-threatening behavior, or who do not cooperate with appropriate medical treatment, present serious challenges for clinicians (Blackwell, 1995; Gunderson & Phillips, 1995). Many clinicians find this challenge similar to that involved in treating patients not yet ready to give up addictions. With such patients, the most useful tool for the therapist is confidence in the therapeutic value of social support, expression of affect, and an accepting and containing environment. Helpful techniques include pointing out the role of the patient's ambivalence in his or her behavior and avoidance of collusion without prematurely attacking the patient's denial. Once an alliance is established with the patient, the therapist can frequently draw attention to the contradiction in the patient's behavior between his or her stated goals of improvement and his or her noncompliant self-destructive behavior. The therapist can invite exploration of this contradiction.

ASSISTANCE FOR FAMILY AND FRIENDS

From time to time, the clinician who provides psychosocial treatment to medically ill patients may find it appropriate to provide assistance to family members and significant others in ways that are not usual for a traditional psychotherapist. When a clinician conducts most types of psychosocial treatment he or she does not usually encourage the development of or interpret negative transference. He or she thus has more leeway in interacting with family members. However, the wishes of the patient need to be respected. The preservation of the therapeutic relationship is the therapist's first priority. If the patient does not want contact between the therapist and the family, another clinician can be of assistance to the family or friends.

Meetings between the clinician, the patient, and the family may help to increase communication concerning medical issues and to minimize distortions and projections. Such meetings should be structured so as not to interfere with the ongoing psychosocial treatment of the medical patient. Clearly stated goals and guidelines for these meetings, including reassurances related to confidentiality, will minimize the potential intrusion into the ongoing relationship with the patient.

COUNTERTRANSFERENCE

Awareness of Countertransference

One of the most important aspects of working with medically ill patients is the clinician's understanding and comfort with his or her own reactions to physical helplessness and mortality, including an understanding of the role of illness in his own individual and family psychological history. As with all psychosocial interventions, the clinician needs to be aware of his or her personal vulnerability to unbearable affects and the characteristic defenses which he or she uses to create affective distance from the patient's experience (Karasu, 1995; Racker, 1968). For example, when combining active, exploratory, and reflective interventions, the clinician may move into action at an inappropriate time, to defend against experiencing unbearable affect stimulated by the patient.

Managing Countertransference

Clinical experience has shown that one of the most effective ways for a clinician to manage his or her countertransference toward medically ill patients is to use the knowledge gained in his or her own psychotherapy and supervision to recognize his or her typical countertransference reactions such as distancing from the patient, colluding with the patient's denial, or initiating inappropriate active interventions. Consulting with colleagues and supervisors is invaluable in helping the clinician maintain vigilance and avoid arrogance.

Using Countertransference to Therapeutic Advantage

A clinician who is aware of individual affective vulnerabilities and who is comfortable reflecting on his or her internal reactions to patients, is in an optimal position to minimize the impact of countertransference on any psychosocial interventions. For most clinicians, any changes in business as usual, such as a decrease or increase in activity or bending or breaking of customary boundaries should be red flags for the possibility of inappropriate action based on countertransference.

TERMINATION

As with all therapeutic interventions, the termination of any psychosocial intervention with medical patients is a vital aspect of treatment.

The decision to terminate a psychosocial intervention is determined by the goals of the intervention. These goals have been determined by the clinician and patient at the time of the initial visit. In the case of time-limited group interventions, the date of termination is determined by the therapist when treatment is commenced and is known to the group members from the outset (Ulman, 2000).

Determining the Termination Date

The process by which the termination is decided has a significant impact on the effectiveness of the intervention. The termination date is one of the therapeutic factors which helps create a sense of clear and firm boundaries for patients.

Frequently, when engaged in a successful time-limited intervention, patients are aware only of their wish to continue to experience the good feelings stirred up by the clinical experience and are unaware of their ambivalence toward the treatment. At times, patients may urge the clinician to extend the agreed-upon time. In individual psychosocial treatment the time of the intervention could be extended after careful attention to the implications of such a decision and exploration of the patient's resistance to working through feelings of loss. However, in the case of a time-limited group, changing the group agreement is a boundary violation which threatens to undermine the effectiveness of the intervention (MacKenzie, 1990). When the clinician determines that continuation of the group experience might be beneficial for the group members, the clearest course of action is to terminate the group at the original date and start another group with a new contract. This group may be made up only of the original members or also might include new members. Regardless, this will be a new group.

For medical patients who are chronically or terminally ill, termination of any psychosocial intervention must be carefully thought out and, at times, may not be appropriate. For those patients for whom a time-limited intervention is not an appropriate intervention, ongoing individual or group supportive interventions may be most appropriate.

Management of Termination

The power of all time-limited psychosocial interventions is enhanced when the termination date is mentioned at the beginning of each meeting (Mohl, 1995). Such clarity helps to set the framework for the intervention. When the intervention passes the halfway mark, the termination may be mentioned more frequently. The last few meetings may be devoted to evaluation of the experience, future treatment planning, and saying good-bye.

In the case of open-ended psychosocial interventions with medical patients, the decision to terminate is managed as it would be in any therapeutic situation. The patient and the therapist will decide when the goals of treatment have been achieved and will evaluate the experience and explore the patient's feelings related to parting (Karasu, 1995). Except in the case of open-ended psychotherapy, the patient's past history of endings will probably not be explored unless the patient brings it into the treatment. As stated earlier, special consideration needs to be given to chronically or terminally ill patients.

SUMMARY

In summary, there are a number of effective psychosocial interventions available for medical patients. The first psychosocial intervention takes place when the health care provider discusses with the patient his or her psychological reactions to his or her illness. With a thorough assessment of the patient's needs and careful treatment planning, psychosocial interventions can have a significant impact on the course of a patient's illness and his or her quality of life. Psychosocial interventions, when they work well, bring about a number of changes which positively influence a patient's medical condition, such as decreased social isolation, increased opportunity to put words to chaotic affect, an increased awareness of the connection between the physical and psychological, an increased sense of control and decreased sense of vulnerability, an occasion to grieve the loss of health with another person, and the development of skills which enhance stress reduction.

In spite of a wide array of research demonstrating that psychosocial interventions are cost effective and impact the course of illness and the medical patient's ability to cooperate in his or her treatment, the availability of such interventions for medical patients is haphazard in our current medical system. Ideally in the future, psychosocial interventions will be considered part of the accepted treatment protocol for most medical problems.

REFERENCES

Agras, W. S. (1995). Behavior therapy. In H. I. Kaplan & B. J. Sadock. (Eds.), *Comprehensive textbook of psychiatry/VI* (Vol. 2, 6th ed.). Baltimore: Williams and Wilkins.

Allen, R., & Scheidt, S. (1981). Group psychotherapy with coronary heart disease. *International Journal of Group Psychotherapy, 48*, 187–214.

Altshuler, K. Z. (1995). Other methods of psychotherapy. In H. I. Kaplan & B. J. Sadock (Eds.), *Comprehensive textbook of psychiatry/VI* (Vol. 2, 6th ed.). Baltimore: Williams and Wilkins.

Baker, R. W. (1996). *Successful surgery: A doctor's mind/body guide to help you through surgery.* New York: Pocket Books.

Beck, A. T., & Rush, A. J. (1995) Cognitive therapy. In H. I. Kaplan & B. J. Sadock (Eds.), *Comprehensive textbook of psychiatry/VI* (Vol. 2, 6th ed.). Baltimore: Williams and Wilkins.

Benson, H., Beary, J. F., & Carol, M. P. (1974). The relaxation response. *Psychiatry, 37*, 37–46.

Benson, H., & Stuart, E. M. (1992). *The wellness book: The comprehensive guide to maintaining health and treating stress-related illness.* New York: Carol Publishing.

Blackwell, B. (1995). Noncompliance. In H. I. Kaplan & B. J. Sadock (Eds.), *Comprehensive textbook of psychiatry/VI* (Vol. 2, 6th ed.). Baltimore: Williams and Wilkins.

Broadhead, W. E., Blazer, D. G., George, L. K., & Tse, C. K. (1990). Depression, disability days, and days lost from work in a prospective epidemiological survey. *Journal of the American Medical Association, 264*, 2524–2528.

Brown, D. P., & Fromm, E. (1987). *Hypnosis and behavioral medicine*. Hillsdale, NJ: Lawrence Erlbaum Associates Publishers.

Caudill, K. A., Galluci, B. B., & Bevus, P. (1996). A psychoneuroimmunologic perspective of resistance: implications for clinical practice. *Mind/Body Medicine, 1*, 192–202.

Coulahan, J. L., Schulberg, H. C., Block, M. R., Janosky, J. E., & Arena, V. C. (1990). Medical comorbidity of major depressive disorder in a primary care medical practice. *Archives of Internal Medicine, 50*, 2363–2367.

Domar, A. D., & Dreher, H. (1996). *Healing mind, healthy woman*. New York: Henry Holt and Co.

Fawzy, F. I., Fawzy, N. W., Arndt, L. A., & Pasnau, R. O. (1995). Critical reivew of psychosocial interventions in cancer care. *Archives of General Psychiatry, 52*, 100–113.

Gick, M., McClelland, D., & Budd, M. (1997). Group treatment of irritable bowel syndrome and implicit motivational predictors of outcome. *Mind/Body Medicine, 2*, 52–61.

Greenfield, S., Kaplan, S., & Ware, J. E. (1985). Expanding patient involvement in care: Effects on patient outcomes. *Annals of Internal Medicine, 102*, 520–528.

Gunderson, J. G., & Phillips, K. A. (1995). Personality Disorder. In H. I. Kaplan & B. J. Sadock (Eds.), *Comprehensive textbook of psychiatry/VI* (Vol. 2, 6th ed.). Baltimore: Williams and Wilkins.

Hellman, C. J. C., Budd, M., Borysenko, J., McClelland, D. C., & Benson, H. (1990). A study of the effectiveness of two group behavioral medicine interventions for patients with psychosomatic complaints. *Behavioral Medicine, 16*, 165–173.

Hoffman, J. W., Benson, H., Arns, P. A., Stainbrook, G. L., Landsberg, L., Young, J. B., et al. (1982). Reduced sympathetic nervous system responsivity associated with the relaxation response. *Science, 215*, 190–192.

House, J. S., Landis, K. R., & Umberson, D. (1988). Social relationships and health. *Science, 241*, 540–545.

Kabat-Zinn, J. (1982). An outpatient program in behavioral medicine for chronic pain based on the practice of mindfulness meditation: Theoretical considerations and preliminary results. *General Hospital Psychiatry, 4*, 373–348.

Karasu, T. B. (1995). Psychoanalysis and psychoanalytic psychotherapy. In H. I. Kaplan & B. J. Sadock (Eds.), *Comprehensive textbook of psychiatry/VI* (Vol. 2, 6th ed.). Baltimore: Williams and Wilkins.

Kiecolt-Glaser, J. K., Glaser, R., Williger, G., et al. (1985). Psychosocial enhancement of immunocompetence in a geriatric population. *Health Psychology, 4*, 25-41.

Lazare. A., & Eisenthal, S. (1979). A negotiated approach to the clinical encounter. I: Attending to the patient's perspective. In A. Lazare (Ed.), *Outpatient psychiatry: Diagnosis and treatment*. Baltimore: Williams and Wilkins.

Lazare, A., Eisenthal, S., & Frank, A. (1979). A negotiated approach to the clinical encounter. II. Conflict and negotiation. In A. Lazare (Ed.), *Outpatient psychiatry: Diagnosis and treatment*. Baltimore: Williams and Wilkins.

Lonergan, E. C. (1985). *Group intervention: How to begin and maintain groups in medical and psychiatric settings*. New York: Jason Aronson.

MacKenzie, K. R. (1990). *Introduction to time-limited group psychotherapy*. Washington, DC: American Psychiatric Press.

Magruder-Habib, K., Zung, W. W. K., Feussner, J. R., Alling, W. C., Saunders, W. B., & Stevens H. A. (1989). Management of general medical patients with symptoms of depression. *General Hospital Psychiatry, 11*, 210–206.

Mohl, P. C. (1995). Brief psychotherapy. In H. I. Kaplan & B. J. Sadock (Eds.), *Comprehensive textbook of psychiatry/ VI* (Vol. 2, 6th ed.). Baltimore: Williams and Wilkins.

Orne, M. T., Dinges, D. F., & Bloom, P. B. (1995). Hypnosis. In *Comprehensive textbook of psychiatry/VI* (Vol. 2, 6th ed.). Baltimore: Williams and Wilkins.

Pennebaker, J. W. (1992). Putting stress into words: Health, linguistic and therapeutic implications. *Behavioral Research Therapy, 31*, 539–548.

Pennebaker, J. W., Kiecolt-Glaser, J. K., & Glaser, R. (1988). Disclosure of traumas and immune function: Health implications for psychotherapy. *Journal of Consulting Clinical Psychology, 56*, 239–245.

Racker, H. (1968). *Transference and countertransference.* Madison, CT: International Universities Press.

Roth, S. (1990). *Psychotherapy: The art of wooing nature.* Northvale, NJ: Jason Aronson Inc.

Rutan, J. S., & Stone, W. N. (1993). *Psychodynamic group psychotherapy* (2nd ed.). New York: Guilford Press.

Simonton, S., & Sherman, A. (2000). An integrated model of group treatment for cancer patients. *International Journal of Group Psychotherapy, 50*, 487–506.

Sobel, D. S. (1995). Rethinking medicine: Improving health outcomes with cost-effective psychosocial interventions. *Psychosomatic Medicine, 57*, 234–244.

Speigel, D., Bloom, J. R., Kraemer, H. C., & Gottheil, E. (1989). Effect of psychosocial treatment on survival of patients with metastatic breast cancer. *Lancet, ii*, 888–891.

Speigel, D. (1993). *Living beyond limits: New hope and help for facing life-threatening illnesses.* New York: Time Books.

Spira, J. L. (1997). *Group therapy for medical patients.* New York: Guilford Press.

Taylor, S. E., & Aspinwall, L. G. (1990). Psychosocial aspects of chronic illness. In G. M. Herek, S. M. Levy, S. R. Maddi, S. E. Taylor, & D. L. Wertlieb (Eds.), *Psychological aspects of serioud illness: Chronic conditions, fatal diseases, and clinical care.* Washington, DC: American Psychological Association.

Toner, B., Segel, Z. V., Emmott, S., Myrar, D., et al. (1998). Behavioral group therapy for patients with irritable bowel syndrome. *International Journal of Group Psychotherapy, 48*(2), 215–244.

Uchino, B., Cacioppo, J., & Kiecolt-Glaser, J. K. (1996). The relationship between social support and physiological processes: A review with an emphasis on underlying mechanisms and implications for health. *Psychological Bulletin, 119*, 488–531.

Ulman, K. (1993). Group psychotherapy with the medically ill. In H. I. Kaplan & B. J. Saddock (Eds.), *Comprehensive group psychotherapy/VI* (Vol. 2, 6th ed.). Baltimore: Williams and Wilkins.

Ulman, K. (2000). An integrative model of stress management groups for women. *International Journal of Group Psychotherapy, 50*, 341–362.

Wells, K. B., Stewart, A., Hays, R. D., Burnham, M. A., Rogers, W., Daniels, M., Berry, S., Greenfield, S., & Ware, J. (1989). The functioning and well-being of depressed patients: Results from the Medical Outcomes Study. *Journal of the American Medical Association, 262*, 914–919.

Summary

12

Summary and Future Directions

HAROLD S. BERNARD
HENRY I. SPITZ
LEON A. SCHEIN
PHILIP R. MUSKIN

We are in a new century, and we are continuing to develop an increasingly so-phisticated understanding of the neuroscience which explains how we experi-ence the world. Neuroscientists are beginning to discover how emotions are generated and are learning more and more about the anatomical and molecular components of cognition. At the same time, mysteries about the functioning of the brain and mind continue to exist, and always will.

The tremendous advances in neuroscience over the past decade have not altered the fact that psychotherapy, and psychosocial interventions more gener-ally, continue to be central components in treating people who experience emo-tional suffering. Since most patients with medical illnesses also suffer psychologically, as a part of and in addition to the biology of their illness, psy-chosocial interventions are often a crucial component in the overall regimen for patients with a wide variety of medical problems. Many medical patients require skilled and compassionate attention to their emotional suffering if they are to recover fully from their medical travail. Even when full medical recovery is un-attainable, or death is likely, it is often the opportunity to share one's experi-ence, the support of a compassionate and understanding mental health professional, and the insights about oneself that a person may develop, that make it possible for a patient to face the inevitable (Eissler, 1955).

Unfortunately, the impact of a managed care environment (see below) and the high costs of medical care have sharply curtailed reimbursement for medi-cal and mental health services. While it is relatively easy to demonstrate the efficacy of an antibiotic or an antidepressant, the benefits of psychosocial inter-ventions are more difficult to isolate and validate. As a result, there has been a decrease in available resources for such interventions for patients with medical problems, as well as for the population at large. This is in spite of the fact that there have been several studies which have demonstrated that participants who have been able to avail themselves of a psychosocial intervention in addition to proper medical treatment do better medically than those who have not had the same opportunities. It is important to note that patients with treated psychiatric disorders utilize fewer medical resources than those who do not receive treatment.

This same managed care environment encourages primary care physicians to spend less and less time with their patients. At the same time, physicians report that the scope of care they provide has increased in the past few years, and a substantial number feel it has become greater than it should be (St. Peter et al., 1999). The burden of treating patients who are medically ill mitigates against physicians having the time to focus on patients' emotional responses to their illnesses. Research demonstrates that on average physicians interrupt patients' opening statements after only 23 seconds (Marvel et al., 1999). There simply is not time for patients to describe their concerns before physicians feel the need to arrive at a diagnosis and to formulate a treatment approach. Even when patients broach their emotional concerns in a direct way, physicians often do not acknowledge what they are hearing; rather, they attempt to redirect patients back to their medical symptoms in order to arrive at a diagnosis (Suchman et al., 1997). Where and when is there the opportunity to describe one's emotions, express concerns about pain and suffering, and explore misinformation that might be creating anxiety that could lead to noncompliance?

Over the course of a mental health professional's career, one can expect to see many patients who have, or will, develop some of the disorders described in this volume. There will always be an important role for psychosocial interventions in dealing with most medical conditions. Individual, group, and family approaches can enable people suffering from medical illnesses to utilize the most effective coping skills within their capability. We can expect the future to reveal a host of secrets about the brain, but such knowledge will never replace the experience of being understood by another person.

There is an emerging realization that training programs in all disciplines must prepare mental health professionals to understand the psychology of human suffering and to minister to those who are struggling with medical difficulties of one kind or another. However, the dualism between mind and body has not been completely overcome. As a result, psychiatric residents, who are exposed to the tremendous increase in knowledge about the neurobiology of psychiatric disorders, and the numerous pharmacological agents available to treat these disorders, are receiving less and less training in how to work with people psychosocially. Conversely, many nonphysician mental health professionals learn little, if anything, about medical disorders and how to work with people who are physically ill. As a result, they often have little knowledge about the impact of medical disorders on psyche and soma, and the effects and side effects of medications. It is clear that this dualism needs to be overcome and that we need a coterie of mental health professionals who have expertise about the medical aspects of various illnesses, their psychosocial sequelae, and how to work with people who are physically ill and suffering emotionally in one way or other.

RESEARCH: CURRENT STATUS AND FUTURE DIRECTIONS

Current Status

The research in this volume demonstrates that psychosocial sequelae associated with a wide variety of medical conditions can affect the course of the disease, patients' responses to their illness, and hence their quality of life (Andersen, Kiecolt-Glaser, & Glaser, 1994; Andrykowski et al., 1996; Bloom, 1982; Drossman et al., 1999; Ell et al., 1992). Specifically, the authors of the preceding chapters have extensively documented the psychosocial sequelae that can positively or adversely affect patients' responses to all of the categories of diseases focused on in Chapters 3–9 of this volume.

Since research about psychosocial sequelae is still relatively new, it is probably prudent to consider the relationships that have been uncovered thus far as hypotheses rather than definitive conclusions. It often happens that subsequent research refines, and occasionally refutes, earlier research. For example, when Friedman and Rosenman (1974) investigated the Type A personality behavior pattern, they concluded that time pressure, free-floating hostility, and observable psychomotor responses led to premature coronary heart disease. Subsequent research by Friedman and Ulmer (1984) expanded the initial formulation of Type A personality to include the influence of diminished self-esteem, insecurity, and the pressure to achieve. Still other studies have focused on the contributions of depression (Frasure-Smith, Lesperance, & Talazic, 1993) and anxiety (Kawachi et al., 1980).

Although numerous psychosocial sequelae are present for any given medical condition, we will cite just a few examples of those detailed throughout this volume. Depression has been found to be associated with most of the medical conditions discussed in this text. Among the specific findings reported in this volume are the following: elevated rates of suicide among AIDS patients, decreased socialization and capacity to work among chronic fatigue syndrome patients, failure to comply with the rigors of dialysis among kidney patients, and low self-esteem among patients with a variety of medical difficulties.

Anxiety is another prevalent psychosocial sequelae in many medical conditions. Among AIDS patients it is frequently manifested in the fear of being shamed or ostracized and in the fear of death. Anxiety often causes an individual to postpone testing, and thus begin treatment, for AIDS and many other serious diseases. It can contribute to panic attacks, myocardial infarctions (sometimes fatal), anticipatory nausea, decreased socialization, and reduced compliance with treatment protocols.

Social support, via its direct and indirect effects, is another crucial variable in many medical conditions. Berkman et al. (1992; Berkman, 1995) explored the relationship between social support and its contribution to survival following a myocardial infarction; Helgeson, Cohen, and Fritz (1998) explored the relationship between social support and adjustment to cancer; and Fawzy et al. (1993) and Spiegel et al. (1989) demonstrated the relationship between social support and survival time among those diagnosed with breast cancer and malignant melanoma. The presence of effective social support seems to influence the patient to obtain medical treatment in a timely fashion, to improve the patient's ability to sustain painful or otherwise uncomfortable treatment, and to increase adherence to necessary medical protocols and lifestyle changes. Conversely, interpersonal conflict may not only adversely affect the immune system (Kiecolt-Glaser et al., 1993), but it also diminishes the motivation to seek necessary medical treatment, lessens optimism and self-esteem, and decreases the willingness to make necessary lifestyle changes. These findings apply to children and adolescents as well as adults.

An often underestimated aspect of social support is the role of the physician's attitude about patient participation in treatment decisions, which generally helps patients in their emotional adaptation to being ill. While the physician's point of view is crucial, some patients are more amenable to participating in decisions about their treatment than are others: age, education, socioeconomic status, race, cultural background, and the capacity to process information all may affect the patient's ability and willingness to participate in treatment decisions (Greenfield et al., 1988; Kaplan et al., 1995; Kaplan et al., 1996). The physician's disposition and pattern of communication are also important determinants of how much support patients feel in coping with their illness and the effect of the illness on their self-esteem.

Other psychosocial sequelae which do not manifest themselves as frequently include reduced capacity to concentrate, lapsed memory, posttraumatic stress disorder, cognitive deficits, decreased capacity to work, and lowered self-esteem.

Future Research

The authors of the chapters in this volume have highlighted psychological sequelae, some of which heighten resilience, and some of which increase vulnerability, to medical conditions. Future research will not only validate or refine what we already know, but will also illuminate more effective psychosocial treatments that will help patients enhance their responses to their illnesses.

As the results of future research emerge, we will undoubtedly come to an increased appreciation of the complex relationship between various medical conditions and their multiple psychosocial sequelae. This section will consider several areas for further inquiry.

First, it will be desirable for the terminology that researchers employ to become increasingly operationalized. This will enable people using the same words to be sure that they are all talking about the same thing. Some of the words commonly used in this area of research are particularly difficult to pin down: apathy, social withdrawal, fear, anxiety. It would be useful to move toward consensual validation of such terms.

It will also be important to achieve greater understanding of the contributions of ethnicity, race, gender, sexual orientation, age, socioeconomic status, and cultural influences to the emergence of particular psychosocial sequelae to various disease entities, as well as differential responses to various treatment interventions. We need to better understand the relationship between these demographic factors and the following: the timeliness of seeking medical treatment; adherence to treatment regimens; expectations of and responses to physicians; and comfort level in disclosing information to physicians and mental health workers.

There is more work to be done concerning the relationship between patients and their physicians. This is a crucial variable when the diagnosis is made and communicated, when a treatment course is suggested, when relapses occur, and throughout the course of the illness. Future investigators should delineate what is required to forge an active partnership between patient and physician at every step in the diagnosis and treatment of the disease in question.

As a disease evolves from acute onset to chronic condition, sustaining medical regimens, and at times lifestyle changes, can be paramount in determining the ultimate treatment outcome. Thus the psychosocial factors that lead to favorable or unfavorable treatment outcomes with different disease entities must be identified and understood. It is also important that we learn as much as possible about which treatment interventions are most useful in working with patients from varying demographic groups, as well as patients with different disease entities.

Research relating to caregivers has not been given sufficient attention. Addressing the experience of the caregiver has the potential to improve the provider's quality of life as well as the quality of care offered to patients.

As we look toward the future, the objective is to avoid both complacency and demoralization about patients with significant medical illnesses. We need to recognize how much we have learned in a relatively short amount of time, and build from here. Understanding more about psychosocial sequelae, and the best ways to respond to them, will ultimately enhance the care offered to patients struggling with the disorders discussed in this text.

THE SPECIAL EFFICACY OF GROUP INTERVENTIONS

While individual, marital, and family interventions are often the best ways to work with people suffering from medical illness, there are some special features of group interventions that make them particularly effective for such patients. A number of the chapters in this volume make mention of group approaches in dealing with the psychosocial sequelae of various medical conditions. What follows is a brief description of some of the factors that make groups the optimal form of intervention when they can be organized. Since they are more difficult to arrange than individual, marital, and family meetings, they are not always a viable option. However, when they can be arranged, what are the special characteristics that make them the intervention of choice?

1. While people who are ill realize intellectually that they are not the only ones struggling with the problem they have, they often feel alone. Suffering from a major medical problem can be very lonely, even when one has the support of loved ones. It is enormously relieving and cathartic to spend time with others dealing with the same or similar problems to your own: talking about the experience of having the illness, coping with it, telling people about it, and dealing with their reactions. A mental health professional can help in a variety of ways; however, there is a special aid and comfort derived from being with others dealing with the same situation.

2. Closely allied but separate from the emotional support derived from being with people who share a common medical problem is the opportunity to learn about the ideas and approaches that others are employing and finding useful. No one can know all there is to know about resources available and the coping strategies that different medical patients employ. Patients with the same or similar medical problems learn a great deal from each other just by spending time together and sharing what they are doing to cope with their illness.

3. It is heartening to meet others with the same problem as you recovering, or at least struggling nobly and not giving in to despair. While a professional can attempt to ameliorate hopelessness, such efforts cannot match the power of empathy and even mentoring from those who are traveling the same arduous path.

4. Patients with medical problems, even more than typical psychotherapy patients, are basically on the receiving end of helping services. While there are often things that people can do to help themselves, and while many people do actively participate in their own treatment, medical patients are first and foremost recipients of professional services. Though this is often necessary, it can have a devastating effect on one's sense of self. Suffering from a major illness often requires that an individual adjust his or her sense of self to incorporate feelings of vulnerability, mortality, and powerlessness. This impact on one's sense of self can last even after the individual recovers medically. A group experience provides the best antidote to this problem, because of the possibility that a participant can give as well as receive help. There may be nothing as ego enhancing as being genuinely helpful to other human beings at a time in one's life when one is feeling frightened, vulnerable, impotent, and perhaps even hopeless and despairing.

As indicated above, it is often not possible to offer a group experience to patients suffering from medical maladies. There may not be enough patients to constitute a viable group, at least not enough who can meet at the same time and place. The mental health professional may not feel proficient in running groups, or may not have (or make) the time to organize a group. There are some patients who are unable or unwilling to talk about their problems in the presence of peers and just want to speak with a mental health professional. Thus groups are not a panacea, anymore than is any other single approach. However, when it is feasible to arrange a group experience for patients suffering from a similar medical malady, the special features of groups enumerated above make it often the best approach for patients, families, and significant others affected by physical illnesses and their psychosocial sequelae.

The Impact of Managed Care

Concerns over open-ended costs of providing medical and mental health services have prompted government, insurers, and others involved with the financing of health care to focus on cost containment while still attempting to provide high-quality patient care. A wide range of alternatives have been instituted to stem the tide of runaway costs. These systems are broadly subsumed under the rubric of managed health care.

Many practitioners fear what they experience as the corporatization of psychosocial treatments and the end of treatments that they have become accustomed to offering. The principles and language of business and economics threaten to shatter time-honored cornerstones of practice such as the provider-patient alliance and the sanctity of patient confidentiality. With financial profit as the engine that drives these new systems, many feel that quality care has suffered and will only get worse.

Although health care reform affects all segments of medicine, it does not affect them equally. Specifically, mental health services are treated as "step children" in many managed care systems. A preferential model has emerged which favors reimbursement for forms of treatment which are brief, documentable, and conducted by practitioners with the lowest fee scales. The current trend is toward biological, cognitive-behavioral, and time-limited outpatient models which are symptom-focused and aim to help patients make a rapid return to a reasonable level of vocational, familial, academic, and interpersonal functioning.

What are the implications for those who work in the psychosocial arena? For one thing, it can result in providers not even mentioning to patients what they believe would be the ideal approach because they know it is not covered by a managed care plan. It is crucial for practitioners to discuss the full range of options available, and what they believe would be optimal, and let their patients decide how they want to proceed. To elucidate the many ways practitioners are affected by our current health care system, group psychotherapy will be used in this discussion as the prototype of a widely practiced form of psychosocial intervention.

Ethical Concerns

Managed care has been in existence long enough for clinicians to have experienced its intrusion into diverse aspects of mental health treatment. Concerns over patient confidentiality, the alteration of the relationship between provider and patient, and decisions regarding what interventions are acceptable to managed care are but a few of the issues which have caused concern for the mental health community and the public.

Despite enlightened attitudes on the part of many, there remains a stigma attached to mental illness and to many medical conditions. Information concerning people who are in treatment for these conditions must be handled in a sensitive way. The clinician's sense of responsibility to patients involves a protective function that includes insuring that data about an individual will not be used for prejudicial purposes. Managed care, which is predicated on sharing information about patients in order to determine eligibility, medical necessity, and authorization for further treatment, is faced with the ethical challenge of getting the needed information about patients from the providers without overstepping the boundaries which violate traditional concepts of confidentiality and the patient's privacy.

Clinicians in managed care programs must inform patients at the beginning of treatment about whatever they know concerning the nature of the information which will be shared about them, with whom it will be discussed, toward what purpose, and what will happen with that information in terms of where it will be stored, to which individuals and organizations it will be accessible, and how long it will be retained. The knowledge that someone has been or is mentally ill, physically ill, or a substance abuser still poses the danger of discrimination in seeking employment, securing housing, and living openly in the community.

In response to these growing concerns and ethical dilemmas resulting from the shifting structure of health care delivery, many private and public efforts are gaining support to insure that the rights of psychiatric and medically ill patients will not be violated. Perhaps the best-known examples are found in the increasing number of bills and proposals being put forth on the Congressional and state legislative levels. Patient Bill of Rights proposals and the interface between health information access and patient information contained in medical records is at the forefront of this movement.

The thrust of these plans is not only to protect patients from biases by new health care insurance plans but to inform them of their legal rights and encourage them to be proactive. In the case of access to information contained in medical records, patients should be made aware of their ability to request, inspect, copy, and, in some instances, amend their records. Consumers of mental health services are becoming more assertive in holding authorities who pay for, administer, provide direct service, or conduct research under managed care accountable in their role as "health information trustees" to insure safeguards against unwanted intrusions into their medical records.

A corollary to this issue is the dilemma a clinician faces in a telephone conversation with a case reviewer. The legitimate requests for details about a patient's condition and state of recovery are an integral part of the managed care scenario. Providers are faced with the choice between two unenviable extremes: revealing too little about the patient and risking possible denial of authorization for ongoing treatment, or divulging more than one would ordinarily and in so doing "pathologizing," or overstating the information in order to influence the reviewer to authorize further treatment.

Impact on Clinical Practice

The managed care model has infringed on the clinician's sense of independence in many ways. A representative sampling of concerns voiced by practitioners in the current managed care culture ranges from administrative conflicts to outright denial of services which seem justified and necessary in the judgment of the provider. Problems involving the selection of providers for inclusion on managed care panels, disputes about credentialing clinicians, low fee schedules, delays in payment for services rendered, and discontents emanating from the review process are additional sources of concern.

These changes have resulted in a shift in the patterns of practice among mental health and medical practitioners. The increased value placed on brevity of treatment has resulted in an expansion of the use of short-term psychosocial interventions. The concern here is not with the broader use of brief therapies, but rather the view of brief therapy as a panacea, which is dangerous. Clinical settings where short-term work is mandated will not provide adequate therapy for many. Despite the conflicts between the economic and therapeutic agendas involved in patient care, there are economically prudent ways to provide quality care for many patients. The increased use of group psychotherapy is a case in point. When clinicians are skilled in assessing patients for group treatment and in leading groups themselves, they can provide treatment to many people formerly relegated to more expensive long-term inpatient or outpatient therapies. Short-term, symptom-focused groups which emphasize specificity of treatment focus, teach skill acquisition, and disseminate accurate information about issues such as a medical condition shared by group members are being expanded to meet the needs of a very wide range of psychological problems.

Another effect of the impact of outside control of treatment is the change in daily practice habits of the clinician in a managed care system. Record keeping has taken on enormous importance. The pressure on therapists to include more than they normally would in a patient's written record and to conform to a standard set by an outside agency are sources of concern. The sheer volume of paperwork associated with the treatment of an individual patient in psychotherapy is burdensome for practitioners.

Managed care's emphasis on standardization of treatment and determining what is commonly accepted practice for given psychiatric conditions has led to an interest in establishing practice guidelines for treating specific psychological conditions. The American Psychiatric Association's Practice Guidelines series is the prototype of this effort. Practice guidelines are, as their name implies, just guides for effective and generally accepted protocols which apply to a given psychiatric entity. They are created by panels of experts in specific sectors of the mental health field who synthesize the best available research concerning therapies for a given entity. Conditions such as depression, bulimia, and substance abuse are a few examples of entities for which therapy guidelines have been established. Authors of guidelines are careful to caution clinicians not to use them as a substitute for individual clinical judgment or to apply them in a wholesale, formulaic manner. Under the best circumstances, clinicians and managed care reviewers can utilize practice guidelines to further the effort to speak a common language of psychosocial treatment.

In a positive sense, the emergence of managed care has spurred pre-existing interest in the development of protocols for treating a broad range of psychosocial problems. Accountability to third-party payers demands distinguishing treatments with documented efficacy from those which are idiosyncratic or only anecdotally reported as beneficial. The trend toward evidence-based psychiatric treatment is an example of confluence between the goals of managed care organizations and clinicians concerned with providing the highest quality patient care.

From the first encounter with a person seeking psychological help, there is an awareness in the provider, and perhaps the patient as well, of the presence of a third party in the treatment. In order to obtain consent and cooperation, providers now have to go through a much more elaborate patient orientation process. This is akin to a psychological Miranda warning, usually associated with the criminal justice system. In order for their agreement to participate to be informed, patients must be made aware of their rights and vulnerabilities.

For many practitioners, this skews the introduction to treatment in ways that work against the kind of provider-patient relationship they are trying to build. Patients often complain of feeling more inhibited or constricted in spontaneous self-disclosure for fear that what they divulge will have negative ramifications for them if the managed care organization has access to it.

Termination of treatment is also often affected by outside influences. No longer can patients and their therapists decide when a working relationship has served its purpose and termination of treatment is in order. Abrupt, involuntary disruptions and terminations of treatment are much more common under managed care. Therapists who find themselves caught in this situation have an added responsibility to find ongoing professional support for patients whose treatment they regard as incomplete.

The shift from conventional psychiatric diagnosis to reporting on the basis of functional impairment is another offshoot of the managed care system. Symptom specificity is the hallmark of reporting case material in the world of managed care. Global goals such as improvement of self-esteem are being discarded in favor of measures of performance in vocational, academic, and family settings. Hence, interventions which are behaviorally oriented, aimed at specific functional difficulties, and circumscribed in their duration are more likely to be approved for reimbursement.

Those in academic and research circles are greatly distressed by the reduction of funding for professional education, training, and clinical investigation. The trend away from invention, teaching, and exploration on a broad scale is troubling in that it foreshadows cuts in areas considered to be essential to the future of the mental health field. By putting a fiscal priority on the immediate, we may be mortgaging our future. There remains the need for refinement and further study of creative ways to control costs without compromising the access to and quality of medical and mental health care.

In summary, it is the responsibility of mental health practitioners to have at least some basic understanding of the biology of medical disorders, as well as the psychological effects of medical illnesses, and of biological and psychological treatments, on the brain and on the mind. Armed with this knowledge and understanding, the mental health practitioner is equipped for the challenge of treating the psychological impact of medical illnesses and treatments. Close collaboration between physicians who are specialists in the various disease entities and knowledgeable mental health professionals is highly desirable in providing optimal treatment to these patients. If mental health professionals do not rise to the challenge of meeting the psychological needs of patients suffering from medical illnesses, there is no one else who can or will provide these desperately needed services.

REFERENCES

Andersen, B. J., Kiecolt-Glaser, J. K., & Glaser, R. (1994). A biobehavioral model of cancer stress and disease course. *American Psychologist, 49*(5), 389–404.

Andrykowski, M. A., Cordova, M. J., Studts, J. L., et al. (1998). Diagnosis of posttraumatic stress disorder following treatment for breast cancer. *Journal of Consulting and Clinical Psychology, 66,* 586–590.

Berkman, L. F. (1995). The role of social relations in health promotion. *Psychosomatic Medicine, 57,* 245–254.

Berkman, L. F., Leo-Summers, L., & Horowitz, R. I. (1992). Emotional support and survival after myocardial infarction: A prospective, population-based study of the elderly. *Annals of Internal Medicine, 117,* 1003–1009.

Bloom, J. R. (1982). Social support, accommodation to stress and adjustment to breast cancer. *Social Science and Medicine, 16,* 1329–1338.

Drossman, D. A., Creed, F. H., Olden, K. W., et al. (1999). Psychosocial aspects of the functional gastrointestinal disorders. *Gut, 45,* 1125–1130.

Eissle, K. R., Jr. (1955). *The psychiatrist and the dying patient.* New York: International Universities Press.

Ell, K., Nishimoto, R., Mediansk, Y. L., et al. (1992). Social relations, social support, and survival among patients with cancer. *Journal of Psychosomatic Research, 36,* 531–541.

Fawzy, F. I., Fawzy, N. W., Hyun, C. S., et al. (1993). Effects of an early structured psychiatric intervention, coping and affective state on recurrence and survival 6 years later. *Archives of General Psychiatry, 15,* 153–160.

Frasure-Smith, N., Lesperance, F., & Talazic, M. (1993). Depression following myocardial infarction. *Journal of the American Medical Association, 270,* 1819–1825.

Friedman, M., & Rosenman, R. H. (1974). *Type A behavior and your heart.* New York: Knopf.

Friedman, M., & Ulmer, D. (1984). *Treating Type A behavior and your heart.* New York: Knopf.

Greenfield, S. Kaplan, S. H., Ware, J. E., et al. (1988). Patient participation in medical care: Effects on blood sugar control and quality of life in diabetes. *Journal of General Internal Medicine, 3,* 448–457.

Helgeson, V. S., Cohen, S., & Fritz, H. L. (1998). Social ties and cancer. In J. C. Holland (Ed.), *Psycho-oncology* (pp. 99–109). New York: Oxford University Press.

Kaplan, S. H., Gandek, B., Greenfield, S. K., et al. (1995). Patient and visit characteristics related to physicians' participatory decision-making style. Results from the Medical Outcomes Study. *Medical Care, 33,* 1176–1187.

Kaplan, S. H., Greenfield, S., Rogers, W., et al. (1996). Characteristics of physicians with participatory decision-making styles. *Annals of Internal Medicine, 124,* 511–513.

Kawachi, I., Sparrow, D., Wokonas, P. S., et al. (1994). Symptoms of anxiety and risk of coronary heart disease. *Circulation, 90,* 2225–2229.

Kiecolt-Glaser, J., Malarkey, W. B., Chee, M., et al. (1993). Negative behavior during marital conflict associated with immunological down-regulation. *Psychosomatic Medicine, 55,* 410–412.

Marvel, M. K., Epstein, R. M., Flowers, K., et al. (1999). Soliciting the patients' agenda: Have we improved? *Journal of the American Medical Association, 281*(3), 283–287.

Spiegel, D., Bloom, J. R., Kraemer, H. C., et al. (1989). Effect of psychosocial treatment on survival of patients with metastatic breast cancer. *Lancet, 2,* 888–891.

St. Peter, R. F., Reed, M., Kemper, P., et al. (1999). Changes in the scope of care provided by primary care physicians. *New England Journal of Medicine, 341,* 1980–1985.

Suchman, A. L., Markakis, K., Beckman, H. B., et al. (1997). A model of empathic communication in the medical interview. *Journal of the American Medical Association, 277*(8), 678–682.

Index

abacavir, 278
Abraham, H.D., 190
absolute threshold, 16
abuse, gastrointestinal disorders and, 190–191.
    See also violence
achalasia, 182
acromegaly, 220–221
acting-out, 382
acute seroconversion syndrome, of HIV, 272–
    273
addiction. *See* substance abuse
Addison, T., 201
Addison's disease (adrenocorticol
    insufficiency), 214–215
Ader, R., 7–8
adjuvant systemic therapy, 355
Adler, G., 382–383
adolescents. *See also* children
    with cancer, 108–110, 113
    smoking among, 37
adrenal disorders, 212–215
adrenocorticotropic hormone (ACTH), 393
affect, 40
affective social support, 102
African American population
    cancer in, 110–111
    coronary heart disease in, 155
    diabetes mellitus in, 202–203
    essential hypertension in, 137
    HIV in, 269–272, 284, 290–291
age factors
    coping with cancer and, 105
    dementia and, 236
    endocrine disorders and, 201
    endometrial cancer and, 360
    end-stage renal disease and, 162
    health screening for women and, 367–368
    hypothyroidism and, 208
    multiple sclerosis and, 244
    Parkinson's Disease and, 243–244
    patient participation in treatment and, 11–
    12

Agras, S., 15
AIDS, defined, 270. *See also* HIV
Alameda County study, 5, 31
alcoholism, 366
Aldwin, J., 384
alendronate sodium, 352
Alexander, F., 40, 45, 181, 184–185, 187
allergies, chronic fatigue syndrome and, 310–
    311
allostasis/allostatic load, 393–395
Almy, T.P., 181
alternative medicine, 315, 364–366
Alzheimer's Disease (AD), 236–237
amantadine, 314–315
amenorrhea, 343–344
American College of Physicians, 368
American Heart Association, 351
American Psychiatric Association's Practice
    Guidelines, 440
amprenavir, 279
anabolic steroid use, 225–226
Andersen, B.L., 9–10, 119
androgens, 349
Andrykowski, M.A., 114–116
Angelica sinensis, 349
anger, coronary heart disease and, 148, 149
angina pectoris, 145
angiography, 260
angioplasty, 153
anorexia nervosa, 300–301, 344–346
antiretroviral medications, 271, 276–279,
    286–287
antithrombolitic medication, 154–155
antithyroid agents, 363
Antonovsky, A., 4–5
anxiety, 433
    brain trauma and, 251–252
    chronic fatigue syndrome and, 315–316
    coronary heart disease and, 148
    esophagus disorders and, 182
    HIV and, 283
    Lyme disease and, 302

anxiety (*continued*)
  Parkinson's Disease and, 243
  poststroke, 235
  in women, 346–347
apraxia, 237
arthritis, 296
Asian population, 11–12
Astrom, M., 235
atherosclerosis, 143–145. *See also* coronary
  heart disease (CHD)
atrophic vaginitis, 335–336
auras, 248, 254
autoimmune thyroiditis, 210
availability heuristic, 14
avoidance, 104, 193–194

baclofen, 245
bacterial vaginosis, 335
Balducci, L., 115
barrier contraceptive methods, 338
Baum, A., 33
Beaumont, William, 181, 185
Beck Depression Inventory (BDI), 188
behavioral medicine, 133–134. *See also*
  psychotherapy
behavioral psychotherapy, 410–411. *See also*
  psychotherapy
Benson, H., 411, 412
Berkman, L.F., 434
Bernstein, L., 35
Berry, J.F., 411
beta-blockers, 138
Bibring, G.L., 387
binge-eating disorders, 344–346
biofeedback, 6, 196, 398
biologic treatments, 365
biomedical advances, 9–10
biopsychosocial model of treatment, 3, 40,
  164, 181
Black Cohosh, 349
bladder incontinence, 352–353
Blanchard, E.B., 193
Bleijenberg, G., 193–194
blood pool imaging, 151
blood pressure, 135–137. *See also* hypertension
bone mineral density (BMD) testing, 351
bone sarcomas, 90
Borrelia burgdorferi, 293–294
  anomalous forms of, 298–299
  chronic fatigue syndrome and, 309, 313
brachytherapy, 81
Bradley, L.A., 183

brain. *See also* cognition; neurological illnesses
  channel capacity of, 12–13
  immune system and, 4
  stress and, 394–395
  trauma to, 250–253
Branch, L.G., 253
BrCa 1 gene, 354, 356
breast cancer, 83, 84, 90–91, 111–112, 354–
  356
  fatigue and, 115
  hormone replacement therapy and, 348
  personality and, 42–45
breast disease, 344
Breuer, Josef, 48
Briquet, Paul, 48
Broekel, J.A., 115
bromocriptine, 220
Brooks,N., 251
Bruhn, J.G., 5
Buie, D.H., 382–383
bulimia, 344–346
Bulloch, K., 8
bypass graft surgery, coronary artery (CABG),
  153

calcium blockers, 138
calcium metabolism disorders, 216–219
Canadian Task Force, 368
cancer, 6, 17, 79–82, 106. *See also individual
  types of cancer*
  children/adolescents with, 108–110
  cognitive dysfunction and, 113–114
  coping with, 98–106
  delirium and, 55–56
  diet and, 34–35
  doctor-patient relationship and, 58–59
  in elderly population, 110
  HIV and, 288–287
  hormone replacement therapy and, 348
  identifying negative psychosocial sequelae
    and, 119–120
  incidence and mortality rates of, 83
  infertility and, 118–119
  open-ended groups for, 419
  positive psychological sequelae and, 120–
    122
  recurrence, 106–108
  response to diagnoses, 91–92
  response to treatment, 92–98
  sexual dysfunction and, 117–118
  side effects from treatment, 114–115
  sleep dysfunction and, 115–116

stress and, 395–396
suicide and, 108
survival rates, 112–113
candidiasis, 334–335
Cannon, R.O., 183
Cannon, Walter, 7
carotid angiography with coronary arteriography, 151
cardiac catheterization test, 151
Carol, M.P., 411
cartotid evaluation, for neurological disorders, 261–262
CD4 cell count, 270
CD4 T helper lymphocytes, 270
Centers for Disease Control, 269
    criteria for AIDS, 276
    criteria for Lyme disease, 294
    on lead exposure, 32
central nervous system (CNS)
    blood glucose levels and, 203
    chronic fatigue syndrome and, 315
    HIV and, 273–275
    Lyme disease and, 295, 297–298, 304–305
    psychoneuroimmunology, 7–9
cerebral tumors, 239–241
cerebrospinal fluid (CSF) analysis, 262, 295
cerebrovascular accident (stroke), 233–236
cerebrovascular disease, 233–236
cervical cancer, 88–89, 357–358
cervical infections, 336–337
Chambers, H., 114
Cheang, A., 44
chemotherapy, 81, 359
    for breast cancer, 355
    cognitive dysfunction and, 97–98
    infertility and, 118
    nausea induced by, 93–94
children. *See also* adolescents
    blood lead levels in, 32
    brain trauma in, 251
    cancer in, 59, 108–110, 113
    family interventions and, 415
    Lyme disease and, 302
    in poverty, 30
    with somatic complaints, 48–49
chlamydia trachomatis, 336–337
cholesterol, 34–35, 350–351
chronic fatigue immune dysfunction syndrome (CFIDS), 306–307. *See also* chronic fatigue syndrome (CFS)
chronic fatigue syndrome (CFS), 267–268, 307–308, 318
    central nervous system and, 315
    diagnoses of, 308, 316
    epidemiology of, 307
    etiology of, 309–313
    immune dysregulation and, 310–311
    Lyme disease and, 308
    psychiatric disorders and, 311–312, 314–316
    psychological issues of, 316–317
    sociocultural issues, 306–307
    treatment for, 313–315, 317–318
Cimicufuga racemosa, 349
cisplatin, 93, 359
clarthromycin, 301–302
clot-dissolving agents, 233–234
Clouse, R.E., 182
cluster headaches, 255
CMV encephalitis, 274
cognition. *See also* brain
    affect and, 40
    in cancer patients, 97–98, 113–114
    channel capacity and, 12–13
    chronic fatigue syndrome and, 312
    Cognitive Motor Disorder, 280
    cognitive triad, 192–193
    disease and, 55–56
    heuristics and, 14
    impaired by renal disease treatment, 160–161
    treatment delay and, 18
cognitive behavioral psychotherapy (CBT), 397
    for gastrointestinal disorders, 192–194
    for vascular dementia, 239
cognitive psychotherapy, 410. *See also* psychotherapy
Cohen, N., 7–8
coherence, sense of, 4
colleagues, consultation with, 422
colonoscopy, 86
colorectal cancer, 86–87
compulsivity, 387–388
computer tomography (CT) scans, 236–237, 258
conception, 339, 340
conceptualization, 10–11
Constitutional Predisposition Model, 41
continuous ambulatory peritoneal dialysis (CAPD), 158, 161, 163
contraception, 337–339
Cooper, C., 44
coping, 408–409
    assessment of, 385–390

coping (*continued*)
  defined, 384–385
  determinants of, 104–106
  improving skills for, 390–392
  resources for cancer patients, 100–103
  response to illness and, 385–386
  strategies, 103–104
  stressors of cancer diagnoses/treatment, 98–100
Corcoran, P.J., 253
coronary artery bypass graft surgery (CABG), 153
coronary heart disease (CHD), 143
  adjunctive psychosocial treatments for, 156
  anatomy and pathophysiology, 143–147
  assessment and management of, 150–154
  management of coronary crisis, 154–156
  personality and, 42
  psychophysiological influences on, 149
  risk factors for, 147–149
  stress and, 394
  Type A Behavior Pattern and, 433
  in women, 350–351
corticotrophin releasing factor (CRF), 393
cortisol, 7, 393
Coster, G., 15
countertransference, 424
Coyne, J.C., 384
Creed, F.H., 194–195
Crowther, D., 114
cryptococcal meningitis, 274
cultural beliefs, 376, 401
Cushing, H., 201
Cushing's syndrome, 202, 212–214, 226
cytomegalovirus (CMV) infection, 271

dacarbazine, 93
Dangerous Behaviors Model, 41
DASH diet (Dietary Approaches to Stop Hypertension), 139
death/dying, 376
  emotional adjustment to, 54
  end-of-life decision making and, 60–61
  HIV and, 290
decision-making, 58–61, 413, 434. *See also* doctor-patient relationship
deep brain stimulation (DBS), 243
defovir, 278
DeJong, G., 253
delavirdine, 278
delirium, 55–56, 97
dementia, 56, 236–239

among cancer patients, 97
HIV-associated dementia, 280
Lyme disease and, 297
demyelinating diseases, 244–247
depression, 433. *See also individual medical conditions*
  Addison's disease and, 215
  assessing, 408
  brain trauma and, 251
  chronic fatigue syndrome and, 311–312, 315–316
  coping strategies and, 384
  coronary heart disease and, 148
  Cushing's syndrome and, 212
  diabetes and, 206–207
  end-stage renal disease and, 161
  esophagus disorders and, 182
  gastrointestinal disorders and, 189–190
  HIV and, 282
  Lyme disease and, 302
  multiple sclerosis and, 245
  Parkinson's Disease and, 243
  in primary care, 54
  spinal cord trauma and, 252
  stroke and, 235
  thyroid disease and, 210–212
Descartes, Rene, 3–4
DeVita, V.T., 82
Devlen, J., 114
dexamethasone suppression test (DST), 213
DHEA/DHEA-S, 349–350
diabetes, 157
  diabetes insipidus, 222
  diabetes mellitus, 202–207
diagnoses. *See also individual illnesses*
  acromegaly, 221
  Addison's disease, 215
  Alzheimer's Disease, 236–237
  brain tumors, 240
  breast cancer, 355
  cancer, 98–106
  cervical cancer, 358
  cervical infections, 336–337
  chronic fatigue syndrome, 308, 316
  coronary heart disease, 148–149
  Cushing's syndrome, 213
  diabetes mellitus, 204
  eating disorders, 345
  emotional adjustment to, 53–54
  endometrial cancer, 359–360
  hirsutism, 226
  HIV staging, 273

hyperprolactinemia, 220
hypoparathyroidism, 218
hypopituitarism, 222
Lyme disease, 294–298
male hypogonadism, 224
malignant cancers, 80
neurological disorders, 257–262
ovarian cancer, 356
pheochromocytoma, 222–223
primary hyperparathyroidism, 217
responses to cancer, 91–92
seizure disorders, 248
stroke, 235
thyroid diseases, 208, 211
tumor markers, 92
vaginitis, 334–336
wellness continuum *vs.*, 10–11
Diagnostic and Statistical Manual (DSM-IV) (American Psychiatric Association), 56, 134, 187
Diagnostic Interview Schedule (DIS), 187
dialysis, 157–158. *See also* end-stage renal disease
didanosine, 278
diet, 34–35
    alternative health issues and, 365–366
    chronic fatigue syndrome and, 313–314
    end-stage renal disease and, 158–159
    essential hypertension and, 139–140
difference threshold, 16
diffuse esophageal spasm (DES), 182
DiMatteo, M.R., 15
DiNicola, D.D., 15
Direct Impact Model, 41
disease. *See also individual medical conditions*
    cognitive factors in, 55–56
    emotional moderators of, 53–54
    personality and, 42–47
    psychological moderators of, 50–53
    recovery from, 6
disseminated mycobacterium avium complex/ intracellurare, 271
diuretics, 138
doctor-patient relationship, 28, 57–62, 422–423, 429–431
    coping ability and, 391
    decision making and, 58–61, 413, 434
    HIV and, 285
    patient preparation, 318
    sick role and, 378–381
    for women, 333–334
Dollard, J., 13

Dong Quai, 349
dopamine agonists, 242
Doppler assessment, 261
Dorgan, J., 35
Dreher, H., 6
Drossman, D.A., 189
Druss, R.G., 385
Dunbar, F., 39–40
Dunbar, J., 15
duodenal ulcers, 185, 186. *See also* peptic ulcer disease (PUD)
dysmenorrhea, 343–344
dysthymia, 206–207, 235

eating disorders, 206, 344–346
efavirenz, 278
elderly population
    cancer in, 110 *See also* age factors
    endocrine disorders in, 201
    patient participation in treatment and, 11–12
    renal disease in, 156–157
electrocardiogram (ECG), 150
electrodiagnostic tests, 260–261
electroencephalogram (EEG), 248, 260
electromagnetic therapies, 365
electromyography (EMG), 261
ELISA, 294–295
Emanuel, E., 57–58
Emanuel, L., 57–58
emotional moderators, of disease, 53–54
emotion-focused coping strategies, 103–104
employment, 164, 375
encephalitis, 256–257, 274, 296
encephalomyelitis, 297
encephalopathy, 297
endocrine disorders, 201–202, 227
    adrenal disorders, 212–215
    anabolic steroid use, 225–226
    calcium metabolism disorders, 216–219
    diabetes mellitus, 202–207
    endocrinology, defined, 202
    hirsuitism, 226–227
    hypoglycemia, 207–208
    male hypogonadism, 223–225
    pheochromocytoma, 222–223
    pituitary function, 219–222
    thyroid disease, 208–212, 361–364
end-of-life decision making, 60–61
endometrial cancer, 88–89, 348, 359–360
end-stage renal disease, 156–157
    dialysis for, 157–158

end-stage renal disease (*continued*)
  intervention approaches, 163–164
  pathophysiology and care of, 157–160
  psychosocial impact of treatment for, 160–162
  transplantation for, 159–160
  treatment compliance in, 158–159, 162–163
Engel, G., 3, 40, 164
environmental factors, 29
Epidemologic Catchment Area, 189
epilepsy, 247–250
Epstein-Barr infection, 309
erythema migrans, 295
esophagus, 182–184
essential hypertension. *See also* hypertension
  blood pressure assessment, 135–137
  lifestyle and, 139–141
  prevalence of, 134–135
  stepped-care approach to management of, 138
estrogen
  lipids and, 350
  vaginitis and, 335
ethical concerns, 438–439
ethnic factors, 11–12. *See also individual ethnic group names*
  cancer and, 110–111
  coronary heart disease and, 155
  endocrine disorders and, 202–203
  HIV and, 269–272, 284, 290–291
  patient participation in treatment and, 11–12
  representativeness in treatment delay and, 18–19
  stress and, 377
euphoria, 246
Evans, E., 44
exercise, 35–36
  for essential hypertension, 140–141
  obesity and, 366
  physical deconditioning in chronic fatigue syndrome, 312–313
  during pregnancy, 340
"existential plight," 91
Eysenck Personality Questionnaire, 45–46

family, 374. *See also* support system
  interventions, 414–415
  sick role and, 380
  therapy groups, 416
Faragher, E., 44

fasting hypoglycemia, 207
fasting plasma glucose test, 204
fatigue, from cancer treatment, 95–96, 114–115
Fawzy, F.I., 434
Feldman, H.A., 18
Fennis, J.F.M., 193–194
fibroadenoma, 344
fibrocystic breast changes, 344
fibromyalgia, 296
finances, 375, 377
Florian, V., 19
fluoxetine, 252
foam cells, 144
Fobair, P., 114
focal seizures, 248
food allergies, 313–314
Freud, Sigmund, 39–40, 48
Friedman, H., 43
Friedman, M., 433

Gallo, Robert, 269
gamma globulin, 313
gastroesophageal reflux disease (GERD), 184
gastrointestinal cancers, 83, 84, 86–87
gastrointestinal disorders, 181–182
  of esophagus, 182–184
  gastroesophageal reflux disease (GERD), 184
  hypnotherapy for, 195–196
  inflammatory bowel disease, 187–188
  irritable bowel syndrome, 189–190
  peptic ulcer disease (PUD), 184–187
  personality and, 42
  psychodynamic psychotherapy for, 194–196
  psychotherapy for, 191–196
  trauma and abuse history and, 190–191
Gelpin, Y., 46–47
gender factors. *See* men; women
"General Adaptation Syndrome," 7
generalized anxiety disorders, 347
generalized seizures, 248
genetic risk, 92, 354, 356
genetics, weight and, 34
genitourinary cancers, 83, 84, 87
Glaser, R., 9–10
glioblastoma multiforme, 241
glucocorticoid-cascade hypothesis, 394
glucose metabolism disorders, 202–208
Goff, D.C., Jr., 18
gonorrhea, 336
Goodwin, P.J., 103

Graves' disease, 202, 209, 363
Greene, B., 193
Greenfield, S., 12
Grinker, R., 40
Grossman, S., 281
group interventions, 415–417
  composition of, 419
  efficacy of, 435–437
group psychotherapy, 439
growth hormone, 220–221
guided imagery, 412
Guthrie, E.A., 194–195
gynecologic cancers, 83, 84, 88–89. *See also
  individual cancer types*
  hormone replacement therapy and, 348
  sexual dysfunction and, 117

HAART (highly active antiretroviral therapy),
  271, 277–279, 281. *See also* antiretroviral
  medications
Hall, C.W., 214
hallucinations, auditory, 248
Hann, D.M., 115
Harvard Alumni Study, 35–36
Hashimoto's disease, 210
Haynes, R., 53
head and neck cancers, 83–85
Health Belief Model (HBM), 50
health care
  attitude toward, 401
  costs, 135, 250, 429–432 *See also* managed
    care
  cultural mistrust of, 375–376
  decision making about, 383–384
  HIV and, 284
  roles in, 378–381
heart disease
  depression following heart attack, 4
  diet and, 34–35
  social support and, 5
  treatment delay and, 18
Helicobacter pylori, 9, 46–47, 185, 186. *See also*
  peptic ulcer disease (PUD)
Helzer, J.E., 187
hematologic cancers, 83, 85–86
hemodialysis, 159. *See also* end-stage renal
  disease
hemophiliacs, 269
herbal supplements, 349, 365
Herpes simplex, 274
heuristics, 14, 18–19
Heyman, D.J., 195–196

high-density lipoproteins (HDL), 350–351
highly active antiretroviral therapy (HAART),
  271, 277–279, 281. *See also* antiretroviral
  medications
hippocampus, 395
hirsuitism, 226–227
Hispanic population, 269–272, 284, 290–
  291
histrionic personality, 388
HIV, 267–269, 292, 318
  antibody testing for, 284–285
  central nervous system infections and, 274–
    275
  clinical course, 272–273
  epidemiology, 269–272
  glossary of medical terms for, 270–271
  high-risk sexual behavior and, 37–38
  Lazarus Syndrome, 289–290
  neuropsychiatric complications of, 279–
    280
  opportunistic infection and malignancies,
    288–289
  pathogenesis, 272
  prevalence of, 269
  psychiatric disorders and, 282–283
  staging of, 272–276
  transmission of, 290–291
  treatment for, 276–279, 286–288
  in women, 361
Hodgkin's disease, 118
Hoerauf, K., 32
Holmes, Oliver Wendell, 58
Holtmann, G., 185
homosexual population, 269, 290–291
hopelessness, 104, 386
hormone replacement therapy (HRT), 348
  ischemic heart disease and, 362
  for osteoporosis, 351–352
hormones. *See also* endocrine disorders; men;
    women
  in cancer treatments, 81
  changes in, during pregnancy, 340
  in contraceptives, 337–338
  elevated lipids and, 350
  growth hormones, 202 *See also* endocrine
    disorders
  menopause and, 347–350
  osteoporosis and, 351–352
  physiologic response to stress and, 393
  system hormonal therapy, 355
  testosterone, 223–225
  vaginitis and, 335

Horton, J., 115
hospitalization, 380–381
hostility complex, 43
Houghton, L.A., 195–196
human papillomavirus, 357
hyperglycemia, 204
hyperparathyroidism, 216–217
hyperprolactinemia, 219–220
hypertension. *See also* essential hypertension
   end-stage renal disease and, 157
   in women, 350
hyperthyroidism, 363–364
hypnosis, 398–399
hypnotherapy, 195–196
hypnotics, 115–116
hypoglycemia, 207–208
hypogonadism, 223–225
hypoparathyroidism, 217–219
hypopituitarism, 221–222, 346
hypotension, 314
hypothalamic-pituitary axis disorders, 224, 393
hypothalamus, 8, 208, 393
hypothyroidism, 208, 210–212, 345–346, 361–363
hysteria, 48

iatrogenesis, 10–11
Illich, I., 10–11
imagery, 6
imaging tests, 236–237
imipramine, 183
immune system. *See also* HIV
   brain and, 4
   conflict and, 5
   overactivation, 313
   psychoneuroimmunology, 7–9
   stress and, 7, 395
incontinence, 352–353
indinavir, 279
infectious diseases. *See* chronic fatigue syndrome (CFS); HIV; Lyme disease
infertility, 118–119, 340–342
inflammatory bowel disease, 187–188
informed consent, 58–60
injecting drug users, 269, 361. *See also* HIV
insight-oriented psychotherapy, 411. *See also* psychotherapy
instrumental social support, 102
interleukin-2 (IL-2), 56
International Headache Society classification, 254

International League Against Epilepsy, 247
intrauterine devices (IUDs), 338
intravenous drug users, 290–291
Ironson, G., 149
irritable bowel syndrome, 189–193
ischemic heart disease, 362

Jacobsen, P.B., 115
Jacobson, A.M., 206
Jakob-Creutzfeldt virus, 275

Kabat-Zinn, J., 412
Kahana, R.J., 387
Kallmann's syndrome, 224
Kaplan, S.H., 12
Kaposi's Sarcoma (KS), 269, 271, 275
Karnofsky Performance Status score, 81
karosh (sudden death from overwork), 31
kidneys. *See* end-stage renal disease
Kiecolt-Glaser, J.K., 9–10
Klinefelter's syndrome, 224, 225
Kornblith, A.B., 117
Kubler-Ross, E., 54

lamivudine, 278
Lazarus, R.S., 384
Lazarus Syndrome, 289–290
L-dopa therapy, 242
legal issues
   of HIV, 284
   informed consent, 58–60 *See also* doctor-patient relationship
Leserman, J., 190–191
leukemia, 83, 85–86
Levenstein, S., 46, 47, 185, 186
levothyroxine (T4), 211, 362
Levy, R.L., 15
lifestyle, 33–34, 366
   coronary heart disease and, 152
   modification difficulties, 401
   stress and, 394
limbic system activation, 393
lipids, elevated, 350–351
local disease, 80. *See also* cancer
Locus of Control Model, 50–51
lopinavir, 279
L-triiodothyronine (T3), 211
L-tryptophan, 349
lumbar puncture (LP), 262
lung cancer, 82–84
Lusardi, P., 31
Lustman, P., 182

Lyman, G.H., 115
Lyme disease, 256–257, 267–268, 318
  diagnosis of, 294–298
  early disseminated disease, 295–296
  early localized disease, 295
  epidemiology of, 293–294
  functional disorders of, 302
  late-stage, 292–293, 296–298
  microbiology of, 298–299
  psychiatric disorders from, 300–303
  psychological issues of, 303–305
  sociocultural issues, 292–293
  treatment for, 299–300, 305
lymphomas, 83, 86, 275
Lynch, S.E., 5

Magill Pain Inventory, 189
magnetic resonance angiography (MRA), 260
magnetic resonance imaging (MRI), 236–237,
  258–259
Maguire, P., 114
Maher, E.J., 11
major depressive disorder, 189–190, 206–207.
  See also depression
male hypogonadism, 223–225
mammography, 354
managed care, 417–418, 437–440. *See also*
  health care
manual healing methods, 365
marital roles, 5, 375
Mark, M.M., 11
masochistic personality, 388
Maudsley Personality Inventory, 45–46
McGovern, P.G., 18
Mechanic, D., 11
Medical Nemesis (Illich), 10–11
medical treatment, 28, 114–115, 318, 407,
  417–419. *See also* managed care;
  pharmacotherapy;   psychotherapy;
  *individual illnesses; individual treatment
  techniques*
  for Addison's disease, 215
  alternative, 364–366
  for anabolic steroid use, 226
  biopsychosocial model of, 3, 40, 164, 181
  for breast cancer, 111–112, 354–355
  compliance, 14–16, 106, 142–143, 158–
  159, 162–164
  control issues and, 378–384
  for Cushing's syndrome, 213–214
  decisions by patient about, 11–13, 58–61,
  413, 434

delay in, 16–20
for diabetes, 205
for gastrointestinal disorders, 191–196
for gynecologic cancers, 357, 358, 360–361
for hirsutism, 226–227
for HIV, 271, 276–279, 287–288
for hyperparathyroidism, 217
for hyperprolactinemia, 220
for hypoparathyroidism, 218–219
for hypopituitarism, 222
for incontinence, 353
infertility from, 118–119
for Lyme disease, 299–300, 305–306
for male hypogonadism, 224–225
for menopause, 348
for neurological disorders, 240–241, 254,
  256–257
noncompliance, 382
for osteoporosis, 351–352
for pheochromocytoma, 222–223
response to cancer, 92–93
for seizure disorders, 248–249
for thyroid diseases, 208, 210–212, 363
Medicare End-Stage Renal Disease Act of 1973,
  157
meditation, 399
medroxyprogesterone acetate, 338
Mekarski, J., 54
melanoma, 83, 84, 89–90
melatonin, 349
Melmed, R., 46–47
men. *See also* homosexual population
  hyperprolactinemia in, 219–220
  infertility in, 340–342
  male hypogonadism, 223–225
meningiomas, 241
meningitis, 256–257, 274
menopause, 347–350
menstruation, 342–344, 347–350
metabolism, 201. *See also* endocrine disorders
Meyer, T.J., 11
migraine headaches, 253–254
Mikulincer, M., 19
Miller, George, 12
Miller, N.E., 13
Million Behavioral Health Index (MBHI),
  184
mind-body connection, 4, 27, 364–365
  biopsychosocial model and, 40
  psychoneuroimmunology, 7–9
Minnesota Multiphasic Personality Inventory
  (MMPI), 46, 185

Minor Cognitive Motor Disorder (MCMD), 280
money, 375, 377
monotherapy, for HIV, 287
Montagnier, Luc, 269
mood disorders
  in epilepsy, 249
  HIV and, 280–281
"morning-after" pill, 338
movement disorders, 241–244
Multidimensional Health Locus of Control scales, 51
Multiple Risk Factor Intervention Trial (MRFIT), 141
multiple sclerosis (MS), 244–247, 297
Murison, J., 9
Murphy, J., 15
muscle biopsy, 261–262
muscle relaxants, 314–315
musculoskeletal disorders, 31–32
myocardial infarction, 145. *See also* coronary heart disease (CHD)
myocardial ischemia, 145. *See also* coronary heart disease (CHD)

narcissistic personality, 389
National Commission of Sleep Disorders Research, 30–31
National Domestic Violence Hotline, 354
National Institutes of Health, 333, 364
natural contraceptive methods, 339
nefazodone, 215
neisseria gonorrhea, 336
nerve biopsy, 261–262
nerve conduction studies, 261
neurally mediated hypotension (NMH), 311, 314
neuroendocrine dysregulation, 311
neurohumeral dysregulation, 311
neurological illnesses, 231–232, 262–263. *See also* cognition; Lyme disease
  from *Borrelia burgdorferi*, 293–294
  brain and spinal cord trauma, 250–253
  cerebrovascular disease, 233–236
  dementia, 236–239
  demyelinating diseases, 244–247
  headaches, 253–255
  infections, 256–257
  movement disorders, 241–244
  seizure disorders, 247–250
  tumors, 239–241
neuropsychiatric disorders

of HIV, 279–281
  multiple sclerosis and, 246
neuropsychological testing, 262
neuroscience, advances in, 431
nevirapine, 278
nonnucleoside reverse transcriptase inhibitors (NNRTI), 271, 278
nonspecific esophageal motility disorders (NSMD), 182
nonspecific vaginitis, 335
North, C.S., 187, 188
nucleoside reverse transcriptase inhibitors, 278
nutcracker esophagus (NE), 182
nutrition
  alternative health issues and, 365–366
  during pregnancy, 340

obesity. *See also* weight
  essential hypertension and, 139–140
  exercise and, 35–36, 366
Oddi dysfunction, 190
olanzapine, 215
open-ended groups, 416–417, 419
opportunistic infections (OI), 270, 288–289
opthalmodynamometry, 261
oral personality, 387
osteroporosis, 351–352
ovarian cancer, 88–89, 356–367
Overmier, B, 9
overt hypothyroidism, 361–362. *See also* hypothyroidism
Ovral, 338

pallidotomy, 243
panic disorder, 347
Pap smear, 357–358
paranoid personality, 389
Parkinson's Disease (PD), 242–244
"passive suicide," 108
Pavlov, Ivan, 7
Paykel Interview for Stressful Life Events, 185
Payne, A., 193
Payne, C., 193
Pearlin, L.I., 384
pelvic inflammatory disease (PID), 336–337
Pennebaker, J.W., 16–17
peptic ulcer disease (PUD), 9, 45–47, 184–187
percutaneous transluminal angioplasty (PCTA), 152–154
personality
  brain trauma and, 251

as cause of somatization, 49
character style, 387
coping and, 101–102, 387–390
disease and, 42–47
illness and, 39–42
Lyme disease and, 303
psychotherapy to change, 420
pharmacotherapy. *See also* chemotherapy;
    medical treatment; *individual drug names*
for Addison's disease, 214, 215
alternative, 365
antiretroviral medication, 271, 276–279,
    286–287
for anxiety disorders in women, 346
for brain trauma, 252
chemotherapy-induced nausea, 93–94
chronic fatigue syndrome and, 311–312,
    314–315
for coronary heart disease, 152, 154–156
for Cushing's syndrome, 212
for dementia, 239
for depression and diabetes, 207
for depression and thyroid disease, 210
for diabetes mellitus, 205
for end-stage renal disease, 159
for essential hypertension, 138, 141–143
for gastrointestinal disorders, 182–183,
    185–186
for headaches, 254, 256
HIV and, 271, 276–279, 282–283
hypnotics, 115–116
for Lyme disease, 299–300
for multiple sclerosis, 245, 246
for neurological infections, 256–257
for osteoporosis, 351–352
for Parkinson's disease, 242, 243
for stress, 400
for stroke, 233–235
pheochromocytoma, 222–223
Philips, P., 114
physical activity. *See* exercise
physical deconditioning, of chronic fatigue
    syndrome, 312–313
physical therapy, 305
phytoestrogens, 349
Pick's disease, 237–238
pills, contraceptive, 337–338
pituitary disorders, 219–222
pneumocystis *carinii* pneumonia (PCP), 269,
    271
polycystic ovary syndrome, 226–227
Polymerase Chain Reaction (PCR), 295

positron emission tomography (PET), 259–
    260
Posluszny, D., 33
postmastectomy radiotherapy, 355
posttraumatic stress disorder (PTSD), 100,
    302–303
poverty, 29–30
pregnancy, 339–340
    HIV and, 361
    hyperthyroidism and, 364
    hypothyroidism and, 362–363
premenstrual syndrome (PMS), 342–343
primary care physicians, 432. *See also* doctor-
    patient relationship
problem-focused coping strategies, 103–104
progressive multifocal leukoencephalopathy
    (PML), 271, 275
prolactin, 219
prostate cancer, 87–88, 117
protease inhibitors (PI), 271, 276
psychodynamic groups, open-ended, 416–417
psychodynamic psychotherapy, 194–196, 421
psychoeducation, 409
psychological reverse deconditioning, 317
psychoneuroimmunology, 7–9
psychosis
    Addison's disease and, 214–215
    brain trauma and, 251
    and epilepsy, 250
    HIV and, 280–281
    Parkinson's disease and, 243–244
psychosocial moderators, of disease, 50–53
psychosocial   treatments.   *See   also*
    psychotherapy; *individual names of*
    diagnoses
assessment for, 408–409
countertransference in, 424
future directions of, 431–437
managed care and, 437–438
problems of, 400–401
psychotherapy vs., 420–422
selection of, 414–417
termination of, 424–425, 440–441, 410–
    412. *See also* psychosocial treatments;
    individual names of diagnoses
attachment and, 19–20
combining interventions for, 413
factors influencing, 412–413
future directions of, 431–437
for lifestyle behaviors, 33–34
for Lyme disease, 305–306
managed care and, 437–438

psychotherapy (*continued*)
   psychodynamic, 194–196
   psychosocial treatment *vs.*, 420–422
   to reduce stress, 396
   termination of, 440–441

racial factors
   cancer and, 110–111
   coronary heart disease and, 155
   diabetes mellitus and, 202–203
   essential hypertension and, 137
   HIV and, 269–272, 284, 290–291
radiation
   for cancer, 81
   infertility and, 118
   nausea induced by, 93
radioiodine therapy, 363
radionuclide ventriculography, 148–149
radiosurgery, 81
radiotherapy, 355
Radmacher, S.A., 15
raloxifene, 352
ranitidine, 186
Rasgon, S., 164
rash, from Lyme disease, 295
reactive hypoglycemia, 207
regional disease, 80. *See also* cancer
regression, 381–382
relaxation techniques, 6, 397, 411–412. *See also* stress
religious beliefs, 39, 105, 375–376, 399
representative heuristic, 14
representativeness, 18–19
ritonavir, 279
Robbins, F., 40
Robertson, M.M., 249
Rogers, W.H., 12
Rosenman, R.H., 43, 433
Roseto Study, 5
Rotter, J.B., 50
Rozanski, A., 148–149

S-adenosyl methionine (SAMe), 315
Safer, M.A., 19
saquinavir, 276, 279
sarcomas, 83, 90
Sarno, John, 317–318
schizoid personality, 389–390
Schooler, C., 384
screening mammography, 354
seizures, 240, 247–250
selegiline, 242

self, illness and, 386, 391–392
self-hypnosis, 398–399
self-image, 376
Selye, Hans, 7, 392
semen analyses, 342
sense of coherence, 4
sensory-evoked potentials, 260–261
seroconversion, 284–285
serum TSH concentration test, 211
sexual dysfunction
   cancer patients, 96–97, 117–118
   spinal cord trauma and, 253
sexually transmitted diseases (STDs), 37–38,
      336, 340–341. *See also* HIV
sexual practices
   cervical cancer and, 357
   high-risk, 37–38
   HIV and, 361
   medical history and, 334
sexual roles, 375, 377
Sheehan, H.L., 201
Sheridan, C.L., 15
Sherman, A., 419
sick role, 378–381. *See also* doctor-patient
      relationship
Simonton, S., 419
single photon emission computer tomography
      (SPECT), 259, 317
skin cancer, 38–39, 89–90
sleep dysfunction, 30–31, 115–116
Smith, M., 51
smoking, 36–37, 52, 350, 401. *See also*
      substance abuse
social class, 376–377
social learning theory, 50–51
social phobia, 347
Social Readjustment Rating Scale, 188
soft tissue sarcomas, 90
somatization, 47–49, 189–190
   abuse and, 334
   Freud on, 39–40
specificity theory, 187
spermicides, 338
Spiegel, D., 419, 434
spinal cord trauma, 250–253
spiritual practices, 39
SSRIs (selective serotonin reuptake inhibitors),
      215
St. Martin, Alexis, 181
stavudine, 278
sterilization, 339
steroidal medications, 214

Strain, J.J., 381

stress, 54–55, 374, 392–396. *See also* medical treatment

associated with cancer diagnosis/treatment, 98–100

of caregivers, 373

control issues and, 378–384

coronary heart disease and, 148, 149

essential hypertension and, 137

management for essential hypertension, 141

peptic ulcers and, 9, 186

personality and, 42

psychosocial risk factors of, 396

relaxation techniques, 396–400, 411–412

socioeconomic status and, 376–377

somatization and, 49

stress echocardiography, 151

stress model, 7

stroke (cerebrovascular accident), 233–236

Strong Memorial Hospital, 59

Stuart, E.M., 412

subclinical hypothyroidism, 362. *See also* hypothyroidism

substance abuse, 36–37. *See also* smoking

alcoholism in women, 366

anabolic steroid use, 225

Transtheoretical Model and, 51–52

sudden coronary death, 146. *See also* coronary heart disease (CHD)

suicide

among cancer patients, 95, 108

HIV and, 281

hyperparathyroidism and, 216

Parkinson's disease and, 242

"passive," 108

seizure disorders and, 249

sundowning, 239

sun exposure, 38–39

support groups

cancer survival rates and, 102–103

for Lyme disease, 305–306

supportive psychotherapy, 410. *See also* psychotherapy

support system, 5, 52–53, 376–377, 434, 435

assistance for, 423

childhood cancer and, 109

coping resources and, 102–103

elderly population and, 110

for end-stage renal disease, 161–162

psychosocial treatment type and, 414–415

response to cancer diagnosis, 91–92

stress on caregivers, 373–377

tragic unexpected illness and, 422–423

surgery

acromegaly, 221

cancer, 81

endometrial cancer, 360–361

hyperprolactinemia, 220

Parkinson's disease, 243

and pheochromocytoma, 222–223

preparation for, 6

and primary hyperparathyroidism, 217

survival rates

among African American cancer patients, 111

for breast cancer, 90–91

cancer recurrence and, 106–108

for coronary heart disease, 148

for different cancer types, 79, 83–84, 112–113, 121

for gastrointestinal cancers, 86

for gynecologic cancers, 89, 359

for head and neck cancers, 85

for hematologic cancers, 85

for prostate cancer, 88

supportive group intervention and, 102–103

Sutton, William, 189

Svedlund, J., 194

Talley, N.J., 190, 196

tamoxifen, 355–356

TB meningitis, 274

temporal lobe epilepsy, 249

Tennant, C., 46

tenofovir, 278

termination, of treatment, 424–425, 440–441

testes, 223–225

testis cancer, 87

testosterone, 223–225

thalamotomy, 243

thallium scan, 150–151

therapeutic relationship. *See* doctor-patient relationship

Thomsen, I.V., 251

thyroid disease, 208–212, 361–364

thyroiditis, 363–364

thyrotoxic crisis (thyroid storm), 364

thyrotoxicosis, 209–210

time-limited groups, 416, 419

tobacco use. *See* smoking

toxic adenoma, 363

toxic nodular goiter, 363

toxic shock syndrome, 14

toxoplasmosis, 271, 274
Transactional Model of Stress and Coping, 100
transient hypothyroidism, 362. *See also*
    hypothyroidism
transient ischemic attacks (TIAs), 233
transitional events, 120–121
Transtheoretical Model, 51–52
trazodone, 182–183
Treatise on Hysteria (Briquet), 48
treatment. *See* medical treatment; psychosocial
    treatments; psychotherapy
trichomoniasis—vaginal infection, 335
tricyclic antidepressants, 156, 314
    Addison's disease and, 215
    for brain trauma, 252
triglycerides (TG), 350–351
Trimble, M.R., 249
tubal ligation, 339
tumor markers, 92
tumors, 239–241
Turner, S., 11
24-h urinary-free cortisol assay, 213
Type A Behavior Pattern (TABP), 41–43, 46,
    148, 433
Type B personality, 44
Type C (Cancer) personality, 44
Type 1/Type 2 diabetes, 202–207

Ulman, K., 412
Ulmer, D., 433
ultraviolet sunlight, 38–39
undetectable viral load, 270
University of Chicago, 30–31
urinary incontinence, 351–352
U.S. Preventive Services Task Force, 368
uterine cancer, 359–360

vacuolar myelopathy (VM), 271, 281
vaginitis, 334–336
Van Dulmen, A.M., 193–194
Van t Spijker, A., 120
varicella zoster virus, 275
vascular dementia, 238–239
vasectomy, 339
Vaughan, H.G., 11
violence, 334, 353–354
viral load, 270
visualization, 412

Walker, E.A., 187, 188
Wallston, K., 51
Ware, J.E., 12
weight, 34–35
    essential hypertension and, 139–140

exercise and, 35–36
    during pregnancy, 340
Weiner, H., 9
Weisman, A.D., 91, 390
wellness continuum, 10–11
Western Blot, 294–295
Western Collaborative Group Study, 43
"white coat hypertension," 136
Whorwell, P.J., 195
Wolf, S., 5
women, 333, 346–347, 364–366, 373, 377.
    See also breast cancer
    breast disease in, 344
    cancer in, 354–360
    cervical infections, 336–337
    contraception used by, 337–339
    coronary heart disease in, 155, 350–351
    doctors chosen by, 333–334
    eating disorders in, 344–346
    endocrine disorders in, 201, 206, 208, 210,
        216, 217
    with end-stage renal disease, 162
    health screening for, 367–368
    hirsutism in, 226–227
    HIV in, 269–272, 290–291, 361
    hyperprolactinemia in, 219–220
    incontinence in, 352–353
    infertility in, 340–342
    Lyme disease in, 3304
    and menopause, 347–350
    and menstruation, 342–344
    multiple sclerosis in, 244
    osteroporosis in, 351–352
    pregnancy, 339–340, 361
    Somatization Disorder and, 48
    thyroid disease in, 361–364
    vaginitis, 334–336
    violence against, 333, 353–354
Women's Health Iniative, 333
Worden, J.W., 91
work environment, 29, 31–32
World Health Organization, 251
Wrezesniewski, K., 46

yeast allergies, 313–314
yoga, 399
Young, J., 11
Young, T., 11

zalcitabine, 278
Zan, 399
zidovudine, 278
Zuckerman, C., 60
Zung Anxiety and Depression Scales, 185